# Comprehensive Cardiac Care

*Edited by*

**Marguerite R. Kinney, R.N., D.N.Sc, F.A.A.N.**

Professor of Nursing
School of Nursing
University of Alabama at Birmingham
Birmingham, Alabama

**Donna R. Packa, R.N., D.S.N.**

Professor of Nursing
Associate Dean of Academic Affairs
University of Mississippi School of Nursing
University of Mississippi Medical Center
Jackson, Mississippi

**Kathleen G. Andreoli, D.S.N, F.A.A.N.**

Vice-President for Nursing Affairs
John L. and Helen Kellogg
Dean of the College of Nursing
Rush-Presbyterian-St. Luke's Medical Center
Chicago, Illinois

**Douglas P. Zipes, M.D.**

Professor of Medicine
Krannert Institute of Cardiology
Indiana University Medical Center
Indianapolis, Indiana

**SEVENTH EDITION**

*with 1075 illustrations*

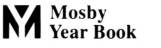

**Mosby
Year Book**

St. Louis   Baltimore   Boston   Chicago   London   Philadelphia   Sydney   Toronto

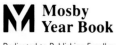
**Mosby**
**Year Book**

Dedicated to Publishing Excellence

Executive Editor: Don Ladig
Developmental Editor: Jeanne Rowland
Project Manager: Patricia Gayle May
Production Editor: Sheila Walker
Designer: Susan Lane

**SEVENTH EDITION**

Previous editions copyrighted 1968, 1971, 1975, 1979, 1983, 1987

Printed in the United States of America

Mosby−Year Book, Inc.
11830 Westline Industrial Drive
St. Louis, Missouri 63146

**Library of Congress Cataloging-in-Publication Data**

Comprehensive cardiac care.—7th ed. / edited by Marguerite Kinney
   . . . [et al.]
     p.   cm.
   Includes bibliographical references.
   Includes index.
   ISBN 0-8016-2770-2
   1.  Heart—Diseases—Nursing.  2.  Coronary care units.  I.  Kinney,
Marguerite Rodgers.
   [DNLM:  1.  Coronary Care Units.  2.  Heart Diseases—nursing.  WY
152.2 C737]
RC674.C65    1991
616.1′2—dc20
DNLM/DLC
for Library of Congress                      90-13636
                                         CIP

GW/VH/VH  9  8  7  6  5  4  3  2

**Erin L. Abramczyk,** R.N., M.S.N., CCRN
Assistant Nursing Coordinator
Cardiovascular Surgical Unit
Georgetown University Hospital
Washington, DC

**Martha Branyon,** R.N., Ed.D.
Associate Professor
School of Nursing
University of Alabama at Birmingham
Birmingham, Alabama

**Lynne T. Braun,** R.N., Ph.D.
Practitioner-Teacher
Department of Medical Nursing
Rush-Presbyterian-St. Luke's Medical Center
Assistant Professor
College of Nursing
Rush University
Chicago, Illinois

**Mary-Michael Brown,** R.N., M.S., CCRN
Nursing Coordinator
Cardiovascular Surgical Unit
Georgetown University Hospital
Washington, DC

**William Combs,** M.S.E.E.
Pacing Systems Group
Medtronic, Inc.
Minneapolis, Minnesota

**Mary Sue Craft,** R.N., M.S.N.
Clinical Nurse Specialist
Cardiovascular Surgical Intensive Care Unit
University of Alabama Hospitals
Birmingham, Alabama

**Barbara A. Erickson,** R.N., Ph.D., CCRN
Codirector
Clinical Education Associates;
President
Specialty Nursing Care, Inc.

**Dorothy K. Gauthier,** R.N., Ph.D.
Associate Professor
School of Nursing
University of Alabama at Birmingham
Birmingham, Alabama

**Doris F. Glick,** R.N., Ph.D.
Assistant Professor
School of Nursing
University of Virginia
Charlottesville, Virginia

**Cathie E. Guzzetta,** R.N., Ph.D., CCRN, F.A.A.N.
Director
Holistic Nursing Consultants
Bethesda, Maryland

**Nancy Houston Miller,** R.N., B.S.
Program Nurse Director
Stanford Cardiac Rehabilitation Program
Stanford University School of Medicine
Stanford, California

**Janine M. Neeley,** R.N., M.S.N.
Formerly, Head Clinician
Cardiovascular Surgical Intensive Care Unit
University of Alabama Hospitals
Birmingham, Alabama

**Marcia Pencak Murphy,** R.N., M.S.
Assistant Unit Leader
Department of Medical Nursing
Rush-Presbyterian-St. Luke's Medical Center
Assistant Professor
College of Nursing
Rush University
Chicago, Illinois

**Joann M. Pillion,** R.N., M.S.N.
Clinical Nurse Specialist
University of Alabama Hospitals
University of Alabama at Birmingham
Birmingham, Alabama

**Patricia C. Seifert,** R.N., M.S.N., CNOR
Operating Room Coordinator
Cardiac Surgery
Department of Surgery
The Arlington Hospital
Arlington, Virginia

**Ruth Stanley,** Pharm. D.
Birmingham Veteran's
Administration Medical Center
Samford University
Birmingham, Alabama

**Nancy L. Stephenson,** B.S.N.
Manager of Physician Relations
Medtronic, Inc.
Minneapolis, Minnesota

**Laurel J. Sutherland,** R.N., M.S.N.
Education Coordinator-Critical Care
Alexandria Hospital
Alexandria, Virginia

**Elizabeth VanBeek Carlson,** R.N., D.N.Sc.
Interim Chairperson
Department of Medical Nursing
Rush-Presbyterian-St. Luke's Medical Center
Assistant Professor
College of Nursing
Rush University
Chicago, Illinois

**Connie White-Williams,** R.N., B.S.N., C.C.T.C.
Senior Cardiac Transplant Coordinator
University of Alabama Hospitals
Birmingham, Alabama

# Preface

While diseases of the heart and blood vessels continue as the number one health problem in the United States, understanding of the mechanisms involved in the disorders, as well as options for diagnosis and treatment, steadily increase. The seventh edition of *Comprehensive Cardiac Care* contains the latest information related to the diagnosis and treatment of atherosclerosis, valvular heart disease, and cardiomyopathies. In keeping with the changes in the health care environment, both rehabilitation and care of the cardiac patient in the home are prominent features of this edition. In this revision, a holistic nursing model is presented as a framework for a comprehensive assessment that can be employed in primary, secondary, and tertiary care settings. The chapter on pacemakers not only focuses on technology available today but also describes systems expected to be useful in controlling dysrhythmias in the future. We believe the reader will find in these pages detailed descriptions of medical and nursing management of cardiac populations that can be readily applied to the care of adults with heart disease.

## ACKNOWLEDGMENTS

Readers acquainted with previous editions will note some changes in the editorial team who revised the text. While Drs. Kathleen G. Andreoli, Marguerite R. Kinney, and Douglas P. Zipes have continued as members of the team, Dr. Andrew G. Wallace and Ms. Virginia Kliner Fowkes have turned their attention to new endeavors. We thank them both for their early contributions, which continue to influence this text. It is our pleasure to welcome to the editorial team an experienced editor and colleague, Dr. Donna R. Packa. We also wish to thank contributors to the previous edition, on whose work we have built: James A. Blumenthal, Ph.D.; Elizabeth Darling, R.N., M.S.N.; Edwin G. Duffin, Jr., Ph.D.; Sue Faust, R.N., M.S.N.; Ruth A. Giebel, R.N., B.S.N.; Susan J. Hasselman, R.N.; James J. Heger, M.D.; Paula Hindle, R.N., M.S.N.; F. Paul Koisch, B.A., B.S; Lori B. Maloy, R.N.; Elaine G. Martin, R.N.; Helen S. Mau, R.N.; John C. McMahon, Ph.D.; Miriam C. Morey, M.A.; Leigh Anne Musser, M.P.H.; Gerald V. Naccarelli, M.D., F.A.C.C.; Akira Nishikawa, M.D.; Debra L. Peeples, R.N., M.S.N.; Eric N. Prystowsky, M.D.; Cynthia M. Schuch, R.N., M.S.N., CCRN; Elizabeth Wagner, R.N.; Jennifer J. Williams, P.A.; and R. Sanders Williams, M.D.

We are especially indebted to the authors who contributed to the present edition. Their dedication to the task resulted in the timely receipt and publication of outstanding manuscripts. Their willingness to share their knowledge and experience is appreciated more than we can adequately express. Chapter 2 authors, Cathie Guzzetta and Patricia Seifert, wish to thank Shelia D. Bunton, R.N., M.S.N., Linda A. Prinkey, R.N., M.S.N., CCRN, and Anita P. Sherer, R.N., M.S.N., CCRN for their review of the cardiovascular assessment content.

Don Ladig, Jeanne Rowland, Patricia Gayle May, and Sheila Walker at Mosby–Year Book deserve our heartfelt thanks for the many ways in which they have contributed to this text and made our work a pleasant experience. We also want to thank June McKaig and Muriel Wright for their assistance with manuscript preparation and their cheerful acceptance of short deadlines. It has been our pleasure to work with all of these individuals, and we look forward to other opportunities to continue these working relationships and friendships. Again, we offer our appreciation to our readers who transfer the words on these pages into skilled and artful patient care, which is of course the ultimate purpose of the text.

**Marguerite R. Kinney**
**Donna R. Packa**
**Kathleen G. Andreoli**
**Douglas P. Zipes**

# Contents in Brief

# Contents

## 6  Coronary Artery Disease, 253

Lynne T. Braun
Marcia Pencak Murphy
Elizabeth VanBeek Carlson

## 7  Care of the Cardiac Patient, 270

Joann M. Pillion

## 8  Valvular Heart Disease, 327

Erin L. Abramczyk
Mary-Michael Brown

## 9  Cardiomyopathy, 343

Connie White-Williams

**10 Cardiovascular Drugs, 354**
Ruth Stanley

**11 Artificial Cardiac Pacemakers and Implantable Cardioverter Defibrillators, 398**
Nancy L. Stephenson
William Combs

Comprehensive
Cardiac
Care

# Anatomy and Physiology of the Heart

Dorothy K. Gauthier

This chapter reviews the anatomy and physiology of the heart and related aspects of the systemic and pulmonary circulations. It is not intended to be a detailed discussion but merely to provide a basis for further study.

## ANATOMY

Cardiac muscle cells are characterized by their branched appearance and the presence of *intercalated discs,* areas where adjacent cells meet end-to-end with partial fusion of their cell membranes. These structures form low-resistance bridges that allow electrical impulses to pass from cell to cell. The anatomical arrangement of cells in cardiac tissue gives it a syncytial appearance (Fig. 1-1, *A*), that is, it resembles a network of cells with no separation between the individual cells. The heart contains an atrial syncytium (the muscle of the two upper chambers) and a ventricular syncytium (the muscle of the two lower chambers), separated by fibrous tissue.

Each individual cardiac muscle cell or fiber contains *myofibrils* (the contractile elements) and mitochondria (the energy-producing units) (Fig. 1-1, *B*). Viewed with a microscope, myofibrils exhibit alternating light and dark bands because of the orderly arrangement and overlap of two protein filaments, the thinner *actin* and the thicker *myosin.* When the muscle is excited, projections on the myosin filaments interact with adjacent actin filaments to form cross-bridges. These cross-bridges use energy released from ATP to bend, sliding the actin filaments over the myosin and causing the myofibrils and the entire muscle fiber to shorten.

In addition to these structures, the muscle fiber also contains two systems of tubules and two regulatory proteins. *T tubules,* or *transverse tubules,* which are extensions of the cell membrane, conduct the impulse to the interior of the cell. *L tubules,* or *longitudinal tubules,* also referred to as the *sarcoplasmic reticulum,* store calcium (Fig. 1-1, *B*). The regulatory proteins, troponin and tropomyosin, normally form a complex with the actin filament to prevent it from forming cross-bridges with myosin. In this state, the muscle is relaxed.

Excitation of the muscle fiber is initiated by passage of an electric impulse over the cell membrane (sarcolemma).

As the impulse passes over the T tubule membrane to the interior of the cell, calcium ions are permitted to enter the sarcoplasm, both from outside the cell through the sarcolemma and T tubule membrane and from the nearby sarcoplasmic reticulum. Calcium ions bind to troponin-tropomyosin, causing an alteration in its position, which now permits the interaction of actin and myosin, and the muscle fiber shortens.[1] Because each muscle fiber membrane is connected to its immediate neighbors by the low-resistance intercalated discs, the excitatory impulse can spread to all cells in the atrial or ventricular syncytium.

When the electrical stimulation is ended, calcium ions are returned to the sarcoplasmic reticulum and the extracellular fluid, lowering the calcium concentration in the sarcoplasm. At the lower calcium level, the regulatory proteins can again interfere with the interaction of actin and myosin; therefore the filaments return to their original position and the muscle relaxes.

The heart has a skeleton consisting of four fibrous rings or annuli arranged as shown in Fig. 1-2. Each annulus is the supporting structure for one of the four valves of the heart and the connecting site for the muscular networks that comprise the four chambers. This fibrous skeleton is nonconductive and insulates the atrial syncytium from the ventricular syncytium. Specialized conduction pathways that are responsible for initiating an impulse and conducting it through the fibrous skeleton from atria to ventricles and within the walls of the chambers will be discussed later in the chapter.

The wall of the heart can be divided into three layers. The inner *endocardium* is composed of endothelial cells supported by fibrous tissue. The endothelial layer is continuous with the endothelial lining of the blood vessels. The middle *myocardium* is mainly cardiac muscle. The outer *epicardium* contains fibrous connective tissue and mesothelial cells. The heart is surrounded by the *pericardium,* a double layer of fibrous tissue and mesothelial cells. The inner layer of the pericardium forms the epicardium. Accumulation of blood or other fluid in the space between the two layers of the pericardium can lead to compression of the heart (cardiac tamponade) and compromise the heart's ability to fill with blood.

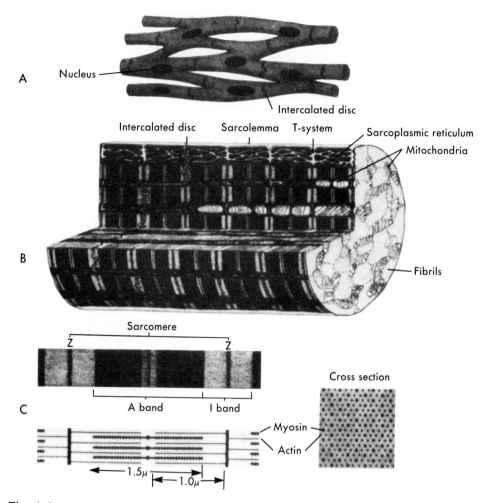

**Fig. 1-1** **A,** Syncytial nature of myocardial tissue, with intercalated discs between cells. **B,** Cardiac muscle fiber. Fibrils = myofibrils. **C,** Arrangement of the protein filaments actin and myosin to produce dark *(A)* and light *(I)* bands. The protein filaments of the myofibril form subunits (sarcomeres) bounded on either end by a dark Z-line. The arrangement of filaments is shown in microscopic, schematic, and cross-sectional views. (Reprinted with permission from Sonnenblick EH: Myocardial ultrastructure in the normal and failing heart. In Braunwald E, editor: The myocardium: failure and infarction, New York, HP Publishing Co, Inc, 1974, p 4.)

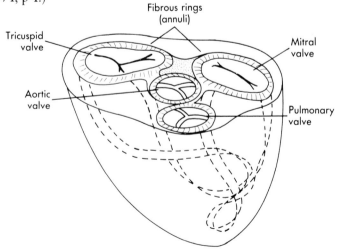

**Fig. 1-2** Fibrous rings connecting the four heart valves.

## BLOOD FLOW

The heart is a double pump, divided anatomically into right and left sides. It receives blood from the venous (return) system and propels it into the arterial (delivery) system (Fig. 1-3). The right atrium receives deoxygenated venous blood from the superior vena cava, which drains the upper half of the body, the inferior vena cava, which drains the lower half of the body, and the coronary sinus (not shown), which drains blood that has nourished the heart, itself. From the right atrium, blood flows through the *tricuspid* valve into the right ventricle. On contraction the ventricle ejects blood through the *pulmonary valve* into the pulmonary artery, which branches and conducts the blood to the lungs for oxygenation. Oxygenated blood returning from the lungs enters the left atrium through four pulmonary veins (only two are shown in Fig. 1-3). It passes from the left atrium through the *mitral valve* to the left ventricle. Contraction of the left ventricle causes ejection of blood through the *aortic valve* into the aorta, which distributes it to the peripheral circulation.

The leaflets of the tricuspid and mitral valves (the atrioventricular, or AV, valves) are attached by fibrous bands, the chordae tendineae, to the papillary muscles, which are anchored in the ventricular walls (Fig. 1-3). Contraction of the papillary muscles during ventricular contraction ensures tight closure of the valves and prevents their leaflets from everting into their respective atria because of the increasing pressure of blood in the ventricles at this time.

The pumping action of the heart can be divided into a period of ventricular relaxation, *diastole,* and a period of ventricular contraction, *systole.* During diastole, the mitral and tricuspid valves are open and the aortic and pulmonary valves are closed. Blood flows freely into the atria and ventricles, filling the ventricles to about 70% of their ultimate *end-diastolic volume.*[2] Toward the end of diastole, the atria contract and propel the remaining volume of blood into the ventricles. At the beginning of systole, ventricular contraction occurs, increasing the pressure within the ventricles and closing the atrioventricular valves. With both sets of valves closed, the pressure in each ventricle increases rapidly until it is sufficient to force the pulmonary and aortic valves open and eject blood into the pulmonary artery and aorta.

With each ventricular contraction, 70 to 80 ml of blood are ejected. This *stroke volume* represents 60% to 75% of the total volume of blood in the ventricle at the end of diastole, producing an *ejection fraction* of 0.60 to 0.75.[1] The *cardiac output,* (the total volume of blood pumped per minute from either ventricle) is the product of stroke volume and heart rate and is approximately 5.6 L/min for a normal supine adult.[3] Use of another value, *cardiac index,* which is cardiac output divided by square meters of body surface area, takes into consideration the fact that stroke volume and cardiac output depend, in part, on the size of the person. Normal cardiac index ranges from 2.8 to 4.2 L/min/m².[1]

The major physiologic roles of the circulatory system are the delivery of oxygen and other essential substrates to the tissues of the body and the removal of carbon dioxide and other products of cellular metabolism. Many of the substances carried to and from the tissues are dissolved in plasma, and their transport depends on the volume of flow. Almost all of the oxygen, however, is transported by hemoglobin in red blood cells, giving importance to the red blood cell and hemoglobin concentrations, as well as to blood flow, for the transport of this nutrient. Carbon dioxide is carried both on hemoglobin and in the plamsa.

As blood from the right side of the heart passes through the pulmonary capillaries, oxygen from air in the pulmonary alveoli enters the blood and attaches to the hemoglobin in red cells. Carbon dioxide diffuses from blood into the alveolar air. As blood from the left side of the heart passes through systemic capillaries, red blood cells surrender a portion of their oxygen (the exact amount depending on the needs of the tissue at the time), and the blood picks up carbon dioxide to be transported away. The rate of metabolism in a specific tissue not only affects the ability of blood passing through this tissue to exchange gases but also affects the diameter of blood vessels in the tissue, thereby regulating blood flow. The local rate of metabolism is probably the most important determinant in the distribution of cardiac output. During exercise, for example, blood flow increases in areas involved in the activity (such

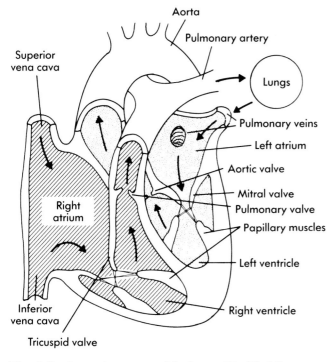

**Fig. 1-3** Internal anatomy of the heart. (Modified from Guyton AC: Function of the human body, ed 3, Philadelphia, 1969, WB Saunders Co.)

as specific skeletal muscle groups and the heart) and decreases in areas of little metabolic activity (such as the kidneys, stomach, and intestines). Blood flow to the brain remains the same at rest or during exercise.

## SYSTEMIC CIRCULATION

The systemic circulation is comprised of the arteries, arterioles, capillaries, venules, and veins. Blood flows through the system because of the downward pressure gradient along these conduits from the aorta to the superior and inferior venae cavae, which lead into the right atrium (Fig. 1-4). When blood is pumped from the left ventricle into the aorta, relatively high pressure is created and the aorta becomes distended. During ventricular diastole, the elastic aorta recoils providing additional pressure to pump blood into the systemic circulation. Blood pressure in the aorta gradually falls as blood flows into peripheral vessels. Pressure in the aorta and large arteries normally fluctuates between approximately 120 mm Hg (the *systolic pressure*) and 80 mm Hg (the *diastolic pressure*). The difference between systolic and diastolic pressures, the *pulse pressure,* can be noted in arteries and arterioles. The *mean arterial pressure* is the arterial pressure averaged during one cardiac cycle (systole and diastole); it can be quite accurately calculated as the diastolic pressure plus ⅓ of the pulse pressure.

The major arteries branch to form smaller ones, which eventually give rise to arterioles. Arterioles have muscular walls that can dilate or constrict, controlling blood flow into capillary beds. The relatively high vascular resistance of arterioles causes a drop in blood pressure to less than 35 mm Hg as the blood enters the capillaries (see Fig. 1-4). Vasodilatation or vasoconstriction in systemic arterioles is controlled, in part by *local conditions*. Arterioles respond to a decrease in oxygen or an increase in carbon dioxide or certain other waste products in the fluid around them by dilating to increase blood flow. This local control of blood vessel size ensures that a tissue that needs extra oxygen can receive increased blood flow. Arterioles in some tissues also respond to changes in pressure. A local increase in blood pressure will cause the arterioles to constrict to protect the smaller vessels in the tissue from the increased pressure. If pressure in arterioles suddenly decreases, the arterioles will dilate to ensure that the tissue receives sufficient blood flow for nutrition. This local regulatory mechanism (sometimes called autoregulation) is believed to be an important factor in maintaining relatively constant

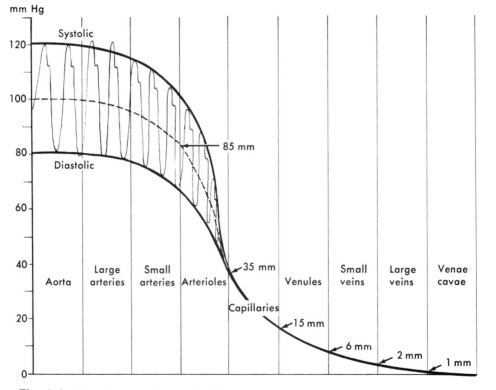

**Fig. 1-4** Blood pressures in vessels of the systemic circulation. The dotted line is an approximation of the mean pressure in arteries and arterioles. A more precise value for the mean pressure would be: diastolic pressure + 1/3 (systolic pressure − diastolic pressure). (Reprinted with permission from Thibodeau GA, and Anthony CP: Structure and function of the body, St Louis, 1988, Mosby–Year Book, Inc, p 271.)

blood flow in both the cerebral and coronary circulations despite fluctuations in mean arterial pressure. One other factor that influences the diameters of arterioles is the *sympathetic nervous system*. Increased sympathetic stimulation to blood vessels usually causes constriction, whereas, decreased sympathetic stimulation results in vasodilatation.

Once the blood is in the capillary bed, its velocity of flow is at its slowest. This allows sufficient time for the blood and the interstitial space to exchange fluid, as well as gases and other nutrients. Capillary walls are very thin and have a large total surface area, permitting rapid exchange of nutrients between the blood and interstitial fluid. Capillaries are unique in displaying an intermittent blood flow. At any given time, some of the capillaries in a tissue are open and others are closed by the constriction of a band of muscle at their proximal end (the precapillary sphincter) or by the constriction of arterioles.[3] The length of time an individual capillary is open or closed depends on the nutrient needs of the tissue.

Blood flows from the capillaries into venules, which converge to form veins. At this level of the systemic circuit, pressure is low (see Fig. 1-4). Venous walls are thin and compliant, yet muscular and contractile, which allows the veins to accommodate a greater or lesser volume of blood. In this manner veins can adjust the total volume of the circulatory system to the amount of blood available to fill it, and thus contribute to the regulation of blood pressure.

## PULMONARY CIRCULATION

Like the systemic circulation, the pulmonary circulation is a continuous circuit. Blood is pumped by the right ventricle into pulmonary arteries, which branch into arterioles and capillaries, where oxygen and carbon dioxide are exchanged. The pulmonary capillaries converge into venules and veins, which return oxygenated blood to the left atrium.

Gas exchange between the blood in pulmonary capillaries and the alveolar air takes place through the *pulmonary membrane,* or respiratory membrane. The pulmonary membrane consists of a thin layer of fluid that lines the alveolar wall, the alveolar wall itself, a thin layer of interstitial fluid, and the wall of the pulmonary capillary. Despite its complex nature, this membrane is only 0.63 micrometers thick. It has a total area (for both lungs) of approximately 160m$^2$ to further facilitate gas exchange. When the body is at rest, blood traverses a pulmonary capillary in about 1 second, but with increased activity and increased cardiac output, this time can be shortened to less than ½ second. However, the exchange of oxygen and carbon dioxide proceeds so fast that even this shortened time is adequate to permit normal exchange of blood gases.

An important feature of the pulmonary circulation is the ability of certain pulmonary vessels to adjust their diameters in response to local conditions. This allows them to regulate the distribution of blood flow in the lungs. Local control of blood vessels in the pulmonary circulation is the opposite of local control in the systemic circulation. Because gas exchange between blood and air is the major reason for blood flow in the pulmonary circulation, vessels in areas of the lung that do not have an adequate oxygen supply (due to bronchiolar obstruction, for example) will constrict, to shunt the blood to a more well-ventilated part of the lung.

Pulmonary blood vessels, which are thin-walled and easily stretched, offer low resistance to blood flow, so blood can flow through the lungs with a smaller pressure gradient than is needed in the systemic circulation. Mean pressure in the pulmonary artery is approximately 15 mm Hg,[4] compared with approximately 100 mm Hg in the aorta. Because the pulmonary and systemic circulations occur in series, the volume of blood flowing through the lungs per unit of time equals that flowing through the systemic circulation. The lungs must be prepared to accept as much as a fivefold increase in blood flow during strenuous exercise without putting undue strain on the right ventricle and without developing a significant increase in blood pressure in the pulmonary vessels, which may cause pulmonary edema. The ability of the pulmonary vessels to stretch to accommodate extra blood flow prevents an excessive increase in pressure in this situation.

## CORONARY CIRCULATION

The function of the coronary artery system is to maintain an adequate blood supply to the myocardium. The two major coronary arteries, the left and right, arise from the aorta immediately above the cusps of the aortic valve. Shortly after its origin, the *left coronary artery* (sometimes called left main coronary artery) divides into two branches (Fig. 1-5), the *anterior descending branch* and the *circumflex branch*. The anterior descending branch passes down the groove between the two ventricles on the anterior surface of the heart. From it arise diagonal branches, which supply the left ventricular wall, and septal perforating branches, which supply the anterior portion of the interventricular septum and the anterior papillary muscle of the left ventricle. The anterior descending branch usually supplies the entire apical portion of the interventricular septum before turning upward at the apex (lower tip) of the heart. The circumflex branch of the left coronary artery passes under the left atrial appendage (one of the earlike flaps that are found on each atrium). It then passes posteriorly in the groove between the left atrium and left ventricle. It gives off several small and one or two large marginal branches that supply the lateral aspects of the left ventricle.

The *right coronary artery* passes in the right atrioventricular groove, giving off several branches to the right ventricle and a large posterior descending branch, which descends in the posterior interventricular groove and supplies the inferior aspect of the septum and the posterior left ventricular papillary muscle. The right coronary artery

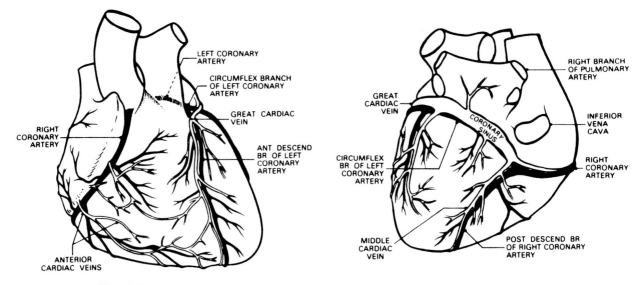

**Fig. 1-5** Coronary arteries supplying the anterior aspect of the heart (left) and the inferior aspect of the heart (right). Major veins which drain the respective aspects of the heart are also shown. (Reprinted with permission from Smith JJ and Kampine JP: Circulatory physiology: the essentials, Baltimore, 1984, Williams & Wilkins, p 188.)

gives off important branches that supply the sinoatrial (SA or sinus) node in 55% of human hearts and the atrioventricular (AV) node in 90%. In the remainder of human hearts, the SA node and the AV node are nourished by branches of the circumflex artery.[5]

Coronary blood flow at rest averages about 250 ml/min, which represents 4% to 5% of the total cardiac output.[4] Blood flow is controlled primarily by the local rate of metabolism, responding especially to myocardial oxygen demand. With normal activity, 65% to 70% of the arterial oxygen content is extracted by the myocardium, the highest rate of extraction of any tissue during normal activity and one that cannot be significantly improved. Thus the only mechanism for the heart to improve its oxygen uptake is to increase coronary blood flow. With strenuous activity, coronary blood flow can increase up to 5 times to ensure adequate oxygen supply to the myocardium.[3]

Impairment of coronary circulation by atherosclerosis constitutes the most frequent cause of heart disease. The atherosclerotic process causes a decrease in the luminal diameters of the coronary vessels, which decreases blood flow to the myocardium. Symptoms of coronary artery disease are not usually manifested, however, until blood flow to an area of the heart is compromised by 60% or more.[6]

## EXCITATION OF THE HEART

The normal cardiac impulse arises in specialized pacemaker cells of the *SA node,* located about 1 mm beneath the right atrial epicardium at its junction with the superior vena cava (Fig. 1-6). A spontaneous change in membrane potential

in these cells (Fig. 1-7) causes a wave of excitation (an impulse) to pass over the atrial myocardium. Spread of the impulse is facilitated by the presence of *internodal pathways,* which conduct faster than ordinary atrial muscle (see Fig. 1-6). Bachmann's bundle (a branch of the anterior internodal tract) conducts the impulse to the left atrium, and the anterior, middle, and posterior internodal tracts conduct the impulse toward the *AV node.* As the impulse spreads over the atrial syncytium, the atria depolarize, producing the P wave on the electrocardiogram (ECG) (see Fig. 1-7). Depolarization results in atrial contraction, which propels extra blood into the ventricles.

Conduction slows markedly when the impulse reaches the AV node (Fig. 1-6), which is specialized for slow conduction. This accounts for the long P-R interval on the ECG and allows sufficient time for blood to flow from the atria into the ventricles before ventricular contraction. After the impulse emerges from the AV node, it enters the rapidly conducting tissue of the *AV bundle* (bundle of His) and the right and left bundle branches. The bundle branches supply the endocardium of their respective ventricles with a profusely branching terminal network of *Purkinje fibers.* The rapid spread of the impulse throughout these structures allows almost simultaneous depolarization of the entire muscle mass of both ventricles, which is necessary for efficient contraction and pumping action. Ventricular depolarization produces the QRS complex on the ECG (Fig. 1-7) and the mechanical contraction of the ventricles that propels blood foward into the pulmonary artery and aorta. The return to resting electric state (repolarization) of the ventricles is recorded on the ECG as

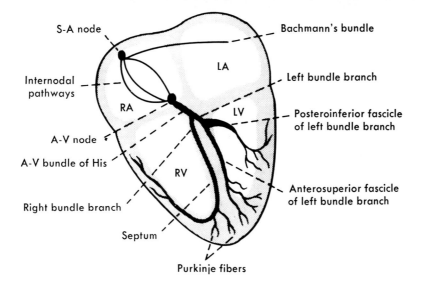

**Fig. 1-6** Transmission of the cardiac impulse from the sinoatrial (SA) node over atrial myocardium, Bachmann's bundle, and internodal pathways, then through the AV node and bundle of His and down the left and right bundle branches to the Purkinje fibers, which distribute the impulse to all parts of the ventricle.

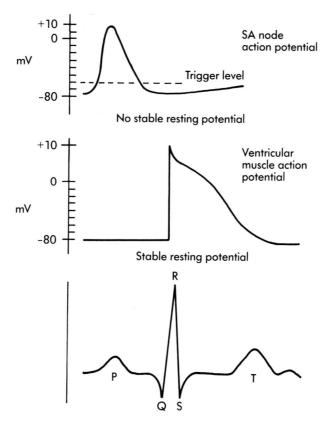

**Fig. 1-7** Changes in membrane potential of SA node cells and ventricular muscle cells when they become excited. The pattern of changes is called an action potential. During the depolarization phase of the action potential, the membrane potential becomes more positive. During the repolarization phase, the membrane potential returns to its resting state. The gradual change in membrane potential during the resting state in SA node cells causes them to depolarize spontaneously, whereas atrial and ventricular muscle cells will not depolarize unless they are stimulated by an impulse transmitted from adjacent cells. A typical ECG tracing is shown at the bottom of the figure, using the same time scale on the horizontal axis as was used for the action potentials above.

the T wave and results in ventricular relaxation. Repolarization of the atria cannot be noted on the ECG because it is masked by depolarization of the ventricles, which occurs at the same time and involves greater tissue mass.

## REGULATION OF CARDIAC FUNCTION

Cardiac function is regulated both by an intrinsic mechanism (the response of the heart to the amount of blood to be pumped) and by nervous reflexes involving the autonomic nervous system. *Intrinsic regulation* of the heart is based on the principle that if cardiac muscle is stretched *before* it contracts, it will contract with greater force. The consequences of this property on cardiac muscle performance are set forth by Starling's law, which states that, within limits, the greater the end-diastolic volume (EDV), the greater will be the force of contraction and the resulting stroke volume. For example, if extra blood returns to the heart every minute from the systemic and pulmonary circulations (increased venous return) as happens during exercise, the ventricles are stretched and contract with greater force, pumping out the extra volume of blood. Thus a healthy heart is able to adjust its force of contraction to handle changes in the amount of blood it receives from the systemic and pulmonary circulations.

The other major regulator of cardiac function is the *autonomic nervous system,* which alters the rate of impulse generation by the SA node, the speed of impulse conduction, and the strength of cardiac contraction. It regulates the heart through both sympathetic and parasympathetic nerve fibers (Fig. 1-8). The sympathetic fibers supply all areas of the atria and ventricles. Parasympathetic fibers, conducted to the heart via the vagus nerves, innervate primarily the SA node, AV node, and atrial muscle mass. At their synapses with cardiac tissue, sympathetic neurons secrete the neurotransmitter norepinephrine, whereas parasympathetic neurons secrete acetylcholine. These neurotransmitters bind to specific receptors on cardiac cells and exert their effects on the heart.

Sympathetic effects on the heart include increased heart rate, increased conduction speed through the AV node (which shortens the P-R interval), and increased force of contraction. Vagal (parasympathetic) stimulation produces decreased heart rate, decreased conduction rate through the AV node (with a longer P-R interval), and decreased force of atrial contraction. There is evidence that parasympathetic fibers invest the ventricles and that they decrease the vigor of ventricular contraction.[3] Whenever sympathetic neurons to the heart are activated, their effect is reinforced by the hormones epinephrine and norepinephrine, which are secreted by the adrenal medulla and reach the heart via the bloodstream.

Sympathetic and parasympathetic control of the heart occurs by reflexes coordinated at the medulla of the brain. Groups of neurons in the medulla that affect heart activity can be referred to as a *cardioacceleratory area* and a *car-*

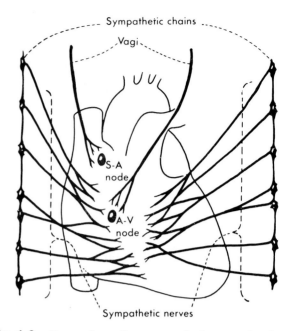

**Fig. 1-8** Connections of parasympathetic nerves (vagi) and sympathetic nerves with the heart. (Modified from Guyton AC: Function of the human body, ed 3, Philadelphia, 1969, WB Saunders Co.)

*dioinhibitory area,* and one that affects blood vessels is referred to as a *vasomotor area.* These three areas are referred to collectively as the *cardiovascular center.* The cardiovascular center can be stimulated by impulses from various nervous receptors. These include pressoreceptors (baroreceptors) located in the walls of the arch of the aorta and the carotid sinuses in the internal carotid arteries. These pressoreceptors alter their rate of impulse generation in response to changes in blood pressure. They transmit impulses to the cardiovascular center via the vagus and glossopharyngeal nerves. A sudden elevation of blood pressure within the aorta or the carotid artery increases impulse transmission to the cardioinhibitory area, which, in turn, inhibits the cardioacceleratory area, producing changes in sympathetic and parasympathetic output to decrease the heart rate and force of contraction. Sympathetic stimulation to blood vessels also is altered, lowering vascular resistance and blood pressure. The opposite reactions occur if the pressoreceptors detect a decrease in blood pressure.

The cardiovascular center also responds to changes in the chemical composition of the blood (a decrease in oxygen, or an increase in carbon dioxide or hydrogen concentrations) and to changes in blood volume. These changes are detected by specific nervous system receptors in varous areas of the body. The cardiovascular center then adjusts sympathetic and parasympathetic output to regulate the heart and blood vessels as needed to bring more oxygen to the tissues and to carry away accumulating waste products.

In addition to the nervous reflexes mentioned above, heart activity is also affected by higher centers in the brain that can stimulate sympathetic or parasympathetic neurons. This is evident when there is a change in heart activity and blood vessel tone in response to fear, pain, or an intense emotional experience. Cardiac and vascular changes, in these cases, are probably initiated by the hypothalamus.[2]

## Control of Cardiac Output

The adequacy of cardiac function is reflected by the cardiac output, which was previously defined as the total volume of blood pumped per minute, and which can be calculated:

$$Cardiac\ output = Heart\ rate \times Stroke\ volume$$

Factors that influence cardiac output, are those that influence its two components. *Heart rate* is determined by the autonomic nervous system, as previously discussed. Stroke volume has three major determinants, preload, afterload, and contractility of the heart.

*Preload* can be thought of as the amount of stress (tension) on the ventricular muscle fibers *before* they contract. This is related to the end-diastolic volume and is often expressed as EDV.[2] As has previously been discussed in relation to intrinsic regulation of the heart, an increase in EDV (preload) causes increases in the stroke volume and the cardiac output. A decrease in EDV has the opposite effect.

*Afterload* is the force that the ventricles must overcome *during* contraction, that is, while they are ejecting blood. The major component of afterload is blood pressure in the aorta. Two additional contributors to afterload are resistance offered by the size of the aortic valve opening (which is an important consideration for persons with aortic stenosis) and resistance in peripheral vessels. Anything that increases afterload increases the work of the heart and decreases stroke volume and cardiac output.

Myocardial *contractility* (inotropy) can be thought of as a change in cardiac performance that cannot be attributed to a change in muscle fiber length (preload), afterload, or heart rate.[7] This property of cardiac muscle is increased by sympathetic stimulation or inotropic drugs and is decreased by a decrease in the "health" of cardiac muscle cells, such as occurs in heart failure. An increase in contractility produces increased stroke volume and cardiac output, whereas a decrease in contractility has the opposite effect.

By making adjustments in the heart rate, preload, afterload, and contractility, the nervous and endocrine systems regulate cardiac output to ensure adequate nutrition of the tissues. Medical interventions used to change or stabilize a patient's cardiac output are also directed at altering these same parameters: heart rate, preload, afterload, and contractility.

## REFERENCES

1. Schlant RC and Sonnenblick EH: Normal physiology of the cardiovascular system. In Hurst JW and others: The heart, arteries and veins, ed 7, New York, 1990, McGraw-Hill, Inc.
2. Guyton AC: Textbook of medical physiology, ed 7, Philadelphia, 1966, WB Saunders Co.
3. Little RC and Little WC: Physiology of the heart and circulation, ed 4, Chicago, 1989, Mosby–Year Book, Inc.
4. Smith JJ and Kampine JP: Circulatory physiology: the essentials, ed 2, Baltimore, 1984, Williams & Wilkins.
5. Conover MB: Understanding electrocardiography: arrhythmias and the 12-lead ECG, ed 5, St Louis, 1988, Mosby–Year Book, Inc.
6. Bullock BL and Rosendahl PP: Pathophysiology: adaptations and alterations in function, ed 2, Glenview, IL, 1988, Scott, Foresman, & Co.
7. Cohn PF: Clinical cardiovascular physiology, Philadelphia, 1985, WB Saunders Co.

# CHAPTER 2

# Cardiovascular Assessment

Cathie E. Guzzetta
Patricia C. Seifert

People who have cardiovascular disease enter the health care system at varying stages of disease progression. Thus to identify patient problems and determine the objectives of care, a thorough patient assessment is needed. The initial assessment phase begins the step of identifying and solving problems, a step that continues throughout the therapeutic relationship.

The purpose of this chapter is to discuss the first step in the nursing process—the assessment phase—emphasizing the assessment from a holistic and nursing point of view.

## Nursing Assessment

A nursing assessment is a logical, systematic, and ordered collection of data used to evaluate the health status of a patient in order to identify body-mind-spirit problems.[1] It includes observation, interviewing, and physical assessment skills, as well as communication. Biopsychosocial data are collected from the patient, family, significant others, members of the health team, previous patient records, and the results of diagnostic and laboratory data.[2]

The kind of assessment tool format used will guide the data collection efforts and will influence the findings and their interpretation. Many nurses throughout the United States are still using a medical database format to guide their assessment.[3,4] A medical database is useful in guiding the collection of data in the physiologic realm but does not provide nurses with a framework for collecting psychosocial data. As a result, a complete physical assessment is generally accomplished, but the psychosocial assessment usually is incomplete. Thus, major obstacles are incurred in trying to identify all of the patient's body-mind-spirit needs because only part of the data is collected. Moreover, it becomes difficult to support the existence of many nursing diagnoses because data to support their existence is not assessed.[3,4]

Over the past decade, there has been a movement in nursing to shift from a biomedical to a holistic model of patient care. Nursing leaders have recommended that conceptual models or frameworks of nursing be used to guide nursing practice and the steps of the nursing process: assessment, nursing diagnosis, patient outcomes, planning,

intervention, and evaluation.[5,6,7] The next sections discuss the development of a holistic nursing database created from a nursing framework.

### NURSING ASSESSMENT USING THE NINE HUMAN RESPONSE PATTERNS

A holistic nursing framework called the *Unitary Person Framework* was developed by the North American Nursing Diagnosis Association (NANDA) to guide the development of nursing diagnoses.[8] This framework focuses on the health of the person who is viewed as an open system in interaction with the environment. Within this framework, each person has unique patterns and organization, which describe their state of health, as manifested by the *nine human response patterns* outlined in the box below.

The patterns described in the box below are believed to reflect all parts of the whole person. Thus, if the nine patterns are assessed, nurses are able to identify all of the patient's body-mind-spirit needs because they are collect-

---

### NINE HUMAN RESPONSE PATTERNS OF THE UNITARY PERSON FRAMEWORK

*Exchanging:* a human response pattern involving mutual giving and receiving

*Communicating:* a human response pattern involving sending messages

*Relating:* a human response pattern involving establishing bonds

*Valuing:* a human response pattern involving the assigning of relative worth

*Choosing:* a human response pattern involving the selection of alternatives

*Moving:* a human response pattern involving activity

*Perceiving:* a human response pattern involving the reception of information

*Knowing:* a human response pattern involving the meaning associated with information

*Feeling:* a human response pattern involving the subjective awareness of information

From the North American Nursing Diagnosis Association, St. Louis, 1988.

## TAXONOMY I REVISED (JUNE 1988)*

**1. EXCHANGING**

1.1 Altered nutrition
    1.1.1.
    1.1.2. [Systemic]
        1.1.2.1. More than body requirements
        1.1.2.2. Less than body requirements
        1.1.2.3. Potential for more than body requirements
1.2. [Altered physical regulation]
    1.2.1. [Immunologic]
        1.2.1.1. Potential for infection
    1.2.2. [Temperature]
        1.2.2.1. Potential altered body temperature
        1.2.2.2. Hypothermia
        1.2.2.3. Hyperthermia
        1.2.2.4. Ineffective thermoregulation
    1.2.3. [Neurologic]
        *1.2.3.1. Dysreflexia
1.3. Altered elimination
    1.3.1. Bowel
        1.3.1.1. Constipation
        *1.3.1.1.1. Perceived
        *1.3.1.1.2. Colonic
        1.3.1.2. Diarrhea
        1.3.1.3. Bowel incontinence
    1.3.2. Urinary
        1.3.2.1. Incontinence
        1.3.2.1.1. Stress
        1.3.2.1.2. Reflex
        1.3.2.1.3. Urge
        1.3.2.1.4. Functional
        1.3.2.1.5. Total
        1.3.2.2. Retention
1.4. [Altered circulation]
    1.4.1. [Vascular]
        1.4.1.1. Tissue perfusion
        1.4.1.1.1. Renal
        1.4.1.1.2. Cerebral
        1.4.1.1.3. Cardiopulmonary
        1.4.1.1.4. Gastrointestinal
        1.4.1.1.5. Peripheral
        1.4.1.2. Fluid volume
        1.4.1.2.1. Excess
        1.4.1.2.2. Deficit
        1.4.1.2.2.1. Actual [1] Actual [2]
        1.4.1.2.2.2. Potential
    1.4.2. [Cardiac]
        1.4.2.1. Decreased cardiac output
1.5. [Altered oxygenation]
    1.5.1. [Respiration]
        1.5.1.1. Impaired gas exchange
        1.5.1.2. Ineffective airway clearance
        1.5.1.3. Ineffective breathing pattern
1.6. [Altered physical integrity]
    1.6.1. Potential for injury
        1.6.1.1. Potential for suffocation

        1.6.1.2. Potential for poisoning
        1.6.1.3. Potential for trauma
        *1.6.1.4. Potential for aspiration
        *1.6.1.5. Potential for disuse syndrome
    1.6.2. Impairment
        1.6.2.1. Tissue integrity
        1.6.2.1.1. Oral mucous membranes
        1.6.2.1.2. Skin integrity
        1.6.2.1.2.1. Actual
        1.6.2.1.2.2. Potential

**2. COMMUNICATION**

2.1 Altered communication
    2.1.1. Verbal
        2.1.1.1. Impaired

**3. RELATING**

3.1. [Altered socialization]
    3.1.1. Impaired social interaction
    3.1.2. Social isolation
3.2. [Altered role]
    3.2.1. Altered role performance
        3.2.1.1. Parenting
        3.2.1.1.1. Actual
        3.2.1.1.2. Potential
        3.2.1.2. Sexual
        3.2.1.2.1. Dysfunction
    3.2.2. Altered family processes
    3.2.3. [Altered role conflict]
        *3.2.3.1. Parental role conflict
3.3. Altered sexuality patterns

**4. VALUING**

4.1. [Altered spiritual state]
    4.1.1. Spiritual distress

**5. CHOOSING**

5.1. Altered coping
    5.1.1. Individual coping
        5.1.1.1. Ineffective
        5.1.1.1.1. Impaired adjustment
        *5.1.1.1.2. Defensive coping
        *5.1.1.1.3. Ineffective denial
    5.1.2. Family coping
        5.1.2.1. Ineffective
        5.1.2.1.1. Disabled
        5.1.2.1.2. Compromised
        5.1.2.2. Potential for growth
5.2. [Altered participation]
    5.2.1. [Individual]
        5.2.1.1. Noncompliance
5.3. [Altered judgment]
    5.3.1. [Individual]
        *5.3.1.1. Decisional conflict
*5.4. Health seeking behaviors (specify)

*Continued.*

---

## TAXONOMY I REVISED (JUNE 1988)*—cont'd

**6. MOVING**

6.1 [Altered activity]
  6.1.1. Physical mobility
    6.1.1.1. Impaired
    6.1.1.2. Activity intolerance
      *6.1.1.2.1. Fatigue
    6.1.1.3. Potential activity intolerance
6.2. [Altered rest]
  6.2.1. Sleep pattern disturbance
6.3 [Altered recreation]
  6.3.1. Diversional activity
    6.3.1.1. Deficit
6.4. [Altered ADL]
  6.4.1. Home maintenance management
    6.4.1.1. Impaired
  6.4.2. Health maintenance
6.5. Self care deficit
  6.5.1. Feeding
    6.5.1.1. Impaired swallowing
    *6.5.1.2. Ineffective breastfeeding
  6.5.2. Bathing/hygiene
  6.5.3. Dressing/grooming
  6.5.4. Toileting
6.6. Altered growth and development

**7. PERCEIVING**

7.1. Altered self concept
  7.1.1. Body image disturbance
  7.1.2. Self esteem disturbance
    *7.1.2.1. Chronic low self esteem
    *7.1.2.2. Situational low self esteem
  7.1.3. Personal identity disturbance
7.2. Altered sensory/perception

7.2.1. Visual
  7.2.1.1. Unilateral neglect
7.2.2. Auditory
7.2.3. Kinesthetic
7.2.4. Gustatory
7.2.5. Tactile
7.2.6. Olfactory
7.3. [Altered meaningfulness]
  7.3.1. Hopelessness
  7.3.2. Powerlessness

**8. KNOWING**

8.1. [Altered knowing]
  8.1.1. Knowledge deficit
8.2.
8.3. Altered thought processes

**9. FEELING**

9.1. Altered comfort
  9.1.1. Pain
    9.1.1.1. Chronic
9.2 [Altered emotional integrity]
  9.2.1. Grieving
    9.2.1.1. Dysfunctional
    9.2.1.2. Anticipatory
  9.2.2. Potential for violence
  9.2.3. Post-trauma response
    9.2.3.1. Rape-trauma syndrome
      9.2.3.1.1. Compound reaction
      9.2.3.1.2. Silent reaction
9.3. [Altered emotional state]
  9.3.1. Anxiety
  9.3.2. Fear

*New Diagnostic categories approved 1988.
From: North American Nursing Diagnosis Association, 1989

---

ing the appropriate data necessary to assess the whole patient.

The nine human response patterns have also been used to classify all the nursing diagnoses approved by NANDA. In the past, the accepted list of nursing diagnoses was organized alphabetically. The alphabetical list has been replaced by *Taxonomy I,* which is organized according to these nine patterns (see the box on pp. 11-12).[9,10,11]

The human response patterns and Taxonomy I were used recently to provide the working categories for developing a holistic nursing database (Cardiovascular Response Pattern Assessment Tool).[3,4] In developing the tool, the nine response patterns were rearranged and became the skeleton of the tool.[4] Next the Standards of Cardiovascular Nursing were included in the tool's skeleton.[12] These standards of practice provide model assessment pa-

rameters to guide the nurse in collecting the data. Specific assessment parameters (signs and symptoms) related to most nursing diagnoses (pertaining to cardiovascular patients) were then added to the appropriate nine human response patterns in the tool (Fig. 2-1).[4]

The tool was developed to group clusters of assessment parameters for a particular patient problem so that a judgment can be made about whether the problem actually exists in the patient being assessed. Within each major category of the tool, subjective data followed by objective data have been included. The case study reported in the box on p. 19 describes a patient admitted to the coronary care unit with infective endocarditis. The Cardiovascular Response Pattern Assessment Tool (Fig. 2-1) illustrates the data that were collected to assess the patient's body-mind-spirit problems. *Text continued on p. 18.*

**CARDIOVASCULAR RESPONSE PATTERN ASSESSMENT TOOL**

Name _Mr. W. J._ Age _45_ Sex _Male_
Address _510 Grove St., Arlington, VA 22006_ Telephone _558·2525_
Significant other _Mrs. P. J. (Wife)_ Telephone _Same_
Date of admission _2/14_ Medical diagnosis _chest pain 2/14; S viridans endocarditis 2/15_
Allergies _None known_

**Nursing Diagnosis**

**COMMUNICATING — A pattern involving sending messages**
(Read,) (write,) (understand) English (circle) _____
Other language _Spanish_
Intubated _No_ Speech impaired _No_
Alternate form of communication _—_

Altered communication
Verbal
Impaired

**KNOWING — A pattern involving the meaning associated with information**
Current health problems _Substernal chest pain with palpitations 2/14 am (10-20 min.) without radiation. No associated N/V, SOB, or diaphoresis. complains of chills, fever, fatigue for 2 weeks_
Previous illnesses/hospitalizations/surgeries _told of existence of heart murmur as child (asymptomatic, functional class I) Periodontal work 1 month ago. Hospitalized for appendectomy at 12 y/o; no other hospitalizations._

History of the following problems:
Heart _murmur; no history of previous chest pain or CAD_
Peripheral vascular _None_
Lung _None_
Liver _None_ Kidney _None_
Cerebrovascular _None_ Rheumatic fever _yes (10 y/o)_
Thyroid _None_
Other _Appendicitis (Appendectomy 12 y/o)_

Current medications _tylenol for fever; penicillin, streptomycin for infective endocarditis._

Knowledge deficit

| Risk factors | Present | Perceptions/Knowledge of |
|---|---|---|
| 1. Hypertension | No | |
| 2. Hyperlipidemia | No | |
| 3. Smoking | No | |
| 4. Obesity | No | |
| 5. Diabetes | No | |
| 6. Sedentary living | No | active lifestyle |
| 7. Stress | moderate | related to job |
| 8. Alcohol use | yes | social drinker |
| 9. Oral contraceptives | — | |
| 10. Family history | _Wife and children in good health; Father died of AMI at age 53; Mother alive and well._ | |

Perception/knowledge of illness/test/surgery _Afraid he has had AMI; unaware of need for prophylactic antibiotics before invasive procedures with hx of heart murmur._
Expectations of therapy _to recuperate, resume activities_
Misconceptions _Worries he suffers from same illness as father._
Readiness to learn _Interested in diagnosis and treatment._
Requests information concerning _As above_
Educational level _College graduate - business school_
Learning impeded by _—_

**Fig. 2-1** Cardiovascular Response Pattern Assessment Tool. (Modified from Guzzetta CE, Bunton SD, Prinkey LA, Sherer AP, and Seifert PC: Clinical assessment tools for use with nursing diagnoses, St Louis, 1989, Mosby–Year Book, Inc.)

<u>Orientation</u>
Level of alertness _fully alert_
Orientation: Person _yes_          Place _yes_          Time _yes_
Appropriate behavior/communication _yes, cooperative_

Altered thought process

<u>Memory</u>
Memory intact: Yes _✓_          No _____          Recent _yes_          Remote _yes_

**VALUING — A pattern involving the assessment of relative worth**
Religious preference _Roman Catholic_
Important religious practices _Sunday mass_
Spiritual concerns _requests visit by priest_
Cultural orientation _Caucasian, American_
Cultural practices _none specific; no restrictions to therapy_

Spiritual distress

**RELATING — A pattern involving establishing bonds**
<u>Role</u>
Marital status _Married 18 yrs._
Age & health of significant other _Wife 43 y/o in good health_

Number of children _2_     Ages _13 y/o boy; 15 y/o boy (John, Bill)_
Role in home _Head of household_
Financial support _Salary from job_
Occupation _Administrator in government office_
  Job satisfaction/concerns _likes to keep busy_
  Physical/mental energy expenditures _mental stress of job_
Sexual relationships (satisfactory/unsatisfactory) _____
  Physical difficulties/effects of illness related to sex _possible difficulties_
  _without treatment_

Altered role performance
  Parenting
  Sexual dysfunction
  Work

Altered family processes
  Parental role conflict

Altered sexuality patterns

<u>Socialization</u>
Quality of relationships with others:
  Patient's description _good relationship with family, friends_
  Significant others' description _wife confirms_
  Staff observations _Pt. and Wife mutually supportive_
  Verbalizes feelings of being alone _NO_
  Attributed to _____

Altered socialization
  Impaired social interaction

Social isolation

**FEELING — A pattern involving the subjective awareness of information**
<u>Comfort</u>
Pain/discomfort: Yes _____          No _None at present, resting_
  Onset _—_                    Duration _—_
  Location _—_          Quality _—_          Radiation _—_
  Associated factors _—_
  Aggravating factors _—_
  Alleviating factors _—_
  Objective manifestations _(with past episode of chest pain, stated he would_
_stop what he was doing, would become pale, alleviated with rest.)_

Altered comfort
  Pain/chronic
  Pain/acute

<u>Emotional Integrity/States</u>
  Recent stressful life events _None_

  Verbalizes feelings of _Anxiety, fear, uneasiness_
  Source _fear of AMI; going through same experience as_
_father_
  Physical manifestations _Becomes quiet, introverted; has darting_
_eye movements, twists sheets in fist._

(Anxiety)
Fear
Grieving
  Dysfunctional
  Anticipatory

**Fig. 2-1, cont'd**  Cardiovascular Response Pattern Assessment Tool.

**MOVING — A pattern involving activity**
Self-care
  Ability to perform self-care (specify level) _Independent - Level 0_
  Specify deficits _recently some deficit related to fatigue_
  Discharge planning needs _none identified related to self-care_

| | Self-care deficit |
| | (Level 0-4) |
| | Feeding |
| | Impaired swallowing |
| | Bathing/hygiene |
| | Dressing/grooming |
| | Toileting |

Activity
  Limitations of movement (specify level) _None - Level 0_

  Limitations in activities _some limitation related to chest pain_
  _and fever._
  Verbal report of fatigue _last 2 wks - with weakness_
  Exercise habits _walks about office during day; yard work,_
  _boating in summer._

Impaired physical mobility
  (Level 0-4)
Activity intolerance
  Fatigue

Rest
  Sleep/rest pattern _8h /night; feels rested in am._
    Sleep aids (pillows, meds, food) _has used 1 extra pillow past 2 wks._
    Difficulty falling/remaining asleep _rare_

Sleep pattern disturbance

Recreation
  Leisure activities _Boating, fishing, yard work_
  Social activities _entertains friends and family; work-_
    _related activities._

Diversional activity deficit

Activities of Daily Living
  Home maintenance management
    Size & arrangement of home (stairs, bathroom) _4 bedroom;_
    _no problem with home._ Safety needs _none._
    Home responsibilities _pays bills, helps wife with food_
    _shopping; occasionally helps with house cleaning._
  Health maintenance
    Health insurance _yes, work_
  Regular physical check-ups _physical once a year; visits dentist_
  _occasionally - recent periodontal work._

Impaired home maintenance
  management

Altered health maintenance

**PERCEIVING — A pattern involving the reception of information**
Body image/Self-esteem
  Perception of self and situation _"I work hard and enjoy life"_
  _not sure if illness will affect ability to work._
  Description of body structure/functioning _"I don't want to die suddenly like_
  _my father; can I continue to take care of my family?"_

Altered self-concept
  Self-esteem disturbance
    Chronic low
    Situational low
  Body image disturbance

Meaningfulness
  Verbalizes hopelessness _No_
  Verbalizes loss of control _No_

Hopelessness
Powerlessness

Sensory/Perception
  History of restricted environment _No_
  Vision impaired _yes_          Glasses _Contact lenses_
  Auditory impaired _No_         Hearing aid _No_
  Kinesthetics impaired _No_
  Gustatory impaired _No_
  Tactile impaired _No_
  Olfactory impaired _No_

Altered sensory/perception
  Visual
  Auditory
  Kinesthetic
  Gustatory
  Tactile
  Olfactory

| Reflexes: | Biceps | R _2+_ | L _2+_ | Triceps | R _2+_ | L _2+_ |
| | Brachioradialis | R _2+_ | L _2+_ | Knee | R _2+_ | L _2+_ |
| | Ankle | R _2+_ | L _2+_ | Plantar | R _2+_ | L _2+_ |

**Fig. 2-1, cont'd**   Cardiovascular Response Pattern Assessment Tool.      *Continued.*

**EXCHANGING — A pattern involving mutual giving and receiving**

Circulation

Cerebral

Neurological changes/symptoms _None_

Complaints of syncope _None_

Altered cerebral tissue perfusion

Pupils

L 2 ③ 4 5 6 mm

R 2 ③ 4 5 6 mm

Reaction: Brisk _X_

Sluggish _____ Non reactive _____

Eye Opening

None (1)

To pain (2)

To speech (3)

Spontaneous ((4))

Fluid volume

Deficit

Excess

Best Verbal

Mute (1)

Incomprehensible sound (2)

Inappropriate words (3)

Confused conversation (4)

Oriented (5)

Best Motor

Flaccid (1)

Extensor response (2)

Flexor response (3)

Semipurposeful (4)

Localized to pain (5)

Obeys commands (6)

Decreased cardiac output

Glasgow coma scale total _15_

Altered cerebral tissue perfusion

Peripheral

Arterial pulses: A = absent    B = bruits    D = Doppler

Altered peripheral tissue perfusion

+3 = bounding    +2 = palpable    +1 = faintly palpable

| | | | | |
|---|---|---|---|---|
| Carotid | R _3+_ L _3+_ | Popliteal | R _2+_ L _2+_ | |
| Brachial | R _3+_ L _3+_ | Posterior tibial | R _2+_ L _2+_ | |
| Radial | R _3+_ L _3+_ | Dorsalis pedis | R _2+_ L _2+_ | |
| Femoral | R _2+_ L _2+_ | | | |

Fluid volume

Deficit

Excess

BP:    Sitting    Lying    Standing

R _120/80_ L _120/80_    R _122/82_ L _122/82_    R _120/80_ L _120/80_

A-Line reading _—_    CVP _—_

Venous pulse _Normal_    Jugular venous distention R _No_ L _No_

Skin temp _warm/hot_    Color _pink_    Cyanosis _No_

Capillary refill _2 seconds_    Clubbing _No_

Edema _Slight pedal edema after standing_

Cardiovascular

PMI _5 ICS, MCL_    Pacemaker _No_

Apical rate & rhythm _120 and regular_

Heart sounds/murmurs _Normal S₁,S₂· No S₃,S₄ or rubs· Grade ii/vi holosystolic murmur at LLSB with_

Dysrhythmias _Sinus tachycardia_    _radiation to left axilla_

Cardiac output _—_    Cardiac index _—_

PAP _—_    PCWP _—_

IV fluids _D 5 W, TKO_

IV medications _—_

Serum enzymes _Normal CPK-MB, LDH_

Altered cardiopulmonary tissue perfusion

(Decreased cardiac output potential)

Dysreflexia

Physical Integrity

Tissue integrity _gums healing_

Skin: rash _none_    Lesions _none_

Petechiae _bilat conjunctival_    Bruises _none_

Abrasions _none_    Surgical incision _RLQ (appendectomy)_

Impaired skin integrity

Impaired tissue integrity

Disuse syndrome

Infection

**Fig. 2-1, cont'd**  Cardiovascular Response Pattern Assessment Tool.

## Oxygenation

Complaints of dyspnea _rare_ Precipitated by _lying down (at night)_
Orthopnea _rare_
Rate _16_ Rhythm _regular_ Depth _normal_     Ineffective breathing patterns
Labored/(unlabored)(circle) Use of accessory muscles _none_
Chest expansion _symmetrical_ Splinting _none_     Ineffective airway clearance
Cough: Productive/nonproductive _none_
Sputum: Color _—_ Amount _—_ Consistency _—_     Impaired gas exchange
Breath sounds _normal breath sounds; no rales, crackles, or wheezes_ Potential for aspiration
Arterial blood gases _—_
Oxygen percent and device _nasal cannula, 6 L/min._
Ventilator _—_

## Physical Regulation

Immune          ⟨~~Potential for infection~~⟩
   Lymph nodes enlarged _NO_ Location _—_     Hypothermia
   WBC count _24,000_ Differential _65% Segs, 15% bands_   ⟨Hyperthermia⟩
Temperature _101.4°F_ Route _oral_     Altered body temperature
_ESR elevated; positive rheumatic factor_     Ineffective thermoregulation

## Nutrition

Eating patterns
   Number of meals per day _3 meals (occasionally skips lunch)_    Altered nutrition
   Special diet _none_      More than body
   Where eaten _home, work, restaurant, friends' house_       requirements
   Food preferences/intolerances _enjoys all foods_      Less than body
   Food allergies _none_       requirements
   Caffeine intake (coffee, tea, soft drinks) _3 cups coffee (decaf) per day;_
_1-2 diet cokes per day_
   Appetite changes _eating less past 3 wks; normal fluid intake_
   Presence of nausea/vomiting _none_
   Condition of mouth/throat _gums inflammed and sore; no dentures_   Impaired oral mucous
_or missing teeth; lips and tongue hydrated._      membranes
   Height _5' 9"_ Weight _162_ Ideal body weight _160_     Altered nutrition
     More than body
      requirements
Current therapy      Less than body
   NPO _—_ NG suction _—_       requirements
   Tube feeding _—_     Potential for aspiration
   TPN _—_

Labs
   Na _140 m Eq/L_ K _4.0 m Eq/L_ Cl _102 m Eq/L_ Glucose _110 mg/dl_
   Cholesterol _175 mg/dl_ Triglycerides _150 mg/dl_ Fasting _yes_
   Hct _42%_ Hgb _13.5 g/dl_
   Other _—_

## Elimination

     Altered bowel elimination
Gastrointestinal/Bowel      Constipation
   Usual bowel habits _daily bowel movement_      Perceived
   Use of laxatives, enemas, and/or suppositories _no_      Colonic
   Alterations from norm _—_     Diarrhea
   Abdominal physical exam _normal size, shape, and symmetry;_     Incontinence
_no masses, pain, or organ enlargement; 2+ bowel sounds._ Altered GI tissue perfusion

Renal/Urinary     Altered urinary elimination
   Usual urinary pattern _voids without difficulty_      Incontinence
   Alteration from norm _none_      Retention
   Bladder distention _none_     Altered renal tissue perfusion
   Color _yellow_ Catheter _—_
   Urine output: 24 hour _> 1440 cc_ Average hourly _> 60 cc_
   BUN _22 mg/dl_ Creatinine _0.7 mg/dl_ Specific gravity _1.010_
   Urine studies _none additional_

**Fig. 2-1, cont'd**   Cardiovascular Response Pattern Assessment Tool.     _Continued._

**CHOOSING — A pattern involving the selection of alternatives**

Coping

Patient's ability to cope _discusses problems and their resolution with wife and/or children_

Family's ability to cope/give support _mutually supportive; share problems with each other._

Patient's acceptance of illness _realizes need for hospitalization; concerned about future well-being._

Patient's adjustment to illness _Demonstrates willingness to participate in therapy._

Ineffective individual coping
  Defensive coping
  Ineffective denial
  Impaired adjustment

Ineffective family coping
  Disabled
  Compromised

Judgment

Decision making ability:
  Patient's perspective _"I can make decisions for myself."_
  Other's perspective _family believes he has good judgment._

Ability to choose from alternatives _able to make choices; understands information provided._

Decisional conflict

Participation

Compliance with past/current health care regimen _No previous specific health regimen recommended or ordered._

Willingness to comply with future health care regimen _States he will comply with recommendations._

Noncompliance

Health Seeking

Express desire to seek higher level of wellness _wants to recover in order to resume former lifestyle._

Health seeking behaviors

Prioritized nursing diagnosis/problem list:

1. _Infection (cardiac valve) R/To invasive dental work._
2. _Potential decreased cardiac output R/To tachydysrhythmia and damage to mitral valve._
3. _Knowledge deficit R/To prophylactic prevention of endocarditis._
4. _Anxiety R/To acute illness, hospitalization, family hx._
5. _____

Signature _Patricia C. Seifert, R.N._          Date _2/15_

**Fig. 2-1, cont'd**  Cardiovascular Response Pattern Assessment Tool.

Because it was not practical to include in the tool all possible signs and symptoms related to each specific nursing diagnosis, summary assessment parameters were developed instead (e.g., limitations of movement and daily activities under "moving pattern" are summary parameters intended to evaluate the nursing diagnoses of impaired physical mobility and activity intolerance). The section on p. 19 outlines the specific data to be extracted from the summary assessment parameters listed in the tool so that the appropriate data can be elicited.[13]

The theory, process, and structure used to develop this tool (for use with cardiovascular patients) also were used in adapting the tool for use with other patient populations (e.g., pulmonary, trauma, renal, transplant, neonatal patients). Twenty-three other assessment tools were thereby developed for a variety of diverse patient groups.[4] The results of this work offer a model for standardizing nursing databases.

## CASE STUDY

Mr. W.J., a 45-year-old government administrator, was admitted to the coronary care unit with substernal chest pain lasting 10 to 20 minutes and associated with chills, elevated temperature, fatigue, and frequent palpitations. When he was 14 years old he had been told he had a heart murmur, but remained asymptomatic without restrictions in activity until recently. A month before admission he had visited the dentist for periodontal care but had not received prophylactic antibiotics before or after the procedure.

On admission, the patient had a sinus tachycardia of 120 beats per minutes and a blood pressure of 120/80 mm Hg. First and second heart sounds were normal; a grade 2/6 holosystolic murmur at the lower left sternal border was present and radiated to the left axilla. A presumptive diagnosis of infective bacterial endocarditis was made during the first day of admission by the physician. The diagnosis of acute mitral regurgitation was later confirmed by echocardiography, which demonstrated mild retrograde flow.

The initial electrocardiogram suggested that the patient had anteroseptal myocardial ischemia, but cardiac serum enzyme values were normal. Serial aerobic and anaerobic blood cultures revealed a heavy growth of *Streptococcus viridans*. The patient was medically treated with penicillin, streptomycin, and bed rest.

## INTERVIEWING TECHNIQUES USED TO ELICIT APPROPRIATE DATA

Interviewing and communicating are essential skills necessary to perform a thorough assessment. Interviewing is a goal-directed method of communication—a medium of interaction between two persons. Its major purpose is to elicit pertinent information about the patient so that body-mind-spirit problems can be assessed. When the interaction between the nurse and the patient is marked by concern and sensitivity, the interviewing process can help to establish a meaningful nurse-patient relationship. The accuracy and completeness of the data gathered during the assessment depends on the nurse's ability to communicate effectively and elicit pertinent information.

A holistic assessment involves more than just collecting the appropriate data. Nurses and patients are both open systems; they exchange energy and information at many levels.[1,7] Their energy fields overlap and are affected by one another. The key to achieving a comprehensive and holistic assessment is to be wholly involved with the patient during the encounter. This means that the nurses need to be relaxed and focused.[5] Astute and sensitive nurses are able to function at their highest level when they are open to subtle cues, environmental exchanges, and intuitive feelings that can have an enormous impact on the data collected and the conclusions formulated during the patient assessment. Nurses who are focused during the assessment and aware of collecting data with purposeful intention become receptive to the encounter, thus allowing the free flow of information to occur at many levels.

To facilitate the assessment, the nurse needs to remember some guidelines for establishing an effective nurse-patient relationship.

## ESTABLISHING A NURSE-PATIENT RELATIONSHIP

1. Provide as much privacy as possible for the assessment.
2. Introduce yourself.
3. Call the patient by his or her preferred name.
4. Tell the patient the purpose of the assessment.
5. Sit at eye level, establish eye contact with the patient, and lean toward the patient.
6. Probe and listen for the patient's concerns and beliefs about his or her condition and health problems.
7. Show caring and concern for the patient as a human being.
8. Be nonjudgmental in your responses to the patient.
9. Use language that is appropriate for the patient's educational, cultural, and psychosocial background.
10. Observe the patient's nonverbal behavior such as facial grimacing or wringing of hands.

In addition to establishing a good nurse-patient relationship, it is important that the nurse be familiar with alternatives in guiding an interview and responding to patients. All to often nurses use only one or two alternatives. The use of the following techniques can help to structure the interview and facilitate more complete and accurate data collection.

### Guiding the Interview

1. Use open-ended questions and statements ("Tell me about your chest pain").
2. Clarify words, phrases, or statements ("What do you mean by 'a little bit'?").
3. Summarize data during and after the interview to ensure accuracy.
4. Reflect words, phrases, statements, and feelings ("You've been having trouble sleeping?").
5. Use silence to organize your thoughts and allow the patient time to answer questions.
6. Use supportive statements and gestures ("That must have been difficult—tell me more"). (Nod head yes.)
7. Focus the interview on the current topic(s) ("Let's talk some more about your chest pain").

## GUIDELINES FOR ELICITING APPROPRIATE DATA WHEN ASSESSING THE NINE HUMAN RESPONSE PATTERNS

The following sections discuss specific information to be extracted from the tool's summary assessment parameters in order to elicit the necessary data to assess the patient's nine human response patterns.* The ordering of these sections follows the assessment parameters outlined in the tool (Fig. 2-1).

Data should be collected within a time period that reflects the gravity of the patient's condition. If the patient is critically ill or easily fatigued, priority sections can be completed first and other sections can be completed later (usually within a 24-hour time frame).

## COMMUNICATING PATTERN

The purpose of the communicating pattern is to determine whether the patient is able to communicate with others and how well. Data are collected regarding speech, languages, and verbal and nonverbal forms of communication. This pattern is evaluated first because the rest of the assessment depends on the ability and reliability of the patient to communicate. Thus it may be necessary initially to obtain the information from the patient's family (significant other) or to validate the data with them.

### Read, Write, and Understand English

Begin the assessment by evaluating the patient's ability to understand, speak, read, and write English. Determine whether there is a physiologic or psychologic reason for any difficulty (e.g., reduced circulation to the brain, stroke, brain tumor, oral anatomic defect, severe anxiety, psychosis, lack of stimuli).

### Other Languages

Identify what primary language is spoken in the home and what other languages are spoken. If the patient's primary language is not English and the nurse finds that communication with the patient is difficult, an interpreter is recommended.

### Intubation/Speech Impairment

Evaluate whether the patient has any barriers in communicating. If the patient is unable to speak, document this information in the assessment and determine the cause. If the patient is intubated or has a tracheostomy, for example, why was the intubation or tracheostomy done and how long ago? Inability to speak may be related to other causes such as severe shortness of breath, facial paralysis, facial laceration or burns, or a mandibular fracture. Assess whether the patient is able to modulate speech, find words, name words, identify objects, and speak in sentences.[14-16]

### Alternate Forms of Communication

When assessing the communication pattern, also recognize whether the patient can use any alternate form of communication such as sign language, sign board, writing, typewriter, or computer.[16]

## KNOWING PATTERN

Assessment of the knowing pattern permits the nurse to determine what the patient knows about the current and past health status. Data are collected regarding knowledge and perception of risk factors, illness, tests, surgery, medications, readiness to learn, misconceptions, and level of orientation.

### Current Health Problems

To determine information about the patient's current health problems, the question—"What brought you to the hospital?"—is generally most effective in focusing this line of inquiry. Attempt to elicit the signs, symptoms, and problems in the order they occurred. This information will provide a focus for collecting more specific data in the associated pattern of concern. For example, for a patient admitted to the coronary care unit with chest pain, a comprehensive assessment of the coronary artery disease risk factors outlined in this pattern and the cardiac and respiratory categories under the exchanging pattern is appropriate. As the patient expresses perceived physiologic or psychologic changes, the nurse reorganizes the patient's words according to the database format to identify the patterns and processes underlying each sign and symptom. For each sign and symptom identified in the pattern of concern, determine when, where, and under what circumstances the sign or symptom occurred. Also determine the location, quality, quantity, and duration of the sign or symptom and any aggravating, alleviating, or associated factors. Within each pattern, it is also important to identify pertinent "negatives" or the absence of certain signs and symptoms that often are involved with the problem, for example, absence of weight gain or dyspnea in a patient suspected of having decreased cardiac output. In the seriously ill patient, priority is given to the information that appears most relevant to the immediate situation.

### Previous Illnesses, Hospitalizations, Surgeries, Problems

Information regarding the patient's previous illnesses, hospitalization, and surgeries is identified. Specifically, the nurse should collect the following data:

1. Identify any history of heart problems including cardiac enlargement, heart failure, murmurs, myocardial infarction, and heart infection.
2. Determine any history of peripheral vascular disease or intermittent claudication (e.g., calf cramping and fatigue that occurs when walking or exercising and is relieved by rest).
3. Inquire about a history of lung disease such as tuberculosis, asthma, lung infections, or bronchitis.
4. Identify any history of liver disease, such as liver

---

*Pp. 19-46 based on material from Guzzetta, CE: General focus questions and parameters for eliciting appropriate data. In Guzzetta CE, Bunton SD, Prinkey LA, Sherer AP, and Seifert PC: Clinical assessment tools for use with nursing diagnosis, St Louis, 1989, Mosby–Year Book, Inc.

enlargement or hepatitis; kidney disease such as infections or stones; cerebrovascular problems, such as dizziness, fainting, strokes, or high blood pressure; rheumatic fever; thyroid problems; gallbladder problems; gastrointestinal problems, or genitourinary problems.

5. Consider also if the patient has a history of drug abuse, and if so what kind, how long it lasted, how long ago it occurred, and how it was treated.

## Current Medications

Identify what medications the patient is taking. Determine the name of the medication, dosage, frequency, how long the patient has been taking the medication, and any side effects. Also determine any over-the-counter medications such as aspirin, acetaminophen, ibuprofen, laxatives, sleeping pills, or diet pills. It may be useful to ask the patient to pick a typical day and describe all medications (physician-prescribed and self-prescribed) taken from morning until bedtime. A medication history is particularly necessary with the elderly patient, who may see more than one health care provider and consume a series of drugs that have synergistic or mutually inhibitory effects.[7]

## Risk Factors

Determine whether the patient has any coronary artery risk factors and assess the patient's perception and level of understanding of each.[7,17] Query the patient about a history of hypertension, hyperlipidemia, smoking, obesity, diabetes mellitus, a sedentary lifestyle, high levels of psychophysiologic stress, alcohol abuse, and use of oral contraceptives, cessation of menses, or the beginning of menopause.

## Family History

The family background also may contribute important information to the assessment. Identify the age, sex, and health status of living family members, including parents, siblings, children, and spouse or significant other. Determine the age, sex, and cause of death for deceased family members. In addition, certain familial diseases that grandparents, parents, and close relatives may have had are pertinent to the assessment, for example, coronary artery disease risk factors (from the list outlined above). Also determine any family history of cancer, other heart diseases, peripheral vascular disease, cerebrovascular disease, hypertension, stroke, respiratory disease, diabetes mellitus, nervous or mental conditions, kidney disease, arthritic conditions, hematologic abnormalities, rheumatic fever, sickle cell anemia, or thyroid disease.

## Perception/Knowledge of Illness and Expectations

It is important to discover the patient's knowledge and perception of the illness, tests, or surgery in the current situation. Query patients about what they perceive as their biggest health problem at the moment. Ask them to discuss the problem and what they believe the cause is. Likewise, evaluate what the patient knows and understands about the tests, procedures, or surgery they are about to undergo. Patients can have diverse expectations about their hospitalization and therapy. Determine how patients expect their health problem to be treated and what they think will be the results of this treatment.

## Misconceptions

Throughout the assessment, evaluate any misconceptions or lack of understanding regarding the patient's hospitalization, illness, tests, surgery, or therapy. Assess the areas of risk factors, perception and knowledge of the current situation, and expectations of therapy. Evaluate the answers given by both the patient and the family. Determine if the information is correct, whether the patient and family have a good understanding of the information, and whether the understanding is realistic for the given situation.

## Readiness to Learn

Within the knowing pattern, readiness to learn is assessed. In the critical care unit, the patient may be requesting information that relates only to the immediate situation. Assess the kinds of questions being asked and evaluate the kind of information being requested. For example, is the patient asking questions about the therapy, treatments, illness, or prognosis? Is the patient acknowledging that a health problem exists or is a state of denial present?[6,7] (Integrate this data with the information associated with coping in the choosing pattern). When assessing the patient's readiness to learn, it is important to determine the patient's educational level so that teaching content and material can be selected appropriately. Evaluate also whether there are any barriers to learning such as pain, environmental distractions, or other physical, emotional, or psychologic conditions that have an impact on learning.

## Orientation/Memory

Evaluate whether the patient is alert, lethargic, comatose, and oriented to person, place, and time. Assess also whether the patient's behavior and communication are appropriate for the situation or whether the patient is confused. Determine if the patient's memory is intact. Assess the patient's *recent memory* by asking the day, month, and year or where the patient lives, and assess *remote memory* by asking if the patient recalls what holidays were celebrated last month or in some other specified month.

## VALUING PATTERN

The valuing pattern is assessed primarily to determine spiritual and cultural values and beliefs that may have an impact on the patient's hospitalization, therapy, and recovery.

## Religious Preference and Practices

Data are collected to identify the patient's religious preference and to evaluate whether the patient practices the religion, how often church or synagogue is attended, and the importance of religion in the patient's life. Determine whether the patient would like to talk to a religious representative and if there are any specific religious items deemed important to have while in the hospital. Also appraise whether the patient's religious beliefs and practices might affect treatment. For example, are there any treatments that are forbidden by the religion?

## Spiritual Concerns

Spiritual concerns are assessed to discover if patients are overly preoccupied with issues of life or death or are expressing excessive concerns about their relationship with God. Illness may cause patients to question the meaning of suffering and illness and may create inner conflicts about beliefs.

## Cultural Orientation/Practices

To determine cultural orientation and practices, identify the patient's cultural background or heritage. Patients may have strong ties to the customs and practices of their country. Identify any special customs that might be important in the current situation. Determine how the culture defines the role of the family in illness. Ask patients whether there are any medical treatments that are unacceptable because of their cultural beliefs.

## RELATING PATTERN

The relating pattern is assessed to determine how the patient relates to others in terms of role performances, and sexual and social relationships.

## Role

**Marital status, age, and health of significant other/ children.** Begin the assessment by determining the patient's marital status. Determine the ages and health of significant others. Inquire about children, their ages, and whether they are living in the home.

**Role in the home.** Focus the line of questioning to determine the patient's role in the home. For example, determine if the patient is responsible for running the household, making the major decisions in the home, and providing discipline for the children. Discover if this current illness might affect the patient's ability to complete the tasks expected at home, and inquire about the patient's feelings about such changes.

**Financial support.** Financial concerns, frequently precipitated by illness, also are assessed in this pattern. Identify whether the patient is the major breadwinner in the family and if the patient believes there is money available to meet current expenses or if financial assistance is needed.

**Occupation.** The patient's occupation is identified.

Note specifically the hours worked per week, the amount of physical or mental energy involved, and the amount of stress perceived. Evaluate whether the patient likes the job, verbalizes any major concerns or problems, or believes that this current illness will affect the ability to return to work.

**Sexual relationships.** The patient's sexual role is appraised. Illness can have an impact on both the patient's ability to perform sexual activity and the patient's interest in the activity. Identify any reports of difficulties, limitations, or changes in sexual behaviors, interests, or activities.[14,16] Assess the patient's risk for human immunodeficiency virus (HIV) infection, that is: Has the patient received blood transfusions? Does the patient have a history of homosexuality, prostitution, or intravenous drug abuse? Does the patient admit to multiple sexual partners or to sexual contact with a person who is HIV positive?

## Socialization

**Quality of relationships with others.** To assess the patient's socialization pattern, discover how the patient relates to others. Ask patients how they relate to others, if they are comfortable in most social situations, and whether they feel a sense of belonging, caring, and interest when they are with family or friends. Determine whether the patient prefers to be alone most of the time or if the patient feels isolated or rejected by family and friends.[16] If it is important to do so, corroborate the patient's perceptions with family or significant others. Observe how the patient interacts with and relates to family, friends, and staff to validate the patient's perceptions.

## FEELING PATTERN

Assessment of the feeling pattern involves an evaluation of how the patient feels both physically and emotionally.

## Comfort

**Pain/discomfort.** Ask the patient about any *pain or discomfort*. Determine if the pain or discomfort is acute or chronic, when it began, whether it was sudden or gradual, and if the patient has ever had the pain before.[6,7] Assess how long the pain lasts, where the pain is located, whether it is intermittent, continuous, dull, sharp, mild, or severe. Identify if the pain travels or radiates to other parts of the body and whether there are any associated, aggravating, or alleviating factors. Explore whether the patient has experienced any *palpitations* that occur with premature beats or other cardiac rhythm disturbances or whether the patient has experienced the subjective sensation of dyspnea or shortness of breath (see also Exchanging Pattern).

**Objective manifestations.** Assess the patient for objective psychophysiologic manifestations of pain or discomfort. Observe for guarding or protective behaviors such as self-focusing (e.g., altered time perception, withdrawal from social contact, impaired thought processes), moaning, crying, restlessness, and grimacing. Evaluate any alteration in muscle tone or autonomic nervous system response to pain such as diaphoresis, or blood pressure, pulse, respiratory rate, and pupillary changes. With chronic pain, observe for fear of reinjury, physical and social withdrawal, anorexia, and weight or sleep pattern changes.

### Emotional Integrity/States

Recent stressful life events. Within the feeling pattern, also assess the patient's emotional integrity. Discover if patients have had any recent stressful life events such as family, financial, or work-related problems or if anything has been particularly upsetting to them lately. Determine whether they have had any feelings of anxiety, fear, or grieving.[10,16]

Verbalizes feeling/source/physical manifestations. When assessing for the presence of *anxiety*, recognize if the patient is experiencing a threat to self-concept, a threat of death, or a threat or change in health status, socioeconomic status, role functioning, environment, or interactional patterns. Evaluate verbal complaints of increased tension, apprehension, uncertainty, inadequacy, or shakiness. Ask patients whether they feel jittery, distressed, rattled, overexcited, or scared. To assess for *fear,* explore feelings of dread related to an identifiable source that can be validated. Also observe for any physical manifestations of anxiety and fear, such as elevated heart rate and blood pressure, darting eye movements, startle reflex to normal sounds, nonpurposeful activity such as picking at sheets, hair, fingernails, or constant leg motion.[10,15,16]

To assess for *grieving,* query patients about any personal or anticipated losses. Is the patient denying the loss or having difficulty expressing the loss? Determine if the patient is having difficulty concentrating, eating, sleeping, or performing normal daily activities.[10]

### MOVING PATTERN

Illness can have an impact on the patient's ability to move, perform activities of daily living, maintain self-care, sleep, and play and can interfere with the ability to sustain environmental and health maintenance.

### Self-Care

Ability to perform self-care. Evaluate the patient's ability to perform *self-care.* Determine if the patient is independently able to feed self, adequately swallow fluids and solids, bathe self, wash hair, brush teeth, dress self, maintain a satisfactory appearance, and use a toilet or commode. Discharge planning needs regarding self-care deficits are identified during this section of the assessment. The following suggested codes can be used to define the level of functional ability. These codes are also used to classify the nursing diagnoses listed under self-care deficits (e.g., feeding, impaired swallowing, bathing/hygiene, dressing/grooming, and toileting deficits), as well as the diagnosis of impaired physical mobility (see next section).

**Suggested codes for functional level classification**[10]

0 = Completely independent
1 = Requires use of equipment or device
2 = Requires help from another person for assistance, supervision, or teaching
3 = Requires help from another person and equipment or device
4 = Dependent, does not participate in activity

### Activity

Limitation of movement. Ask the patient about any limitations in movement (physical mobility) including the ability to get in and out of a chair and bed. Determine if the patient has observed any decrease in muscle size, tone, strength, or control. Observe the patient for any limitations of movement such as a reluctance to move, limited range of motion, or impaired coordination; and identify if the patient has any perceptual, cognitive, neuromuscular, or musculoskeletal impairments. To classify the patient's functional level, use the functional code outlined above.

Limitation in activities. Ask if the patient has noticed any pain or discomfort when performing activities (activity intolerance). Has the patient observed any decreased strength or endurance? Are there any activities that can no longer be performed? Observe the patient's psychophysiologic response to activity and identify any symptoms associated with or precipitated by such activity.

Verbal reports of fatigue. Fatigue can have an enormous impact on the moving pattern. Fatigue, a subjective feeling, is common in the elderly patient and can be associated with cardiac complications, particularly congestive heart failure. Ask patients if they have felt constantly tired, weak, or exhausted. Determine if patients verbalize a lack of energy, irritability, listlessness, or an inability to concentrate or maintain usual routines that might validate the diagnosis of fatigue.

Exercise habits. Determine if the patient is involved in any type of exercise program; ask about the type of program, the number of times per week the exercise is performed, and the duration of each exercise session. Because illness can interfere with normal exercise patterns, inquire about the importance of the exercise to the patient's psychophysiologic well-being. A marathon runner who has suddenly developed angina during exercise may be devastated if the daily exercise routine is curtailed. Query the patient also about the amount of exercise involved with job, outside activities, sports, and household or yard work.

### Rest

Sleep/rest pattern. When assessing the patient's sleep/rest pattern, inquire about the patient's usual bed time, number of hours slept per night, and if any rest periods are routinely set aside for naps, relaxation, or meditation. Ask the patient about use of sleep aids, such as alcohol, tranquilizers, hypnotics, warm showers, music, or food. Explore whether the patient has trouble falling asleep, remaining asleep, returning to sleep once awakened, or has any recurring nightmares. Ask patients if they usually feel rested after sleeping. If the patient verbalizes difficulty sleeping, inquire about changes in behavior such as irritability, restlessness, lethargy, or listlessness and observe the patient for signs of sleep pattern disturbances such as mild fleeting nystagmus, light hand tremor, ptosis of eyelids, expressionless face, dark circles under eyes, frequent yawning, or changes in posture.

### Recreation

Leisure activities. Recreation, including leisure and social activities, is assessed as part of the moving pattern. Ask patients what they do in their leisure time (e.g., participating in sports, reading, listening to music, or playing cards). Inquire about any hobbies. Explore any complaints of boredom and evaluate if the patient's environment, condition, or treatments prohibit involvement in diversional activities. Is it possible for the patient to engage in any usual hobbies or activities while in the hospital?

Social activities. Discover if the patient is involved in any social activities such as church groups, clubs, or organizations. Determine the extent of the involvement and the importance of the activities to the patient.

### Activities of Daily Living

Home maintenance management. Included in the moving pattern is environmental maintenance. The size and arrangement of the home may impose obstacles for the patient. Explore any difficulty entering the home because of entrance steps and determine whether the kitchen, bedroom, and bathroom are accessible. Will steps make movement inside the home difficult? Inquire about any safety needs such as a safety rail in the bath and repair of frayed electrical cords or torn carpets. Determine what activities the patient engages in on a typical day—including meal preparation, shopping, cleaning, child care, bill paying, and household chores—and whether the current illness might interfere with such activities. (Also integrate this data with information listed under "role in home" in the relating pattern.)

Health maintenance. Inquire if the patient routinely sees a physician for regular physical check-ups. Does the patient visit other physicians or nurses for any other reason? How often does the patient visit the dentist? Evaluate whether the patient demonstrates an understanding of basic health practices, such as the need for prophylactic antibiotics following invasive procedures when the patient has a history of a heart murmur; and determine whether the patient accepts responsibility for meeting basic health needs. Does the patient express an interest in improving health behaviors, and if so, does the patient indicate a need for special equipment or personal resources? Identify whether the patient has health insurance or is in need of any financial medical assistance.[10,16,17]

## PERCEIVING PATTERN

Within the perceiving pattern, data are collected to evaluate the patient's self-perception. The assessment focuses on self-concept as manifested by self-esteem and body image. The perceiving pattern also includes an evaluation of perceived hopelessness and powerlessness and an assessment of the patient's sensory perception.[4]

### Self-Concept

Perception of self and situation. Body image and self-esteem can be dramatically altered because of the effects of illness. To assess *self-esteem,* ask patients to describe themselves, how they feel about themselves, and whether they are comfortable about the way they look, feel, and function. Evaluate the effects of illness or surgery on the patient's self-esteem. Ask patients to describe what the illness/surgery means to them and their families.

Observe to see if patients express self-negating talk, shame, or guilt. Determine if patients feel they are unable to deal with events, project blame on to others, or rationalize positive and exaggerate negative feedback about self. Distinguish whether negative verbalization about self is of a *chronic* nature or is *situational* in response to the illness.

Description of body structure/functioning. To assess for *body-image* disturbance, assess the patient for verbal or nonverbal expressions of an actual or perceived change in body structure or functioning.[16] For example, if the patient has a missing body part, does he or she refuse to look in a mirror? Refuse to look at a body part? Hide or overexpose a body part? Ignore, neglect, or traumatize a body part?[14] Refuse to discuss the illness, injury, or surgery? Have negative feelings about the body or a preoccupation with a change or loss of a body part?[16] Observe whether the patient demonstrates responsibility for self-care or demonstrates self-neglect.

### Meaningfulness

Hopelessness. Depending on the perception of the patient, illness may produce feelings of hopelessness and powerlessness. It is important to diagnose such problems because of the potentially profound effects they can produce on the patient's illness and recovery. To assess for *hopelessness,* ask patients to describe possible solutions to the problem, how they feel about the future, and what plans they have. Observe the patient for negative feelings, passivity, decreased verbalization, flat affect, a lack of initiative, decreased appetite or response to stimuli, increased sleep, lack of involvement in care, and sighing or verbal clues such as "I can't."[10] Synthesize this data with that found under "emotional integrity states" in the feeling pattern.

Powerlessness. To evaluate powerlessness, observe for verbalization that indicates a perceived loss of control. Ask patients to describe what can be done to change, improve,

---

## TESTING FOR DEEP TENDON REFLEXES

*Biceps:* The patient's arm is flexed at 45-degree angle at the elbow. Palpate the biceps tendon in the antecubital fossa. Place your fingers over the biceps muscle and your thumb over the tendon. With the reflex hammer, strike your thumb. Flexion of the elbow should occur.

*Brachioradialis:* The patient's arm is flexed up to a 45-degree angle and rests on your arm with the hand slightly pronated. With the reflex hammer, directly strike the brachioradialis tendon. Observe for flexion and supination of the forearm.

*Triceps:* The patient's arm is flexed up to a 90-degree angle, with the patient's hand resting against the side of your body. Palpate the triceps tendon and strike it directly with the relfex hammer just above the elbow. Contraction of the triceps muscle causes extension of the elbow.

*Knee:* The patient's knee is flexed up to a 90-degree angle, wtih the lower leg loosely hung. Support the patient's upper leg with your hand without allowing it to rest against the side of the table. With the reflex hammer, strike the patellar tendon just below the patella. The lower leg will extend when the quadriceps contract.

*Ankle:* With the patient sitting, flex the knee and dorsiflex the ankle up to a 90-degree angle holding the heel of the foot in your hands. Strike the Achilles tendon at the level of the ankle malleoli. Contraction of the gastrocnemius muscle causes plantar flexion of the foot at the ankle. Note also the speed of relaxation after muscular contraction.

*Plantar:* The patient's ankle is held in one hand while a sharp object is stroked from the lateral surface of the sole, starting at the heel of the foot and going to the base or the foot, curving medially across the ball and ending beneath the great toe. The normal response is flexion of all toes (negative Babinski's reflex). Extension or dorsiflexion of the great toe and fanning of the others represents a positive Babinski's reflex, which may reflect upper motor neuron disease.[6,8]

---

From Guzzetta CE and others: Clinical assessment tools for use with nursing diagnosis, St Louis, 1989, Mosby–Year Book, Inc.

or help the current situation or problem. Does the patient verbalize perceived physical deterioration despite total compliance with the medical regimen? Determine whether the patient perceives a loss of control regarding self-care and the outcomes of medical and nursing care. Verify whether the patient chooses not to participate in decision making even when opportunities are provided or whether dissatisfaction or frustration is expressed because of an inability to perform previous tasks or activities.[10,16]

### Sensory/Perception

**History of restricted environments.** The perceiving pattern also includes an assessment of the patient's sensory perception. Investigate if the patient has experienced any restricted environments such as an incubator, isolation, surgery, intensive care, prolonged bed rest, traction, or confining illness.[16]

**Senses.** Evaluate the status of the patient's senses. Observe if the patient has difficulty seeing and determine whether the patient has cataracts, a false eye, contact lenses, or glasses. Assess the patient's ability to hear normal conversation. Determine if the patient wears a hearing aid and whether it improves hearing. Assess the patient's degree of demonstrated coordination while walking or during other activities (kinesthetics). Does the patient maintain a sense of balance? Inquire about any loss or impairment of taste (gustatory). Does the patient describe a metallic or unusual taste? Question the patient regarding any loss in the sense of touch (tactile impairment). Can the patient distinguish between dull, sharp, and light touches? Explore any complaints of numbness, tingling, hypersensitivity, or decreased sensation. Query patients regarding their sense of smell. Are they able to recognize the smell of rubbing alcohol after closing their eyes?

**Reflexes.** To complete the assessment of the perceiving pattern, the deep tendon reflexes are assessed (see the box above). Compare the responses on corresponding sides and grade the responses using the following code:[18,19]

> 0 = No response
> 1 = Sluggish or diminished
> 2 = Active or expected response
> 3 = More brisk than usual
> 4 = Brisk or hyperactive

## EXCHANGING PATTERN

In the exchanging pattern, data are collected to assess the patient's physical condition. Physical assessment, interviewing, communicating, and listening skills are needed. The assessment focuses on the cerebral, peripheral, cardiovascular, respiratory, nutritional, gastrointestinal, and renal subsystems, as well as laboratory values.

### Cerebral Circulation

**Neurologic changes/symptoms.** When assessing the cerebral circulation, ask the patient about any difficulty walking or complaints of dizziness, loss of balance, falls, weakness, numbness, or development of tremors. Investigate whether the patient's family reports any changes in personality.[1]

**Syncope.** Explore whether the patient has experienced syncope. Syncope is a temporary loss of consciousness caused by inadequate oxygen supply to the brain. Heart block, cardiac asystole, severe sinus bradycardia or arrest, or ventricular tachydysrhythmias may be the cause.

Pupils. Assess the pupils for size, shape, and equality. Determine whether the pupillary reaction to light is brisk, sluggish, or nonreactive.[1]

Glasgow coma scale. Determine the patient's level of consciousness using the Glasgow Coma Scale. The three categories of this scale—eye opening, best verbal response, and best motor response—are scored and totaled.[1] The patient who is completely awake will score 15.

## Peripheral Circulation

Arterial pulses. Determine the patient's pulse rate and evaluate each set of peripheral pulses. If the presence of a pulse is questionable, Doppler ultrasonography can be used to determine its audible quality, symmetry, and the presence of bruits.[20,21]

The arterial pulse is a propagated wave of arterial pressure resulting from left ventricular contraction. The pulse wave begins with the opening of the aortic valve and the ejection of blood from the left ventricle (Fig. 2-2). The pressure in the aorta rises sharply, since blood enters the vessel more rapidly than it runs off to the peripheral vessels. An *anacrotic notch* may appear during the sharp rise in the central arterial pressure curve. After peak pressure has been reached, aortic pressure decreases, ventricular ejection slows, and blood continues to flow to peripheral vessels. As the ventricles relax, there is a brief reversal of flow (from the central arteries back toward the ventricle) and the aortic valve closes. This produces the *dicrotic notch* on the peripheral pressure pulse tracing. Following this, aortic pressure increases slightly and then decreases as diastole continues and blood flows to the periphery. In the graphic recording of aortic pressure in Fig. 2-2 the peak of the pulse wave represents systolic pressure and the lowest point on the wave represents diastolic pressure.

The pulse wave changes in shape as it travels to the periphery. The height, or amplitude, of the wave (the systolic reading) increases as it moves from the aortic root to the peripheral arteries, with a slight decrease in the diastolic pressure. The ascending part of the wave becomes steeper and the peak becomes sharper.

The examination covers the carotid, brachial, radial, femoral, popliteal, dorsalis pedis, and posterior tibial pulses. These pulses can best be evaluated with the patient in a reclining position and the trunk of the body elevated about 30 degrees.

The pulse is examined for *rate and rhythm, equality of corresponding pulses, contour,* and *amplitude.* The pulses should be palpated on both sides and simultaneously at the brachial and femoral arteries. To obtain information about *rate and rhythm,* the pulse should be palpated for 30 seconds in the presence of a regular rhythm and for 1 to 2 minutes in the face of an irregular rhythm. If an irregularity exists, the apical and radial pulses should be checked for deficits (see Apical Rate, p. 34).

The *character of the arterial wall,* which normally feels soft and pliable, is noted by palpation. With significant atherosclerotic disease the vessel may be resistant to compression and feel much like a rope.

The pulse *contour* is assessed by extending the patient's arm and palpating the radial or brachial pulse or the carotid pulse in the neck. The artery should be compressed lightly with a finger while the examiner ascertains the contour of the pulse wave.[22] Variations in the contour of the arterial pulse are depicted in Fig. 2-3.

The *normal arterial pulse* (Fig. 2-3, *A*) has a pulse pressure of about 30 to 40 mm Hg; the systolic pressure is measured by the peaks of the waves, and the diastolic pressure measured by the troughs. One can feel a sharp upstroke and a more gradual downstroke (the dicrotic notch of the descending slope of the wave is too weak to be palpable). The contour of the normal pulse is smooth and rounded.

With *large bounding pulses* (Fig. 2-3, *B*), the pulse pressure is increased and one feels a rapid upstroke, a brief peak, and a fast downstroke. This type of pulse wave is encountered most often with exercise, anxiety, fear, hyperthyroidism, anemia, aortic regurgitation, and hypertension. It is also found as a result of generalized arteriosclerosis and rigidity of the arterial system in elderly people.

*Small weak pulses* (Fig. 2-3, *C*) are characterized by diminished pulse pressure and pulse contour that is felt as a slow gradual upstroke, a delayed systolic peak, and a prolonged downstroke. This pulse is found in severe cases of left ventricular failure as a result of decreased stroke volume and in moderate or severe cases of aortic stenosis as a result of slow ejection of blood through the narrowed orifice.

*Pulsus alternans* (Fig. 2-3, *D*) refers to a pulse pattern in which the heart beats with a *regular* rhythm, but the pulses alternate in size and intensity.

The *bigeminal pulse* (Fig. 2-3, *E*) is usually produced by a premature ventricular extrasystole that occurs regularly following a normally conducted beat. The stroke volume of the premature beat is less than that of the normal beat, since contraction occurs before complete ventricular filling. The rhythm is *irregular,* since the time between the normal beat and the premature beat is shorter than the time between the pairs. The irregularity may be consistent. Simultaneous arterial palpation and cardiac auscultation assist in diagnosing this cardiac irregularity.

The *amplitude* of pulses is categorized into levels using the following code and compared bilaterally:

| | |
|---|---|
| 0 = Not palpable | +3 = Bounding |
| +1 = Faintly palpable | |
| +2 = Palpable | |

In patients with significant vascular disease it is useful to draw a small stick figure ○ and label the amplitude of pulses accordingly.

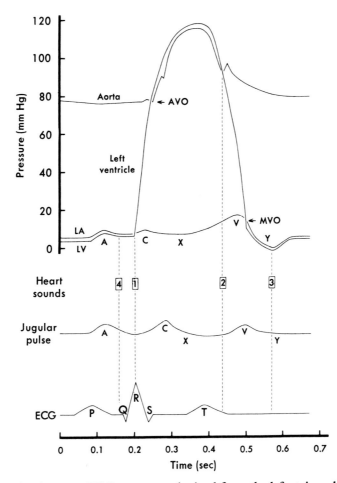

**Fig. 2-2**  **Simultaneous ECG pressures obtained from the left atrium, left ventricle, and aorta, and the jugular pulse during one cardiac cycle.** For simplification, right-sided heart pressures have been omitted. Normal right atrial pressure closely parallels that of the left atrium, and right ventricular and pulmonary artery pressures time closely with their corresponding left-sided heart counterparts, only being reduced in magnitude. The normal mitral and aortic valve closure precedes tricuspid and pulmonic closure, respectively, whereas valve opening reverses this order. The jugular venous pulse lags behind the right atrial pressure.

During the course of one cardiac cycle, note that the electrical events *(ECG)* initiate and therefore precede the mechanical *(pressure)* events, and that the latter precede the auscultatory events *(heart sounds)* they themselves produce. Shortly after the P wave, the atria contract to produce the a wave; a fourth heart sound may succeed contraction. The QRS complex initiates ventricular systole, followed shortly by left ventricular contraction and the rapid buildup of left ventricular *(LV)* pressure. Almost immediately LV pressure exceeds left atrial *(LA)* pressure to close the mitral valve and produce the first heart sound. When LV pressure exceeds aortic pressure, the aortic valve opens *(AVO),* and when aortic pressure is once again greater than LV pressure, the aortic valve closes to produce the second heart sound and terminate ventricular ejection. The decreasing LV pressure drops below LA pressure to open the mitral valve *(MVO)* and a period of rapid ventricular filling commences. During this time a third heart sound may be heard. The jugular pulse is explained under the discussion of the venous pulse. (Modified with permission from Hurst JW and others: The heart: arteries and veins, ed 6, New York, 1986, McGraw-Hill Book Co.)

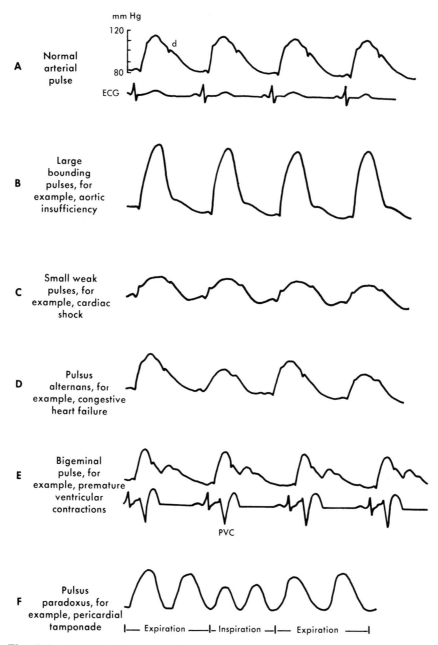

**Fig. 2-3** Variations in contour of the arterial pulse with correlated ECGs. See text for description.

*Pulsus paradoxus* (Fig. 2-3, *F*) refers to the phenomenon in which the pulse diminishes perceptibly in amplitude during normal inspiration.[23] Although the differences in pulse volume can be palpated, they can be more precisely demonstrated with sphygmomanometry. Under normal conditions of rest the systolic blood pressure ordinarily decreases by 3 to 10 mm Hg. The procedure for detecting pulsus paradoxus is as follows:

1. Have the patient breathe *normally*.
2. Pump up the sphygmomanometer, then lower the pressure until the first sound (systolic) is heard.

3. Observe the patient's respirations. The systolic sound may disappear during normal inspiration.
4. Slowly deflate the cuff until all systolic sounds are heard, regardless of phase in the respiratory cycle.

The change (in millimeters of mercury) from the point at which systolic sounds were first heard to the point where they are heard during the entire respiratory cycle represents the millimeters of paradox observed. A paradox greater than 10 mm Hg is usually abnormal.

To be significant, a paradoxical pulse must occur during normal cardiac rhythm and with respirations of normal rhythm and depth. In short, it is an exaggeration of a normal response during respiration. Pulsus paradoxus is found in cases of pericardial tamponade, adhesive pericarditis, severe lung disease, advanced heart failure, and other conditions.

**Auscultation of arteries.** Arteries are normally silent when auscultated with the stethoscope. Occlusive arterial disease, such as arteriosclerosis, will interefere with normal blood flow through the artery, resulting in a blowing sound called a *bruit*. Auscultation of the carotid arteries should be done with the patient holding the breath so that the bruits can be distinguished from the sounds of respiration. Often these abnormal arterial vibrations can be felt as *thrills*. Auscultation is also done over the abdominal aorta and femoral arteries to detect the presence of bruits.

**Arterial blood pressure.** Determine the patient's systolic and diastolic blood pressure. The arterial blood pressure is an overall reflection of ventricular function.

Normal blood pressure in the aorta and large arteries, such as the brachial artery, varies between 100 and 140 mm Hg systolic and between 60 and 90 mm Hg diastolic. Pressure in the smaller arteries is somewhat less, and in the arterioles, where the blood enters the capillaries, it is about 35 mm Hg. The difference between the systolic and diastolic pressures is called the *pulse pressure;* it represents the range of pressure in the arteries. The *mean arterial pressure,* in contrast, is the average pressure that exists in the aorta and its major branches during the cardiac cycle.[24]

Wide variations of normal blood pressure exist and the value may fall outside the normal range in healthy adults. The normal range also varies with age, sex, and race. A pressure reading of 100/60 mm Hg may be normal for one person but hypotensive for another. Blood pressure trends, rather than absolute numbers, must be analyzed and treated in light of the patient's clinical situation.

Arterial blood pressure can be measured indirectly or directly. *Indirect blood pressure monitoring* can be achieved manually or by automated devices. The most convenient and noninvasive method of measuring *manual indirect blood pressure* is auscultatory monitoring using a stethoscope and a sphygmomanometer. For routine indirect blood pressure monitoring the patient may be either sitting or reclining. In some cases, blood pressure may change with body position, and in this situation the pressure should be recorded with the patient lying, sitting, and standing. Severe decreases in pressure from the lying to sitting or standing position, indicate postural hypotension. If this type of decrease occurs, assess the patient for the cause; possible causes are dehydration, hemorrhage, medications, neurologic impairment, or prolonged bedrest associated with decreased muscle tone. The patient's blood pressure is checked in both arms and any differences are noted. Normally, there may be a 5 to 10 mm Hg difference between the two arms.

The collapsed cuff is affixed snugly to the patient's arm, with the distal margin of the cuff at least 2.5 cm above the antecubital fossa. The cuff width should be 40% of the circumference of the arm, and the length of the bladder should encircle half the arm.[25] The patient's arm should be resting on a table or bed at heart level, and the brachial artery is then palpated. Pressure in the cuff is rapidly increased to a level about 30 mm Hg above the point at which the palpable pulse disappears. As the cuff is deflated, observations may be made by either palpation or auscultation. For *palpation,* the point at which the pulse can be felt is recorded as the palpable systolic pressure.

The *auscultatory method* is usually preferred to palpation. With the auscultatory method, turbulence, vibrations, and sound occur (Korotkoff's sounds) as indicators of blood pressure. The stethoscope is placed over the brachial artery while the cuff is slowly deflated (2 to 3 mm Hg per heartbeat). As intermittent blood flow returns, sounds become audible. The *systolic pressure* is the point at which at least two consecutive beats can be heard. As the cuff is further deflated, the sounds become louder for a brief period, then become muffled, and finally disappear. The *diastolic pressure* is the point at which the sounds disappear although there is conflict as to whether the point of muffling is a more accurate indicator of the diastolic pressure.[25] If the diastolic sound continues until 0 mm Hg, as can occur with aortic regurgitation, the systolic, muffled, and zero values should all be recorded, for example, 120/70/0 mm Hg.

Although the sounds may disappear at a certain reading on the sphygmomanometer, one must continue listening to the zero pressure to detect the possible presence of an *auscultatory gap*. In this situation the nurse may first detect systolic sounds at a high level, only to have the sounds suddenly disappear and then reappear at a lower level. The silent period is called the auscultatory gap and is usually 20 to 40 mm Hg in length (Fig. 2-4). If the gap is not recognized, incorrect systolic and diastolic pressures may be recorded.

Another primary method of measuring indirect blood pressure is use of *automated blood pressure monitors*. There are several devices available. One type uses a microphone to detect infrasound waves associated with arterial wall motion. Another type uses a double air bladder cuff that is applied in the same manner as a conventional cuff. The bladder senses the arterial wall oscillations and records the systolic, mean, and diastolic pressures.

The *Doppler method* of recording systolic blood pressure is similar to the auscultatory method. The Doppler technique is commonly used during low-flow, hypotensive states to augment the Korotkoff's sounds when they cannot be heard by auscultation. As the blood pressure cuff is slowly deflated, the Doppler device is applied with conduction gel over the brachial artery. The device uses amplified reflected ultrasound to audibly identify the systolic pressure.

**Arterial line.** *Direct blood pressure monitoring* is accom-

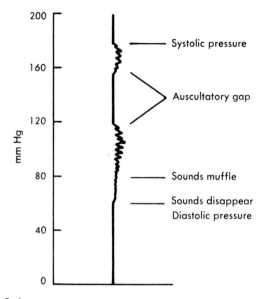

**Fig. 2-4** Detection of auscultatory gap in blood pressure measurement. The systolic sounds are first heard at 180 mm Hg. They disappear at 160 mm Hg and reappear at 120 mm Hg; the silent interval is called the auscultatory gap. Korotkoff's sounds muffle at 80 mm Hg and disappear at 60 mm Hg. The blood pressure is recorded as 180/80/60 with auscultatory gap.

plished by inserting a catheter or needle into an artery and attaching the catheter to plastic tubing filled with heparinized saline solution. The tubing is connected to a transducer, which converts the mechanical energy that the blood exerts on the recording membrane into electrical voltage or current that can be calibrated in millimeters of mercury (mm Hg). The electrical signal is then transmitted to an electronic recorder and an oscilloscope, which continually record and display the pressure waves (see Fig. 2-3, *A*).

In some situations, there are major discrepancies between direct and indirect blood pressure measurements. Such inconsistencies suggest that when a high degree of accuracy is required, direct monitoring should be used. Thus in patients whose Korotkoff's sounds might be diminished or absent, making auscultatory techniques unreliable, direct arterial measurements should be employed. Such patients include those who are in shock, those who have high peripheral vascular resistance, and those who are hypothermic, obese, or edematous. Direct blood pressure monitoring is also indicated when titrating intravenous drugs, especially those used for hypertension or hypotension. An arterial catheter is also beneficial in providing continuous pressure monitoring without disturbing the patient, and it allows for frequent arterial sampling to determine blood gas levels and pH in patients on ventilators or those with cardiogenic shock or respiratory insufficiency.[25]

**Venous pulse.** Assess the patient's venous pulse by examining the neck veins to gather information about right heart functioning. For this clinical evaluation, one must study the waveform of the venous pulsations, correlate them with the cardiac rhythm, and determine the venous pressure.

The examination begins with observation of the external and internal jugular veins. For accurate evaluation of the venous waveform the *right internal jugular vein* is usually selected. If the venous pressure is relatively normal, the patient can assume a comfortable recumbent position with the head and trunk elevated to about a 30-degree angle without flexing the neck. If the venous pressure is greatly elevated, the pulses can be examined better with the patient in a completely upright position so that the pulsations appear at the jugular level.

The patient's head should be gently rotated away from the examiner. A light shined tangentially across the area being examined may help detect a slightly distended vein. A series of undulant waves that are more clearly seen than felt characterize the venous pulse, a graphic recording of which is shown in Fig. 2-5.

**a Wave.** The a wave is produced by right atrial contraction and the retrograde transmission of the pressure pulse to the jugular veins. It occurs at the time of the fourth heart sound, preceding the first heart sound. The a wave can be easily identified by placing the index finger on the carotid pulse opposite the side being inspected. Because of the compliance of the great veins and the low pressures in the right side of the heart, the a wave will be seen to start just slightly before the carotid pulse is palpated. The a wave is absent during atrial fibrillation. Giant a waves reflect an elevated right atrial pressure and may be seen in pulmonary hypertension and pulmonic and tricuspid stenosis.

**c Wave.** The c wave begins shortly after the first heart sound and may result from the pressure generated by the bulging tricuspid valve during right ventricular systole. The c wave is often difficult to visualize by inspecting the neck veins.

**v Wave.** Continued atrial filling during ventricular systole produces the v wave, which peaks just after the second heart sound, when the tricuspid valve opens. Tricuspid insufficiency causes a very large v wave.

**x Descent.** The x descent is the downslope of the a and c waves; it results from right atrial diastole plus the effects of the tricuspid valve being pulled downward during ventricular systole.

**y Descent.** The y descent represents the fall in the right atrial pressure from the peak of the v wave following tricuspid valve opening; it occurs during the period of rapid atrial emptying in early diastole.

**Venous pressure.** Information about the right side of the heart also can be obtained by determining the venous pressure. Venous pressure refers to the pressure exerted within the venous system by the blood. It is highest in the

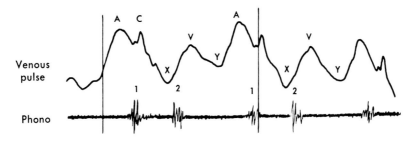

**Fig. 2-5** Relationship of jugular venous pulse to right atrial activity.

venules of the extremities and lowest at the point where the vena cava enters the heart. Venous blood flow is continuous rather than pulsatory. In the arm venous pressure ranges from 5 to 14 cm $H_2O$, and in the inferior vena cava it ranges from 6 to 8 cm $H_2O$.

The external and internal jugular veins are inspected to estimate venous pressure, right atrial pressure, and right ventricular function. The internal jugular veins are preferred for observation because the external jugular veins are smaller and do not adequately transmit pressure changes.[6,7] When evaluating the *internal jugular vein,* the patient's trunk is elevated to an optimum angle to observe the venous pulse. The highest point of visible pulsation is determined and the vertical distance between this level and the level of the angle of Louis is recorded. The patient's angle of elevation is also recorded (Fig. 2-6). The *angle of Louis,* or sternal angle, is located at the junction of the sternum with the second rib; it lies approximately 5 cm above the right atrium for all positions between supine and 90 degrees upright. Pressures of more than 5 cm above the angle of Louis are considered to be elevated.

It is important to note that the sternal angle is used as a bedside reference point for the sake of convenience. The ideal reference level for venous pressure measurement is the midpoint of the right atrium. This level is established by running an imaginary anteroposterior line from the fourth interspace halfway to the back. A horizontal plane through this point is the zero level for the venous pressure measurement. The vertical distance from this plane to the head of the blood column, or the meniscus, approximates the venous pressure (Fig. 2-7). Elevations of pressure above 10 cm $H_2O$ measured from the right atrial midpoint are considered abnormal.

**Central venous pressure.** Direct measurement of central venous pressure (CVP) is indicated if there is doubt about the venous pressure value estimated by using the indirect method and when precise measurements are needed to monitor critically ill patients. The CVP indicates right atrial pressure, which primarily reflects alterations in right ventricular pressure and only secondarily reflects changes in pulmonary venous pressure or the pressures in the left side of the heart. The CVP provides valuable information about blood volume, right ventricular function, and central venous return.

The CVP is obtained by cannulating a vein and threading the catheter into the vena cava. The pressure can be measured in centimeters of water by a water manometer or in millimeters of mercury by a pressure transducer. The normal CVP ranges from 4 to 15 cm $H_2O$ or 3 to 11 mm Hg.[6,7] Centimeters of water can be converted to millimeters of mercury by dividing the former by 1.36 because 1 mm Hg = 1.36 cm $H_2O$. Elevated CVPs may indicate right

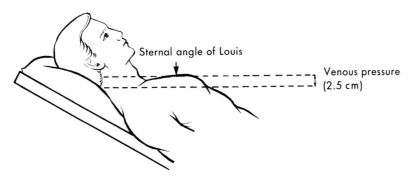

**Fig. 2-6** Angle of Louis, or sternal angle, as a reference point for measuring venous pressure. Height of the distended fluid column in the internal jugular vein is less than 3 cm above the sternal angle.

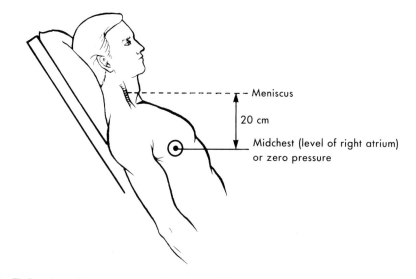

**Fig. 2-7** Estimation of venous pressure is accomplished by elevating the head until the meniscus is visualized. Venous pressure is measured as the vertical distance between the meniscus and midchest, or right atrial level, in this case 20 cm and elevated above normal.

ventricular failure, pulmonary disease such as pulmonary hypertension or embolism, or cardiac tamponade. A low CVP may indicate hypovolemia or peripheral blood pooling, as in septic shock. Serial measurements must be interpreted according to the patient's clinical situation and correlated with other physical findings.

**Skin temperature and color.** Evaluate the patient's skin temperature to determine if it is normal, warm, hot, cool, clammy, or moist. Also evaluate the patient's skin color. Does the patient exhibit pink, pale, or red coloring? Does the patient exhibit pallor, jaundice, mottling, increased pigmentation, or blanching?

**Cyanosis.** Determine if the patient is cyanotic. *Cyanosis* is a bluish discoloration of the extremities and lips caused by poor circulation. It is brought on by cold temperatures or some severe dysfunction, such as pulmonary disease or shock. Examine the color of the earlobes, nose, lips, nail beds, and mucous membranes. *Central cyanosis* occurs with low arterial oxygen saturation associated with congenital right-to-left shunts or pulmonary diseases such as pneumonia. It is observed in the mucous membranes such as the conjunctiva and the inside of the lips and cheeks. With *peripheral cyanosis* the arterial oxygenation saturation may be normal, but the oxygen within the peripheral vascular bed is inadequate. This may occur with heart failure and shock.[26]

**Capillary refill.** Describe whether the patient's capillary refill is normal. Capillary refill is assessed by pressing the nail bed, earlobe, or forehead so it blanches; releasing the pressure; and observing whether the skin color returns to normal within 2 seconds.[26]

**Clubbing.** Determine whether the patient exhibits any clubbing of the nail beds.[7] With clubbing, the proximal nail beds are convex and rise above the flat plane of the finger. The skin proximal to the nail bed feels spongy in clubbing, and in some cases the fingernails pulsate and flush. Clubbing is associated with certain pulmonary and cardiac diseases[22,23] (Fig. 2-8).

**Edema.** Determine whether the patient has any edema. Edema tends to accumulate in the dependent areas of the body: the hands and feet in the ambulatory patient and the sacral area of the bedridden patient. Edema accompanies right-sided heart failure. Edema is assessed by firmly indenting the skin with the finger tips. The degree of pitting that occurs is quantified and described by the following scale:[20]

```
 0 = None present
+1 = Trace—disappears rapidly
+2 = Moderate—disappears in 10 to 15 seconds
+3 = Deep—disappears in 1 to 2 minutes
+4 = Very deep—present after 5 minutes
```

Sudden weight gain may be a sign of edema. In examining the bedridden patient for edema, it is important to press over the sacrum, buttocks, and posterior thighs.

**Cardiovascular Circulation**

**Point of maximum impulse (PMI).** Begin the cardiac assessment by inspection and palpation of the precordium. The anterior part of the chest is inspected with the patient in a supine position and the trunk elevated to an angle of about 30 degrees.

The approach should be made from the patient's right side. Certain landmarks on the anterior chest wall are useful as points of reference in describing the location of the heart. The heart rests on the diaphragm and is located beneath and to the left of the sternum. The base of the heart is situated approximately at the level of the third rib; the apex

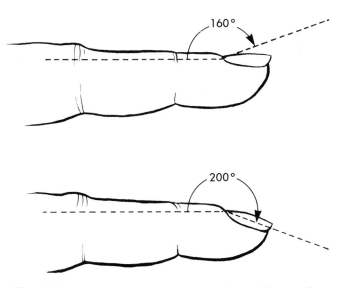

160°

200°

**Fig. 2-8** Early clubbing is sometimes evidenced by a nail-to-nail bed angle of more than 180 degrees. Top view is normal; bottom view is abnormal. (From Thompson DA: Cardiovascular assessment: guide for nurses and other health professionals, St Louis, 1981, Mosby—Year Book, Inc.)

of the heart lies approximately at the level of the fifth rib in the midclavicular line (Fig. 2-9). The anterior surface of the chest closest to the heart and aorta is called the *precordium.*

Inspect the precordium for abnormal pulsations. Tangential lighting is helpful to detect these pulsations. Any visible impulse medial to the apex and in the third, fourth, or fifth, intercostal space generally originates in the right ventricle and is usually abnormal. The point of maximal impulse is normally visible between the fourth and sixth intercostal spaces just medial to the left midclavicular line. However, it is also normal not to see this impulse. In pronounced right ventricular enlargement, the lower sternum can be observed to heave with each heart beat. It is important to determine when the movements occur by correlating them with the heart sounds or carotid artery pulsations.

Following inspection, palpation of the precordium is performed to confirm the findings of inspection and to locate other impulses or thrills. The palmar bases of the fingers are used because this area is most sensitive to feeling vibrations. First, palpate the areas where pulsations are visible, then feel specific areas of the precordium systematically (Fig. 2-10). The *point of maximum impulse* (PMI) is palpated at the left midclavicular line in the fifth intercostal space. Palpation of other precordial areas and abnormal findings are described in the box on p. 34.

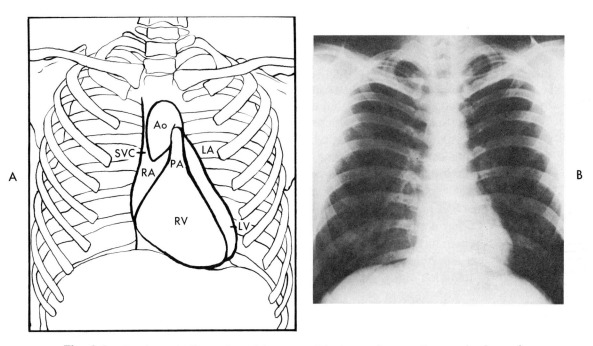

**Fig. 2-9** **A,** schematic illustration of the parts of the heart whose outlines can be detected in *B. Ao,* Aorta; *SVC,* superior vena cava; *RA,* right atrium; *PA,* pulmonary artery; *LA,* left atrium; *RV,* right ventricle; *LV,* left ventricle. **B,** Frontal projection x-ray film of the normal cardiac silhouette.

Pacemaker. Observe for an internal or external pacemaker. If an internal pacemaker is present, record the type and how it is functioning. If an external pacemaker is present, record the type, settings, and how it is functioning.

Apical rate and rhythm. Determine the patient's apical heart rate. Evaluate if the rhythm is regular or irregular. If irregular, is it regularly irregular or irregularly irregular? If the rhythm is irregular, determine if a peripheral pulse deficit is present. An *apical-radial deficit* indicates that the apical heart rate (counted by auscultation) exceeds the radial pulse rate (counted by palpation). A deficit means that not every cardiac systole is forceful enough to produce a palpable radial pulse. This may occur in the presence of premature extrasystoles or atrial tachydysrhythmias such as atrial fibrillation.

Heart sounds/murmurs. Auscultate the heart to identify the normal first ($S_1$) and second ($S_2$) heart sounds and to determine if there is a third ($S_3$) or fourth ($S_4$) heart sound or whether there are any ejection sounds, midsystolic clicks, opening snaps, or heart murmurs.

Selection and use of the appropriate stethoscope can influence the dependability of the findings. The stethoscope should have properly fitting earpieces and should be equipped with both a diaphragm and a bell. The diaphragm is used to evaluate high-pitched sounds, such as $S_1$ and $S_2$, and it is pressed firmly against the skin. The bell is used to detect low-pitched sounds, such as $S_3$ and $S_4$, and it is placed lightly on the skin, with just enough pressure to seal the edge of the bell. The environment and the patient's position also are important during the auscultation process. The room should be quiet with the patient resting comfortably on a bed or table that will easily accommodate lying flat, turning to the side, or sitting up.

Auscultation of the heart is never performed as an isolated event. The findings are correlated with the data collected in other categories of the exchanging pattern, such as the arterial pulse contour, venous pulse waves, and precordial movements, to validate the judgments derived during this portion of the assessment.

Auscultation of the heart requires selective listening for each component of the cardiac cycle as the nurse inches the stethoscope over the five main topographic areas for cardiac auscultation (Fig. 2-11). Note that these auscultatory areas do not correspond to the anatomic locations of the valves, but rather to the sites at which the particular valve sounds are best heard. Accordingly, one listens with the stethoscope over the following areas:

1. *Aortic area* at the base of the heart in the second right intercostal space close to the sternum
2. *Pulmonic area* at the second left intercostal space close to the sternum
3. *Third left intercostal space* where murmurs of both aortic and pulmonic origin may be heard
4. *Tricuspid area* at the lower left sternal border
5. *Mitral area* at the apex of the heart in the fifth left intercostal space just medial to the midclavicular line

## PALPATING PRECORDIAL AREAS

### AORTIC AREA

The second interspace to the right of the sternum is felt for a pulsation, thrill, or vibration of aortic valve closure. A vibratory thrill is associated with aortic stenosis. Thrills at the base can best be palpated with the patient sitting up and leaning forward.

### PULMONIC AREA

The second and third left interspaces are evaluated for abnormalities in the pumonary artery or valve. A forceful pulsation of the pulmonary artery may be felt in mitral stenosis and primary pulmonary hypertension. A palpable sustained pulse and a thrill are associated with pulmonary stenosis.

### RIGHT VENTRICULAR AREA

The lower left sternal border, incorporating the third, fourth, and fifth intercostal spaces, is palpated. Abnormal pulsations here are most commonly found in conditions associated with right ventricular enlargement. When the sternum can be felt to move anteriorly during systole, this movement is termed a *substernal heave* or *lift*.

### APICAL AREA

The *point of maximum impulse* (PMI) is evaluated for its location, diameter, amplitude, and duration. In normal adults the PMI is located at or within the left midclavicular line in the fifth intercostal space (Fig. 2-10). The impulse is normally less than 2 cm in diamter and often is smaller. It is felt as a light tap, beginning approximately at the time of the first heart sound, and it is sustained during the first one third and one half of systole.

### EPIGASTRIC AREA

The upper central region of the abdomen can have visible or palpable pulsations in some normal individuals. Abnormally large pulsations of the aorta may be produced by an aneurysm of the abdominal aorta or by aortic valvular regurgitation. In right ventricular hypertrophy, right ventricular pulsations may also be detected in this area.

Auscultation is conducted in a systematic fashion. By beginning the process at the aortic area, one can determine the heart rate and the cardiac cycle time by identifying the first and second heart sounds. This will serve as a frame of reference as the examiner moves to other auscultatory areas of the precordium. At each site the procedure is as follows:

1. Listen to the first heart sound, noting its intensity and splitting.
2. Listen to the second heart sound, noting its intensity and splitting.
3. Note extra sounds in systole, identifying their timing, intensity, and pitch.

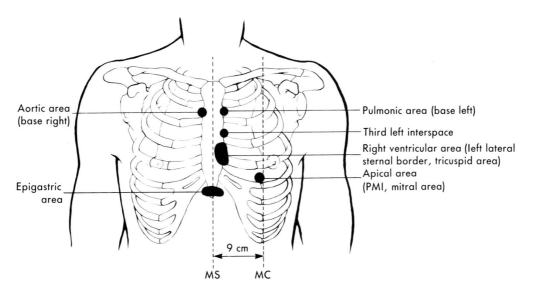

**Fig. 2-10**  Palpation areas on the precordium for detecting normal and abnormal cardiac pulsations. See text for description.

4. Note extra sounds in diastole, identifying their timing, intensity, and pitch.
5. Listen for systolic and diastolic murmurs, noting their timing, intensity, quality, pitch, location, and radiation.
6. Listen for extracardiac sounds, such as a pericardial friction rub.

If an abnormal sound is detected, the surrounding area is carefully explored to evaluate the radiation of the sound. The patient's position should be changed for better evaluation of abnormal sounds. For example, an aortic murmur may be heard best by having the patient sitting, leaning forward, exhaling, and holding the breath. Changes with respiration or during Valsalva maneuver may be important.

Changes in the intensity of heart sounds may be clinically significant. The first sound heard at the mitral area (apex) may become softer at the aortic area (base). Similarly, the second sound loses intensity as the stethoscope is moved toward the apex. The diagrams in Fig. 2-12 indicate the intensity and splitting of the first and second heart sounds, their relationship to the third and fourth heart sounds, and the auscultatory areas where these sounds can be heard best.

**First heart sound ($S_1$).** $S_1$ is associated with the closure of the mitral and tricuspid valves. It is synchronous with the apical impulse and corresponds to the onset of ventricular systole (Fig. 2-13). It is louder, longer, and lower pitched than the second sound at the apex (Fig. 2-12, *A*).

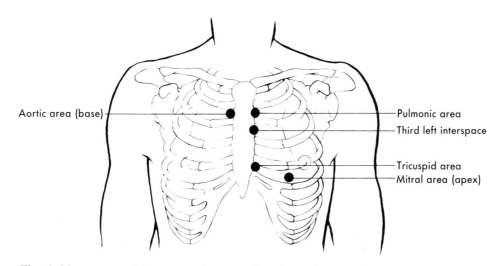

**Fig. 2-11**  Topographic areas on the precordium for cardiac auscultation. Auscultatory areas do not correspond to the anatomic locations of the valves but to the sites at which the particular valves are heard best. See text for description.

HEART SOUNDS                    AREA HEARD BEST

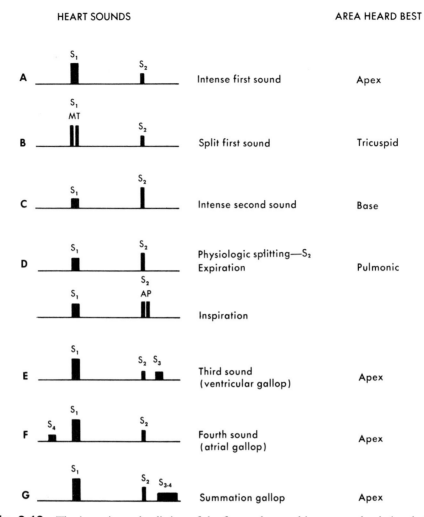

**Fig. 2-12** The intensity and splitting of the first and second heart sounds, their relationship to the third and fourth heart sounds, and the auscultatory areas where these sounds are heard best.

As the ventricles begin to contract and pressure rises within, the tricuspid and mitral valves close. Valvular sounds of the left side slightly precede those of the right and are of higher intensity; the mitral valve closes before the tricuspid valve. *Splitting* of the first sound may therefore be heard, particularly in the tricuspid area (Fig. 2-12, *B*). When the PR interval is prolonged, the intensity of the first heart sound is decreased, and when the PR interval shortens, $S_1$ is increased.

As the pressure within the ventricles continues to rise and exceeds the pressure within the pulmonary artery and aorta, the pulmonic and aortic valves open. Opening of these valves is usually inaudible. If opening of the aortic valve is heard, this is called an aortic ejection sound or click. The same is true for the pulmonic valve. *Early systolic ejection clicks* occur shortly after $S_1$, as depicted in Fig. 2-13. Aortic ejection clicks are associated with aortic ste-

nosis, dilatation of the aorta, and hypertension and are heard at both the base and the apex.

**Second heart sound ($S_2$).** $S_2$ is associated with the closure of the aortic and pulmonic valves. With the completion of ventricular contraction, the pressure within the ventricles and great vessels decreases. The ventricular pressure decreases more rapidly than the pressures within the aorta and pulmonary arteries, causing the aortic and pulmonic valves to close. This is followed by the start of ventricular diastole. At the aortic area, or base, the second sound is almost always louder than the first sound (Fig. 2-12, *C*).

The aortic component is widely transmitted to the neck and over the precordium. It is, as a rule, entirely responsible for the second sound at the apex. The pulmonary component is softer than the aortic and is normally heard only at and around the second left interspace (pulmonic area).

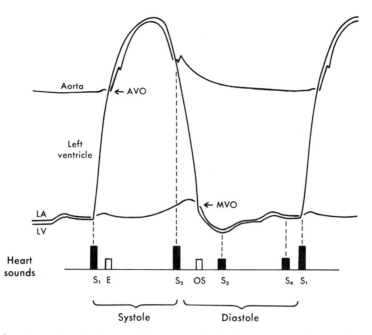

**Fig. 2-13** **Normal and abnormal heart sounds during one complete cardiac cycle** as correlated with left-sided heart pressure waves. Right-sided heart pressures have been omitted for simplification. At the onset of ventricular systole, left ventricular *(LV)* pressure exceeds left atrial *(LA)* pressure to close the mitral valve, producing $S_1$ (in association with tricuspid valve closure). When LV pressure exceeds aortic pressure, the aortic valve opens *(AVO)*. With valvular disease and hypertension, aortic valve opening may be audible and heard as an early ejection click *(E)*. When aortic pressure exceeds LV pressure, the aortic valve closes to produce $S_2$ in association with pulmonic valve closure. When LV pressure drops below LA pressure, the mitral valve opens *(MVO)*. With thickening of the mitral valve as a result of rheumatic heart disease an opening snap *(OS)* is produced in early diastole. During rapid ventricular filling, an $S_3$ or ventricular gallop, is produced in patients with myocardial failure. Late in diastole an $S_4$, or atrial gallop, is produced in association with atrial contraction, owing to increased resistance to ventricular filling.

Splitting of the second sound is therefore usually heard best in this region.

Again, events of the left side of the heart occur before those on the right, and aortic valve closure slightly precedes that of the pulmonic valve. Transient *splitting* of the second sound may be demonstrated in most normal people during inspiration. Closure of the aortic and pulmonary valves during expiration is synchronous because right and left ventricular systoles are approximately equal in duration. With inspiration, venous blood rushes into the thorax from the large systemic venous reservoirs. This action increases venous return and prolongs right ventricular systole by temporarily increasing right ventricular stroke volume, which delays pulmonary valve closure. At the same time, venous return to the left heart diminishes because of the increased pulmonary capacity during inspiration, which decreases left ventricular stroke volume and shortens left ventricular systole. Thus the aortic valve tends to close earlier. These two factors combine to produce transient *physiologic splitting* of the second sound (Fig. 2-12, *D*).

As the pressure in the ventricles decreases below the pressure in the atria, the atrioventricular valves open. The opening of these valves is characteristically silent. However, when either the mitral or the tricuspid valve is altered, as by rheumatic heart disease, it produces an *opening snap* in early diastole (Fig. 2-13). The opening snap of the mitral valve is differentiated from a third heart sound at the apex because it occurs earlier, is sharper and higher pitched, and radiates more widely.

**Third heart sound ($S_3$).** $S_3$ occurs early in diastole during the phase of rapid ventricular filling after $S_2$ (Fig. 2-13). It is a low-pitched sound, heard best with the bell of the stethoscope pressed lightly over the apex and the patient in the left lateral decubitus position (Fig. 2-12, *E*). When $S_3$ is heard in healthy children and young adults, it is called a *physiologic third heart sound* and usually disappears with age. When an $S_3$ is heard in an older person with heart disease, it usually indicates myocardial failure and is called a *ventricular gallop*. In patients with cardiac disease, one should search carefully for the presence of a ventricular gallop, since it is a key diagnostic sign for the presence of congestive heart failure from any cause.

**Fourth heart sound ($S_4$).** $S_4$ occurs late in diastole, prior to $S_1$, and is related to atrial contraction (Fig. 2-13). It is a low-pitched sound heard best at the apex with the bell (Fig. 2-12, *F*). It is uncommon to hear this sound in normal individuals. $S_4$, or *atrial gallop,* is associated with increased resistance to ventricular filling and is frequently heard in patients with hypertensive cardiovascular disease, coronary artery disease, myocardiopathy, and aortic stenosis. It is a common finding in patients who have had a myocardial infarction.

**Summation gallop.** In adults with severe myocardial disease and tachycardia, summation of $S_3$ and $S_4$ may occur, producing the so-called summation gallop (Fig. 2-12, *G*).

**Murmurs.** Murmurs are carefully evaluated and described in a manner that provides maximum information. Murmurs are usually characterized in relation to the following criteria:

1. *Timing.* Does the murmur occur during systole, during diastole, or continuously through both? A murmur may be easily differentiated as systolic or diastolic by palpating the carotid pulse. If the murmur occurs simultaneously with the pulse, it is systolic; if it does not, it is diastolic. If a murmur occupies all the time period measured, it is described as holosystolic (pansystolic) or holodiastolic (pandiastolic).

2. *Intensity.* How loud is the murmur? A graded point system is generally accepted to describe the intensity of murmurs, as follows:

    *Grade 1:* Softest audible murmur

    *Grade 2:* Murmur of medium intensity

    *Grade 3:* Loud murmur unaccompanied by thrill

    *Grade 4:* Murmur with thrill

    *Grade 5:* Loudest murmur that cannot be heard with the stethoscope off the chest, thrill associated

    *Grade 6:* Murmur audible with the stethoscope off the chest, thrill associated

3. *Quality.* What is the tonal characteristic of the murmur? Is it harsh? Musical? Blowing? Rumbling? The configuration or shape of a murmur further defines its quality. It may be a crescendo (increasing intensity), decrescendo (decreasing intensity), or crescendo-decrescendo (diamond-shaped) type. Fig. 2-14 depicts these configurations.

4. *Pitch.* What is the sound frequency of the murmur? Is it high? Medium? Low? If the murmur is heard best with the diaphragm of the stethoscope, it is high pitched. If it is heard best with the bell, it is low pitched. If it is heard equally well with either the bell or the diaphragm, it is medium pitched.

5. *Location.* Over what area on the precordium is the murmur heard best? The aortic area? The pulmonic area? The tricuspid area? The mitral area?

6. *Radiation.* Is there transmission of the murmur elsewhere in the body? Does it radiate across the chest? Into the axilla? Into the neck? Down the left sternal border?

In addition, each of these characteristics is further evaluated as it is influenced by the patient's position and respiration. Asking the patient to sit up, exhale, lean forward and hold his or her breath may make aortic murmurs easier to hear. The left lateral decubitus position makes mitral murmurs more easily heard.

*Systolic murmurs.* Systolic murmurs are the most common murmurs and generally are either ejection or regurgitant murmurs. *Functional* or innocent systolic murmurs are commonly heard in young people and should be distinguished from those murmurs that represent valvular heart disease. Functional murmurs occur during ejection, are short (less than two thirds of systole), are grade 2 or less in intensity (they may become inaudible if the patient raises from a supine to a sitting position), and are heard best over the pulmonary outflow tract.

*Midsystolic (ejection) murmurs.* Aortic stenosis and *pulmonic stenosis* produce systolic ejection murmurs that begin after the first sound, swell to a crescendo in midsystole, then decrease in intensity, and terminate before $S_2$, generated by closure of the appropriate valve (Fig. 2-14, *A*). The murmur may be harsh or musical and is usually high pitched because of the high velocity of blood flow. Aortic valve murmurs frequently radiate from the second right interspace to the cardiac apex and the carotid arteries. A systolic thrill may be present. Characteristically, pulmonic stenosis murmur is heard better at the second left interspace.

*Holosystolic (regurgitant) murmurs.* Holosystolic murmurs last throughout ventricular systole (Fig. 2-14, *B*), and no interval can be heard between $S_1$ and $S_2$. *Tricuspid* and *mitral regurgitation* and *ventricular septal defects* produce holosystolic murmurs owing to the backflow of blood from the ventricle (high pressure) to the atrium (low pressure) through an incompetent tricuspid or mitral valve or from a higher-pressure ventricle (left) to a low-pressure ventricle (right). The murmurs may be blowing, musical, or harsh and are often high pitched. The tricuspid regurgitation murmur is best heard along the lower left sternal border, and the intensity commonly increases during inspiration. Mitral regurgitation is best heard at the apex with the patient lying on his or her left side and often radiates to the left axilla or back.

Myocardial infarction may produce *papillary muscle rupture,* with subsequent mitral insufficiency and predominantly left-sided heart failure. Abnormalities of the chordae tendineae may produce clicking sounds that occur in the middle of ventricular systole and are referred to as *midsystolic clicks.* These may occur with or without a late systolic murmur.

*Diastolic murmurs.* Diastolic murmurs generally can be classified into two types: the high-pitched decrescendo

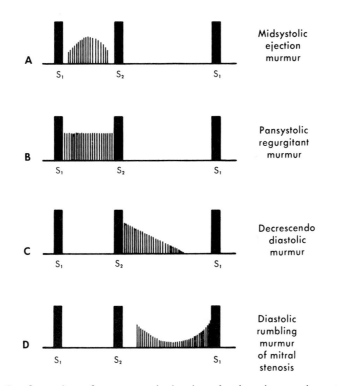

A [Midsystolic ejection murmur]
S₁   S₂   S₁

B [Pansystolic regurgitant murmur]
S₁   S₂   S₁

C [Decrescendo diastolic murmur]
S₁   S₂   S₁

D [Diastolic rumbling murmur of mitral stenosis]
S₁   S₂   S₁

**Fig. 2-14** **Configuration of murmurs.** **A,** Aortic and pulmonic stenosis produce systolic ejection murmurs that begin after the $S_1$, swell to a crescendo in midsystole, then decrease in intensity (decrescendo), and terminate before the $S_2$. **B,** Tricuspid and mitral regurgitation and ventricular septal defects produce pansystolic (holosystolic) murmurs that last throughout ventricular systole; usually no interval can be heard between $S_1$ and $S_2$. **C,** Aortic and pulmonic regurgitation produce murmurs that begin early in diastole immediately after the $S_2$ and then diminish in intensity (decrescendo). **D,** Mitral and tricuspid stenosis produce murmurs that begin during early diastole, have a rumbling or rolling quality, and terminate in late diastole with a crescendo effect.

murmurs of aortic and pulmonic regurgitation and the lower-pitched murmurs of mitral and tricuspid stenosis.

*Murmurs of aortic and pulmonic regurgitation* begin early in diastole, immediately after the $S_2$, and then diminish in intensity (decrescendo), as shown in Fig. 2-14, *C.* They are high pitched and blowing and may vary in intensity roughly according to the size of the leak. The murmur of aortic regurgitation may be heard best at the second right or third left interspace along the left sternal border with the patient holding his or her breath in expiration while leaning forward. The murmur of pulmonic regurgitation is heard at the upper left border of the sternum and cannot be distinguished from its aortic counterpart by auscultation alone.

*Mitral stenosis* characteristically produces a low-pitched, localized apical, diastolic rumble, which may be accentuated in late diastole (Fig. 2-14, *D*) when atrial systole causes increased flow across the narrowed mitral valve. A sharp mitral "opening snap" frequently initiates the murmur in early diastole. In addition, a loud, sharp $S_1$ and accentuation of the $S_2$ often accompany mitral stenosis. The murmur of mitral stenosis is usually confined to the apex and may be enhanced by mild exercise or by the patient lying on his or her left side. The *tricuspid stenosis* murmur is heard near the tricuspid area and is often accentuated along the left sternal border by inspiration.

*Continuous murmurs.* Murmurs audible in both systole and diastole are usually caused by connections between the arterial and venous or systemic and pulmonary circulations. A patent ductus arteriosus produces such a murmur. Table 2-1 summarizes the characteristics of the most common heart murmurs.

*Pericardial friction rub.* An extracardiac sound that may be detected during auscultation is the pericardial friction rub. It is a sign of pericardial inflammation, and in its complete form it exhibits three components. One is associated with ventricular systole, the second with the phase of rapid ventricular filling early in diastole, and the third with atrial systole. If only the systolic component of the rub is present, it may be misinterpreted as a scratchy murmur. With the patient lying flat, the pericardial friction rub is best heard in the third or fourth interspace to the left of the sternum, although the location may be variable. There is little radiation, and the quality of the sound is a

**TABLE 2-1** Characteristics of types of valvular heart disease

| | | | Description of Murmurs |
|---|---|---|---|
| **Time** | **Quality** | **Pitch (Frequency)** | **Location of maximum intensity** |
| Systolic (ejection) | Crescendo-decrescendo (diamond shaped) Harsh Rough | Variable pitch | Second interspace (aortic area) |
| Diastolic | Blowing loudest just after $S_2$—diminishes during diastole (decrescendo) | High pitch | Second right interspace; third left interspace or along left sternal border with patient leaning forward and holding breath |
| Diastolic | Rumbling, presystolic accentuation in sinus rhythm | Low pitch | Well localized to apex, best heard in left lateral decubitus position |
| Holosystolic | Blowing | High pitch | Apex, best heard in left lateral decubitus position |
| Variable Late systolic can become holosystolic | Crescendo-decrescendo whooping, honking | High | Apex with patient in left lateral decubitus position Decreased venous return (sitting, standing, and Valsalva's maneuver) will cause murmur earlier in systole Increased venous return (squatting, lying down, elevating legs) causes murmur later in systole |

leathery, high-pitched, multiphasic, scratchy rub, which sounds like two pieces of sandpaper being rubbed together.

**Dysrhythmias.** Assess the patient for any dysrhythmias including tachydysrhythmias; bradydysrhythmias; atrial, junctional, or ventricular dysrhythmias; first-, second-, or third-degree heart blocks; and premature atrial, junctional, or ventricular beats. Investigate any hemodynamic symptoms associated with the dysrhythmia such as hypotension, dizziness, confusion, or decreased cardiac or urinary output.

**Cardiac output and cardiac index.** Patients in critical care units sometimes require cardiac output monitoring. Normal cardiac output is 5 L/min[7] (see Chapter 1). Also evaluate the patient's cardiac index. Normal cardiac index is 3.5 L/min/m$^2$ and ranges from 2.5 to 4.5 L/min/m$^2$. The cardiac index is derived by dividing the cardiac output by the body surface area[17] (see Chapter 1).

**Pulmonary artery and pulmonary capillary wedge pressures.** Evaluate the patient's pulmonary artery pressure (PAP) and pulmonary capillary wedge pressure

| Radiation or transmission | Other Signs | Condition | Causes |
|---|---|---|---|
| Radiates to carotid arteries and apex | Slow rising "anacrotic" Sustained pulse Left ventricular lift Systolic thrill Ejection "click" Diminished aortic closing sound | Aortic stenosis (narrowing of valve) | Rheumatic Calcification Congential |
| | Wide pulse pressure Left ventricular lift Brisk, quick pulses (water hammer) Tambour aortic closing sound | Aortic regurgitation (blood flows back from aorta into left ventricle) | Rheumatic Syphilitic Calcification Cystic medial necrosis |
| | Atrial fibrillation often develops Loud $S_1$ Opening snap | Mitral stenosis (narrowing of valve; blood flows through valve during diastole) | Rheumatic Congenital Tumor (myxoma) |
| Axilla and back | $S_3$ common | Mitral regurgitation ("leaky" valve—blood reenters left atrium from left ventricle during systole) | Rheumatic Congenital Papillary muscle dysfunction/rupture Chordae tendineae dysfunction/rupture Heart failure associated with left ventricular dilatation from any cause |
| | Loud mitral component of $S_1$, early midsystolic or late systolic nonejection click, intermittent atrial and ventricular dysrhythmias | Mitral valve prolapse syndrome-billowing upward and backward of one or both valve leaflets into the left atrium during systole | Marfan's syndrome Rheumatic endocarditis Mitral valve surgery Trauma Lupus erythematosus Congestive cardiomyopathy. |

(PCWP). Normal PAP is less than 25 mm Hg systolic and 5 to 10 mm Hg diastolic, with a mean pulmonary pressure of less than 13 mm Hg.[7] Normal PCWP ranges from 4 to 12 mm Hg (see Chapter 3).

**Intravenous fluids and medications.** Determine the type, amount, and rate of administration of all intravenous fluids the patient is receiving. Record all intravenous medications noting the name, dosage, and rate of administration.

**Serum enzymes.** Evaluate the levels of the patient's serum cardiac enzymes including CPK, CPK-MB isoenzyme, LDH, and LDH isoenzymes,[7,27] (see Chapter 3). Refer to your institution's designated normal values.

## Physical Integrity

**Tissue integrity.** Explore whether the patient has any corneal, mucous membrane, integumentary, or subcutaneous tissue damage such as a crushing injury or intravenous infiltration.

**Skin integrity.** Assess the patient's skin integrity in terms of hydration, vascularity, elasticity, texture, turgor, mobility, and thickness. Does the patient have any skin rashes, lesions, petechiae, bruises, abrasions, or surgical incisions? Also investigate other causes of disrupted skin surfaces such as invasive hemodynamic lines, stomas, or tubes.[18,19]

## Oxygenation

*Dyspnea/orthopnea.* Explore whether the patient has any complaints of dyspnea. Dyspnea is labored or difficult breathing; it accompanies a number of cardiac conditions and is a manifestation of congestive heart failure. Commonly, this occurs with exertion and may be affected by position. Dyspnea varies in degree; the amount of exertion required to cause it and the amount of rest necessary to relieve it should be quantified carefully. *Paroxysmal nocturnal dyspnea* occurs at night; the patient awakens with a terrifying sensation of suffocating. The distress diminishes after sitting up for a few minutes. *Orthopnea* is associated with congestive heart failure; the patient has difficulty breathing when lying flat in bed and requires two or more pillows for sleep. Thus when evaluating dyspnea, determine when the dyspnea occurs, what precipitates it, what alleviates it, and what body position is associated with it.

*Respiratory rate, rhythm, depth, and expansion.* Determine the patient's rate, rhythm, and depth of respirations. Under normal conditions, the adult breathes comfortably about 16 to 20 times per minute. Observe the depth of breathing to determine if it is shallow, moderate, or deep. Investigate if the breathing is labored or unlabored and if the patient is expending a great deal of energy to breathe. Observe whether the patient is using accessory muscles to breathe and whether the chest expands symmetrically. Normally the entire rib cage uniformly moves laterally and upward with respiration. Evaluate any abnormal breathing patterns such as asymmetric, obstructive, or restrictive breathing. Variations in the normal rate and character of respirations are outlined in the box at right.

*Cough and sputum.* If the patient has a cough, observe if it is productive or nonproductive. Is the patient's cough effort effective or ineffective and is it weak or strong? What is the color, amount, odor, and consistency of the sputum? Investigate any hemoptysis, or coughing up blood, which may be associated with pulmonary edema or a pulmonary embolus.

*Breath sounds.* Auscultate the patient's breath sounds on deep inspiration with the mouth open. Auscultation is accomplished in an ordered sequence beginning with the upper lung fields; one side is auscultated, then the other side, and then both are compared down to the level of the diaphragm. All portions of the lung fields—posterior, anterior, and lateral—must be systematically auscultated. The nurse first concentrates on normal breath sounds and then on abnormal sounds.

*Normal breath sounds* can be categorized as vesicular, bronchial, and bronchovesicular. *Vesicular* breath sounds

---

## VARIATIONS IN RESPIRATION

**tachypnea** Rapid shallow breathing that may indicate pain, cardiac insufficiency, anemia, fever, or pulmonary problems.

**bradypnea** Slow breathing as a result of opiates, coma, excessive alcohol, and increased intracranial pressure

**hyperventilation** Simultaneous rapid, deep breathing found in extreme anxiety states, in diabetic acidosis, and after vigorous exercise.

**Cheyne-Stokes respiration** Periodic breathing with *hyperpnea* (increased depth of breathing) alternating with *apnea* (cessation of breathing), encountered in cardiac failure and central nervous system disease.

**sighing respiration** Normal respiratory rhythm interrupted by a deep inspiration, followed by a prolonged expiration accompanied by an audible sigh. This variation is often associated with emotional depression.

**dyspnea** Conscious difficulty or effort in breathing. When the patient assumes an elevated position of the trunk at rest to breathe more comfortably, this is called *orthopnea*. Dyspnea is a cardinal sign of left ventricular failure and may also occur in certain lung disorders.

**obstructive breathing (air trapping)** In obstructive pulmonary diseases such as emphysema and asthma, it is easier for air to enter the lungs than for it to leave. During rapid respiration, sufficient time for full expiration is not available and air becomes trapped in the lungs. The patient's chest overexpands and breathing becomes more shallow. Expiratory wheezes may be present.

---

occur over most of the lungs and have a prominent inspiratory component and a brief expiratory phase. *Bronchial* breath sounds, also called tracheal breath sounds, are normally heard over the trachea and main bronchi. These sounds are hollow, tubular, and harsh and are heard best during expiration. *Bronchovesicular* breath sounds are heard over the main stem of the bronchi and represent an intermediate stage between bronchial and vesicular breathing.

Diminished breath sounds occur with bronchial obstruction and with pleural disease associated with the presence of fluid, air, or scar tissue. With airways narrowed, the breath sounds are characteristically wheezing and whistling in nature, with a prolonged expiratory and a short inspiratory phase, as heard in patients with asthma.

*Rales* are abnormal sounds that occur when air passes through bronchi that contain fluid of any kind. They are subdivided into crackling sounds, termed *moist rales,* and continuous coarse sounds, called *rhonchi.* Rhonchi suggest a pathologic condition in the trachea or larger bronchi, whereas moist medium and fine rales imply bronchiolar and alveolar disease. *Fine rales* are short and high pitched and can be simulated by rubbing a strand of hair between the thumb and forefinger next to the ear. *Medium rales* are louder and lower pitched.

In left ventricular failure the presence of rales is one of the earliest physical findings. Rales occur as a result of the transudation of edema fluid into the pulmonary alveoli. At first the alveolar fluid is dependent in location, and rales are present at the base of the lungs. As the failure becomes increasingly severe, the rales become more generalized. The rales of left ventricular failure are typically fine and crepitant, but as failure progresses, they may become moist and coarse.

**Pleural friction rub.** Inflammation of the visceral and parietal pleurae may result in loss of lubricating fluid so that opposing pleural surfaces rub together, producing a low-pitched, coarse, grating sound with respiration. When patients hold their breath the rub disappears.

Arterial blood gases and oxygen. Evaluate the patient's arterial blood gases. Describe any type of oxygen therapy and the percentage delivered. If the patient is on a mechanical ventilator, describe the type, settings, and the patient's psychologic reaction to the ventilator.

### Physical Regulation

Lymph nodes. Determine the size, shape, mobility, tenderness, and enlargement of the lymph nodes. Assess lymph nodes in the head, neck, axillae, inguinal, and pelvic areas.

WBC count/differential. Elevation of the total white blood cell (WBC) count (leukocytes) usually indicates infection. The differential count is performed to determine the percentage of the types of leukocytes, that is neutrophils, lymphocytes, monocytes, eosinophils, and basophils in the blood. Elevation of the percentage of neutrophils indicates a bacterial infection. Elevation of the lymphocytes and monocytes indicates either a bacterial or viral infection.[19,27]

Temperature. Assess the patient's temperature. Although there are several routes to assess temperature, rectal temperatures are the most accurate. Normal rectal temperatures range from 36.1° C (97° F) to 37.0° C (99.6° F). In the past, rectal temperatures were avoided in patients with acute myocardial infarction as a precaution against undue vagal stimulation. However, recent studies suggest that taking rectal temperatures in such patients is no longer contraindicated.[28] Temperature is measured on a Fahrenheit or centigrade scale. The formula for converting centigrade measurement to Fahrenheit and vice versa follows:

$$\text{Fahrenheit} = 1.8 \ (^\circ\text{C}) + 32$$

$$\text{Centigrade} = \frac{^\circ\text{F} - 32}{1.8}$$

### Nutrition

Eating patterns. The patient's nutritional status can have a profound impact on illness and recovery. Collect data to determine how many meals the patient eats each day. Ask patients to describe what they eat or drink in a typical day. Investigate any dietary needs or restriction such as low-sodium, low-fat, low-calorie, low-sugar, or low-protein diets. Find out if most of the meals are eaten at home or in restaurants. Identify types of foods the patient prefers. Explore whether there are foods that the patient does not tolerate and whether there are any food allergies. Determine how many caffeinated beverages (including caffeinated coffee, teas, or soft drinks) are consumed each day and identify the amount of chocolate intake per day.

Appetite changes. Query the patient about any change in appetite such as eating or drinking more or less. Does the patient have an explanation for this change in eating pattern? Has the patient experienced any nausea or vomiting?

Mouth and throat. Assess the condition and function of the patient's mouth, lips, buccal mucosa, teeth, hard and soft palate, and throat. Is the patient able to bite, chew, taste, and swallow? Does the patient have any oral pain or odor?

Height and weight. Assess the patient's height and weight and calculate the patient's ideal body weight. For men, 5 feet equals 106 pounds; for each additional inch, add 6 pounds. For a man 5 feet 10 inches tall, ideal body weight is 166 pounds. For women, 5 feet equals 100 pounds; for each additional inch, add 5 pounds. For a woman 5 feet 4 inches, ideal body weight is 120 pounds.[13]

Current nutritional therapy. Identify whether the patient is currently receiving nothing by mouth; nasogastric suctioning; tube feedings, including the type, amount, and frequency; or total parenteral nutrition (TPN), including the type, additives, and rate.

Laboratory data. Assess the patient's laboratory data, which may include blood sodium, potassium, chloride, glucose, cholesterol, and triglycerides (determine if these were drawn under fasting conditions), hematocrit, and hemoglobin. Other laboratory data might include a blood coagulation profile or drug toxicity screening.

### Elimination

Usual bowel habits. Investigate the patient's usual bowel habits and whether the patient uses any laxatives, enemas, suppositories, bran, or fruits to regulate bowel movements.

**Alterations in bowel habits.** Does the patient complain of difficulty with constipation, hemorrhoids, bowel cramping, diarrhea, or bowel incontinence? Does the patient have pain or bleeding with defecation? Does the patient have a colostomy or ileostomy? What is the reason, and for how long?[14]

Abdominal physical examination. Inspect the abdomen

for rashes, scars, lesions, striae, or dilated veins. Observe if the patient has *ascites* or edema of the abdominal cavity. Note the size, shape, and contour of the abdomen. Auscultate the abdomen for bowel sounds and determine their frequency, quality, and pitch. Auscultation is done before palpation so bowel sounds will not be altered. Use the following code for classifying bowel sounds:

0  = Absent
1+ = Hypoactive
2+ = Normal
3+ = Hyperactive

Percuss the abdomen to determine liver borders, gastric air bubbles (in left upper quadrant), splenic dullness, air, fluid, or masses. Palpate the abdomen to determine organ enlargement, muscle spasm or rigidity, masses, involuntary guarding, rebound tenderness, or pain.[6]

Usual urinary pattern. How many times per day does the patient urinate? Determine if the patient limits fluid during the day or night or whether excessive amounts of fluid are consumed.

**Alterations in urinary patterns.** Investigate any complaints of incontinence or retention of urine. Ask the patient to describe any frequency, burning, pain, dribbling, urgency, hematuria, nocturia, oliguria, or polyuria. Determine if the patient has a urostomy or is receiving dialysis including type, frequency, and cause. Observe whether the bladder is distended.

**Characteristics of urine.** Observe the color of the urine. Is there any blood? Determine if the patient has a urinary catheter, including type, how long, and any problems. Determine the patient's 24-hour urinary output or hourly output as indicated.

**Urine studies.** Record the patient's blood urea nitrogen (BUN) and creatinine levels. Assess the specific gravity of the urine and evaluate any additional urine studies, such as urine culture, acetone, glucose, blood, or protein.[6,26]

## CHOOSING PATTERN

The choosing pattern is assessed to determine whether the patient is successfully selecting alternatives that are consistent with the medical regimen, as well as health promoting activities. The assessment includes an evaluation of the patient's coping abilities, judgment, participation, and wellness behaviors.

### Coping

Patient's ability to cope. Evaluate the patient's *individual coping* behaviors. Question patients as to whether they satisfactorily solve problems, who helps them to solve problems, and if it is easy or hard for them to accept needed help. Also ask patients how they deal with a major problem. For example, do they become depressed, anxious, or nervous; eat food, drink alcohol, take drugs, ask someone for help, call the family, or try to solve the problem? Inquire about activities that are used to reduce stress, such as listening to music, exercising, or using relaxation techniques.

Verify the patient's perceptions by asking the family whether the patient asks others for needed help.[10]

Evaluate any *defensive coping behaviors.* Assess whether the patient is denying obvious problems or weaknesses. Observe whether the patient blames others for health or functioning. Does the patient rationalize failures or project a falsely positive self-evaluation?[10]

Family's ability to cope/give support. When evaluating *disabling family coping,* observe whether a family member or significant other is neglectful of the patient regarding basic needs, attention, or treatment. Do they deny the patient's health problem and its extent and severity? Do they demonstrate rejection, intolerance, or abandonment? Evaluate whether the family member or significant other makes decisions or demonstrates behavior that is detrimental to the patient's psychophysiologic, social, or economic well-being.[10]

To assess *compromised family coping,* determine whether the patient expresses concerns regarding the family member's response to the illness. Discover inadequate knowledge of the patient's illness, treatment, or recovery that interferes with the family member's ability to support and assist the patient.[10]

Acceptance and adjustment to illness. Evaluate the patient's degree of *denial.* Patients who are denying frequently fail to recognize the importance and danger of symptoms, minimize symptoms, or displace the source of symptoms to other organs, for example, chest pain may be dismissed as gastrointestinal gas. Such patients also tend to delay seeking health care assistance when symptoms appear and often dismiss distressing events even when it is dangerous to their health to do so.[10]

Investigate the patient's level of *adjustment* to the illness. Does the patient accept the change in health status brought about by the illness? Observe whether the patient demonstrates an unwillingness to become involved in problem solving or goal planning for the future. Does the patient exhibit a prolonged period of shock, disbelief, or anger regarding the current health status?[10] Evaluate the patient's movement toward independence.

### Judgment

Decision-making ability—patients' perspectives. To evaluate patients' *decision-making abilities,* query patients about whether they usually make good decisions. Investigate the circumstances under which they have difficulty making a decision or whether they find it difficult to decide what to do. If the patient is faced with a decision regarding treatment, observe whether the patient verbalizes uncertainty regarding the possible choices, vacillates between the possible alternatives, or demonstrates an unusual delay in making the decision.[10]

Decision-making ability—others' perspectives. To validate the patient's perspective, ask the family about the soundness of the patient's decisions and whether the patient usually is able to make timely decisions.

## Participation

**Compliance with past and current health care regimens.** Assess the patient's past and current compliance with the medical regimen that could affect the patient's plan and treatment for recovery. Ask patients whether they have had difficulty in the past remembering to take their medication, following their diet, or adhering to a prescribed exercise program. Also ask patients what problems they have had and why they believe such problems occurred.[10]

**Willingness to comply with future health care regimen.** Determine the patient's motivation and willingness to comply with the newly prescribed health care regimen. Ask patients whether they believe they will have difficulty following their new diet, exercise program, prescribed activities, and treatments, or taking their medications. Observe whether patients express an interest in following the medical regimen and whether they foresee any problems. Ask the patient if there is anything that is particularly unpleasant or difficult regarding the medical regimen instructions.[10,16] Evaluate also whether the patient has the motivation to comply.

Ask the family how they believe the patient will comply with the medical regimen. Determine whether the family understands the regimen and will support the patient in compliance.

## Health-Seeking Behaviors

**Expresses desire to seek higher level of wellness.** Evaluate the patient's level of health-seeking behaviors. Explore whether the patient is interested in finding ways to alter personal health habits or the environment to move toward a higher level of wellness. Does the patient express a need to change unhealthy habits such as smoking or overeating, and is the patient familiar with programs or resources that can be used for health promotion?[10]

## FORMULATING NURSING DIAGNOSES

Diagnosis is defined as a statement or conclusion concerning the nature or cause of some phenomenon. The term *diagnosis* has most commonly been applied to the discipline of medicine.[29] Medicine is guided by the biomedical model, which asserts that all disease is caused by a malfunction of specific molecules or organs.[30] As a result, medicine is involved with the pathology, diagnosis, and cure of disease. The purpose of a *medical diagnosis* is to identify the cause of the disease and the treatment is directed toward the cause.[7]

Nurses also collect and organize systematic data about patient problems and form conclusions or judgments appropriate to their domain of expertise. Nursing practice, however, is guided by a holistic framework that reflects the interconnections of the body and mind. Holistic frameworks convey the oneness and unity of the individual. From this framework, the purpose of a nursing diagnosis is to identify human responses to stressors or other factors that adversely affect the attainment of optimum health.[7] Thus a *nursing diagnosis* is defined as a judgment about the health of the person based on the data collected from the nine human response patterns.[8] Characteristics of a medical versus a nursing diagnosis are outlined in the boxes below and on p. 46.

---

### MEDICAL DIAGNOSIS DETERMINATION

**OBSERVATION**

Includes history, physical examination, and routine laboratory studies.

**DESCRIPTION**

Includes ordering these findings into logical clusters and eliminating irrelevant material.

**INTERPRETATION**

Compares data with a known body of knowledge; that is, the information is synthesized into integrated concepts compatible with known diseases.

**VERIFICATION**

A course of action is determined and discussed with the patient. Differential diagnostic test results are analyzed and further patient observations are made.

**DIAGNOSIS**

A final label, which is disease oriented, is determined. The most likely diagnosis that explains the present illness is recorded in descending order with other active problems. Examples of medical diagnoses include angina pectoris, myocardial infarction, pulmonary edema, and congestive heart failure.

**ACTION**

A course of treatment based on the diagnosis is initiated.

## NURSING DIAGNOSIS DETERMINATION

Just as medicine has identified diagnoses that reflect that discipline's area of concern, nursing has also begun to identify patient problems or concerns in which nurses are uniquely involved. These nursing diagnoses are statements of the patient's actual or potential health states that focus on human responses or reactions to that state. These human responses may be any observable manifestation, need, condition, concern, event, dilemma, occurrence, or fact within the target area of nursing practice. A nursing diagnosis is *not* a diagnostic test (e.g., cardiac catheterization), a piece of equipment (e.g., Swan-Ganz catheter), or a surgical procedure (e.g., pacemaker insertion). It is important that nursing diagnoses be derived from data collected by nurses. This nursing database should describe the whole patient, not just medical problems. The nursing diagnosis consists of three components: the problem title, etiology, and signs and symptoms.

### PROBLEM TITLE

The title or label gives a concise description of the health state of the patient. The title can be derived from the list from the North American Nursing Diagnosis Association (NANDA) or a new diagnostic category may be developed by the nurse. If may be described as actual, possible, or potential. A possible nursing diagnosis indicates that more data must be collected to be certain of the label. A potential diagnosis is a problem that may occur if the nurse does not initiate nursing measures to prevent it. Examples of problem titles are decreased cardiac output, fear, and impaired skin integrity.

### ETIOLOGY

Etiology refers to the probable cause of the problem. It can be environmental, psychologic, spiritual, physiologic, socio-cultural, or developmental. The term *related to* is used as the connecting link from the title to the etiology, for example, fear related to inadequate knowledge concerning the cardiac catheterization procedure.

### SIGNS AND SYMPTOMS

These are the defining characteristics, derived from the assessment, that support the problem title and etiology. These signs and symptoms can be used to evaluate the patient's progress. For example, the patient states that he is fearful because he has never had a cardiac catheterization before and he does not know what to expect. Assessment indicates that the patient keeps asking patients and staff questions about the procedure; he is pacing his hospital room and has an increased heart rate. Nursing diagnoses help to define independent functions of the nurse and distinguish nursing from medicine. A nursing diagnosis describes a health state for which the nurse can legally provide primary assistance to the patient; the nursing diagnosis may change more frequently than the medical diagnosis.

The Cardiovascular Response Pattern Assessment Tool was developed so that the data necessary to formulate nursing diagnoses could be collected. It elicits data about holistic responses rather than eliciting information that almost exclusively reflects medical patterns. It provides a new approach to collecting and synthesizing the data to understand patterns and processes that form the whole person. Thus the tool is different from the assessment formats that most nurses are accustomed to using. Nurses become familiar with the tool's organization after it is used several times to assess patients. With practice, nurses will become comfortable with the new ways of clustering and synthesizing data.

Nursing diagnoses are formulated after the data have been synthesized and analyzed.[31] As a learning aid, the nursing diagnoses associated with a cluster of signs and symptoms are listed in the right-hand column of the Cardiovascular Response Pattern Assessment Tool. Some of these diagnoses are repeated because of the need to synthesize several clusters of assessment parameters to make a judgment about whether the diagnosis exists. The diagnoses were included in the tool to focus thinking but were not intended to be static.

When a particular diagnosis is suspected based on the data collected, the diagnosis is circled in the right-hand column. Although a circled diagnosis does not indicate that a diagnosis has been made, it does indicate that a problem might exist and a more thorough assessment of the problem and its critical defining characteristics is necessary.

If the problem is potential rather than actual, write the word "potential" in the right-hand column before circling the diagnosis. Not all possible diagnoses have been listed in the right-hand column. If the data collected support the existence of a new diagnosis, label the problem, and write the new diagnosis in the right-hand column.[4]

After the assessment is complete, scan the circled problems and synthesize the data to determine if other clusters of data also support the existence of a specific problem, and then make a judgment as to whether the diagnosis actually applies. After the nursing diagnoses have been identified, their etiologies are formulated, and the problem statements (composed of the problem and the etiology) are prioritized and written at the end of the tool. Patient outcomes, a plan of care, and a method of evaluation are identified for the most critical nursing diagnoses, and these are written on the patient's care plan.[31] Other less important diagnoses can be considered at a later date or referred to other health team members as appropriate.

## REFERENCES

1. Guzzetta CE: Nursing process. In Dossey BM, Guzzetta CE, and Kenner CV: Critical care nursing: body-mind-spirit, ed 3, Philadelphia, JB Lippincott Co (in press).
2. Sanford SJ and Disch JA: American Association of Critical-Care Nurses standards for nursing care of the critically ill, ed 2, East Norwalk, CT, 1989, Appleton & Lange.
3. Guzzetta CE and others: Unitary person assessment tool: easing problems with nursing diagnoses, Focus Crit Care 15:12, 1988.
4. Guzzetta CE and others: Clinical assessment tools for use with nursing diagnoses, St Louis, 1989, Mosby–Year Book, Inc.
5. Dossey BM and others: Holistic nursing: a handbook for practice, Rockville, MD, 1988, Aspen Publishers, Inc.
6. Guzzetta CE: Nursing assessment and diagnosis. In Kenner CV, Guzzetta CE and Dossey BM: Critical care nursing: body-mind-spirit, ed 2, Boston, 1985, Little, Brown & Co, Inc.
7. Guzzetta CE and Dossey BM: Cardiovascular nursing: biobehavioral interventions, St Louis, Mosby–Year Book, Inc., (in press).
8. Roy C: Framework for classification systems development: progress and issues. In Kim MJ, McFarland GK, and McLane AM, editors: Classification of nursing diagnoses: proceedings of the fifth conference, St Louis, 1984, Mosby–Year Book, Inc.
9. Aydelotte MK and Peterson KH: Keynote address: nursing taxonomics—state of the art. In McLane AM, editor: Classification of nursing diagnoses: proceedings of the seventh conference, St Louis, 1987, Mosby–Year Book, Inc.
10. Carroll-Johnson RM, editor: Classification of nursing diagnoses: proceedings of the eighth conference, Philadelphia, 1989, JB Lippincott Co.
11. Kritek PB: Development of a taxonomic structure for nursing diagnoses: a review and update. In Hurley M, editor: Classification of nursing diagnoses: proceedings of the sixth conference, St Louis, 1986, Mosby–Year Book, Inc.
12. American Nurses' Association Division of Medical-Surgical Nursing Practice and American Heart Association Council of Cardiovascular Nursing: Standards of cardiovascular nursing practice, Kansas City, MO, 1981, American Nurses' Association.
13. Guzzetta CE: General focus question and parameters for eliciting appropriate data. In Guzzetta CE and others: Clinical assessment tools for use with nursing diagnoses, St Louis, 1989, Mosby–Year Book, Inc.
14. Carpenito LJ: Nursing diagnoses: application to clinical practice, ed 3, Philadelphia, 1989, JB Lippincott Co.
15. Gordon M: Manual of nursing diagnosis, St Louis, 1989, Mosby–Year Book, Inc.
16. Kim MJ, McFarland GK, and McLane AM: Pocket guide to nursing diagnoses, ed 3, St Louis, 1989, Mosby–Year Book, Inc.
17. Underhill SL and others: Cardiac nursing, Philadelphia, 1989, JB Lippincott Co.
18. Malasanos L and others: Health assessment, ed 4, St Louis, 1990, Mosby–Year Book, Inc.
19. Seidel HM and others: Mosby's guide to physical examination, St Louis, 1987, Mosby–Year Book, Inc.
20. Bates B: A guide to physical examination, Philadelphia, 1983, JB Lippincott Co.
21. Swartz MH: Physical diagnosis: history and examination, Philadelphia, 1989, WB Saunders Co.
22. Braunwald E: Heart disease: a textbook of cardiovascular medicine, ed 3, Philadelphia, 1988, WB Saunders Co.
23. Hurst JW and others, editors: The heart, ed 7, New York, 1990, McGraw-Hill Information Services Co.
24. Daily EK and Schroeder JS: Techniques in bedside hemodynamic monitoring, ed 4, St Louis, 1989, Mosby–Year Book, Inc.
25. Henneman EA and Henneman PL: Intricacies of blood pressure measurement: reexamining the rituals, Heart Lung 18:263, 1989.
26. Kinney MK, Packa DR, and Dunbar SB, editors: AACN's clinical reference for critical-care nursing, ed 2, St Louis, 1988, Mosby–Year Book, Inc.
27. Thompson J and others: Mosby's manual of clinical nursing, ed 2, St Louis, 1989, Mosby–Year Book, Inc.
28. Kirchhoff KT: An examination of the physiologic basis for "coronary precautions," Heart Lung 10:874, 1981.
29. Guzzetta CE and Kinney MR: Mastering the transition from medical to nursing diagnosis, Prog Cardiovasc Nurs 1:41, 1986.
30. Dossey L: Space, time, and medicine, Boulder, 1982, Shambhala Publications, Inc.
31. Alfaro R: Application of nursing process: a step-by-step guide, Philadelphia, 1986, JB Lippincott Co.

# CHAPTER 3

# Patient Assessment: Diagnostic Studies

Laurel J. Sutherland

Diagnostic studies used in the assessment of patients with cardiovascular disease are important adjuncts to the history and physical examination. Noninvasive studies are those that do not involve the insertion of vascular instruments; noninvasive studies include exercise stress testing with or without nuclear imaging, echocardiography, cardiac Doppler, long-term ECG recording (Holter monitoring), and serum enzyme analysis. Invasive studies involve the vascular insertion of catheters, electrodes, or bioptomes; invasive studies include Swan-Ganz monitoring, cardiac catheterization, electrophysiology studies, and endoymyocardial biopsy. The purpose of this chapter is to review the use of these diagnostic studies.

In evaluating study results for which there is a standard, the sensitivity of a test measures its ability to select patients with disease while specificity is a measure of its ability to select patients without disease. The predictive value of a test measures its ability to determine the probability of disease in a given patient. The ideal study is not available but would theoretically offer complete sensitivity and specificity and have a predictive value of 100%.

## EXERCISE STRESS TESTING

The treadmill exercise stress test is one of the most commonly used noninvasive techniques to detect coronary artery disease. Physical or emotional stress typically precipitates myocardial ischemia in patients who have a fixed coronary artery obstruction. Exertional stress can induce ischemia by causing myocardial oxygen demand to exceed available supply. During the exercise stress test, an attempt is made to provoke and electrocardiographically document exercise-induced myocardial ischemia and to correlate these electrocardiographic changes with the patient's symptoms.

The treadmill stress test is performed as follows. A baseline ECG, heart rate, and blood pressure are obtained, and these parameters are monitored during exercise. An ECG is repeated following hyperventilation of the patient to screen for nonischemic ST-T wave changes. Although stress testing may be performed with the patient supine or upright using a bicycle ergometer, it is usually performed in the upright position on a treadmill. The rate and incline at which the patient exercises on the treadmill are progressively increased, depending on the protocol, until the patient achieves a target heart rate. The target heart rate used is greater than 85% of the predicted maximum heart rate for the patient's age and sex.[1] In some situations other predetermined heart rates may be used. The exercise stress test may be terminated before this target heart rate is achieved because of hypotension, malignant ventricular dysrhythmias, marked ST segment changes, or severe chest pain.[2]

A positive exercise stress test can be defined as being greater than 1 mm of horizontal or down-sloping ST segment depression occurring 80 msec after the J point (Fig. 3-1). Increasing the criteria to at least 2 mm of ST segment depression increases the specificity but decreases the sensitivity of the test. However, the pretest likelihood of coronary artery disease[3,4] (Fig. 3-2) affects the sensitivity and the specificity of stress testing significantly. The magnitude of ST segment depression and the level of exercise at which ST segment depression occurs provides an indication of the severity of coronary artery disease.[5] For example, 3 mm of down-sloping ST depression developing at a heart rate of only 100 beats/min would suggest multivessel coronary artery disease, severe proximal left anterior descending artery stenosis, or left main coronary artery stenosis. Prolonged persistence of ischemic changes in the recovery period also correlates with the severity of coronary disease.[5] ST elevation in anterior ECG leads usually indicates left anterior descending coronary artery disease while inferior lead ST elevation indicates posterior descending coronary artery obstructions. The development of ventricular dysrhythmias during exercise is a less specific marker of coronary artery disease than the development of ST segment abnormalities. The development of hypotension, inverted U waves, or anginal chest pain may provide additional information.[6]

The box below lists accepted indications for stress testing.[7-9] The most frequent use of stress testing is to evaluate

---

**INDICATIONS FOR STRESS TESTING**

Evaluation of chest pain
Evaluation of dysrhythmias
Stratification of high-risk patients
Assessment of cardiac reserve and functional capacity

---

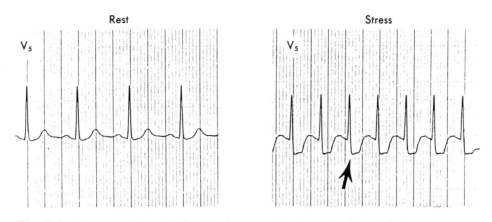

**Fig. 3-1**  Electrocardiographic lead $V_5$ demonstrating 4 mm horizontal ST segment depression *(arrow)* during exercise stress test.

the patient who has chest pain that is suggestive of angina. In this setting an attempt is made to induce the patient's symptoms during exercise and to correlate these symptoms with electrocardiographic evidence of myocardial ischemia. Since the initial manifestation of coronary disease in many individuals is sudden death or acute myocardial infarction, the exercise stress test is often used as a means of screening high-risk individuals in an attempt to make an earlier diagnosis of latent ischemic heart disease.

Stress testing is also useful to evaluate the patients with known coronary artery disease, such as those who have suffered myocardial infarction, angioplasty, or coronary artery bypass surgery. The exercise stress test can objectively evaluate an individual's functional capacity. This application of the stress test is especially important for the

patient who has angina or valvular heart disease because the patient's functional status may determine the timing of medical and surgical intervention.[10] Exercise testing may be used in conjunction with cardiac rehabilitation programs for the patient who has stable coronary artery disease; in this case it is used to assess the cadiovascular effects of exercise. The presence of angina, dyspnea, or exercise-aggravated dysrhythmias at a certain reproducible workload can be useful in prescribing physical restrictions for the above patients.

A stress test may be performed in patients with ventricular rhythm disturbances. Stress testing is more sensitive than the routine 12-lead electrocardiogram because of the longer sampling period and the induction of stress-related dysrhythmias. The stress test can be used to cor-

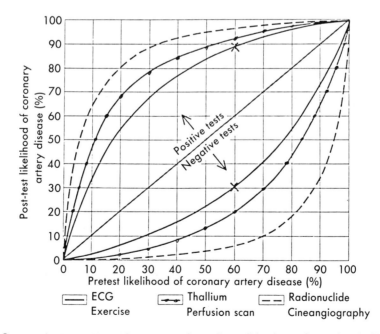

**Fig. 3-2**  Sensitivity and specificity curves for radionuclide cineangiography, thallium scan, and exercise stress tests. (From Cohn PF: Hosp Pract 18:125, 1983.)

relate ischemic ST segment changes with the occurence of potentially malignant dysrhythmias. In addition, it is useful in documenting exercise-aggravated or exercise-induced ventricular tachycardia.[11] In these patients the efficacy of the treatment may be monitored by serial stress tests.[12] Some investigators[13,14] believe that stress testing is useful in evaluating some patients with preexcitation syndromes.

Stress testing can aid in stratifying patients' risk after a myocardial infarction. Several studies have documented that the occurrence of angina, ventricular dysrhythmia and diagnostic ST segment changes in the postmyocardial infarction period identifies patients at increased risk for developing future angina, myocardial infarction, and sudden death.[15] Patients found to be in high-risk categories with the above screening may need early cardiac catheterization with appropriate treatment to decrease this risk.[16] Data from a recent study showed the predictive accuracy for coronary events during the first year after myocardial infarction was 72% using data from predischarge exercise testing.[9]

The interpretation of ST segment shifts during exercise is difficult in patients with baseline ST segment abnormalities. Such patients include those taking digitalis, those with bundle branch block or left ventricular hypertrophy with associated ST-T changes, and those with the Wolff-Parkinson-White syndrome.[5] In addition, during stress testing many patients with mitral valve prolapse may have ST segment shifts that represent a false positive response.[5] In those patients thallium stress testing is more accurate. Likewise, medications that may produce false positive test results include sympathetic nervous system blocking agents, diuretics, nitroglycerin, nifedipine, quinidine, procainamide, atropine, tricyclics, and lithium.[17]

## RADIONUCLIDE TECHNIQUES
### Thallium 201 Myocardial Imaging

Thallium 201 is a radionuclide whose biologic activity closely parallels that of potassium in normal myocardium. When thallium is injected into the bloodstream, it is concentrated in viable heart muscle in a ratio proportional to regional coronary blood flow. The major factors determining thallium uptake in myocardium are coronary blood flow and myocardial cellular viability.[18] Normal thallium images in the anterior and left anterior oblique projections appear in a horseshoe or doughnut configuration representing thallium uptake in the walls of the left ventricle.

Resting thallium imaging is useful in determining the location and extent of myocardial infarctions. Different areas of the myocardium for imaging with thallium are represented diagrammatically in Fig. 3-3. However, thallium imaging cannot distinguish acute from previous myocardial injury.[18]

Myocardial imaging with thallium 201 is used primarily in conjunction with exercise stress testing. In response to exercise, coronary blood flow normally increases 4 to 5

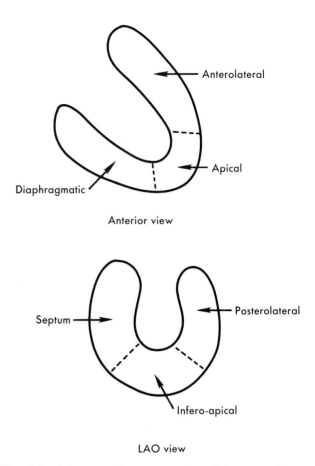

**Fig. 3-3**  Diagrammatic representation of the myocardium demonstrating regions that can be imaged in anterior and 60 to 70 degree LAO view.

times that of resting values. The presence of a significant coronary artery stenosis prevents this increase. Myocardial segments supplied by a stenotic coronary artery demonstrate a perfusion defect compared with normal segments (Fig. 3-4). Because both coronary flow and tissue viability are necessary for myocardial uptake of thallium, either exercise-induced ischemia or previous myocardial infarction with nonviable scar could cause a perfusion defect. Because a single thallium myocardial perfusion image cannot reliably distinguish transient myocardial ischemia from previous myocardial infarction, a redistribution myocardial image is typically obtained 4 hours after the exercise.[19] During this time, ischemic viable myocardium demonstrates an increase in thallium content despite the presence of a severe coronary artery stenosis. Exercise-induced ischemia typically produces transient perfusion defects immediately following exercise (Fig. 3-4), whereas myocardial infarction, with resulting scar formation, results in a perfusion defect that remains during redistribution (Fig. 3-5).

Myocardial perfusion imaging combined with stress testing offers a number of advantages over the conventional

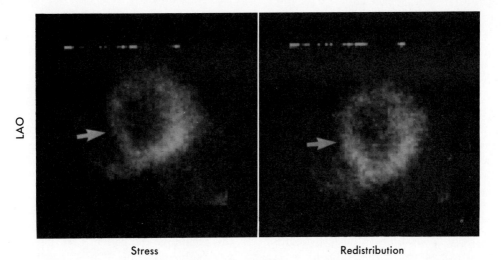

**Fig. 3-4**   Thallium images (LAO view) demonstrating septal *(arrow)* hypoperfusion during stress that redistributes with rest consistent with septal ischemia.

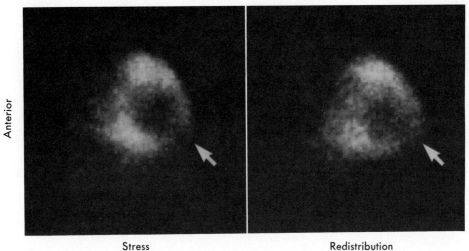

**Fig. 3-5**   Anterior view of stress and redistributed thallium scan demonstrating persistent apical *(arrow)* hypoperfusion consistent with myocardial scar.

exercise stress test. First, the sensitivity and specificity of thallium myocardial imaging in detecting significant coronary artery disease during exercise is 85% and 80% respectively compared with only 65% sensitivity and 85% specificity with a conventional treadmill exercise stress test.[20,21] Second, myocardial perfusion imaging provides a means of detecting ischemia in the patient in whom left bundle branch block, digitalis, or left ventricular hypertrophy may hamper interpretation of the electrocardiogram recorded during stress testing. Although myocardial perfusion imaging with stress testing cannot predict the number of diseased coronary vessels, it can be helpful in evaluating the functional and hemodynamic significance of a given coronary artery lesion. Thallium imaging with single

photon emission computerized tomography (SPECT) allows better imaging of regional myocardial perfusion.

In patients who are unable to exercise, intravenous infusion of dipyridamole may be used. Dipyridamole causes coronary vasodilatation of normal arteries but not of stenotic vessels resulting in the nonhomogeneity of thallium distribution, which reflects the pattern of underlying coronary artery disease.

### Myocardial Infarct Imaging

Technetium-99m pyrophosphate has been shown to concentrate in acutely necrotic myocardium because of the binding of the radiopharmaceutical to calcium within damaged myocardial cells.[11] This technique may be useful in a clinical setting in which a diagnosis of acute myocardial infarction may be difficult to establish by electrocardiographic and serum enzyme methods.

Infarct imaging is generally useful between 2 and 10 days after the onset of infarct symptoms,[18] and it is not sensitive in detecting small or subendocardial infarctions. Consequently, it generally adds little to the early diagnosis of acute myocardial injury or the detection of small areas of infarction. In addition, false positive uptake of pyrophosphate can occur with multiple cardioversions, chest wall trauma, rib fractures, calcified valve structures, left ventricular aneurysm, and cardiac tumors.[22]

### Radionuclide Angiocardiography

One of the most useful applications of nuclear medicine techniques for the patient who has cardiac disease has been in the evaluation of ventricular performance. Radionuclide angiography is a reproducible method of assessing global and regional left ventricular performance.

Global left ventricular systolic pump performance is termed *ejection fraction*. With radionuclide techniques, the ejection fraction is calculated as the percentage of total ventricular radioactive counts ejected from the ventricle during each contraction (Figs. 3-6 and 3-7). A normal ejection fraction calculated by this technique is greater than 50%. Ejection fractions obtained by nuclear techniques correlate well with standard biplane angiographic measured ejection fractions (r = 0.92).[23]

The most commonly used radionuclide technique for assessing ventricular performance is gated cardiac blood pool imaging with multiple gated analysis (MUGA). With this technique the patient's red blood cells are labeled in vivo with technetium-99m. Changes in radioactive counts are therefore proportional to changes in blood volume

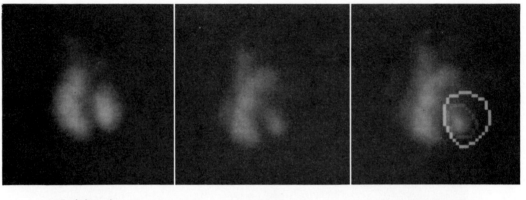

End-diastole        End-systole        Superimposed

**Fig. 3-6**   Gated nuclear ventriculogram demonstrating end-diastole and end-systole and superimposed views of both in a normal patient with an ejection fraction of 53%.

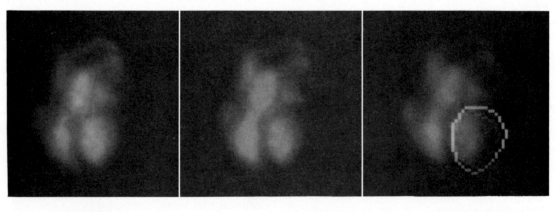

End-diastole        End-systole        Superimposed

**Fig. 3-7**   Gated nuclear ventriculogram demonstrating end-diastole and end-systole and superimposed views of both in a patient with diffuse hypokinesis and an ejection fraction of 17%.

within a cardiac chamber. The study is gated to the patient's ECG, which provides a timing reference within the cardiac cycle.

Information is obtained over a period of several hundred heartbeats, and the individual beats are then added together and averaged to create a representative cycle of the patient's ventricular performance. In some systems, cardiac performance is measured from the initial transit of radionuclide (first pass studies). In addition to measuring ejection fraction, gated cardiac blood pool imaging provides an excellent means of evaluating left ventricular regional wall motion.[23] Thus one can determine whether a wall of the left ventricle is hypokinetic or akinetic, or if a left ventricular aneurysm is present. Relative cardiac chamber size and dilatation of the aorta or pulmonary artery also can be qualitatively assessed with this technique. In addition, right ventricular performance can be evaluated using radionuclide angiography and intracardiac shunting of blood can be assessed by comparing right and left ventricular outputs.[24]

Radionuclide angiocardiography with gated cardiac blood pool imaging can be used in conjunction with exercise stress testing. Because the heart is continuously scanned during the exercise period, a treadmill cannot be used and the patient usually exercises using a supine or erect bicycle ergometer. Normal patients demonstrate at least a 6% increase in left ventricular ejection fraction during exercise stress.[25] In contrast, most patients with coronary artery disease who develop ischemia during exercise either fail to increase ejection fraction or actually demonstrate a decrease in ejection fraction during exercise. In addition to an abnormal ejection fraction response, the patient with exercise-induced ischemia may also develop abnormalities in regional wall motion that can localize the site of exercise-induced ischemia. Therefore gated cardiac blood pool imaging with stress provides an alternative radionuclide technique for the detection of coronary artery disease and has a sensitivity comparable to myocardial perfusion imaging with thallium. Radionuclide angiocardiography is also useful as a noninvasive test for screening patients who might have left ventricular dysfunction after myocardial infarction since patients with large infarctions and markedly diminished ejection fractions are at increased risk for sudden and nonsudden death.[25] In addition, it is important to quantify the presence or absence of left ventricular dysfunction in patients being evaluated for potentially lethal ventricular dysrhythmias because the left ventricular dysfunction identifies patients at higher risk and alerts one to avoid antiarrhythmic medications with significant negative inotropic activity. If the patient has atrial fibrillation with a very irregular ventricular response or frequent spontaneous premature complexes, the gating of the heartbeats can be inaccurate and lead to gross errors in ejection fraction assessment.[23] In addition to patients with coronary artery disease, failure of the radionuclide

ejection fraction to increase with exercise also may be seen in patients with cardiomyopathy, valvular disease, hypertension, or patients receiving beta-blocking medications.[26]

## LONG-TERM ECG RECORDING

Long-term ECG recording has had widespread application as a noninvasive tool since Holter[27] originally demonstrated the use of this technique. Lightweight, battery-powered recorders, worn continuously for 24 hours or more can collect one- or two-lead ECG data for subsequent analysis. A two-lead system is preferred since the extra lead is more sensitive in documenting ST segment abnormalities, identifying aberrancy and screening out artifacts. Attached to a belt or shoulder strap, these recorders can be used in or out of the hospital. A clock on the recorder correlates electrocardiographic events with the patient's log of symptoms, activity, and medications.

Computer-based systems scan and analyze the record with the technician's input for interpretation. Data are reported by mounting representative printout strips of abnormalities (Fig. 3-8) or those corresponding with patient-log entries. An hourly quantitative analysis of the frequency of premature atrial or ventricular complexes, hourly heart rate, and any shifts in ST segment changes can be displayed either on a table or in graphic format. The physician must correlate data from long-term ECG reports with the total patient picture, since it is common for a 24-hour recording to show various abnormalities, even in patients with normal cardiac function. Marked sinus bradycardia, sinus pauses, premature atrial and ventricular complexes, transient AV block, and short runs of atrial tachycardia have been recorded in the normal population.

In general, ambulatory electrocardiography is used to document abnormal cardiac electrical activity, which may occur randomly or in relation to sleep, stress, or emotions.[28] The indications for long-term ECG recording are listed in the box below. Since dysrhythmias can be episodic, one must keep in mind that the detection of complex ventricular dysrhythmias will vary with the duration of the recording. The detection of the highest premature ven-

---

### INDICATIONS FOR LONG-TERM ECG RECORDINGS

Evaluation of patients with suspected or known cardiac rhythm disorders

Evaluation of symptoms suggestive of a dysrhythmic disorder

Evaluation of clinical syndromes where dysrhythmias may increase the risk of sudden death

Evaluation of pacemaker function

Evaluation of patients with chest pain

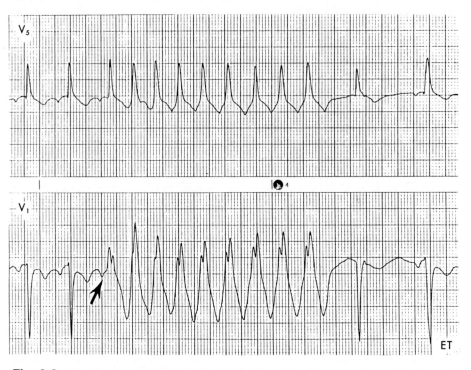

**Fig. 3-8** Simultaneous modified Holter leads $V_5$ and $V_1$ demonstrating a 9-beat run of ventricular tachycardia in patient ET during diary-documented palpitations.

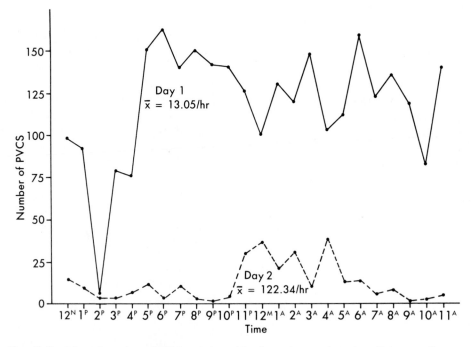

**Fig. 3-9** Plot of number of PVCs per hour/day in patient undergoing 48 hours of consecutive Holter monitoring while off medication. Note the marked variability in the number of PVCs decreasing from a mean of 122/hour on day 1 to 13/hour on day 2.

tricular contraction (PVC) grade can usually be determined within 18 to 36 hours in 95% of the patients.

Long-term ECG recordings may be used in a serial fashion to judge the efficacy of drug treatment. However, there are several limitations to this approach. First, there is a large amount of spontaneous variability in the occurrence of a patient's dysrhythmia[29,30] (Fig. 3-9). Patients may have a low frequency of complex ventricular ectopic activity in between rare episodes of life-threatening dysrhythmias even without any therapy. In one study,[3] infrequent spontaneous ventricular ectopic activity was noted in up to 25% of patients with a history of sustained ventricular tachydysrhythmias.

Because of spontaneous variability, drug effect can be mimicked by a patient spontaneously having a low incidence of dysrhythmias on a given day. Although in an individual patient the definition of drug effect (statistical reduction in the number of dysrhythmic events during dysrhythmic drug treatment) may vary, pooled data suggest that an 80% to 90% reduction in the number of PVCs over a 24-hour period can define this endpoint ($p < .05$).[29,32] If longer recording periods are used before and after drug treatment, the spontaneous variability of the dysrhythmia can be minimized and lower reduction of baseline dysrhythmia can define a drug effect. Although no unequivocal criteria for drug effectiveness are known, in high-risk patients with high-density ventricular dysrhythmias, elimination of spontaneously occurring runs of ventricular tachycardia, at least a 90% reduction of ventricular couplets, and at least a 50% reduction of the number of PVCs every 24-hour period seems to be predictive of a favorable therapeutic response.[32] Limitations of the above endpoints were demonstrated in one study in patients who appeared to have drug effectiveness by long-term ECG recordings. Despite acceptable dysrhythmia suppression documented by these recordings, 71% of patients still had ventricular tachycardia induced by programmed stimulation during drug therapy.[33]

Long-term ECG recording is often used for screening patients with symptoms such as syncope and dizziness, possibly caused by a tachydysrhythmia, patients with suspected sinus node or AV node conduction abnormalities. Although these recordings are frequently used to correlate symptoms with the occurrence of dysrhythmia, the test is more helpful in a negative correlative sense. A previous study[34] demonstrated that syncope or near-syncope occurred during a 24-hour recording in 46% of patients studied. In 14% the symptoms correlated with an ECG abnormality, and in 32% symptoms occurred without any dysrhythmia. In the latter group of patients nondysrhythmic causes for symptoms need to be considered. In patients with syncope or suspected conduction disturbances, documenting a dysrhythmic abnormality correlating with symptoms prior to definitive therapy is critical.[35]

Although long-term ECG recordings can be useful in correlating episodes of chest pain with diagnostic ST-segment abnormalities, there are some limitations. First, since only two ECG leads usually are represented, significant ST-segment changes can occur during an episode of chest pain but ST-T wave changes from the area of the heart involved are not being recorded. Second, false positive ST-segment shifts with changes of position, hyperventilation, or heart rate can occur.[36] Despite these limitations in patients with typical effort angina, it is possible that these recordings may be more useful than stress testing for patients with suspected coronary artery spasm. These patients have episodes of chest pain that cannot be induced routinely by stress testing. Long-term ECG recording can be useful in screening for ST segment elevation and dysrhythmias that occur during spontaneous episodes of chest pain.[36]

Long-term ECG recordings can also be used to screen patients who have clinical syndromes associated with an increased risk of sudden death. Long-term recordings have been found to be superior to treadmill testing in identifying dysrhythmias in patients after myocardial infarction[37] and in patients with hypertrophic obstructive cardiomyopathy. These recordings may also be useful in screening for dysrhythmias in patients with mitral valve prolapse syndrome[36] and in patients with Wolff-Parkinson-White syndrome.[13] Evaluation of suspected pacemaker malfunction can be accomplished through long-term recordings since intermittent failure of pacemaker sensing (Fig. 3-10) or oversensing problems may be difficult to document during short periods of observation.

## Event Recorders

In patients with rare episodes of dysrhythmias, noncontinuous forms of ambulatory recording are useful. These techniques include recorders that can be intermittently activated by an event (for example, by bradycardia or tachycardia) or by the patient during symptoms. Some of these devices have the ability to telephonically transmit an ECG by recording and converting an ECG signal into an audiotone. This transmitted tone is then converted back to an electrocardiographic signal by the receiving unit. In addition to screening patients with infrequent symptoms, these devices can be used to document dysrhythmia recurrences in treated patients[38] and to screen patients at high risk for dysrhythmias, such as those who have recently suffered myocardial infarction.[39] Therefore event recorders may be more useful for patients with infrequent symptoms, but they are limited by short storage capabilities and by their dependence on the patient's perceiving a dysrhythmia.

## ECHOCARDIOGRAPHY

Echocardiography uses ultrasound to visualize cardiac structures. This technique can assess the anatomy, motion and function of the cardiac valves and chambers noninvasively, thereby aiding in the diagnosis of a variety of cardiac abnormalities.

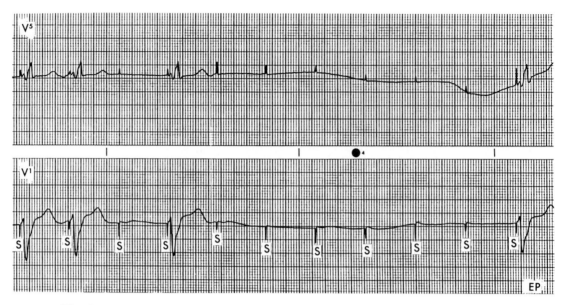

**Fig. 3-10** Simultaneous modified Holter leads V₅ and V₁ in patient EP documenting multiple pacing stimuli *(S)* with failure to capture. Above findings occurred during diary-noted symptom of dizziness.

## Techniques

Currently there are three techniques by which an echocardiogram can be obtained: M-mode echocardiography; two-dimensional, or cross-sectional, echocardiography; and Doppler echocardiography. All these techniques employ the transmission of high-frequency sound waves into the chest. These sound waves are reflected to the transmitter, which also receives sound waves from the cardiac structures. The resultant signals are recorded either on a strip chart recorder or on videotape.

M-mode (or motion) echocardiography uses a single ultrasound beam to record over time cardiac structures by their distance from the transducer. This beam is swept across the cardiac structures, and the resulting time-motion information is displayed on a strip chart recording with the ECG of the patient (Fig. 3-11).

Two-dimensional, or cross-sectional, echocardiography uses a planar beam of ultrasound (Fig. 3-11) that can be transmitted by a single crystal that oscillates or rotates throughout a given plane or by a series of crystals with each crystal transmitting ultrasound through a different point on the chest. The resulting "echo" information is recorded on videotape for subsequent interpretation.

The M-mode and two-dimensional approaches to echocardiography both have advantages and disadvantages, which will be discussed further.

## Applications

**The normal heart.** Figs. 3-12 and 3-13 show normal M-mode and two-dimensional echocardiograms in two different patients. Of importance is the relative size and position of the cardiac chambers and the motion of the cardiac valves during systole and diastole.

**Cardiac chamber size and functions.** The size of the various cardiac chambers can be assessed by echocardiography. The diameter of the left ventricle (Fig. 3-12, *A*), left atrium, and aortic root (Fig. 3-13, *B*) can be measured. Measurements of the right ventricle are less reliable because of its shape and the fact that it varies in size at various patient positions. Two-dimensional echocardiography allows a more accurate visualization of the cardiac chambers and valves, their motion during the cardiac cycle, and their spatial relationships (Fig. 3-14). In addition, the aorta, pulmonary artery, and vena cavae can be visualized.

With the two-dimensional method, segmental wall motion of the left ventricle can be assessed via various views.[40] Ischemic segments may show hypokinesis, akinesis, or dyskinesis. Echocardiography may be performed with exercise to induce wall motion abnormalities that may not be seen at rest.[41] Two-dimensional echocardiography also is useful in identifying the presence of mural thrombi,[42] ventricular aneurysms,[43] intracardiac masses,[44] and the existence and degree of left and right ventricular hypertrophy.

Hypertrophic cardiomyopathy is characterized by the presence of asymmetric hypertrophy, usually of the intraventricular septum. Systolic anterior motion of the mitral valve suggests associated left ventricular outflow obstruction, which may be dynamic. Generalized depression of ventricular function suggests cardiomyopathy, diffuse ischemia, a negative inotropic drug effect, or severe valvular disease. Conversely, regional left ventricular dysfunction suggests infarction, ischemia, or infiltrative processes.[45]

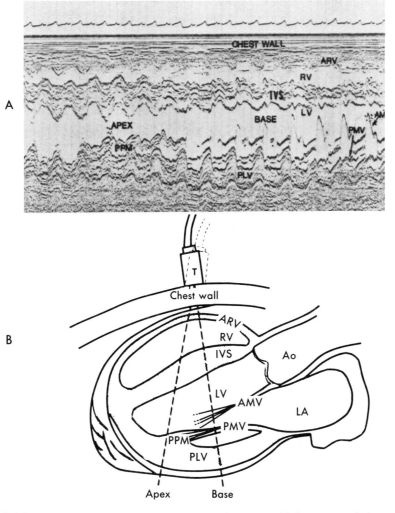

**Fig. 3-11** **A,** Typical M-mode sweep. **B,** Two-dimensional left parasternal view of heart. (From Corya BC and others: Cardiovasc Clin 2:113, 1975.)

**Valvular functions.** Echocardiography can be used to evaluate patients with various types of valvular heart disease. Echocardiography is most commonly used in the diagnosis of patients with suspected mitral valve prolapse, stenosis or regurgitation, in addition to those with suspected aortic stenosis or regurgitation. Specific criteria for each of these are discussed below.

**Mitral valve.** M-mode echocardiographic features of mitral stenosis include the presence of a thickened or calcified mitral valve, a decrease in the size of the valvular opening, a decrease in the EF slope of the valve, and, most importantly, parallel motion of the fused mitral valve leaflets during diastole (Fig. 3-15). Commissural fusion with doming of the leaflets on two-dimensional echocardiography is also indicative of mitral stenosis. The severity of the mitral valve stenosis can be assessed using two-dimensional echocardiography because the size of the orifice can be measured directly from the image in the short-axis view. Moreover, changes in chamber size, such as the dilatation

of the left atrium, can further suggest the severity of stenosis. Mitral valve regurgitation, on the other hand, is not directly assessed with echocardiography. Its presence may be suggested by increases in the size of the left ventricle and left atrium. Hemodynamic assessment of mitral stenosis and the semiquantitative evaluation of mitral regurgitation are further discussed in the section on Doppler echocardiography.

Mitral valve prolapse can be reliably diagnosed with echocardiography by finding the abrupt posterior motion of the mitral valve apparatus in middle or late systole (Fig. 3-16).

A flail mitral valve secondary to infective endocaditis or a ruptured chorda tendineae can be identified from the echocardiogram. The flail leaflet may appear to displace posteriorly but to a much greater degree than mitral valve prolapse. Also, the motion of the mitral valve leaflets may be in an irregular pattern. With two-dimensional echocardiography the leaflet may be seen to prolapse entirely into

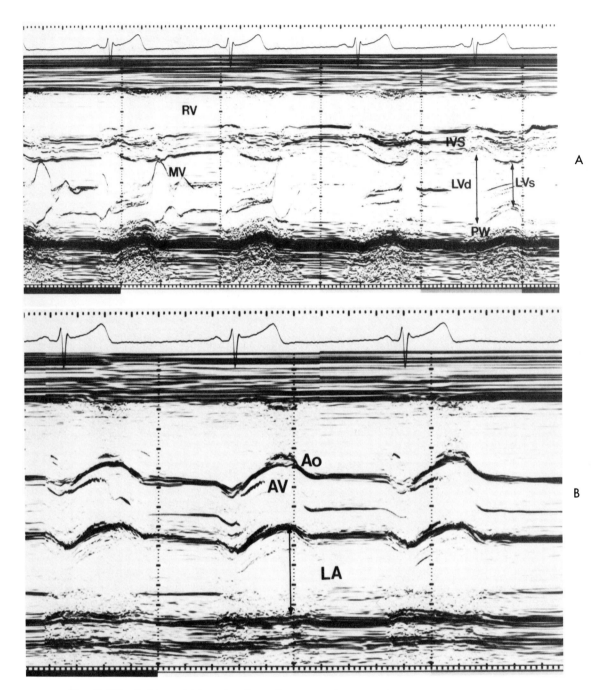

**Fig. 3-12 A,** Normal M-mode echocardiogram at the level of the ventricles and the mitral valve *(MV)* leaflet. **B,** Normal M-mode echocardiogram at the level of the aorta *(Ao),* aortic valve *(AV)* leaflets, and left atrium *(LA).* Abbreviations: *IVS*—interventricular septum; *LVd*—left ventricular diastolic dimension; *LVs*—left ventricular systolic dimension; *PW*—posterior wall; *RV*—right ventricle.

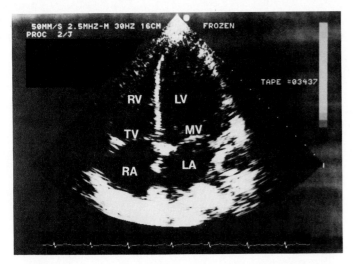

**Fig. 3-13** Apical four-chamber two-dimensional echocardiographic view in a normal patient. Abbreviations as in Fig. 3-12. *RA*—Right atrium; *TV*—tricuspid valve; *LV*—left ventricle.

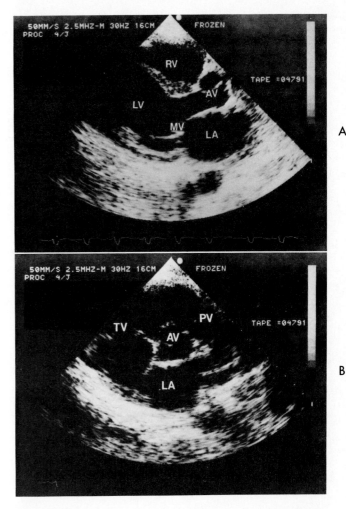

**Fig. 3-14** Two-dimensional echocardiographic view of a patient with dilated left ventricle and left atrium. **A,** Long-axis parasternal view. **B,** Short axis view. Abbreviations as in Figs. 3-12 and 3-13. *PV,* Pulmonic valve.

the left atrium during systole. By using M-mode echocardiography, various hemodynamic states, such as low cardiac output and decreased ventricular compliance, may be manifested by a diminished amplitude of the mitral valve opening or by delayed mitral valve closure.[47]

**Aortic valve.** Echocardiography is useful in determining whether the aortic valve is tricuspid or bicuspid and thickened and/or calcified. Some echocardiographers think that a decreased and restricted opening of a valve is related to the severity of aortic stenosis (Fig. 3-17). The indirect estimation of the severity of aortic stenosis can be made by measuring the extent of left ventricular hypertrophy.[48] However, the severity of aortic stenosis can be judged most accurately by Doppler echocardiography.

Aortic regurgitation cannot be directly assessed through echocardiography. Indirectly, fine fluttering of the anterior mitral valve leaflet during diastole caused by the regurgitant jet flowing into the left ventricle is indicative of aortic regurgitation. Other indirect evidence of aortic valve regurgitation includes left ventricular dilatation and exaggerated left ventricular wall motion. Premature closure of the mitral valve is suggestive of severe, acute aortic regurgitation.[49]

**Tricuspid and pulmonic valve.** The tricuspid and pulmonic valves are not usually as well visualized as the mitral and aortic valves. Tricuspid valve stenosis is identified by noting abnormalities similar to those previously described with mitral stenosis. Tricuspid valve regurgitation manifests itself predominantly with signs of right ventricular overload, such as right ventricular dilatation and paradoxical septal motion. Pulmonic valve stenosis appears as an early opening of the pulmonic valve caused by the right

atrium contracting and ejecting blood into an overloaded right ventricle.[50] The presence of pulmonary hypertension can be diagnosed by a change in the typical contour of the pulmonic valves on M-mode study with notching during systole and the loss of an "a" dip.

**Pericardial disease.** Pericardial disease can be easily assessed with echocardiography. The existence of a pericardial effusion is determined by the presence of an echo-free space between the pericardium and the epicardium (Fig. 3-18). Furthermore, assessment of ventricular wall motion in the presence of pericardial effusion yields useful information regarding the possibility of cardiac tamponade. An echocardiogram with a moderately sized pericardial effusion and compression of the right ventricular free wall in early diastole suggests cardiac tamponade.[51] A collapse of the right atrial wall on the two-dimensional study may also be seen.[52] Constrictive pericarditis is indicated by

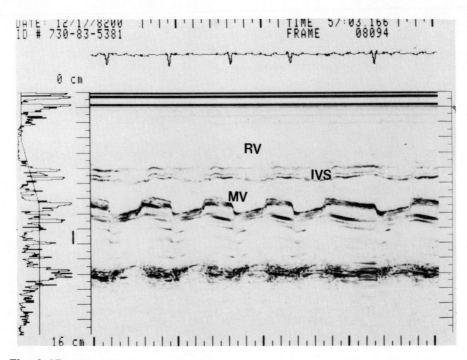

**Fig. 3-15** M-mode echocardiogram demonstrating decreased amplitude, flattened EF slope, and anterior motion of the posterior mitral valve leaflet consistent with mitral stenosis.[74,75]

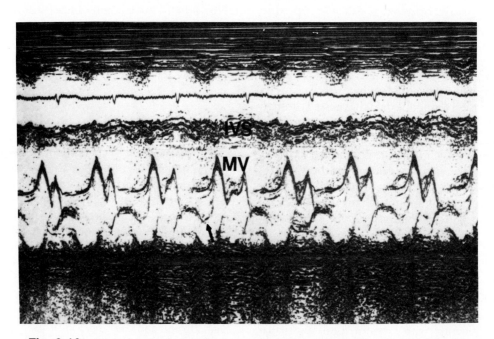

**Fig. 3-16** M-mode echocardiogram demonstrating late systolic posterior displacement *(arrow)* of the posterior mitral view *(MV)* leaflet consistent with mitral valve prolapse.

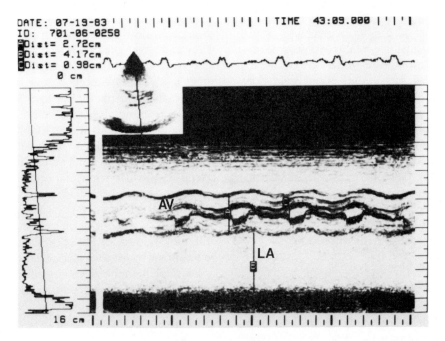

**Fig. 3-17**  M-mode echocardiogram demonstrating thickened aortic valve *(AV)* leaflets and decreased aortic valve opening *(C)* consistent with aortic stenosis. Abbreviations as in Fig. 3-12.

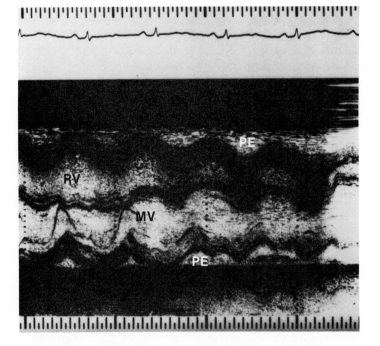

**Fig. 3-18**  M-mode echocardiogram demonstrating anterior and posterior pericardial effusion *(PE)* with diminished right ventricular dimension during inspiration. Abbreviations as in Fig. 3-12.

a thickening of the pericardium and a flat diastolic slope of the posterior left ventricular wall.[51]

**Other applications.** Echocardiography plays an important role in the assessment of congenital heart disease. The relative spatial arrangement of the cardiac structures as well as specific chamber abnormalities combine to provide useful information and identification of various congenital lesions. Intracardiac masses such as tumors and vegetations are frequently identified through echocardiography. Two-dimensional echocardiography is superior to M-mode study in these applications.

Rarely, a technically adequate study cannot be obtained because of chest wall configuration, surgery, or radiation, or because of underlying pulmonary disease. In such instances, or for intraoperative imaging, transesophageal echocardiography may be performed by having the patient swallow an adapted transducer and scanning the heart from the esophagus instead of the anterior chest wall.[52]

## Doppler Echocardiography

The difference between reflected frequency and transmitted frequency is called a *Doppler shift*. By identifying this Doppler shift, the forward or backward velocity and the flow characteristics of blood can be determined. Doppler echocardiography provides information about the flow of blood within the heart, throughout its chambers, across the valves, and in the great vessels. It is a valuable adjunct to the conventional echocardiographic examination for a more complete noninvasive evaluation of cardiac function. Doppler echocardiography allows the quantitation of stenotic gradients, intracardiac pressures, and blood flow as well as a semiquantitative assessment of valvular regurgitation. Doppler echocardiography can allow the hemodynamic assessment of cardiac function, which supplements the anatomic assessment obtained by the M-mode and two-dimensional echocardiography.

Techniques of Doppler echocardiography may use either pulsed wave or continuous wave. Each technique can be used independently or in combination with simultaneously interrupted two-dimensional imaging capabilities. With the pulsed wave Doppler technique, one crystal emits short bursts of ultrasound and also receives the ultrasound reflected from moving red blood cells. The pulsed wave Doppler is combined simultaneously with two-dimensional echocardiography so that the exact location of the sample volume within the chamber can be visually displayed. Because this sample volume can be positioned in various cardiac chambers and vessels, it can be used to localize abnormal blood flow within cardiac structures. However, this technique has a disadvantage in that it cannot quantitate high-velocity flow. Continuous wave Doppler has one crystal that continuously emits the ultrasound signal and another that continuously receives the reflected signal. It has the capability of measuring high-velocity flow but cannot specify the location from which the flow is obtained.

The problem of indicating directional blood flow using Doppler and the two-dimensional echocardiographic image was solved by adding color to the Doppler scan. Current systems arbitrarily have designated red Doppler signals to indicate flow toward the transducer and blue to indicate flow away from the transducer.[50] With color-flow Doppler superimposed on the two-dimensional echocardiographic image, one can follow blood flow through all cardiac chambers throughout the cardiac cycle. Color-flow Doppler is useful in scanning the heart before selective application of pulse and continuous wave Doppler.[53]

**Clinical applications.** Doppler echocardiography is used to evaluate five major cardiac conditions: valvular stenosis, valvular regurgitation, blood flow, intracardiac pressures, and intracardiac shunts.

**Valvular stenosis.** The peak gradient and the valvular area across a stenotic valve can be obtained by measuring the peak velocity of blood flow across the valve by using continuous wave Doppler techniques.[54] For example, a peak velocity in the ascending aorta in patients with aortic stenosis of 4 meters/second yields a calculated peak pressure gradient of approximately 64 mm Hg across the aortic valve by using the modified Bernoulli equation:

$$P = 4 \times V^2, \text{ where}$$
$$P: \text{pressure gradient in mm Hg}$$
$$V: \text{peak velocity in meters/second.}$$

In a similar manner, gradients also can be calculated across prosthetic heart valves. Mitral valve area can be approximated from the Doppler flow pattern. These areas correlate well with two-dimensional and cardiac catheterization, but Doppler calculated aortic valve correlates less well.[54]

**Valvular regurgitation.** The presence of valvular regurgitation is detected as retrograde flow across the valve. Mapping of the extent of regurgitation flow in the receiving cardiac chamber allows semiquantitative assessment of severity and can be done with either pulsed wave or color-flow Doppler.[55] For example, in patients with mild aortic insufficiency, a turbulent flow is detected in the upper left ventricle during diastole (Fig. 3-19). The further away from the aortic valve that turbulence is detected, the more severe the amount of regurgitation. Mitral regurgitation, tricuspid regurgitation, pulmonic regurgitation and prosthetic valve regurgitation can all be evaluated in the same way.

**Blood flow.** Measurement of blood velocity, as well as the area through which blood flows, provides an estimate of volumetric blood flow. This estimate can be applied clinically as a noninvasive method of determining cardiac output, which can be calculated by measuring the mean velocity of the blood flow. The area can be calculated by measuring the diameter of either ascending aorta or pulmonary artery, and less accurately by measuring the inflow tract of the left ventricle. CO = V × A × 60, where CO: cardiac output; V: mean velocity of the blood flow; and

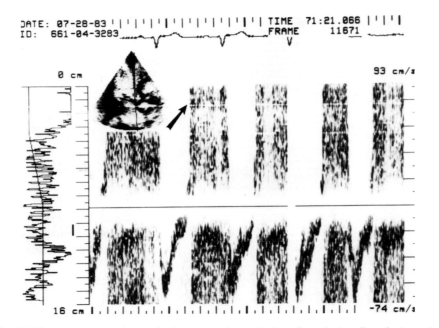

**Fig. 3-19** Pulsed Doppler study demonstrating turbulent flow during diastole *(arrow)* with the sample volume being recorded from the left ventricular outflow tract. This is consistent with aortic regurgitation.

A: the area of the cylinder where the blood flow is obtained.[56]

**Intracardiac pressures.** In the presence of valvular regurgitation, the peak velocity of abnormal blood flow is proportional to the difference in pressure between the two cardiac chambers. Thus in tricuspid regurgitation if the pressure in the right atrium has been calculated by clinical estimation of the jugular venous pressure, the pressure in the right ventricle can be derived, and a rough approximation of pulmonary artery pressure will be established, providing there is no obstruction in the right ventricular outflow tract.

**Intracardiac shunts.** The presence of an intracardiac shunt will result in abnormal velocity and patterns of blood flow on the lower pressure side of the shunt and can usually be seen by color-flow Doppler scanning. In addition, by obtaining the amount of blood flow in the pulmonary artery and aorta, the ratio of the pulmonic versus systemic flow can be approximated.

In summary, two-dimensional and M-mode electrocardiography along with Doppler echocardiography provide a sensitive, noninvasive means of assessing various cardiac conditions such as valvular heart disease, pericardial disease, congenital heart disease, cardiomyopathy, and coronary artery disease.

## RIGHT-HEART CATHETERIZATION USING SWAN-GANZ TECHNIQUE

Right-side heart catheterization can be performed at the bedside in the intensive care unit with the use of a Swan-Ganz thermodilution catheter. Continuous bedside hemodynamic monitoring provides a valuable adjunct to the assessment and management of a variety of cardiovascular disorders. In general, Swan-Ganz catheterization is indicated in any situation in which evaluation and management of intravascular volume and hemodynamic parameters substantially aid in choosing the best therapeutic modality for the patient.[58] While a Swan-Ganz catheter may yield important information, its insertion and chronic placement involve risks such as infection, thrombosis, dysrhythmias, and vascular perforation.

The Swan-Ganz technique involves inserting a balloon-tipped, flow-directed sterile catheter through a protective sterile sheath or directly into an exposed vein. The catheter is advanced blindly while intracardiac pressure is monitored, until it is thought to be near the right atrium. The catheter balloon is then inflated and the catheter is advanced further, carried by the bloodstream across the tricuspid valve directly into the right ventricle. The catheter is then advanced across the pulmonic valve into the pulmonary artery until the balloon becomes wedged in an arterial branch. Pressure recordings should be obtained in each chamber as the catheter is being inserted, and pulmonary artery pressure should be recorded after the balloon has been deflated (Fig. 3-20).

The Swan-Ganz catheter has two pressure lumens and one lumen for balloon inflation. The distal lumen located on the tip of the catheter is first used to record entry pressures and then to record the pulmonary artery and pulmonary capillary wedge pressure. The pressure obtained through the distal lumen when the balloon is wedged in the pulmonary artery is referred to as the *pul-*

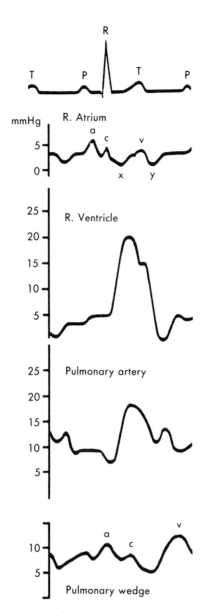

**Fig. 3-20** Simultaneous normal right atrial ventricular, pulmonary artery, and pulmonary wedge tracings timed during cardiac cycle with surface electrocardiogram.

*monary capillary wedge pressure* and reflects the left ventricular end-diastolic pressure, provided there is no obstructive disease present in the pulmonary circulation or at the level of the mitral valve, which might affect the pressure readings. The proximal lumen, located 30 cm from the tip of the catheter, is used to record the right atrial pressure and is the injection port in the thermodilution cardiac output procedure. Normal pressure values for the anatomic sites mentioned above are shown in Table 3-1.

Cardiac output can be easily assessed after the Swan-Ganz thermodilution catheter is in position by using the thermodilution technique,[59] which involves the injection of a known volume of cold fluid into the proximal lumen. A thermistor located near the catheter tip detects the change in temperature as the cold fluid flows through the pulmonary artery. The change in temperature is inversely proportional to cardiac output, that is, the greater the temperture change, the lower the cardiac output.

Once the right atrial (RA) pressure, pulmonary artery (PA) pressure, pulmonary capillary wedge pressure (PCWP), and cardiac output (CO) have been obtained, calculations of stroke volume (SV), systemic vascular resistance (SVR), and pulmonary vascular resistance (PVR) can be made using the equations shown in Table 3-2. These measures provide further information regarding the hemodynamic status of the patient.

Elevated filling pressures (PCWP) suggest heart failure or vascular volume overload, and depressed filling pressures suggest volume depletion. Elevated and approximately equal filling pressures (RA = PCWP) suggest problems of cardiac filling such as tamponade, constriction, or restrictive cardiomyopathy. A very dominant v wave in the wedge position is indicative of relatively acute mitral insufficiency or increased left ventricular end-diastolic pressure. Elevated right heart pressures might suggest right ventricular injury in the presence of a myocardial infarction. Additional information can be obtained by measuring oxygen saturations from the RA and PA, looking for a possible oxygen saturation increase, or step up, consistent with a left-to-right intracardiac shunt.

**TABLE 3-1** Range of normal resting hemodynamic values (mm Hg)

| Pressures | a Wave | v Wave | Mean | Systolic | End-diastolic |
|---|---|---|---|---|---|
| Right atrium | 2-10 | 2-10 | 0-8 | | |
| Right ventricle | | | | 15-30 | 0-8 |
| Pulmonary artery | | | 9-16 | 15-30 | 3-12 |
| Pulmonary capillary wedge (left atrium) | 3-15 | 3-12 | 1-10 | | |
| Left ventricle | | | | 100-140 | 3-12 |
| Systemic arteries | | | 90-105 | 100-140 | 60-90 |

TABLE 3-2 Equations and normal values

| | Equation | Nomal values |
|---|---|---|
| Cardiac index (CI) | $CI = \dfrac{CO}{\text{Body surface area}}$ | 2.5 − 4.2 liter/min/M² |
| Stroke volume (SV) | $SV = \dfrac{CO}{\text{Heart rate}}$ | |
| Stroke index (SI) | $SI = \dfrac{SV}{\text{Body surface area}}$ | 45 ± 13 ml/m² |
| Systemic vascular resistance (SVR) | $SVR = \dfrac{80\,(\overline{AO} - \overline{RA})}{Q_s}$ <br> $\overline{AO}$: mean aortic pressure <br> $\overline{RA}$: mean right atrial pressure <br> $Q_s$: systemic blood flows | 770 − 1500 dynes/sec/CM⁵ |
| Pulmonary vascular resistance (PVR) | $PVR = \dfrac{80\,(\overline{PA} - \overline{LA})}{Q_p}$ <br> $\overline{PA}$: mean pulmonary artery pressure <br> $\overline{LA}$: mean left atrium pressure <br> $Q_p$: pulmonary blood flow | 20 − 120 dynes/sec/CM⁵ |

## CARDIAC CATHETERIZATION AND CARDIAC ANGIOGRAPHY

Cardiac catheterization and angiography are the definitive techniques for establishing the cause and severity of cardiac diseases. These techniques provide physiologic data regarding cardiovascular hemodynamics as well as the angiographic evaluation of cardiac chambers and structures that can be visualized on x-ray film by the injection of radiopaque contrast media.

Cardiac catheterization involves passing a catheter through a vein or artery to the right or left cardiac chambers so that pressures and oxygen saturations within the chambers can be measured, and gradients across stenotic cardiac valves can be determined. In addition, radiopaque contrast media can be injected to visualize the cardiac chambers, great vessels, and coronary arteries on fluoroscopy and x-ray film. Through these laboratory techniques the presence of regional wall motion abnormalities and the severity of valvular regurgitation can be accurately assessed. Complications of myocardial infarction, such as acquired ventricular septal defect with a left-to-right shunt, can be detected and quantitated through measurement of oxygen saturations in the right cardiac chambers.

The most commonly performed angiographic procedure in the patient who has known or suspected coronary artery disease is coronary arteriography. With this technique selective catheterization of the coronary arteries is performed either by a brachial arteriotomy (Sones technique) or by a percutaneous femoral puncture (Judkins technique). Coronary arteriography involves placing a specially designed catheter in the ostia of the left and right coronary arteries and injecting contrast media to visualize the coronary arterial circulation. Typically, several injections of both the left and right coronary arteries are performed in multiple left and right caudal and cranial views to ensure adequate visualization of the proximal and distal portion of each vessel. A hemodynamically significant coronary artery stenosis is defined as a reduction in luminal diameter compared with that of a normal segment of the same vessel of greater than or equal to 50% in the left main coronary artery and 60% in the major branches, such as left anterior descending, circumflex, and right coronary arteries (Fig. 3-21). Quantitative coronary arteriography can be obtained more accurately by using a computerized analysis.[60] By this method measurement of the exact area of the stenosis, percent reduction, and coronary flow reserve in the diameter or the area can be obtained for each stenotic lesion. In addition to atherosclerotic coronary artery lesions, conditions such as idiopathic hypertrophic subaortic stenosis or coronary artery spasm, which often mimic ischemic heart disease in their clinical presentations, can be diagnosed with cardiac catheterization and coronary arteriography.

Serious complications occur in approximately one in every 1000 cardiac catheterizations and include death, stroke, myocardial infarction, loss of peripheral pulse, and

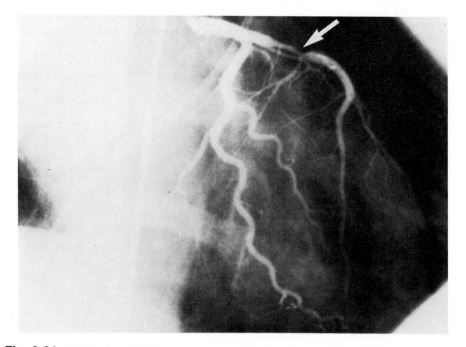

**Fig. 3-21**  RAO view of left coronary artery injection demonstrating high-grade stenosis of the left anterior descending artery *(arrow)* at the lead of the first septal perforator.

allergic reaction to contrast media.[61] More common complications include nausea and vomiting or a transient fall in blood pressure after the injection of contrast material. After cardiac catheterization, there are concerns that must be addressed. Patients who have had a femoral approach must remain supine in bed with the affected leg immobilized for several hours. Heart rate and blood pressure must be monitored and special attention must be given to venous entry sites to note any sign of hemorrhage. The contrast media used often causes an osmotic diuresis; therefore the patient should receive sufficient oral or intravenous fluids after cardiac catheterization.[62]

The indications for cardiac catheterization and coronary arteriography vary slightly among institutions. Moreover, the indications for these procedures have changed as data about the natural history of coronary artery disease and valvular heart disease and the effects of interventional therapy on these lesions have become available. The measurement of valve areas or gradients and the assessment of indices of left ventricular performance such as end-diastolic pressure or cardiac output are often required to determine the optimum timing for surgical intervention.

Traditionally, coronary angiography has been performed in the patient who has classic angina in order to delineate the anatomic sites and the degree of coronary artery stenosis prior to considering aortocoronary bypass surgery or percutaneous transluminal coronary angioplasty (PTCA). For example, patients with left main coronary artery stenosis have been shown to improve long-term survival with aortocoronary bypass surgery.[63] Coronary angiography can be performed in the setting of acute myo-

cardial infarction or unstable angina to determine whether acute interventional therapeutic modalities are indicated. Intracoronary use of a thrombolytic agent such as streptokinase or tissue plasminogen activator (TPA) or PTCA with or without thrombolytic therapy, or coronary artery bypass surgery, are all therapeutic modalities that may be considered. Coronary angiography may be indicated for patients having atypical chest pain for whom noninvasive tests such as exercise with thallium imaging have been equivocal or nondiagnostic. For the patient who develops myocardial ischemia following aortocoronary bypass surgery or PTCA, coronary arteriography may be required to assess the patency of the graft or the status of the previously dilated lesions, or to determine if new coronary artery stenoses have developed in other vessels. Vasospastic angina such as Prinzmetal's variant angina may be diagnosed through the use of angiography in conjunction with the use of provocative agents such as ergonovine.

In summary, coronary angiography and cardiac catheterization are the techniques best able to assist in the precise evaluation of the etiology and severity of cardiac diseases and in the determination of the prognosis and potential therapy for a given patient. The benefits, however, must be balanced against the increased risks and costs of these invasive procedures when compared with noninvasive studies such as stress testing and echocardiography.[63]

## SERUM ENZYMES IN ACUTE MYOCARDIAL INFARCTION

The diagnosis of acute myocardial infarction is typically confirmed by the patient's clinical history, electrocardiographic changes, and elevation of serum enzymes released from the heart muscle after myocardial injury. Necrosis can cause an increased permeability of cellular membranes, which allows these enzymes to leak into the bloodstream. Three major enzymes that occur in abnormal levels in the serum following myocardial injury are creatinine phosphokinase (CPK), lactic dehydrogenase (LDH), and serum glutamic oxaloacetic transaminase (SGOT). Creatinine phosphokinase (CPK) is present in cardiac and skeletal muscle and in the brain and gastrointestinal tract. Abnormal elevation in serum CPK begins to appear in the blood about 4 to 6 hours after the onset of acute myocardial infarction. Peak levels of this enzyme typically appear 16 to 30 hours after the onset of the infarction and return to normal within 3 to 4 days. However, the elevation of serum CPK is nonspecific for cardiac injury. For example, if the patient had received an intramuscular injection of analgesic, this enzyme level may rise secondary to skeletal muscle injury. To determine the precise source of the elevated CPK, electrophoresis or radioimmunoassay can be used to separate CPK into three isoenzymes. The MB isoenzyme is primarily found in cardiac muscle, the MM isoenzyme is found in skeletal muscle, and the BB isoenzyme is primarily found in brain tissue. The MB isoenzyme, like total serum CPK, appears in the serum about 4 hours after the onset of myocardial necrosis and peaks in about 18 to 20 hours (Fig. 3-22).[64] However, if reperfusion occurs either spontaneously or with interventional therapy, such as with the use of a thrombolytic agent and/or PTCA, the peak value occurs sooner and may be higher than without reperfusion.[65] Following acute interventions, peak levels are reached in about 6 to 8 hours for MB isoenzyme and in about 12 hours for the total CPK, presumably because of the rapid washout of the enzymes.

Another enzyme that is released after myocardial infarction is LDH, which appears in abnormal amounts in peripheral blood about 24 to 48 hours after the onset of infarction. Peak levels occur in 3 to 6 days, and the enzyme levels return to normal 7 to 10 days after infarction. LDH is widely distributed throughout such body organs as heart, kidney, skeletal muscle, lung, liver, and red blood cells. LDH can be separated into five isoenzymes. Cardiac muscle is particularly rich in the isoenzymes of $LDH_1$; therefore after myocardial damage, the predominant isoenzyme found in the serum is $LDH_1$. Because the $LDH_1$ value is usually less than that of $LDH_2$, if there are higher levels for $LDH_1$ than $LDH_2$ (known as *$LDH_1$ flip*), or if the percentage of $LDH_1$ exceeds 40% of the total of LDH values, it is considered sensitive for myocardial injury.[66]

A third enzyme that appears in elevated levels in the serum is SGOT. Elevation of SGOT occurs about 12 to 18 hours after the onset of infarction, and peak levels occur about 24 to 48 hours after the onset of infarction. However, elevated levels of SGOT can also occur in patients who have pulmonary embolism, myocarditis, pericarditis, or skeletal muscle and hepatic disease. Because there are

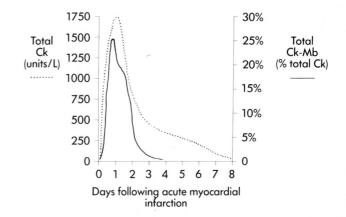

**Fig. 3-22**  The pattern of total creatine kinase (CK) and creatine kinase-MB (CK-MB) activity following acute myocardial infarction (MI). Total CK peaks at 6 to 30 hours after onset of symptoms and persists after the disappearance of CK-MB. The isoenzyme CK-MB peaks at approximately 21 hours after the MI and disappears at 24 to 72 hours. (From Goe MR: Prog Cardiovasc Nurs 2:44-55, 1987.)

no specific isoenzymes of SGOT for myocardial tissue, this enzyme is not especially indicative of myocardial necrosis and the clinical usefulness of obtaining SGOT levels is debatable.[67]

If the patient is admitted within 24 hours of the onset of the suspected myocardial infarction, the total CPK and MB isoenzymes levels of the serum are considered to be the most informative laboratory tests in detecting myocardial cell injury. If those values do not rise in the first 24 hours it is highly indicative of the absence of myocardial necrosis. However, in rare cases, patients with myocardial infarctions may have small elevations in total CPK still within the normal range. In these patients the diagnosis can be confirmed by documenting an elevation in the MB isoenzyme.[68] If the patients are admitted more than 24 hours after the onset of the infarction or if the time of onset is not known, the evaluation of the total LDH and $LDH_1$ isoenzyme becomes important.

## ELECTROPHYSIOLOGIC STUDIES

Electrophysiologic studies are widely used tools in the evaluation and treatment of specific cardiac dysrhythmias. These studies are invasive and generally involve the insertion of intravenous and possibly intraarterial catheters or electrodes, positioned in sites in the atria and ventricles, and occasionally in the coronary sinus and pulmonary artery.[69,70] The electrodes can be used to record electric activity from these sites or to stimulate electric activity with pulses of delivered current.

Electrophysiologic properties of the heart such as automaticity, conduction, refractoriness, and origin and inducibility of tachycardias can be evaluated. In addition, responses to medical or surgical antidysrhythmic therapy can be assessed.[71] Therapeutic interventions such as catheter ablation of dysrhythmogenic foci or conduction pathways can be performed during the course of the study.[72] Electrophysiologic studies are generally modified according to the needs of the individual patient. They are usually performed in a fluoroscopy suite, but variations of electrophysiologic testing may be performed at the bedside or in the operating room at the time of surgery.[73]

Electrophysiologic studies carry the risks of any invasive procedure, including vascular trauma, infection, heart block, and perforation. In addition, either through electrode placement or myocardial stimulation, dysrhythmias can be induced that may prove refractory to either antidysrhythmics or electric shock. Subsequent mortality, while rare, has been reported. The patient is usually awake during the procedure and may experience discomfort associated with prolonged studies or procedures requiring electric cardioversion or defibrillation. The studies are also expensive in terms of personnel and equipment,[74] thus it is important that there be clear clinical indications for the use of electrophysiologic studies. Whether noninvasive testing (ECG, stress testing, Holter testing) is sufficient or electrophysiologic studies of dysrhythmias are necessary is controversial. It is likely, however, that one answer will not apply to all situations, and many patients may require both forms of assessment.[75]

Electrophysiologic studies are usually indicated in evaluating patients who have survived sudden cardiac death particularly if a tachydysrhythmia has been documented.[76] In addition, they may be useful in assessing conduction abnormalities or sinus node function in patients with syncope or near-syncope where a causal cardiac source cannot be found by noninvasive means.[77] Electrophysiologic studies also may be useful in assessing the nature of the tachycardia and prognosis in patients with symptomatic and/or sustained (duration greater than 30 seconds) supraventricular or ventricular tachycardias.[78,79] Electrophysiologic studies with or without catheter ablation techniques may be used in the evaluation and treatment of some patients with symptomatic preexcitation syndromes such as Wolff-Parkinson-White syndrome. Electric mapping of the heart for dysrhythmogenic foci is useful before or during cardiac surgery to treat dysrhythmias. In addition, electrophysiologic study with electric stimulation may aid in assessing the prognosis of a dysrhythmia, the efficacy of possible antidysrhythmic therapies,[80] and the need for implantation of an internal defibrillator.[81]

## ENDOMYOCARDIAL BIOPSY

Endomyocardial biopsy is a procedure that would seem to offer invaluable information in the assessment of underlying cardiac disease. The promise of heart biopsy, however, has thus far gone largely unfilled.[82] The primary indication for this procedure at the current time remains the monitoring of patients after heart transplant for evidence of rejection. It has been used to monitor patients on chemotherapy agents for incipient cardiac toxicity.[83] Heart biopsy can also be useful in the pretransplant evaluation of patients. It has been used in the detection and monitoring of myocarditis, but at this time, it remains uncertain what therapeutic responses might be indicated by these biopsy results.[84] Biopsy also may be helpful in the diagnosis of certain myocardial infiltrative processes and in the differentiation of restrictive cardiomyopathy from constrictive pericarditis. The routine use of endocardial biopsy in idiopathic cardiomyopathy, however, remains controversial.[85]

The biopsy specimens are usually obtained from the right ventricular endocardium, though rarely biopsies may be obtained from the left ventricle. The right ventricle is generally preferred because of the venous access and the risk of arterial embolization of left heart biopsies. The right ventricle may be approached from the right internal jugular vein, using the Stanford-Schultz bioptome, or from the femoral vein, using a long flexible bioptome.[86] The biopsy specimens are then sent for examination by a pathologist with expertise in the evaluation of endoymyocardial tissue. Because venous access is used, the procedure is usually done on an outpatient basis. The procedure is usually performed with fluoroscopic guidance although echocardiographic imaging has also been used.[87] Complications are rare, but they include perforation, possibly with tamponade, dysrhythmias, heart block, vascular trauma, hypotension, and infection.

## REFERENCES

1. Koner RA: Exercise testing and ambulatory monitoring, Cardiovas Rev & Reports 10:47, 1989.
2. Bruce RA: Methods of exercise testing, Am J Cardiol 33:715, 1974.
3. Epstein SE: Implications of probability analysis on the strategy used for noninvasive detection of coronary artery disease: role of single or combine use of exercise electrocardiographic testing, radionuclide cineangiography and myocardial perfusion imaging, Am J Cardiol 46:491, 1980.
4. Cohn PF: Silent myocardial ischemia: to treat or not to treat? Hosp Pract 18:125, 1983.
5. Goldman S, Tselos S, and Cohn K: Marked depth of ST-segment depression during treadmill exercise testing: indicator of severe coronary artery disease, Chest 69:729, 1976.
6. Mark DB and others: Localizing coronary obstructions with the exercise treadmill test, Ann Intern Med 106:53, 1987.
7. Council on Scientific Affairs: Indications and contraindications for exercise testing, JAMA 246:1015, 1981.
8. DeBusk RF and others: Identification and treatment of low-risk patients after acute myocardial infarction and coronary artery bypass graft surgery, N Engl J Med 314:161, 1986.
9. Senaratne MPJ and others: Exercise testing after myocardial infarction: relative values of the low level predischarge and postdischarge exercise test, J Am Coll Cardiol 12:1416, 1988.
10. Weiner DA and others: Prognostic importance of a clinical profile and exercise test in medically treated patients with coronary artery disease, J Am Coll Cardiol 3:772, 1984.
11. Woelfel A and others: Reproducibility and treatment of exercise-induced ventricular tachycardia, Am J Cardiol 53:751, 1984.

12. Podrid PJ and others: The role of exercise testing in evaluation of arrhythmias, Am J Cardiol 62:24H, 1988.
13. Force T and Graboys TB: Exercise testing and ambulatory monitoring in patients with preexcitation syndrome, Arch Intern Med 141:88, 1981.
14. Klein GJ and Gulamhusein SS: Intermittent preexcitation in the Wolff-Parkinson-White Syndrome, Am J Cardiol 52:292, 1983.
15. Cohn PF: The role of noninvasive cardiac testing after an uncomplicated myocardial infarction, N Engl J Med 309:90, 1983.
16. Epstein SE, Palmeri ST, and Patterson RE: Evaluation of patients after acute myocardial infarction: indications for cardiac catheterization and surgical intervention, N Engl J Med 307:1487, 1982.
17. Kloner RA: Exercise testing and ambulatory monitoring, Cardiovasc Rev & Reports 10:49, 1989.
18. Braunwald E and others: Heart disease, ed 3, Philadelphia, 1988, WB Saunders Co.
19. Pohost GM and others: Differentiation of transiently ischemic from infarcted myocardium by serial imaging after a single dose of thallium-201, Circulation 55:294, 1977.
20. Beller GA: Noninvasive assessment of myocardial ischemia, Balor Cardiology Series 12:9, 1989.
21. Okada RD and others: Exercise radionuclide imaging approaches to coronary artery disease, Am J Cardiol 46:1188, 1980.
22. Holman BL, Tanaka TT, and Lesch M: Evaluation of radiopharmaceuticals for the detection of acute myocardial infarction in man, Radiology 121:427, 1976.
23. Okada RD and others: Observer variance in the qualitative evaluation of left ventricular wall motion and the quantitation of left ventricular ejection fraction using rest and exercise multigated blood pool imaging, Circulation 61:128, 1980.
24. Treves S: Detection and quantitation of cardiovascular shunts with commonly available radionuclides, Semin Nucl Med 10:16, 1980.
25. The Multicenter Postinfarction Research Group: Risk stratification and survival after myocardial infarction, N Engl J Med 309:331, 1983.
26. Rozanski A and others: Declining specificity of exercise radionuclide ventriculography, N Engl J Med 309:518, 1983.
27. Holter NJ: Radioelectrocardiography: a new technique for cardiovascular studies, Ann NY Acad Sci 65:913, 1957.
28. Knoebel SB and others: Guidelines for ambulatory electrocardiography: a report of the American College of Cardiology/American Heart Association task force on assessment of diagnostic and therapeutic cardiovascular procedures. JACC 13:251, 1989.
29. Michelson EL and Morganroth J: Spontaneous variability of complex ventricular arrhythmias detected by long-term electrocardiographic recording, Circulation 61:690, 1980.
30. Pratt CM and others: Analysis of the spontaneous variability of ventricular arrhythmias: consecutive ambulatory electrocardiographic recordings of ventricular tachycardia, Am J Cardiol 56:67, 1985.
31. Sokoloff N and others: Utility of ambulatory electrocadiographic monitoring for predicting recurrence of sustained ventricular tachyarrhythmias in patients receiving amiodarone, J Am Coll Cardiol 7:938, 1986.
32. Graboys TB and others: Long-term survival of patients with malignant ventricular arrhythmia treated with antiarrhythmic drugs, Am J Cardiol 50:437, 1982.
33. Heger JJ and others: Comparison between results obtained from electrocardiographic testing, exercise testing, and ambulatory ECG recording. In Wenger NK, Mock MB, and Ringquist I, editors: Ambulatory electrocardiographic recording, St Louis, 1981, Mosby–Year Book, Inc.
34. Zeldis SM and others: Cardiovascular complaints: correlation with cardiac arrhythmias on 24-hour electrocardiographic monitoring, Chest 78:456, 1980.
35. Clark PA, Glasser SP, and Spoto E: Arrhythmias detected by ambulatory monitoring: lack of correlation with symptoms of dizziness and syncope, Chest 77:722, 1980.
36. Knoebel SB and others: Guidelines for ambulatory electrocardiography: a report of the American College of Cardiology/American Heart Association task force on assessment of diagnostic and therapeutic cardiovascular procedures, JACC 13:257, 1989.
37. DeBusk RF and others: Serial ambulatory electrocardiography and treadmill testing after uncomplicated myocardial infarction, Am J Cardiol 45:547, 1980.
38. Pritchett ELC and others: Electrocardiogram recording by telephone in antiarrhythmic drug trials, Chest 81:473, 1982.
39. Tuttle WB and Schoenfeld CD: ECG phone monitoring of the convalescing MI patients, Prim Cardiol Clin 1:13, 1984.
40. Moynihan PF, Parisi AF, and Feldman CL: Quantitative detection of regional left ventricular contraction abnormalities by two-dimensional echocardiography, Circulation 63:752, 1981.
41. Bairey CN, Rozanski A, and Berman DS: Exercise echocardiography: ready or not? JACC 11:1359, 1988.
42. Reeder GS, Tajik AJ, and Seward JB: Left ventricular mural thrombus: two-dimensional echocardiographic diagnosis, Mayo Clin Proc 56:82, 1981.
43. Barrett MJ, Charuzi Y, and Corday E: Ventricular aneurysm: cross-sectional echocardiographic approach, Am J Cardiol 46:1133, 1980.
44. Perry LS and others: Two-dimensional echocardiography in the diagnosis of left atrial myxoma, Br Heart J 45:667, 1981.
45. Sanfilippo AJ and Weyman AE: The role of echocardiography in managing critically ill patients: part 1, J Crit Illness 3:27, 1988.
46. Feigenbaum H: Echocardiography, ed 3, Philadelphia, 1981, Lea & Febiger.
47. Sweatman T and others: Echocardiographic diagnosis of mitral valve regurgitation due to ruptured chordae tendineae, Circulation 46:580, 1972.
48. Reichek N and Devereux RB: Reliable estimation of peak left ventricular systolic pressure by M-mode echocardiographic-determined end-diastolic relative wall thickness: identification of severe valvular aortic stenosis in adult patients, Am Heart J 103:202, 1982.
49. Botuirick EH and others: Echocardiographic demonstration of early mitral valve closure in severe aortic insufficiency: its clinical implications, Circulation 51:836, 1975.
50. Lee RT, Bahatia SJS, and St John Sutton, MG: Assessment of valvular heart disease with Doppler echocardiography, JAMA 262:2131, 1989.
51. Armstrong WF and others: Diastolic collapse of the right ventricle with cardiac tamponade: an echocardiographic study, Circulation 65:1491, 1982.
52. Gillam LD and others: Hydrodynamic compression of the right atrial free wall, a new highly-sensitive echocardiographic sign of cardiac tamponade, Am J Cardiol 49:1010, 1982.
52. Seward JB and others: Transesophageal echocardiography: technique, anatomic correlations, implementation, and clinical applications, Mayo Clin Proc 63:649, 1988.
53. Duncan WJ: Color doppler in clinical cardiology, Philadelphia, 1988, WB Saunders Co.
54. Richards KL and others: Calculation of aortic valve area by Doppler echocardiography: a direct application of the continuity equation, Circulation 73:964, 1986.
55. Abbasi AS and others: Detection and estimation of the degree of mitral regurgitation by range-gated pulsed Doppler echocardiography, Circulation 61:143, 1980.
56. Huntsman LL and others: Noninvasive Doppler determination of cardiac output in man: clinical validation, Circulation 67:593, 1983.
57. Yock PG and Popp RL: Noninvasive estimation of right ventricular systolic pressure by Doppler ultrasound in patients with tricuspid regurgitation, Circulation 70:657, 1984.

58. Swan HJC: The role of hemodynamic monitoring in the management of the critically ill, Crit Care Med 3:83, 1975.
59. Forrester JS and others: Thermodilution cardiac output determination with a single flow-directed catheter, Am Heart J 83:306, 1972.
60. Kloner RA: The guide to cardiology: cardiac catheterization, Cardiovasc Rev & Reports 11:56, 1990.
61. Grossman W: Complication of cardiac catheterization: incidence, causes and prevention. In Grossman W, editor: Cardiac catheterization and angiography, ed 2, Philadelphia, 1980, Lea & Febiger.
62. Kloner RA: The guide to cardiology: cardiac catheterization, Cardiovasc Rev & Reports 11:74, 1990.
63. Ross J and others: Guidelines for coronary angiography: a report of the American College of Cardiology/American Heart Association task force on assessment of diagnostic and therapeutic cardiovascular procedures, JACC 10:935, 1987.
64. Irvin RG, Cobb FR, and Roe CR: Acute myocardial infarction and MB creatinine phosphokinase: relationship between onset of symptoms of infarction and appearance and disappearance of enzymes, Arch Intern Med 140:329, 1980.
65. Neuhaus KL and others: High-dose intravenous streptokinase infusion in acute myocardial infarction, Z Kardiol 70:791, 1981.
66. Weidner N: Laboratory diagnosis of acute myocardial infarct: usefulness of determination of lactate dehydrogenase (LDH)-1 level and of ratio LDH-1 to LDH, Arch Pathol Lab Med 106:375, 1982.
67. Fisher MC and others: Routine serum enzyme tests in the diagnosis of acute myocardial infarction: cost effectiveness, Arch Intern Med 143:1541, 1983.
68. McQueen MJ, Holder D, and El-Maraghi NRH: Assessment of the accuracy of serial electrocardiograms in the diagnosis of myocardial infarction, Am Heart J 105:258, 1983.
69. Josephsen ME and Wellens HJJ: Tachycardias: mechanisms, diagnosis, treatment, Philadelphia, 1985, Lea & Febiger.
70. Kim SG: The management of patients with life-threatening ventricular tachyarrhythmias: programmed stimulation or Holter monitoring (either or both)? Circulation 76:1, 1987.
71. Mitchell LB and others: A randomized clinical trial of the noninvasive and invasive approaches to drug therapy of ventricular tachycardia, N Engl J Med 317:1681, 1987.
72. Morady F and others: Catheter ablation of ventricular tachycardia with intracardiac shocks: results in 33 patients, Circulation 75:1037, 1987.
73. Cassidy DM and others: The use of programmed electrical stimulation in patients with documented or suspected ventricular arrhythmias, Heart & Lung 13:602, 1984.
74. Gettes LS and others: Personnel and equipment required for electrophysiologic testing. Report of the committee on electrocardiography and cardiac electrophysiology, Council on Clinical Cardiology, The American Heart Association, Circulation 69:1219A-1221A, 1984.
75. Zipes DP: Cardiac electrophysiology: promises and contributions, JACC 13:1329, 1989.
76. Wilber DJ and others: Out-of-hospital cardiac arrest: role of electrophysiologic testing in prediction of long term outcome, N Engl J Med 318:19, 1988.
77. Denes P and Ezri MD: The role of EPS in the management of patients with unexplained syncope, PACE 8:424, 1985.
78. Gettes LS and others: Use of electrophysiologic studies to establish the diagnosis, mechanism, and site of tachyarrhythmias, Circulation 75(suppl III):III-116, 1987.
79. Wellens HJ, Brugada P, and Bar FW: Indications for use of intracardiac electrophysiologic studies for the diagnosis of site of origin and mechanism of tachycardias, Circulation 75(suppl III):III-110, 1987.
80. Kowey PR and Friehling TD: Uses and limitations of electrophysiology studies for the selection of antiarrhythmic therapy, PACE 9:231, 1986.
81. Zipes DP and others: Guidelines for clinical intracardiac electrophysiologic studies: a report of the American College of Cardiology/American Heart Association task force on assessment of diagnostic and therapeutic cardiovascular procedures, Circulation 80:1925, 1989.
82. Mason JW and O'Connell JB: Clinical merit of endocardiac biopsy, Circulation 79:971, 1989.
83. Torti FM and others: Cardiotoxity of epirubicin and doxorubicin: assessment by endocardial biopsy, Cancer Res 46:3722, 1986.
84. Lie JT: Myocarditis and endomyocardial biopsy in unexplained heart failure: a diagnosis in search of a disease, Ann Intern Med 109:525, 1988.
85. Chow LC, Dittrich HC, and Shabetai R: Endomyocardial biopsy in patients with unexplained congestive heart failure, Ann Intern Med 109:535, 1988.
86. Anderson JL and Marshall HW: The femoral venous approach to endomyocardial biopsy: comparison with internal jugular and transarterial approaches, Am J Cardiol 53:833, 1984.
87. Miller LW and others: Echocardiography-guided endomyocardial biopsy: a 5-year experience, Circulation, 78(suppl III):III-99, 1988.

# CHAPTER 4

# Introduction to Electrocardiography

Barbara A. Erickson

This chapter explains basic principles and use of electrocardiography (ECG) and introduces common ECG findings in patients with cardiac disease. Additional electrocardiographic disorders are presented in Chapter 5.

## BASIC CONSIDERATIONS

The electrocardiogram (ECG) is a graphic recording of the electrical activity generated by the functioning heart. The first ECG was introduced by Willem Einthoven, a Dutch physiologist, in 1901. From the monopolar lead recorded by Einthoven's string galvanometer, the ECG's progression has included the unipolar leads added by Frank N. Wilson and his associates in 1933 to the present electrocardiogram, which includes 12 leads.

The ECG is one of the most valuable of the diagnostic tools available for the recognition of various cardiac diseases or abnormalities. It is especially significant when combined with the total cardiac assessment, which includes a history and physical examination. Changes in the ECG may be either in pattern, rhythm, or both. Any changes noted on the ECG need to be correlated with clinical findings. Variations from the normal ECG may be found in an individual with a healthy heart. Conversely, cardiac disease may not be reflected by changes in an ECG. Thus a normal ECG does not guarantee a normal heart and vice versa. One of the essential roles of the ECG is in the recognition of cardiac dysrhythmias.

In addition to individual variations, numerous other extrinsic factors may alter the ECG. These include but are not limited to drugs, metabolic changes, electrolyte imbalances, technical factors such as incorrectly applied electrodes, and the patient's age and body build. The ECG's precision of interpretation increases when the greatest amount of clinical information is available. It is essential to compare new with previous tracings.

### Standardization

The ECG is recorded on graph paper that is divided into small and large boxes. The small boxes are 1 millimeter square (1 mm²), and the large boxes, designated by heavy lines, contain 25 small boxes, 5 across and 5 down (Fig. 4-1). Horizontally, the paper measures time, and vertically, it measures voltage. The ECG paper moves at 25 mm sec. Therefore horizontally each small box is equal to 0.04

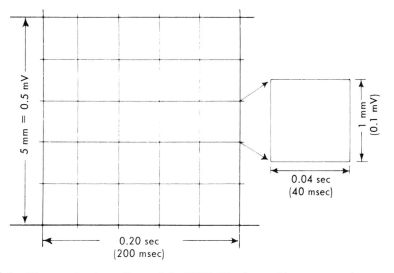

**Fig. 4-1  Time and voltage lines of the ECG.** The interval between two heavy vertical lines is 0.20 second (200 msec); and between each light line, 0.04 second (40 msec). The voltage between each heavy horizontal line is 0.5 mV.

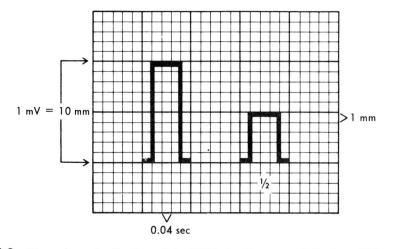

**Fig. 4-2** **Normal standardization of the ECG.** 1 mV causes a deflection of 10 mm. For large ECG deflections the standard must be halved so that 1 mV = 5 mm. For small ECG deflections the standard may be doubled so that 1 mV = 20 mm. Any changes in standardization must be noted on the ECG recording.

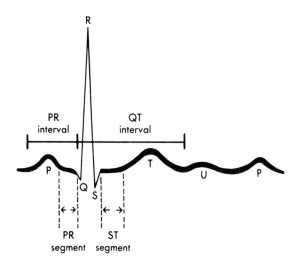

**Fig. 4-3** The deflections in a normal ECG are the P wave (atrial depolarization), QRS complex (ventricular depolarization), and T wave (ventricular repolarization). The U wave is sometimes present and follows the T wave. The PR segment is the interval between the end of the P wave and the beginning of the QRS complex. The ST segment is the interval between the end of the QRS complex and the beginning of the T wave. Sometimes atrial repolarization, the Ta wave, can be recorded (see Fig. 4-7). The PR interval is from the onset of the P wave to the onset of the QRS complex. The QT interval is from the onset of the QRS complex to the end of the T wave.

seconds; each large box (5 mm) is equal to 0.20 seconds (5 × 0.04). Read vertically, the ECG measures voltage or amplitude of the deflections. The exact voltage can be measured because the ECG is set, or standardized, so that 1 millivolt (1 mV) of electric current causes a deflection 10 mm in amplitude (Fig. 4-2). The deflection may be modified by being set at *one-half standard,* which means that 1 mV of electric current causes only a 5 mm deflection or *twice standard,* which means that 1 mV of electric current causes a deflection of 20 mm. When very large deflections are present, it is advisable to record the ECG at one-half standard; when the deflections are very small, the ECG may be recorded at twice standard. Any change in "standardization" must be indicated on the ECG.

### Deflections

In describing the amplitude of the deflections inscribed on the ECG, the following terms are used: *baseline, wave, segment, interval,* and *complex.* The *baseline* is the starting or resting line of the ECG. Any deflection from the baseline is called a *wave.* A wave above the baseline is considered *positive;* one below the baseline is considered *negative.* If the deflection has both positive and negative components, it is called *biphasic* or *diphasic.* A deflection, or wave, that rests on the baseline is called *isoelectric.* A *segment* is a straight line connecting waves, as in the ST segment. An *interval* is a wave plus a straight line, as in the PR interval. A *complex* is a group of waves, as in the QRS complex.

The six major deflections of the normal ECG are designated by the letter P, Q, R, S, T, and U (Fig. 4-3). These waves are produced by the electrical energy caused by the movement of charged particles across the membranes of myocardial cells (depolarization and repolarization).

## ELECTROPHYSIOLOGIC PRINCIPLES

The membrane surrounding a cell is a semipermeable two-layered lipid envelope that maintains a high concentration of potassium ($K^+$) and a low concentration of sodium ($Na^+$) inside the cell and a high concentration of $Na^+$ and a low concentration of $K^+$ outside the cell. The voltage inside a resting (polarized) cardiac cell is negative with respect to the outside of the cell, in large part because of the cell membrane's relative premeability to $K^+$ and impermeability to $Na^+$ during diastole. The ratio of extracellular to intracellular potassium concentrations primarily determines the resting potential of the cell; when the cell becomes depolarized the cell membrane alters its permeability so that it becomes more permeable to $Na^+$ and less permeable to $K^+$. $Na^+$ rushes into the cell, making the voltage inside the cell positive with respect to the voltage outside the cell. These events occur in atrial and ventricular muscle and the His-Purkinje system. In the normal sinus and AV nodes, and possibly in other fibers if they become damaged and lose membrane potential, calcium appears to play a prominent role in the depolarization process. Calcium (and possibly sodium in some instances) enters the cell through the "slow channel," producing the *slow response*. It is called the slow response because the time to activate and inactivate the channel (in essence, turn it on and off) is slow, compared with the sodium, or "fast channel," which is active in muscle and in His-Purkinje fibers (Fig. 4-4).

Understanding these ionic mechanisms is clinically important because of the development of drugs such as ver-

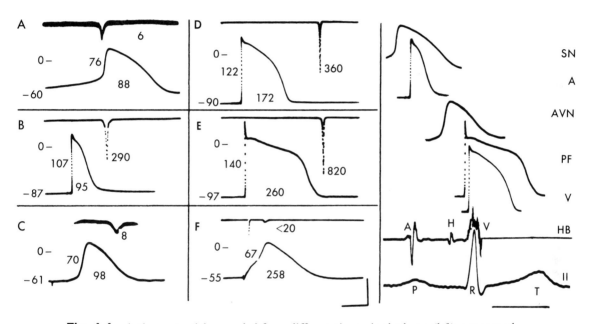

**Fig. 4-4** Action potentials recorded from different tissues in the heart *(left)*, remounted with a His bundle recording and scalar ECG from a patient *(right)* to illustrate the timing during a single cardiac cycle. In **A** to **F** the top tracing is dV/dt of phase 0 and the second tracing is the action potential. For each panel the numbers *(from left to right)* indicate maximum diastolic potential (mV), action potential amplitude (mV), action potential duration at 90 percent of repolarization (msec), and Vmax (maximum rate of rise in volts/second of cardiac action potential) of phase 0 (V/sec). Zero potential is indicated by the short horizontal line next to the zero on the upper left of each action potential. **A,** Rabbit sinoatrial node; **B,** canine atrial muscle; **C,** rabbit atrioventricular node; **D,** canine ventricular muscle; **E,** canine Purkinje fiber; **F,** diseased human ventricle. Note that the action potentials recorded in **A, C,** and **F** have reduced resting membrane potentials, amplitudes, and Vmax compared with the other action potentials. In right panel, *SN* = sinus nodal potential; *A* = atrial muscle potential; *AVN* = atrioventricular nodal potential; *PF* = Purkinje fiber potential; *V* = ventricular muscle potential; *HB* = His bundle recording; *II* = lead II. Horizontal calibration on left: 50 msec for **A** and **C,** 100 msec for **B, D, E,** and **F.** Vertical calibration on left: 50 mV. Horizontal calibration on right: 200 msec. (From Gilmour RF, Jr, and Zipes DP: Basic electrophysiology of the slow inward current. In Antman E and Stone PH, editors: Calcium blocking agents in the treatment of cardiovascular disorders, Mt Kisco, NY, 1983, Futura Publishing Co, Inc.)

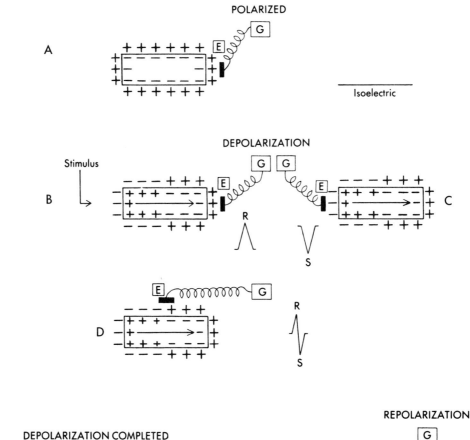

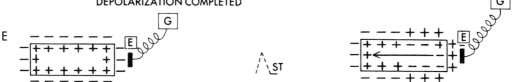

**Fig. 4-5**   **A,** A schematic illustration of a polarized (resting) myocardial muscle cell maintaining a negative charge on the inside of the cell membrane and a positive charge on the outside of the membrane. An electrode *(E)* facing the right side of the polarized cell and attached to an ECG machine (*G,* galvanometer) will record no current, and an isoelectric line results. **B,** The cell is stimulated from the left, and depolarization proceeds from left to right in the direction of the arrow. The depolarized left end of the cell becomes electrically negative, whereas the right end of the cell is still polarized and electrically positive. There now exists a difference of electric potentials (negative and positive ions), and an electric current is flowing. The electrode facing the positive side of this current and attached to an ECG machine will record a positive deflection, and in the case of ventricular depolarization, this deflection is called an R wave. **C,** The same myocardial cell is stimulated again from the left; however, the electrode is facing the negative side of the current, and will therefore record a negative deflection. In the case of ventricular depolarization, this deflection is called an S wave. **D,** Once again the cell is activated from the left. The electrode facing the center of the cell will first write a positive and then a negative deflection. In the case of ventricular depolarization, this deflection is called an RS complex. **E,** With the completion of depolarization, the outer surface of the myocardial cell becomes electrically negative; the flow of electric current ceases, and the R wave returns to the isoelectric line. The short period following complete ventricular depolarization is recorded as the ST segment. **F,** In the previous illustration, the myocardial muscle cell was depolarized from left to right. Now the cell returns to the resting state, repolarization, in the opposite direction, from right to left. The right end of the cell becomes positive first and an electrode facing this site will inscribe a positive deflection. In the case of ventricular repolarization, this deflection is termed a *T Wave.*

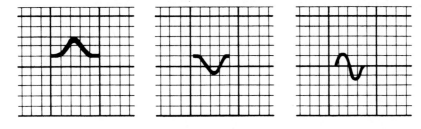

**Fig. 4-6**  The P wave is gently rounded in contour, may be normally positive, negative, or diphasic in different ECG leads, and should not exceed 2 or 3 mm.

apamil that fairly specifically block the slow channel. These drugs are often called "calcium channel or calcium entry blockers."

The cell in a resting, *polarized* state can be represented by negative and positive charges lining, respectively, the inside and outside of the cell membrane (Fig. 4-5, *A*). If an electrode of an ECG machine (galvanometer) were attached to this polarized cell, no electrical potential would be registered because no net change in ionic composition would occur. Hence, there would be no voltage shift and no deviation from the isoelectric baseline (Fig. 4-5, *A*).

When a cell or, more likely, a group of cells is stimulated, and the change in membrane permeability permits sodium ions to migrate rapidly into the cell making the inside positive with respect to the outside *depolarization,* an electric field is generated between the depolarized and polarized areas of myocardium. The P wave represents atrial depolarization, and the QRS complex represents ventricular depolarization (Fig. 4-5, *B* to *D*).

A slower movement of ions across the membrane restoring the cell to the polarized state is termed *repolarization.* Movement of potassium ions out of myocardial cells primarily accounts for repolarization. In late diastole, after most of the repolarization has occurred, potassium and sodium reverse positions to restore ionic concentrations to the polarized state. The Ta wave, representing atrial repolarization, generally lies buried in the QRS complex and ST segment. The ST segment is an isoelectric line extending from the end of the QRS complex to the beginning of the T wave, during which early ventricular repolarization is beginning very slowly (Fig. 4-5, *E*). The T wave represents ventricular repolarization (Fig. 4-5, *F*).

## WAVES AND COMPLEXES
### P Wave

As previously mentioned, the P wave represents atrial depolarization, and begins as soon as the impulse leaves the sinus node (sinoatrial, or SA, node) and initiates atrial depolarization. Because the sinus node is situated in the right atrium, right atrial activation begins first and is followed shortly thereafter by left atrial activation. As left atrial activation begins, before the end of right atrial ac-

tivation, the two processes overlap. This close overlap of the forces results in a gently rounded P wave. As will be discussed later in this chapter, the P wave normally may be positive, negative, or diphasic, depending on which lead of the ECG is recorded. Whatever the case, the amplitude of the P wave should not exceed 2 or 3 mm in any lead (Fig. 4-6).

Although usually not visible on the ECG, the Ta wave of atrial repolarization occurs in a direction opposite to that of the P wave and is recorded after the first portion of the P wave and continues through the PR interval. It is usually not identified unless the P wave occurs independently of the QRS, as in complete AV block (see Chapter 5). When the P wave is large, the Ta wave is also generally large and may be seen to extend beyond the QRS complex, resulting in a distortion of the initial portion of the ST segment. This may cause a depression of the ST segment that may be mistaken to have a pathologic significance. To make a correct interpretation in the setting of a depressed ST segment, one must (1) observe the configuration of the atrial repolarization wave (smooth curve with upward concavity), (2) recognize a similar deviation of the baseline before the QRS is recorded, and (3) recognize a large P wave (Fig. 4-7).

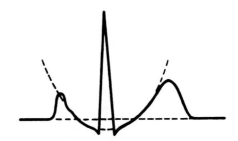

**Fig. 4-7**  Atrial repolarization as a cause of ST segment deviation. Note that the PQ (PR) and ST segments can be connected by a smooth curve, and that the direction of the deviation is opposite in direction to the P wave. (Modified from Hurst JW and others: The heart: arteries and veins, ed 6, New York, 1984, McGraw-Hill Book Co.)

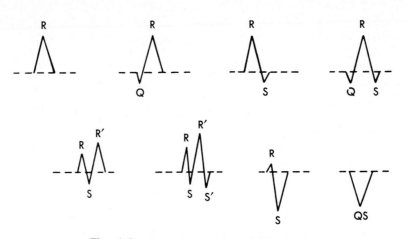

**Fig. 4-8** Components of the QRS complex.

## QRS Complex

The QRS complex representing ventricular depolarization may have various components, depending on which lead of the ECG is recorded. These components are illustrated in Fig. 4-8 and described as follows:

R wave: The first positive deflection

Q wave: The initial negative deflection preceding an R wave

S wave: The negative deflection following an R wave

R' wave: The second positive deflection

S' wave: The negative deflection following the R' wave

QS wave: The totally negative deflection

The QRS complexes should be examined for the following:

1. The *duration* of the complex
2. The *amplitude* of the components
3. The general *configuration* of the complex, including the presence and location of any slurred component (see Chapter 5 discussion of bundle branch block and Wolff-Parkinson-White syndrome)
4. The presence of abnormal *Q waves* (discussed under myocardial infarction in this chapter)
5. The timing of the *intrinsicoid deflections* in precordial leads $V_1$ to $V_6$

**Amplitude.** The amplitude of the QRS complex has wide normal limits; however, it is generally agreed that if the total amplitude (above and below the baseline) is 5 mm or less in all three standard leads, it is abnormally low. Such low voltage may be seen in patients who have cardiac failure, diffuse coronary disease, pericardial effusion, myxedema, primary amyloidosis, or any other conditions producing widespread myocardial damage. Furthermore, it may be found in patients who have emphysema, generalized edema, and obesity. The minimum normal QRS amplitude in precordial leads varies from right to left across the chest, being generally accepted as 5 mm in $V_6$ and $V_6$, 7 mm in $V_2$ and $V_5$ and 9 mm in $V_3$ and $V_4$.

Upper limits for normal QRS voltage (amplitude) have been difficult to set. Diagnostic evaluation is important when QRS amplitudes reach the following upper limits: $V_1$ an R wave of 5 mm; $V_1$, $V_2$ an S wave of 30 mm; $V_5$, $V_6$ an R wave of 30 mm; and in the limb leads an R or S wave of 20 mm.

**Intrinsicoid deflection.** Ventricular activation time is the interval between the beginning of the QRS complex and the onset of the intrinsicoid deflection. The time of onset of the intrinsicoid deflection is measured from the beginning of the QRS complex to the peak of the R wave, and it is measured in the precordial leads (Fig. 4-9). In right-sided precordial leads ($V_1$ or $V_2$) the time of onset for the intrinsicoid deflection is normally 0.03 second or less. In left-sided precordial leads ($V_5$ or $V_6$) the time of onset is normally 0.05 second or less in adults. If the time of onset for the intrinsicoid deflection exceeds 0.03 or 0.05 second in right- and left-sided leads respectively, it is taken to indicate that the impulse arrived late at the epicardial sur-

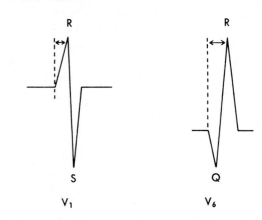

**Fig. 4-9** The time of onset of the intrinsicoid deflection is measured from the beginning of the QRS complex to the peak of the R wave.

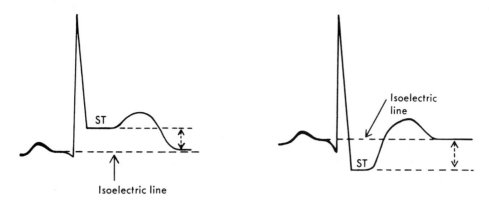

**Fig. 4-10** Elevation of the ST segment is measured from the upper edge of the isoelectric line to the upper edge of the ST segment; depression is measured from the lower edge of the isoelectric line to the lower edge of the ST segment.

face of the ventricle under the electrode. Such delay may be caused by thickening or dilatation of the ventricular wall or a block in the conducting system to the ventricle involved (bundle branch block).

## ST Segment

The interval that occurs between the end of the QRS complex and the beginning of the T wave is called the ST segment. It represents the time during which the ventricles have been completely depolarized and are beginning ventricular repolarization. Usually, the ST segment is isoelectric (see Fig. 4-3), but it may normally deviate between − 0.5 and + 1.0 mm from the baseline in the standard and unipolar leads (ECG leads are presented in the next section). In some instances, upward displacement of 2 or 3 mm may be normal, provided that the ST segment is concave upward and the succeeding T wave is tall and upright. This is called *early repolarizaton.* Downward displacement in excess of 0.5 mm generally is abnormal. In all situations, depression caused by a depressed PR segment must be considered. More important are ST segments, elevated or depressed, that vary temporarily (see discussions of myocardial infarction, pericarditis). Correlation with the clinical condition of the patient is often necessary to determine the significance of ST segment displacement.

Elevation of the ST segment is measured from the upper edge of the isoelectric line to the upper edge of the ST segment; depression is measured from the lower edge of the isoelectric line to the lower edge of the ST segment (Fig. 4-10).

## T Wave

The T wave, normally slightly rounded and slightly asymmetric, represents the electrical recovery period (repolarization) of the ventricles. Upright T waves are measured from the upper level of the baseline to the summit of the T wave, whereas inverted T waves are measured from the lower level of the baseline to the lowest point of the T wave. Diphasic T waves are measured by adding the amplitudes above and below the baseline. T waves normally do not exceed 5 mm in any standard lead or 10 mm in any precordial lead. T wave contour is often very labile and, as with the ST segment, correlation with the clinical status of the patient, often in serially repeated ECGs, is necessary for correct interpretation.

## U Wave

The U wave is a small wave of low voltage sometimes observed following a T wave and in the same direction as its preceding T wave; that is, when the T wave is upright, the U wave normally will be upright. It is best observed in the chest leads, although it is present, but barely detectable, in the limb leads.

Relatively little is known about the U wave. Although the cause and clinical significance of the U wave are uncertain, the appearance of U waves or an increase in their magnitude is seen in certain disorders (see Chapter 5 discussion of hypokalemia). The U wave is generally upright in the precordial leads. A negative U wave may occur in patients who have left ventricular hypertrophy, hypertension, or coronary artery disease. An upright (positive) U wave that becomes inverted (negative) during an exercise stress test often indicates the presence of significant coronary artery obstruction in the main left or left anterior descending coronary artery.

## ELECTROCARDIOGRAM LEADS

As previously mentioned, the deflections on the ECG are produced by the electrical energy caused by the movement of charged ions across the membranes of myocardial cells (depolarization and repolarization). This movement of charged particles results in a flow of electrical current. The pressure behind the flow of electrical current is called *electrical potential,* and it creates an electrical field. This electrical field extends to the body surface, where the electrical potential can be measured by the ECG.

By convention, 12 lead recordings comprise the ECG. Each lead has a positive and negative pole (electrode), and the location of these poles determines the polarity of the lead. A hypothetic line joining the poles of a lead is known as the *axis* of the lead. Moreover, every lead axis is oriented in a certain direction, depending on the location of the positive and negative electrodes.

Six of the twelve ECG leads measure cardiac forces in the frontal plane (the standard limb leads and the augmented leads, I, II, III, $aV_R$, a $V_L$, and a $V_F$); the remaining six leads ($V_1$ to $V_6$) measure the cardiac forces in the horizontal plane.

## Standard (Bipolar) Limb Leads (I, II, III)

The standard limb leads, designated leads I, II, and III, were developed by Willem Einthoven (1860-1927), physiologist and inventor of the string galvanometer. Using the principle that the heart is situated in the center of the electric field it generates, Einthoven placed the electrodes of the three standard leads as far away from the heart as possible, that is, on the extremities—the right arm, left arm, and left leg.* These three electrodes, therefore, are considered to be electrically equidistant from the heart. Consequently, the heart may be viewed as a point source

*The right leg serves as a ground electrode, thereby providing a pathway of least resistance for electric interference in the body. Actually, the ground electrode can be placed at any location on the body.

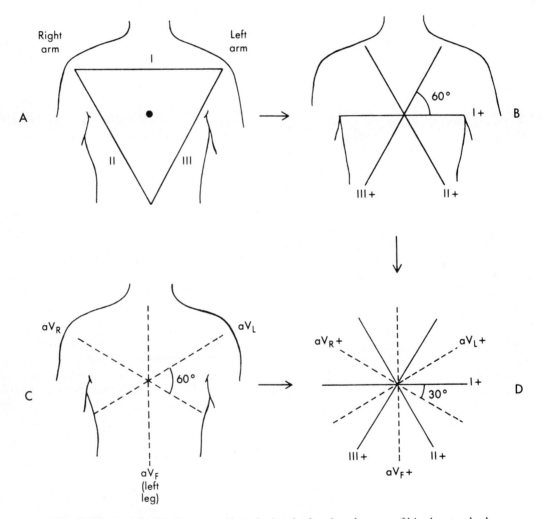

**Fig. 4-11**  **A,** The Einthoven equilateral triangle showing the axes of bipolar standard limb leads I, II, and III. The heart is at the center or zero point. **B,** The axes of the standard limb leads are shifted to the center of the triangle (zero point of the electric field), forming a triaxial figure. **C,** The axes of the unipolar augmented leads. **D,** The axes of the standard and augmented limb leads are combined to form a hexaxial figure. Each lead is labeled at its positive pole.

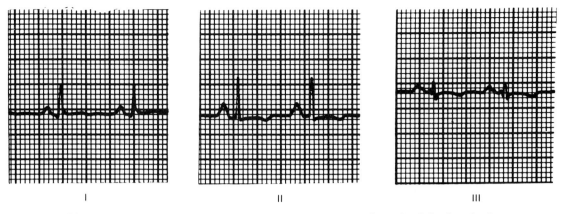

**Fig. 4-12**  Einthoven's law states: lead I + lead III = lead II. The deflections in the ECG leads demonstrate this law.

in the center of an equilateral triangle, whose apices are the right arm, left arm, and left leg. This is called Einthoven's triangle (Fig. 4-11, *A*).

The standard bipolar limb leads measure the difference between two recording sites. The actual potential under either of the electrodes is not known as it is for the unipolar leads. For lead I, the negative electrode is placed on the right arm and the positive electrode on the left arm. For lead II, the negative electrode is on the right arm and the positive electrode on the left leg. For lead III, the left arm electrode is negative, and the left leg electrode is positive (Fig. 4-11, *A*). This is summarized as follows:

| Lead | Location |
|------|----------|
| I | Right arm ($-$) to left arm ($+$) |
| II | Right arm ($-$) to left leg ($+$) |
| III | Left arm ($-$) to left leg ($+$) |

Because of the established relationship of the standard limb leads to each other, at any given instant during the cardiac cycle the sum of the electrical potentials recorded in leads I and III equals the electrical potential recorded in lead II. This is Einthoven's law, and it applies to a triangle of any shape. Stated mathematically, the law is as follows:

$$\text{Lead I} + \text{Lead III} = \text{Lead II}$$

Einthoven's law may be used to detect errors in electrode placement. Furthermore, it may clarify perplexing findings in one or another lead. If, for example, the deflections of lead II are obscured by muscular or electric interference or by a wandering baseline, the characteristics of the other two leads may be used to determine the presence of a Q wave or ST segment deviation in lead II. Einthoven's law also is helpful in evaluating serial tracings. For example, if in a given tracing the T wave in lead I appears to be more negative than in the previous tracing,

changes must be present in the T waves of the other two limb leads as well, so that $T_1 + T_3 = T_2$ (Fig. 4-12).

To prevent confusion about polarities the ECG machine records a positive deflection in the bipolar leads when in lead I the left arm is in the positive portion of the electric field, in lead II the left leg is in the positive portion of the electric field, and in lead III the left leg is in the positive portion of the electric field.

**Triaxial reference figure.** The three lead axes of the equilateral triangle can be shifted without changing their direction so that their midpoints intersect at the same point. Thus the triaxial reference figure is formed with each of the lead axes separated from one another by 60 degrees (Fig. 4-11, *B*).

### Augmented (Unipolar) Leads (aV$_R$, aV$_L$, aV$_F$)

All unipolar leads are called V leads and consist of extremity (limb) leads and precordial (chest) leads. The augmented leads a V$_R$, aV$_L$, and aV$_F$ use the same electrode locations as the standard limb leads. Therefore the positive electrode is attached to the right arm (aV$_R$), left arm (aV$_L$), or left leg (aV$_F$). The negative electrode, however, is formed by combining leads I, II, and III, whose algebraic sum is zero. Because the electric center of the heart is at zero potential, the augmented leads measure the difference in potential between the limbs and the center of the heart.

The axis for each augmented lead is a line drawn from the extremity, where the positive electrode is placed, to the zero point of the electric field of the heart, which is at the center of the equilateral triangle (Fig. 4-11, *C*). These three unipolar lead axes also form a triaxial reference system with the axes 60 degrees apart.

**Hexaxial reference figure.** When the triaxial figure of the standard leads and the triaxial figure of the augmented leads are combined, they form a hexaxial reference figure in which each augmented lead is perpendicular to a standard limb lead (Fig. 4-11, *D*). The hexaxial figure is a useful

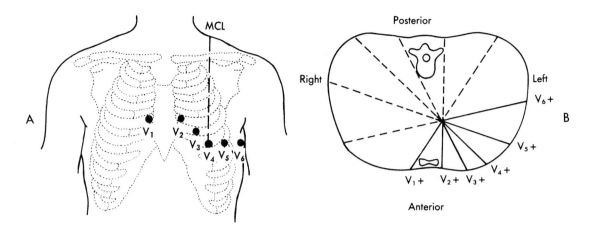

**Fig. 4-13** **A,** Electrode positions of the precordial leads: $V_1$, fourth intercostal space at the right sternal border; $V_2$, fourth intercostal space at the left sternal border; $V_3$, halfway between $V_2$ and $V_4$; $V_4$, fifth intercostal space at the midclavicular line; $V_5$, anterior axillary line directly lateral to $V_4$; $V_6$, midaxillary line directly lateral to $V_5$. **B,** The precordial reference figure. Leads $V_1$ and $V_2$ are called *right-sided precordial leads;* leads $V_3$ and $V_4$, *mid-precordial leads; and leads $V_5$ and $V_6$, left-sided precordial leads.*

reference for plotting mean cardiac forces in the frontal plane.

### Precordial (Unipolar) Leads ($V_1$ to $V_6$)

In the horizontal plane, precordial leads are used to determine how far anteriorly or posteriorly from the frontal plane the electric forces of the heart are directed. The standard precordial ECG consists of six unipolar leads, $V_1$ through $V_6$. In Fig. 4-13, *A*, the V leads are shown with reference to their electrode positions on the anterior chest wall. These chest electrodes represent a positive pole (unipolar). Any electric force traveling toward one of these leads will produce a positive deflection; traveling away from it will produce a negative deflection. For descriptive purposes, leads $V_1$ and $V_2$ are called right-sided precordial leads; leads $V_3$ and $V_4$, midprecordial leads; and leads $V_5$ and $V_6$, left-sided precordial leads.

**Precordial reference figure.** A transverse representation of the chest wall and the V leads results in the precordial reference figure (Fig. 4-13, *B*). This figure is a useful reference for plotting mean cardiac forces in the horizontal plane.

### THE VECTOR APPROACH TO ELECTROCARDIOGRAPHY

The electrical potentials generated during the cardiac cycle can be described and measured. To adequately characterize such an electric potential or force, both the magnitude and the direction of the force must be specified; this can be done by a *vector*. Briefly stated, a vector is a quantity of electric force that has a known magnitude and direction. A vector may be illustrated graphically by an arrow, the length of the arrow representing the magnitude of the force

and the direction of the arrow indicating the direction of the force. The arrowhead depicts the location of the positive field.

Representing electric forces of the heart by vectors more easily explains the relationship between the electric activity generated by the heart and the recording of this electric activity by a specific lead. When an electric force (and therefore the vector that represents it) establishes a direction *parallel* to the lead that records it, this electric force causes the *largest deflection* to be inscribed by that lead. An electric force perpendicular to the recording lead produces no deflection in that lead. Forces in between these extremes generate deflections according to their directions: the more nearly parallel the force (and vector) to the recording lead, the larger the deflection produced in that lead; the more nearly perpendicular the force to the recording lead, the smaller the deflection. When the positive and negative forces on a lead are equal, the net area of the deflection is zero. This results in a biphasic or transitional deflection (Fig. 4-14).

### Sequence of Electric Events in the Heart

In the normal heart, depolarization of the ventricle is a sequential process. The process can be represented by *instantaneous vectors,* each of which corresponds to all the heart's electric forces at a given moment in time. A diagram of successive instantaneous vectors depicting ventricular depolarization is shown in Fig. 4-15, *A.* Initial depolarization passes from left to right across the interventricular septum. During the second phase, depolarization of subendocardial muscle occurs near the apex. The last phase of depolarization occurs in the posterior free wall of the left ventricle.

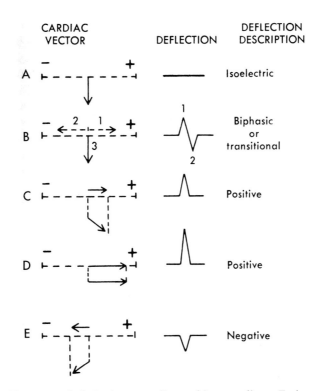

**Fig. 4-14** **Vectors and their electrocardiographic recordings.** Each arrow represents the vector generated by an electric force. This force produces an electrocardiographic deflection, shown on the right. **A,** Because the vector is perpendicular to the axis of the recording lead, no projection appears on that lead. The absence of a deflection establishes an uninterrupted isoelectric line. **B,** The mean vector (number 3) is perpendicular to the axis of the recording lead when the positive and negative forces are equal (the net area of the deflection is zero). A biphasic or transitional deflection is recorded because the initial forces moved rightward (vector 1) at the same distance that the later forces moved leftward (vector 2). The instantaneous vectors have equal magnitude but opposite direction. **C,** The vector projects on the positive side of the axis of the recording lead to inscribe a small positive deflection. **D,** When the vector is parallel with the lead axis, the projection onto the recording lead has its maximum magnitude. **E,** The vector projects on the negative side of the lead axis, and a small negative deflection is recorded.

The deflection recorded by any given lead results from the projection of the cardiac vector generated during depolarization onto the axis of the lead. Thus arrow 1 (Fig. 4-15, *B*), depicting depolarization of the septum, usually causes a small negative deflection in lead I, resulting in a Q wave and a larger positive deflection in lead III, resulting in an R wave. Arrow 2, illustrating depolarization of the apical region of the heart, usually produces a very small positive deflection (R wave) in lead I because of its leftward orientation and an R wave in lead III. Late depolarization of the heart, being from right to left in the posterior free wall of the left ventricle, causes a large positive deflection in lead I (the major part of the R wave) and an S wave in lead III. Following the completion of depolarization of ventricles, the electric wave returns to the baseline. Therefore the three arrows have generated a small initial Q wave

followed by a large R wave in lead I and an R wave followed by an S wave in lead III (Fig. 4-15, *D*).

As previously discussed, each ECG lead has a different orientation to the heart. Therefore the instantaneous vectors of ventricular depolarization will produce a different deflection in each lead. This is also true of ventricular repolarization and atrial depolarization.

In this chapter, detailed consideration is given to the vectors of the QRS complex. However, the positions of the P wave and T wave in the frontal plane are also important. Normally the P wave is upright in leads I and II and may be biphasic, flat, or inverted in lead III; inverted in lead $aV_R$; upright, biphasic, or inverted in lead $aV_L$; and upright in lead $aV_F$.

Normally the T wave is upright in leads I and II, flat, biphasic, or inverted in lead III, and inverted in lead $aV_R$.

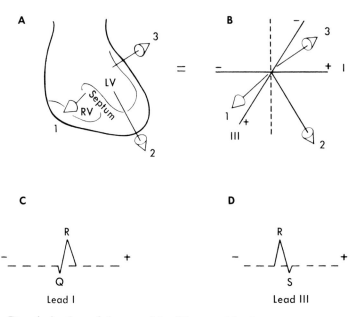

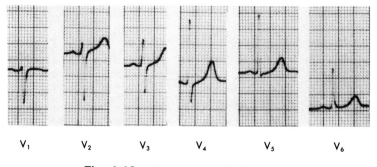

**Fig. 4-15** **Depolarization of the ventricles illustrated by instantaneous vectors.** Arrow 1 depicts depolarization of the septum from left to right and is directed to the right and somewhat anteriorly. Arrow 2 illustrates depolarization of the apical region of the heart and is directed to the left and inferiorly. Arrow 3 represents depolarization of the posterior aspect of the left ventricle and is directed to the left and posteriorly. **B,** The instantaneous vectors representing ventricular depolarization are inscribed on lead I and lead III. **C,** and **D,** Arrow 1 causes a small negative deflection in lead I, resulting in a Q wave, and a larger positive deflection in lead III, resulting in an R wave. Arrow 2 produces a small positive deflection (R wave) in lead I and an R wave in lead III. Arrow 3 causes a large R wave in lead I and S wave in lead III.

In lead $aV_L$, the T wave may be upright, flattened, or biphasic, according to the QRS pattern. It may also be inverted, provided that the T wave in lead $aV_R$ is also inverted. In lead $aV_F$ the T wave is usually upright; however, it can be normally flattened, biphasic, or inverted, provided that the T wave in lead $aV_R$ is also inverted.

In the horizontal plane the P wave is normally upright in all precordial leads, but it may be inverted in $V_1$ and $V_2$ without being abnormal. The normal QRS complex is transitional at some point between $V_3$ and $V_4$. The precordial transition zone is characterized by the transition from the RS complexes recorded by the leads oriented to the right ventricle to the QR complexes recorded by the leads oriented to the left ventricle (Fig. 4-16). The normal T wave is upright in leads $V_2$ through $V_6$. The T wave may be flat or inverted in $V_1$ and still be normal.

**Mean Cardiac Vector**

The mean cardiac vector, which is the average of all the instantaneous vectors, can be expressed accurately on the hexaxial reference figure. Furthermore, since the hexaxial reference system divides the frontal plane into 30-degree

**Fig. 4-16** Normal precordial lead ECG.

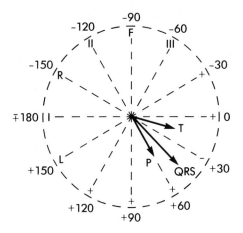

**Fig. 4-17** The hexaxial reference system, which is formed by combining standard limb leads, (I, II, III) with augmented leads (aVR, aVL, aVF), divides the frontal plane into 30-degree intervals. The inside of the hexaxial circle represents leads and their positive and negative poles. The outside of the circle is arbitrarily labeled with a negative value for the degrees in the upper hemisphere and a positive value for those in lower hemisphere. The mean P vector normally lies along +60-degree axis. The mean QRS vector normally lies anywhere between 0 and +90 degrees; in this Fig. the mean QRS vector lies on +45-degree axis. The mean T vector normally lies between −10 and +75 degrees; in this Fig. the mean T vector lies on +15-degree axis. The mean frontal plane QRS axis and T wave axis are usually similarly directed, and the angle between them normally does not exceed 60 degrees.

intervals, the leads have been classified as follows: all degrees in the upper hemisphere of the hexaxial figure are labeled as negative degrees, and all degrees in the lower hemisphere are labeled as positive degrees. Accordingly, commencing at the positive end of the standard lead I axis (labeled 0 degrees and progressing counterclockwise), the leads are successively at −30, −60, −90, −120, −150, and −180 degrees. Progressing clockwise, the leads are successively at +30, +60, +90, +120, +150, and +180 degrees* (Fig. 4-17).

The position of the mean cardiac vector provides information about the electric "position" of the heart, also expressed as the mean electric axis, and it is influenced by the anatomic position of the heart within the chest, the anatomy of the heart itself, and the pathway traveled by the depolarizing wave. If the P vector is projected on the hexaxial figure, the mean electric axis of the P in the frontal plane lies approximately along the +60-degree axis (Fig. 4-17). The mean QRS vector lies normally between 0 and +90 degrees, whereas the mean electric axis of the

*The conventional labeling of the hexaxial reference figure as positive and negative units should not be confused with the positive and negative poles of the lead axis.

T wave lies between −10 and +75 degrees. The mean frontal plane QRS axis and T wave axis are usually similarly directed, and the angle between them normally does not exceed 60 degrees (Fig. 4-17).

**Mean QRS Axis**

The remainder of this section discusses the significance and determination of the mean electric force, or axis, of the QRS. The principles used to determine the QRS axis also may be applied to the determination of the P and T axis.

**Determination of the frontal plane projection of the mean QRS vector.** In the standard ECG the average of the electric forces, or axis, can be determined in either the frontal plane or horizontal plane leads. However, for practical purposes the axis is usually determined from leads of the frontal plane, or leads I, II, III, aVR, aVL, or aVF.

The hexaxial reference system (see Fig. 4-17) and the following principles are used in the determination of the electric axis.

1. An electric force perpendicular to a lead axis will record a small or biphasic complex in that ECG lead.
2. An electric force parallel to a given lead will record its largest deflection in that lead.
3. An electric force going toward a positive electrode will record an upright or positive deflection.

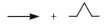

4. An electric force going away from a positive electrode will record a downward or negative deflection.

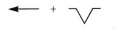

Although there are many methods to determine axes, method A, which follows, is one of the easiest.

**Method A.** Use the frontal plane leads of an ECG (I, II, III, aVR, aVL, aVF) and the hexaxial reference circle to determine the direction of the axes in leads I and aVF. This indicates the quarter of the hexaxial circle in which the axis falls.

1. Find the *main* direction of the QRS in lead I (the algebraic sum of the positive and negative QRS deflections).
   a. If positive, or upright, ⋀ the axis is going toward the positive pole of lead I. Therefore it cannot be in the shaded area of the circle.

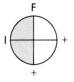

   b. If negative, or downward, ⋁ the axis is going away from the positive pole of lead I. Therefore it cannot be in the shaded area of the circle.

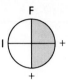

2. Find the *main* direction of the QRS in aVF.
   a. If positive, or upright,  the axis is going toward the positive pole of aVF, or toward the bottom of the hexaxial reference circle. Therefore it cannot be in the shaded area of the circle.

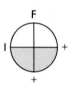

   b. If negative, or downward,  the axis is going toward the negative pole of aVF, or toward the top of the hexaxial reference circle. Therefore it cannot be in the shaded half of the circle.

3. The above two determinations locate the average electric forces, axis, in one quarter of the circle and eliminate three fourths of the circle as a possible location.
   Example:

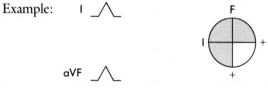

4. Having located the quadrant, the one fourth of the circle in which the average electric force is located, determine what other leads are in that quadrant.
   Example:

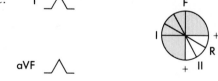

Other leads in the quadrant are II and aVR.

5. Look at the leads in the identified quadrant, that is I, aVF, II, and aVR, and determine in which lead the largest deflection is found. The electric axis is parallel to the lead with the largest deflection. Draw an arrow from the center of the circle along this axis. The tip of the arrow should point toward the outside of the circle.

6. As a final check, the lead axis that is perpendicular to the arrow should contain the smallest deflection.

Use method A to determine the axis of the QRS in the ECG in Fig. 4-18, *A*. To make method A even more precise, note that the lead in which the smallest deflection was found, aVL, is not an algebraic zero but a negative 3. This implies that the true QRS axis is more toward the negative pole of aVL, or about +75, rather than +60 as originally calculated (see Fig. 4-18, *C*).

**Method B.** Another way to determine axes is method B (see Fig. 4-18, *D*).
   1. Calculate the algebraic sum of the QRS in two leads (leads I and III are convenient.)
   2. Plot these values on the hexaxial reference system. Perpendicular lines dropped from the plotted points of leads I and III will produce a crossing point between the two lines.
   3. The line formed by connecting the center point of the circle and the plotted crossing point is the QRS axis in the frontal plane.

### Clinical Significance of Axis

The determination of axis provides one additional piece of ECG information. Taken alone the information may not be significant but combined with the total clinical picture, the axis may clarify a diagnosis. Although there is no universal agreement regarding what are normal and abnormal axes, the following criteria have been used (Fig. 4-19):
   A. General—convenient and realistic boundaries.
   B. Marked left axis between −30 and −90.
   C. Extreme left axis or extreme right axis between ±180 and −90. The ECG axis should be interpreted in conjunction with the patient's clinical background.

The ECG axis may help to determine the presence of normal sinus rhythm when the mean axis of the P wave is within the normal limits of 0 to +90. A wide QRS-T angle almost always means cardiac disease. However, it should be noted that there are a number of causes of axis deviation, some of which are normal variations (see the box on p. 87).

### Electric Heart Positions and Electric Axis

There is a close relationship between electric axis and electric heart positions. The electric position customarily divided into five positions, with their corresponding axes are: horizontal (−30), semihorizontal (0), intermediate (+30), semivertical (+60), and vertical (+90). Because electric positions give little additional clinical information, they are usually not mentioned on a routine ECG interpretation.

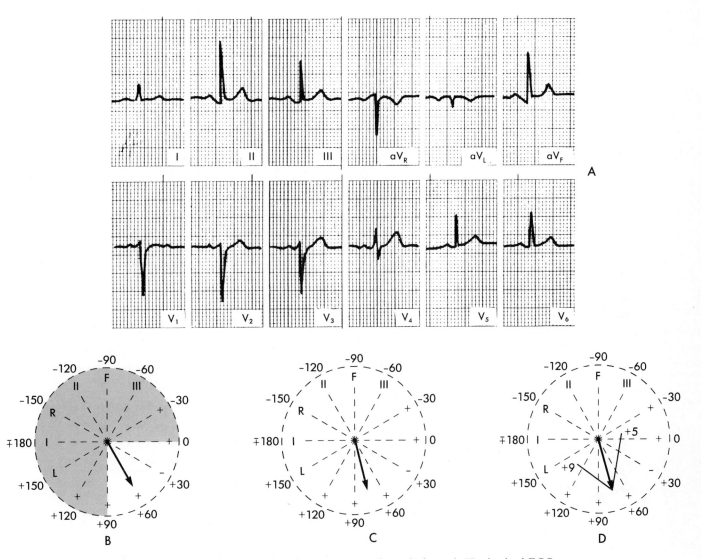

**Fig. 4-18** **Determination of mean QRS axis in frontal plane. A,** Twelve-lead ECG.
**B,** Method A for axis determination. The QRS in lead I is mainly upright, therefore, the
axis is toward the positive pole of lead I. The QRS in lead aVF is mainly upright, therefore,
the axis is toward the positive pole of aVF. The quadrant in which the axis falls is between
0 and +90, or the unshaded area of circle **B.** Leads II and aVR are also found in this
quadrant. The largest deflection is found in lead II; the smallest deflection is found in aVL.
The mean QRS axis is about +60 degrees. **C,** Method A—more precisely used. Because
aVL is negative 3 and not algebraic zero, the true mean QRS axis would be toward the
negative pole of aVL or about +75 degrees. **D,** Method B for axis determination. The algebraic sum of lead I is +5; the algebraic sum of lead III is +9. Plot these two values on the
hexaxial circle. Perpendicular lines dropped from these plotted points produce a crossing
point. The line formed by connecting the center point of the circle and the crossing point is
the mean QRS axis in the frontal plane or +75-degrees.

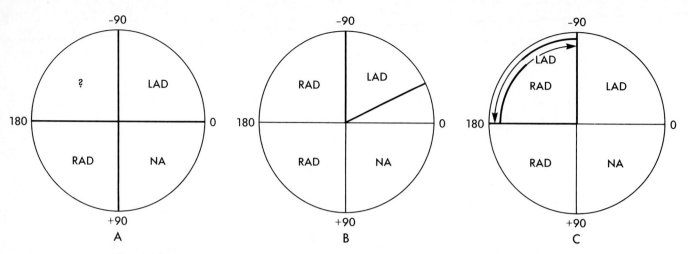

**Fig. 4-19** Hexaxial reference circles indicating values for axis deviation. **A,** Convenient and realistic boundaries: 0 to +90, normal axis (NA); 0 to −90, left axis deviation (LAD); +90 to +180, right axis deviation (RAD); +180 to −90, questionable axis. (Axis of ventricular ectopy may fall in this quadrant.) **B,** Marked left axis deviation between −30 and −90; right axis +90 to −90. **C,** Extreme left axis deviation or extreme right axis deviation, ±180 to −90.

Other terms that may be used are "clockwise rotation" and "counterclockwise rotation." "Clockwise rotation" occurs when the transitional zone is shifted toward the left precordial leads (V$_{5-6}$); it means that there is a posterior axis deviation. "Counterclockwise" rotation occurs when the transitional zone is shifted toward the right (V$_{1-2}$); it

means anterior axis deviation. Anterior and posterior axis deviation are not routinely calculated because they are derived by determining electric axis from the horizontal plane in the precordial leads. Horizontal plane axes are not determined for routine ECG interpretation.

### Determination of the Horizontal Plane Projection of the Mean QRS Vector

1. Identify the precordial lead with the transitional QRS deflection in Fig. 4-20, *A.*
2. Lead V$_4$ is transitional.
3. The QRS vector is perpendicular to the transitional lead (V$_4$).
4. The vector should be directed toward the positive sides of the leads with positive deflections, and on the negative sides of the leads with negative deflections, as shown in Fig. 4-20, *C.*
5. When the horizontal plane direction of the mean QRS is noted, an arrowhead may be placed on the mean QRS frontal plane vector to indicate the vector's anterior or posterior direction, as shown in Fig. 4-20, *B.*

### LEFT VENTRICULAR ENLARGEMENT

It is not usually possible in the ECG to differentiate ventricular dilatation and hypertrophy. The term *hypertrophy* is commonly used; however, this presentation will use *enlargement,* since it includes both dilatation and hypertrophy.

Hypertension, aortic valvular disease, mitral insufficiency, coronary artery disease, and congenital heart disease (for example, patent ductus arteriosus and coarctation of

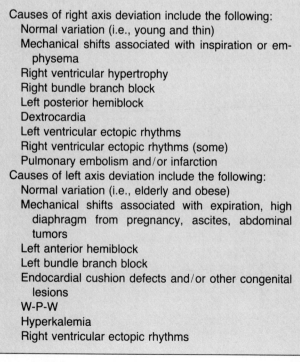

**CAUSES OF AXIS DEVIATION**

Causes of right axis deviation include the following:
  Normal variation (i.e., young and thin)
  Mechanical shifts associated with inspiration or emphysema
  Right ventricular hypertrophy
  Right bundle branch block
  Left posterior hemiblock
  Dextrocardia
  Left ventricular ectopic rhythms
  Right ventricular ectopic rhythms (some)
  Pulmonary embolism and/or infarction
Causes of left axis deviation include the following:
  Normal variation (i.e., elderly and obese)
  Mechanical shifts associated with expiration, high diaphragm from pregnancy, ascites, abdominal tumors
  Left anterior hemiblock
  Left bundle branch block
  Endocardial cushion defects and/or other congenital lesions
  W-P-W
  Hyperkalemia
  Right ventricular ectopic rhythms

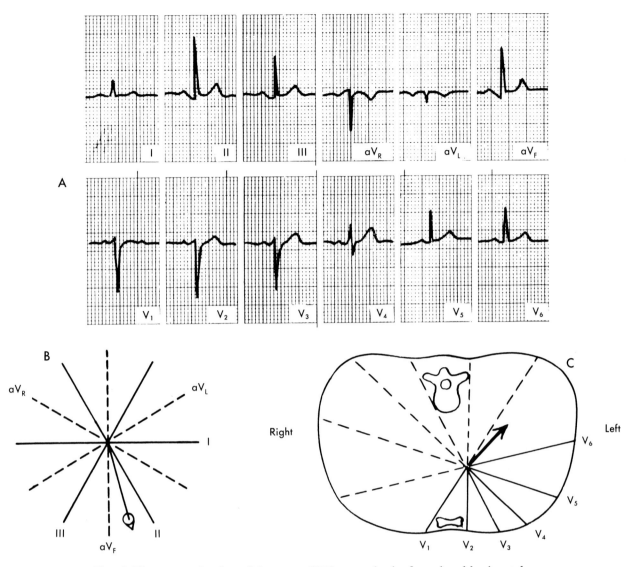

**Fig. 4-20** Determination of the mean QRS vector in the frontal and horizontal planes. **A,** Twelve-lead ECG. **B,** The mean QRS vector in the frontal plane is located at +70 degrees. The arrowhead indicates that the mean QRS vector points posteriorly in the horizontal plane. **C,** The horizontal plane projection of the mean QRS is drawn in a posterior direction on the precordial reference figure. This calculation gives information for the direction of the arrowhead in the frontal plane (**B**).

the aorta) commonly produce left ventricular enlargement. Under these circumstances the wall of the left ventricle is thicker or more dilated than normal. Furthermore, this increase in muscle mass results in increased voltage of those QRS deflections that represent left ventricular potentials. Accordingly, the QRS interval may increase in duration to the upper limits of normal; the intrinsicoid deflection may be somewhat delayed over the left ventricle; and the voltage of the QRS complex will increase—producing deeper S waves over the right ventricle (leads $V_1$ and $V_2$) and taller R waves over the left ventricle (leads $V_5$, $V_6$, I, $aV_L$).

Leads oriented to the left ventricle may also demonstrate a *strain* pattern, that is, depressed ST segments and inverted T waves. "Strain" is a useful, noncommital term and its mechanism is not understood. It is known, however, to develop in patients who have long-standing left ventricular enlargement, and the pattern intensifies when dilatation and failure set in. Myocardial ischemia and slowing of intraventricular conduction are some of the important factors that probably contribute to the pattern.

In general, the voltage criteria proposed for the diagnosis of left ventricular enlargement are unreliable. However, the best approach so far is the Estes scoring system.

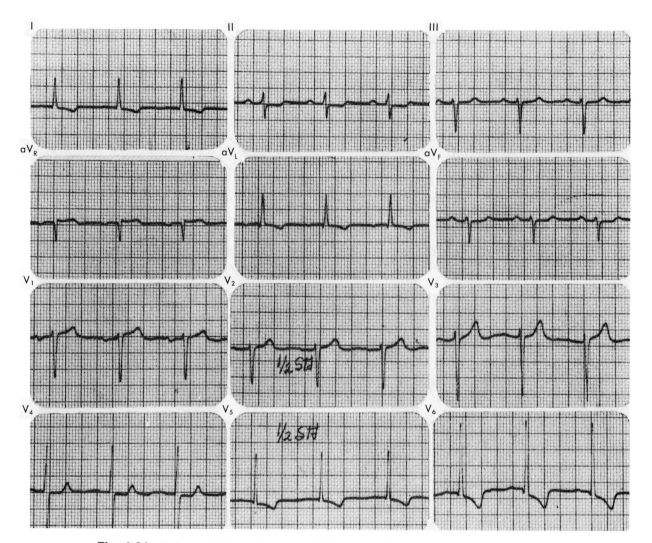

**Fig. 4-21** **Left ventricular enlargement.** This tracing illustrates left ventricular hypertrophy using the Estes criteria: S wave in $V_2$ and R wave in $V_5$ and $V_6$ (note half standard in $V_2$ and $V_5$) exceed 30 mm (3 points); ST segment depression in the absence of digitalis (3 points); terminal negativity of P wave in $V_1$ (1 point). A score of 5 or more points is interpreted as indicating left ventricular hypertrophy. The "score" for this ECG is 7 points.

which is as follows (compare with Fig. 4-21):

1. R wave or S wave in limb lead = 20 mm or more; or S wave in $V_1$, $V_2$, or $V_3$ = 30 mm or more; or R wave in $V_4$, $V_5$, or $V_6$ = 30 mm or more
2. Any ST segment shift opposite to mean QRS vector (without digitalis). Typical "strain" segments T wave (with digitalis).
3. Left axis deviation: − 30 degrees or more
4. QRS interval: 0.09 second or more
   Intrinsicoid deflection in $V_{5-6}$: 0.05 second or more
5. Left atrial enlargement

*Definite left ventricular enlargement* is present with a *point score of 5 or more.* *Probable left ventricular enlargement* is present if the *point score is 4.*

It should be noted that left ventricular enlargement may be present without concomitant left axis deviation. Left axis deviation supports the diagnosis of left ventricular enlargement only when the voltage criteria are fulfilled. The voltage criteria just listed, however, include a small percentage of both false positive and false negative diagnoses. Therefore, in making an electrocardiographic diagnosis of left ventricular enlargement, it is wise to evaluate such factors as body build, the thickness of the chest wall, and the presence of complicating disease. Echocardiography has eliminated many uncertainties about the presence of ventricular enlargement.

## LEFT ATRIAL ENLARGEMENT

Left atrial abnormality occurs frequently in left ventricular enlargement, but this is not always the case. For example,

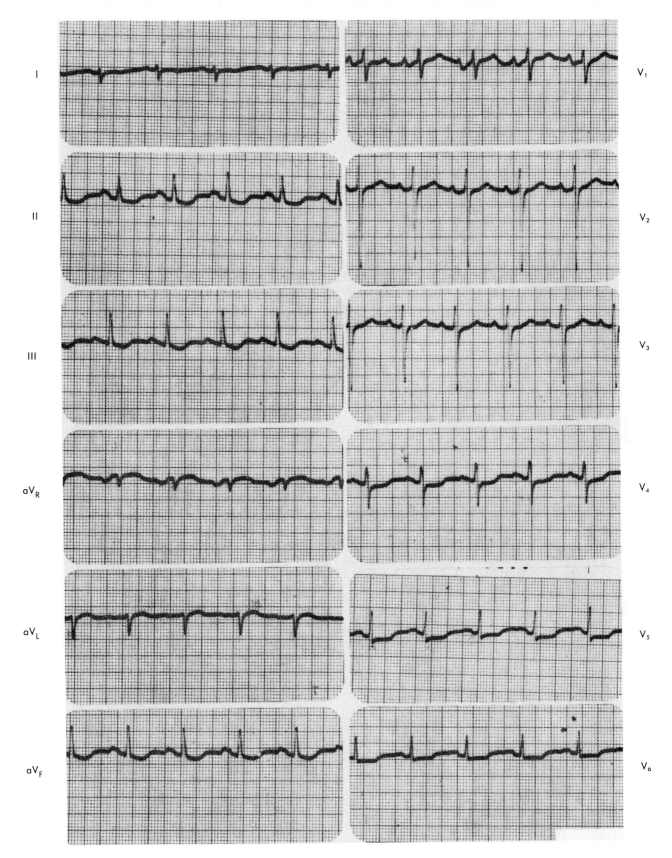

**Fig. 4-22  Left atrial enlargement.** In this example, left atrial enlargement may be diagnosed by the P terminal force abnormality seen in $V_1$. The negative portion of the diphasic P wave is approximately 0.04 second in duration and 1 mm in amplitude. The M-shaped broad contour seen prominently in leads I, II, III, and $aV_F$ and the lateral precordial leads are also found in left atrial enlargement. In addition, right axis deviation of approximately +110 degrees exists in this patient with mitral stenosis.

left atrial enlargement caused by mitral stenosis is not associated with left ventricular enlargement unless there is mitral insufficiency or concomitant aortic valvular disease.

The following criteria are used in the ECG diagnosis of left atrial enlargement (Fig. 4-22):

1. The duration of the P wave is often widened to 0.12 second or more. (Normal P wave duration is 0.11 second.)
2. The contour of the P wave is *notched* and slurred in leads I and II *(P mitrale)*. (Notching per se is not abnormal unless the P wave shows increased voltage or duration or both, or the summits are more than 0.03 second apart.)
3. The right precordial leads ($V_1$, $V_2$) reflect diphasic P waves with a wide, deep, negative terminal component. The duration (in seconds) and amplitude (in millimeters) of the terminal component are measured and the algebraic product determined. A more negative value than $-0.03$ second is considered abnormal.
4. The mean electric axis of the P wave may be shifted left, to between $+45$ and $-30$ degrees.

## RIGHT VENTRICULAR ENLARGEMENT

Right ventricular enlargement is commonly seen with mitral stenosis, some forms of congenital heart disease, and chronic diffuse pulmonary disease such as pulmonary hypertension, emphysema, and bronchiectasis. For right ventricular enlargement in the adult to become evident electrocardiographically, however, the right ventricle must enlarge considerably, since the normal adult ECG reflects left ventricular predominance. This accounts for the relative frequency of a normal ECG in the presence of right ventricular enlargement.

Most of the criteria for diagnosing right ventricular enlargement focus on the QRS pattern in the right precordial leads. As the right ventricle enlarges, the height of the right precordial R waves increases, with a concomitant decrease in the depth of the S wave. When right ventricular enlargement becomes fully developed, the normal precordial pattern is completely reversed so that tall R waves (QR or RS) are recorded in $V_1$ with deep S waves (RS) in $V_6$.

Prolongation of the QRS interval does not develop unless an intraventricular conduction defect develops with the enlarged right ventricle. The time of onset of the intrinsicoid deflection, however, may be delayed in the right precordial leads because the vectors representing activation of the right ventricle usually occur later in the QRS interval than they do normally and are of increased magnitude.

Right axis deviation is the most common sign of right ventricular enlargement. The diagnosis of right ventricular enlargement, however, should not be made on this finding alone unless other causes for right axis deviation have been ruled out. Furthermore, right ventricular enlargement may occur without abnormal right axis deviation.

A right ventricular strain pattern is manifested in ST and T wave alterations, with T wave changes similar to those seen in left ventricular enlargement. The ST segment is depressed and the T wave is inverted in the right-sided precordial leads and often in leads II, III, and a $V_F$, as well. This is a nonspecific abnormality.

Right bundle branch block is seen in right ventricular enlargement, especially of the volume-overload variety. In the younger person, right ventricular enlargement is commonly associated with right bundle branch block, either complete or incomplete. In the older age group (40 years and up) coronary artery disease is the most common cause. The surface ECG is less useful than the vectorcardiogram in the assessment of the degree of right ventricular enlargement in cases of incomplete or complete right bundle branch block. Further elaboration on the vectorcardiogram is beyond the scope of this presentation; therefore the reader is encouraged to refer to other textbooks on this subject. See Chapter 5 for a discussion of right bundle branch block.

A summary of the features of right ventricular enlargement is given here; these should be compared with the example in Fig. 4-23.

1. Reversal of precordial lead pattern with tall R waves over the right precordium ($V_1$, $V_2$), and deep S waves over the left precordium ($V_5$, $V_6$); the R to S ratio in $V_1$ becomes greater than 1.0
2. Duration of QRS interval within normal limits (if no right bundle branch block)
3. Late intrinsicoid deflection in $V_1$, $V_2$
4. Right axis deviation
5. Typical strain ST segment T wave patterns in $V_1$, $V_2$, and in leads II, III, and a$V_F$

## RIGHT ATRIAL ENLARGEMENT

In the presence of right ventricular enlargement, it is not unusual to find an enlarged right atrium. Moreover, right atrial enlargement is often an indirect sign of right ventricular enlargement.

The following criteria are used in the ECG diagnosis of right atrial enlargement (Fig. 4-24):

1. The duration of the P wave is 0.11 second or less.
2. The contour of the P wave is tall, *peaked (P pulmonale)*, and measures 2.5 mm or more in amplitude in leads II, III, and a$V_F$.
3. The right precordial leads reflect diphasic P waves, often with increased voltage of the initial component.
4. The mean electric axis of the P wave may be shifted right to $+70$ degrees or more.

It should be noted that abnormal P waves may occur in healthy patients. For example, acceleration of the heart rate alone may cause peaking and increased voltage of the P wave. Conversely, normal P waves may be identified in the presence of atrial disease.

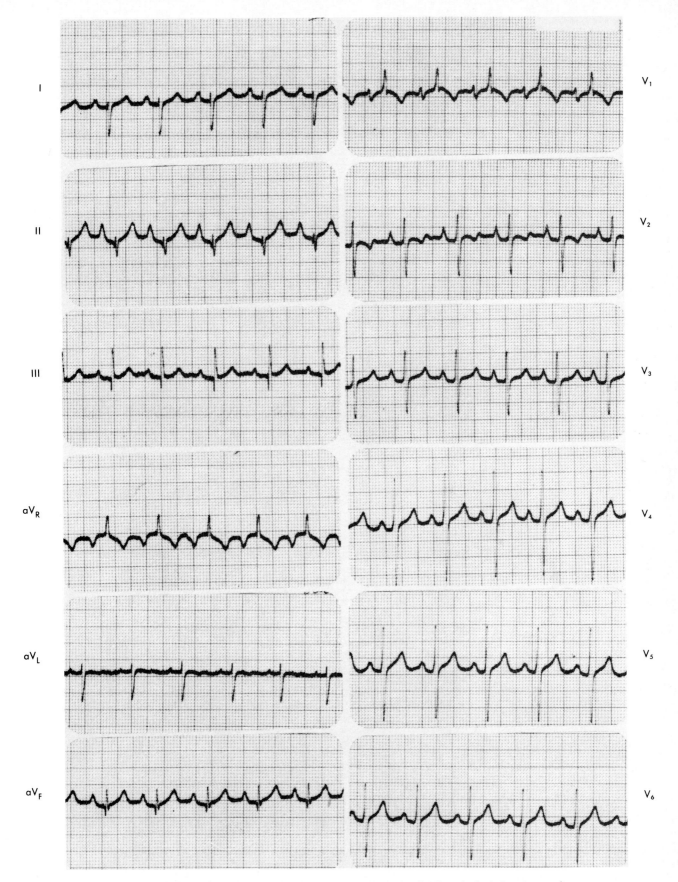

**Fig. 4-23  Right ventricular enlargement.** The presence of right axis deviation (approximately +160 degrees), an R wave in $V_1$ that exceeds 5 mm, and an R:S ratio in $V_1$ that exceeds 1.0 are all diagnostic of right ventricular hypertrophy. In addition, the totally upright R wave in $V_1$ suggests that the pressure in the right ventricle equals or almost equals the pressure in the left ventricle. The P waves suggest right atrial enlargement.

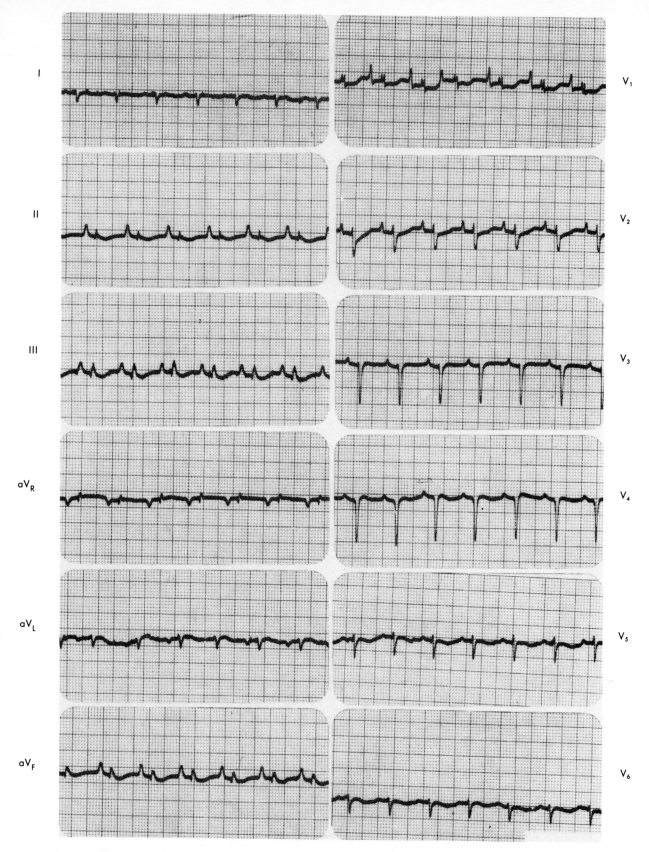

**Fig. 4-24** **Right atrial enlargement.** The large peaked P waves in leads II, III, aV_F, and V_1, with an amplitude that exceeds 2.5 mm in leads II and III, characterize right atrial enlargement. The mean P axis is more positive than +60 degrees, another criterion for right atrial enlargement. The patient has pulmonic stenosis.

## MYOCARDIAL INFARCTION

To diagnose myocardial infarction, the ECG should be used to confirm the clinical impression. Because the ECG may not be diagnostic in many instances, if a patient is suspected clinically of having experienced a myocardial infarction, he should be treated accordingly, regardless of what the ECG shows.

Only Q wave changes (necrosis) are diagnostic of infarction, but changes in the ST segments (injury) and T waves (ischemia) may be suspicious and provide presumptive evidence. These changes are illustrated in Fig. 4-25.

### Q Wave

The Q wave is one of the most important, and sometimes most difficult to interpret assessors of myocardial infarction on the ECG. For example, with normal intraventricular conditions, small Q waves are present in leads $V_5$, $V_6$, $aV_L$, and I, particularly with a horizontal heart position or left axis deviation. Furthermore, with a vertical heart position or right axis deviation, small Q waves may be present in leads II, III, and $aV_F$. Finally, deep wide Q waves or QS complexes are normally present in $aV_R$ and may be present in lead $V_1$.

Major importance is placed on the development of *new* Q waves in ECG leads where they previously were not present.

Accordingly, the *appearance* of abnormal Q waves must be considered in light of the overall picture, considering that pathologic Q waves have the following features:

1. Q waves are 0.04 second or longer in *duration*.
2. Q waves are usually greater than 4 mm in *depth*.
3. Q waves appear in *leads* that do not normally have deep, wide Q waves, $V_1$ and $aV_R$ normally record Q

waves. Pathologic Q waves are usually present in several leads that are oriented in similar directions (e.g., II, III, and $aV_F$, or I, $aV_L$).

### Vector Abnormalities

In acute myocardial infarction, electric and anatomic death of the myocardium occurs in the region of the infarct; hence the initial forces of depolarization tend to point away from the infarcted area, producing Q waves in the ECG leads facing the involved site. The mean T vector also tends to point away from the site of infarction, presumably because of electric ischemia in the tissues surrounding the infarct. The ST vector represents the effect of injury current. When the injury current is in the epicardial layers of the myocardium, as in myocardial infarction and pericarditis, the ST segment is elevated in leads facing the injury and the ST vector points toward the injured area. When the injury current is located in the subendocardial layers, as in angina pectoris, coronary insufficiency, and subendocardial infarction, the ST segment is depressed in leads facing the injury, and the ST vector points away from the site of injury (see Fig. 4-25). The ST displacement in subendocardial infarction persists longer than that of angina pectoris and coronary insufficiency.

Thus with an acute myocardial infarction the ST vector is opposite in direction to the Q vector and the mean T vector, resulting in ST segment elevation in those leads that have Q waves and inverted T waves. The relationship of these three vectors to one another is diagrammed in Fig. 4-26, *B*.

From animal studies, loss of resting membrane potential in the ischemic cells occurs first and is responsible for T-Q segment depression in the scalar ECG. Reduction in action potential duration and amplitude follows and causes

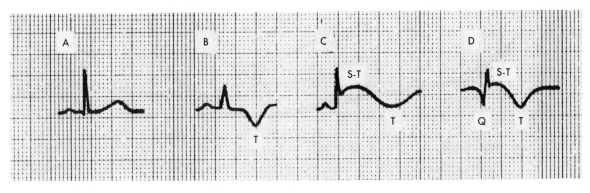

**Fig. 4-25** **ECG wave changes indicative of ischemia, injury, and necrosis of the myocardium. A,** Normal left ventricular wave pattern. **B,** Ischemia indicated by inversion of the T wave. **C,** Ischemia and current of injury indicated by T wave inversion and ST segment elevation. The ST segment may be elevated above or depressed below the baseline, depending on whether or not the tracing is from a lead facing toward or away from the infarcted area and depending on whether epicardial or endocardial injury occurs. Epicardial injury causes ST segment elevation in leads facing the epicardium. **D,** Ischemia, injury, and myocardial necrosis. The Q wave indicates necrosis of the myocardium.

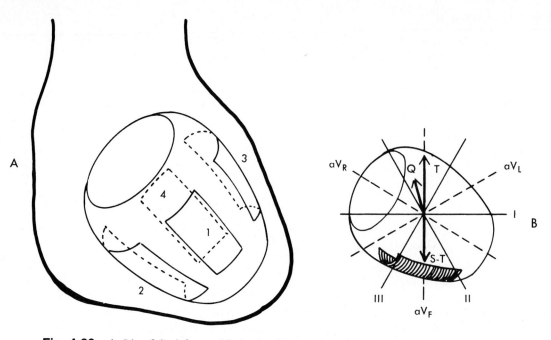

**Fig. 4-26** **A,** Lie of the left ventricle in the chest as viewed frontally. The left ventricle has been divided into four topographic regions where infarctions may occur: (1) anterior, (2) diaphragmatic or inferior, (3) lateral, and (4) posterior (pure). **B,** Vectors of a diaphragmatic myocardial infarction. Hexaxial reference figure is superimposed on the left ventricle as viewed in **B,** The mean vector for the initial 0.04 second of the QRS complex points *away* from the infarcted area and indicates the dead zone. This produces Q waves in the leads "looking at" the infarction. The mean T vector indicates the ischemic zone surrounding the infarct and points *away* from the infarcted area. The ST vector indicates the injury zone and in the event of myocardial infarction, the ST vector points *toward* the injured area. In this example of a diaphragmatic myocardial infarction, leads II, III, and aV$_F$ will exhibit the Q waves, ST segment elevation, and T wave inversion shown in Fig. 4-25, *D.*

ST segment elevation. Delayed repolarization in the ischemic area results in T wave inversion.

## Localization of Infarction

Localization of infarcts may be important for several reasons, including prognosis. Localization is based on the principle that diagnostic ECG signs of myocardial infarction (Fig. 4-25) occur in leads whose positive terminals face the damaged surface of the heart. To facilitate localization, the left ventricle has been divided into four topographic regions where infarctions may occur (Fig. 4-26, *A*). Although these locations represent electric rather than anatomic sites of infarction, anatomic correlations occur with reasonable frequency, particularly for the first myocardial infarction.

An *anterior infarction* produces characteristic changes in leads V$_1$, V$_2$, and V$_3$; a *diaphragmatic* or *inferior infarction* affects leads II, III, and aV$_F$; a *lateral infarction* involves leads I, aV$_L$, V$_5$, and V$_6$. In strictly *posterior infarction,* there are no leads whose positive terminals are directly over the infarct. However, the changes of the electric field produced

by any infarction still apply; hence in purely posterior infarction the initial forces of the QRS complex and the T wave point anteriorly away from the site of the infarct, and the ST segment is directed posteriorly. This is recognized in the ECG as tall broad initial R waves, ST segment depression, and tall upright T waves in leads V$_1$ and V$_2$. In other words, a mirror image of the typical infarction pattern of an anterior myocardial infarction is recorded. Stated another way, infarction of the true posterior surface of the heart must be inferred from reciprocal (opposite) changes occurring in the anterior leads. These locations are summarized in Table 4-1.

It should be noted that although diagnostic signs of myocardial infarction appear in leads facing the infarcted heart surface, *reciprocal changes* occur concomitantly in leads facing the diametrically opposed surface of the heart. These changes include absence of a Q wave, some increase of the R wave, depressed ST segment, and upright tall T wave.

Reciprocal changes, therefore, in an anterior infarction will occur in leads II, III, and aV$_F$. In a diaphragmatic or inferior infarction, reciprocal changes occur in leads I, $aV_L$, and some of the precordial leads. In lateral wall infarction, lead $V_1$ may show reciprocal changes.

Frequently the localization of an infarction is not as strict as just described. If the anterior and lateral walls of the left ventricle are both involved in the process, it is called an *anterolateral infarction*. If the limb leads indicate an inferior infarction and diagnostic changes are also present in leads $V_5$ and $V_6$, then it is called an inferior infarction with lateral extension or an *inferolateral infarction*, and so on.

### Evolution of a Myocardial Infarction

The evolution of a myocardial infarction is a sequential process, and it is important to record the time relationships in the diagnosis. Within the first few hours after infarction, sometimes referred to as the hyperacute state, elevated ST segments and tall (hyperacute) upright T waves appear in those leads facing the infarction. Q waves may appear early or may not develop for several days. Within several days of the infarct the ST segment begins to return to baseline, whereas the T waves develop progressively deeper inversion. After weeks or months the T waves become shallower and may finally return to normal. The Q waves are most likely to remain as a permanent record of the myocardial scar (Fig. 4-27). Persistent ST segment elevation (beyond 6 weeks) suggests the possibility of ventricular aneurysm (Table 4-2). The different locations of myocardial infarction in different stages of clinical evolution are shown in Figs. 4-28 to 4-35.

*Figs. 4-27 to 4-35 follow.*

**TABLE 4-1** Location of myocardial infarction

| Area of Infarction | Leads Showing Wave Changes |
|---|---|
| Anterior | $V_1$, $V_2$, $V_3$ |
| Diaphragmatic or inferior | II, III, $aV_F$ |
| Lateral | I, $aV_L$, $V_5$, $V_6$ |
| Posterior (pure) | $V_1$ and $V_2$: tall broad initial R wave, ST segment depression, and tall upright T wave |

**TABLE 4-2** Time relationships in the evolution and resolution of a myocardial infarction

| ECG Abnormality | Onset | Disappearance |
|---|---|---|
| ST segment elevation | Immediately | 1 to 6 weeks |
| Q waves >0.04 second | Immediately or in several days | Years to never |
| T wave inversion | 6 to 24 hours | Months to years |

| I | II | III | aV_R | aV_L | aV_F | V_1 | V_2 | V_3 | V_4 | V_5 | V_6 |

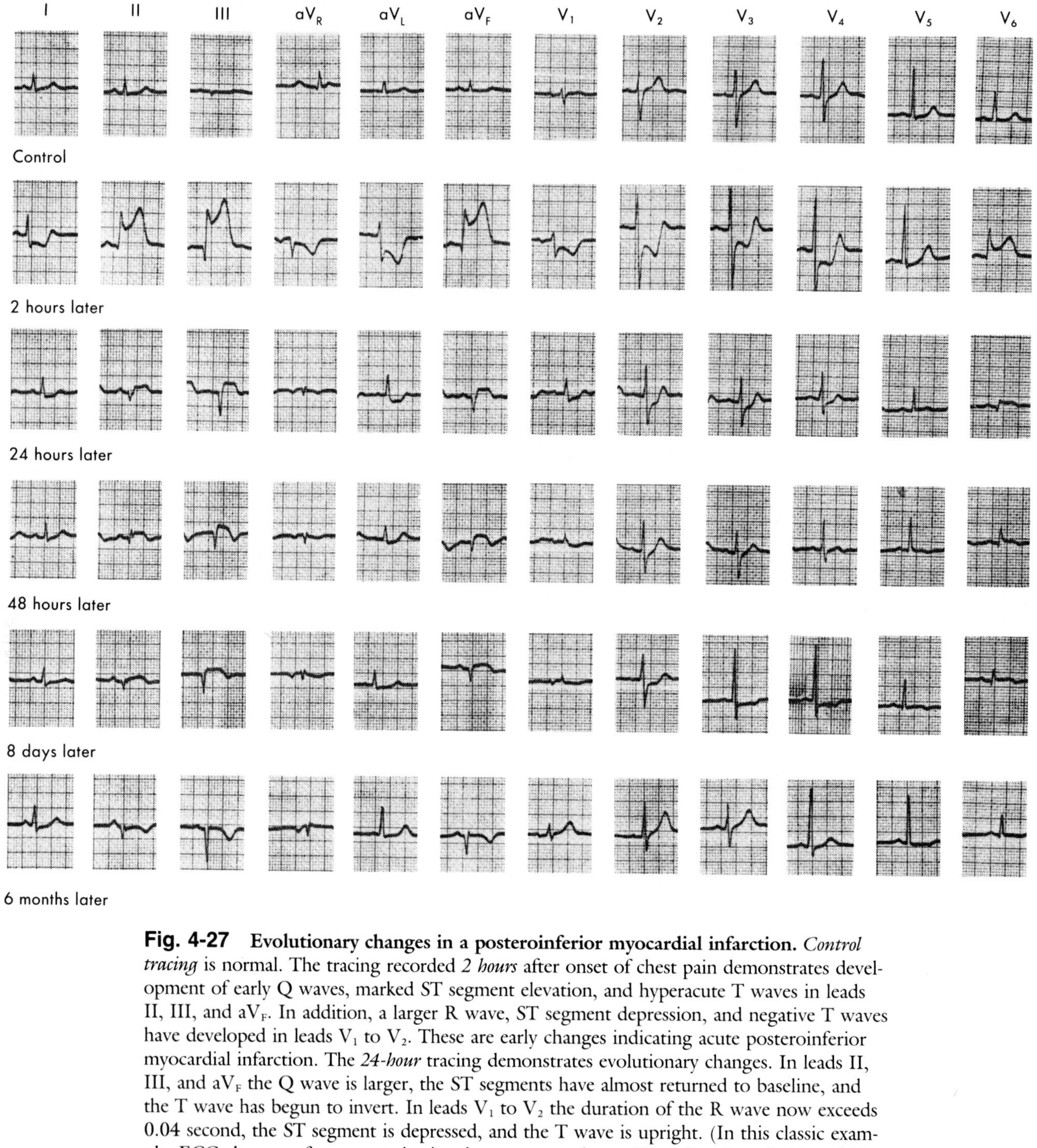

Control

2 hours later

24 hours later

48 hours later

8 days later

6 months later

**Fig. 4-27   Evolutionary changes in a posteroinferior myocardial infarction.** *Control tracing* is normal. The tracing recorded *2 hours* after onset of chest pain demonstrates development of early Q waves, marked ST segment elevation, and hyperacute T waves in leads II, III, and aV_F. In addition, a larger R wave, ST segment depression, and negative T waves have developed in leads V_1 to V_2. These are early changes indicating acute posteroinferior myocardial infarction. The *24-hour* tracing demonstrates evolutionary changes. In leads II, III, and aV_F the Q wave is larger, the ST segments have almost returned to baseline, and the T wave has begun to invert. In leads V_1 to V_2 the duration of the R wave now exceeds 0.04 second, the ST segment is depressed, and the T wave is upright. (In this classic example, ECG changes of true posterior involvement extend past V_2; ordinarily only V_1 and V_2 may be involved.) Only minor further changes occur through the *8-day* tracing. Finally, *6-months later* the ECG illustrates large Q waves, isoelectric ST segments, and inverted T waves in leads II, III, and aV_F, large R waves, isoelectric ST segments, and upright T waves in V_1 and V_2 indicative of an "old" posteroinferior myocardial infarction.

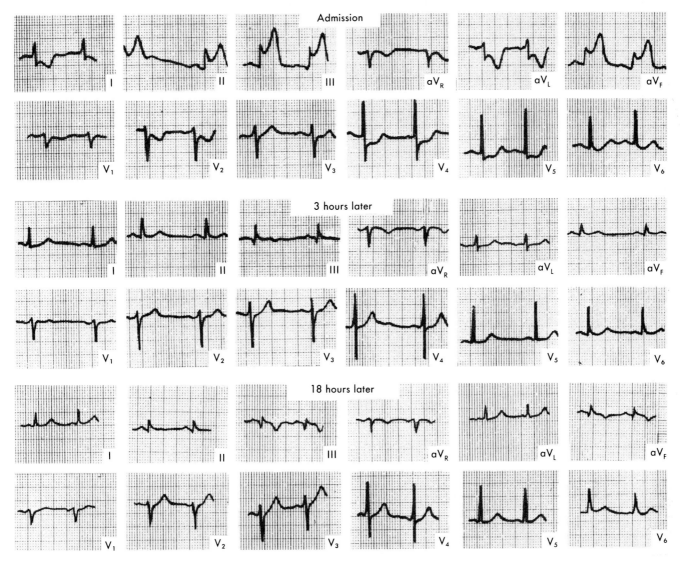

**Fig. 4-28**    These three 12-lead ECGs obtained at different time intervals from a patient who had an unequivocal myocardial infarction demonstrate that at one point during the electrocardiographic evolution of a myocardial infarction, the ECG may appear almost normal. Note the hyperacute T wave changes and unquestionable injury current portrayed in the admission ECG. Hyperacute T wave changes are normally upright; these enlarged T waves can occur very early after infarction, preceding the more characteristic T wave inversion. Three hours later, the ST segment has returned almost completely to the baseline, significant Q waves have not yet appeared, and the T waves remain fairly normal. This ECG is at most "nonspecifically" abnormal. Eighteen hours after admission, classic changes in an acute diaphragmatic myocardial infarction have evolved. This illustration serves to deemphasize the value of a single ECG in diagnosing an acute myocardial infarction. The patient quite possibly would have been sent home if the determination for admission to the CCU had been based solely on a single ECG, that is, the second tracing.

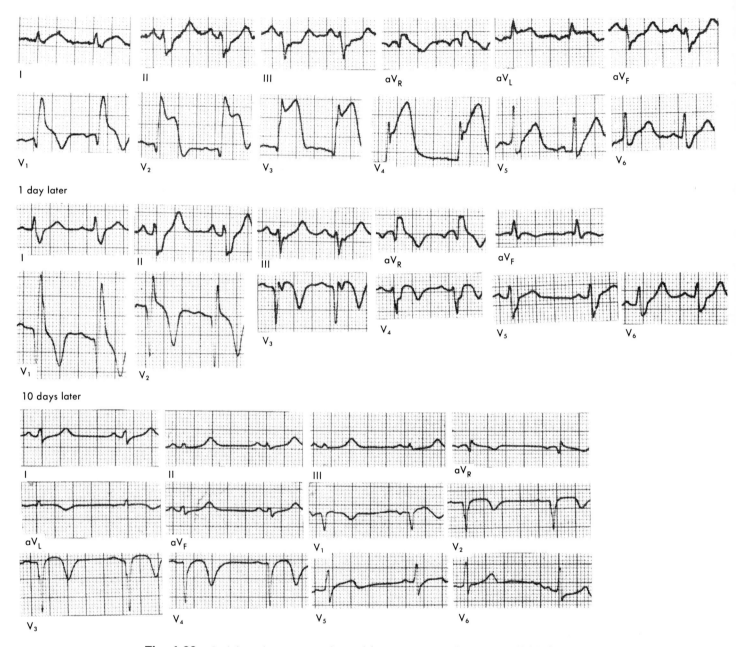

1 day later

10 days later

**Fig. 4-29** **Serial tracings on a patient with an acute anterior myocardial infarction.**
On admission the patient's ECG showed left axis deviation (left anterior hemiblock) and
right bundle branch block, thus supporting the presence of bifascicular block (see Chapter
5). Terminal T wave inversion in $V_1$ to $V_2$ and profound ST segment elevation are present
in $V_1$ to $V_5$. These changes are not masked by the presence of the right bundle branch
block. One day later the ST segments have returned toward the baseline, the Q waves in the
anterior precordial leads have enlarged greatly, and there is now T wave inversion in these
leads. Left anterior hemiblock and right bundle branch block are still present. In the tracing
recorded 10 days later the right bundle branch block and left anterior hemiblock have disappeared, leaving the electrocardiographic changes of an anteroseptal myocardial infarction
with Q waves in $V_1$ to $V_3$ and T wave inversion in $V_1$ to $V_4$.

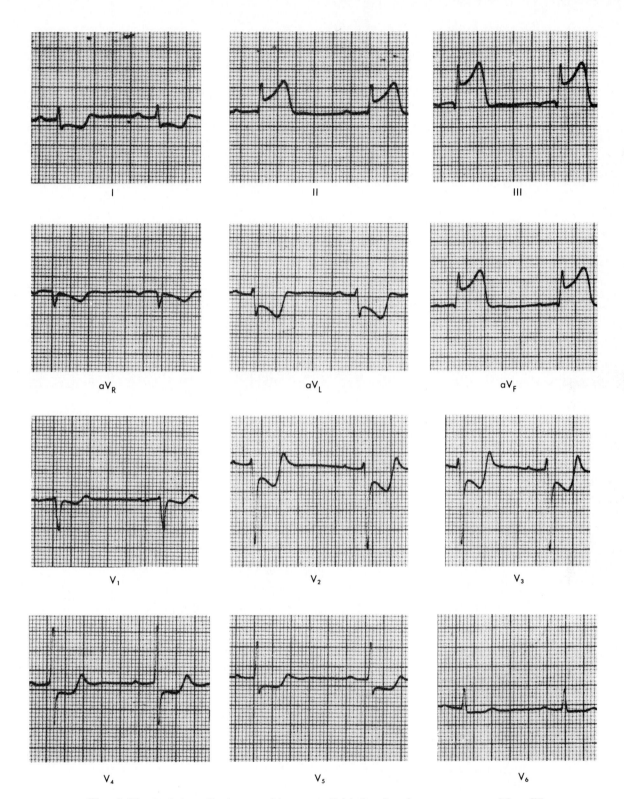

**Fig. 4-30**  **Inferior (diaphragmatic) myocardial infarction, hyperacute stage.** Note ST segment elevation in leads II, III, and aV$_F$ with reciprocal ST depression in the anterior precordial leads. The T waves in leads II, III and aV$_F$ are still upright and pointed and indicate the hyperacute stage of myocardial infarction. Note the development of only very small Q waves in leads II, III, and aV$_F$. Subsequent evolution of this ECG will demonstrate the progressive development of significant (greater than 0.04 second) Q waves and T wave inversion in leads II, III, and aV$_F$; the ST segment will return to an isoelectric position.

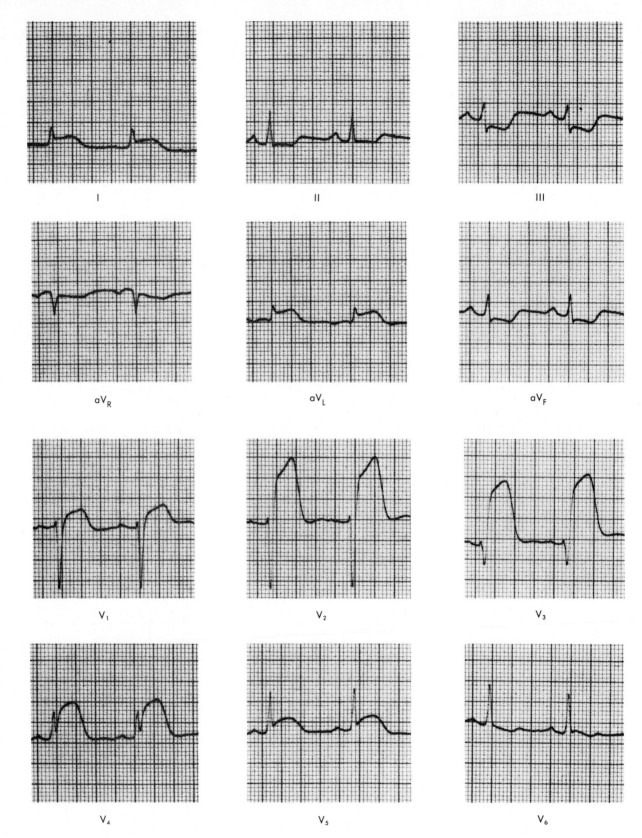

**Fig. 4-31** **Anterolateral myocardial infarction, acute.** ST segment elevation in leads I, aV$_L$, and V$_1$ to V$_5$ indicate an acute anterolateral myocardial infarction. During the evolution of this tracing, one would expect the development of Q waves and T wave inversion in leads I and aV$_L$ and the precordial leads, with the ST segment returning to baseline.

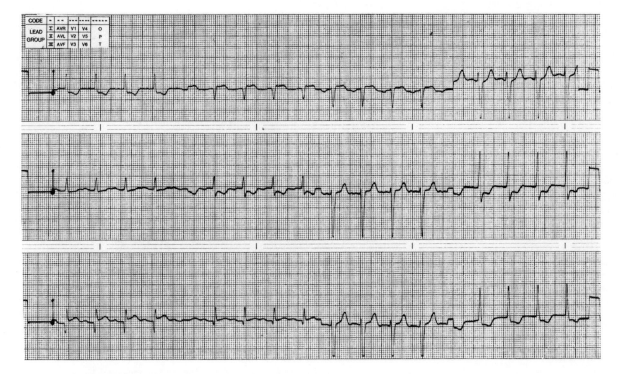

**Fig. 4-32    Sinus tachycardia.** Q waves in III and aV_F, along with ST segment elevation, suggest evolving inferior myocardial infarction.

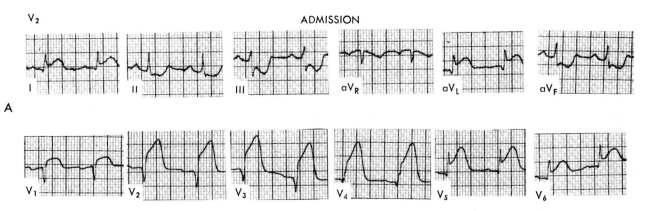

**Fig. 4-33    Anterolateral myocardial infarction, acute.** The 12-lead ECG on admission, **A,** demonstrates ST segment elevation in leads I, aV_L and V_1 to V_6 indicating the anterolateral injury current of an acute anterolateral myocardial infarction.

*Continued.*

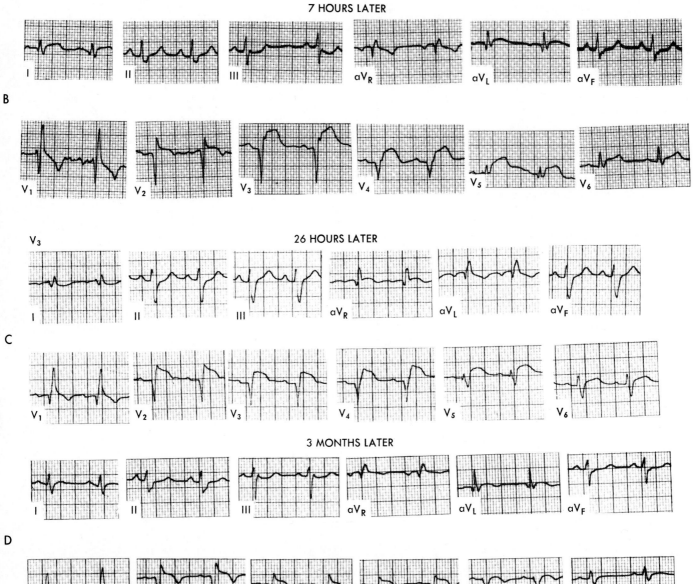

**7 HOURS LATER**

**26 HOURS LATER**

**3 MONTHS LATER**

**Fig. 4-33 cont'd**   **Anterolateral myocardial infarction, acute. B,** Seven hours later. The patient has developed right bundle branch block with abnormal Q waves in leads I, aV$_L$ and V$_2$ to V$_5$. **C,** Twenty-six hours later. In addition to the right bundle branch block, the patient has now developed left anterior hemiblock. **D,** Three months later. The left anterior hemiblock and right bundle branch block are still present. The Q waves in leads I and aV$_L$ are not as prominent as the Q waves in V$_1$ to V$_5$. Persistent ST segment elevation for a duration greater than 6 weeks after the myocardial infarction raises the possibility of a left ventricular aneurysm.

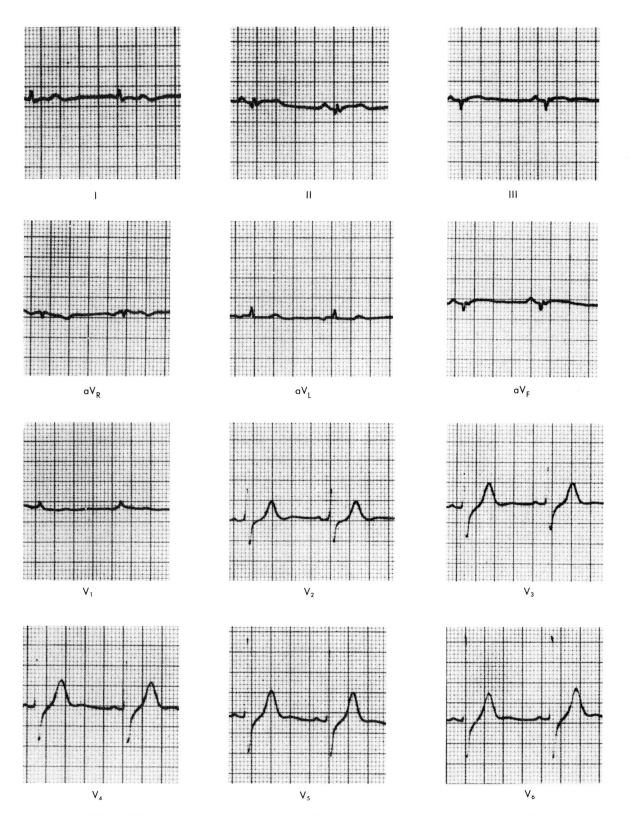

**Fig. 4-34   Posteroinferior myocardial infarction, date indeterminant.** Q waves in II, III, and aV$_F$ are consistent with an old inferior myocardial infarction. The large R wave in V$_1$ signifies true posterior infarction as well. Compare with Fig. 4-27 (at 6 months).

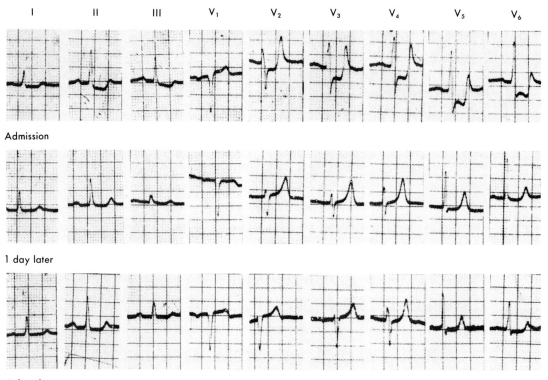

Admission

1 day later

4 days later

**Fig. 4-35** **Subendocardial myocardial infarction.** Note slight ST segment depression in leads I, II, and III with marked ST segment depression in leads $V_2$ to $V_6$ on admission. One day later the ST segments have returned to normal and there is diminution of the height of the R wave in the precordial leads but no other changes. The tracing 4 days later is essentially unchanged. Note failure to develop the classic Q waves of a transmural myocardial infarction. The patient died and at autopsy had an extensive subendocardial myocardial infarction.

## SUGGESTED READINGS

Braunwald E, editor: Heart disease, a textbook of cardiovascular medicine, ed 2, Philadelphia, 1984, WB Saunders Co.

Chung EK: Principles of cardiac arrhythmias, ed 4, Baltimore, 1989, Williams & Wilkins.

Constant J: Essentials of bedside cardiology, Boston, 1989, Little, Brown & Co, Inc.

Hurst JW and others, editors: The heart, ed 6, New York, 1986, McGraw-Hill Book Co.

Ward DE and Camm AJ: Clinical electrophysiology of the heart, London, 1987, Edward Arnold.

Zipes DP: Progress in cardiology, Philadelphia, 1988, Lea & Febiger.

# CHAPTER 5

# Dysrhythmias

Barbara A. Erickson

## NORMAL CARDIAC CYCLE

Before discussing electrocardiographic interpretation of cardiac dysrhythmias, a review of the normal electric events that occur during a cardiac cycle, as well as a discussion of basic electrophysiologic principles is necessary.[1] During normal sinus rhythm the cardiac impulse originates in the sinus node and then travels to right and left atria. Sinus node discharge and conduction from the sinus node to the atria are not recorded from the body surface, and therefore these events are not seen on the ECG. In response to the sinus node impulse, the atria depolarize and generate the P wave; atrial repolarization (Ta wave) is generally obscured by the QRS complex and is therefore not usually seen. Atrial conduction probably proceeds through both atria in a more or less radial fashion (like spreading ripples caused by a rock thrown into still water), eventually reaching the AV node and His bundle. Some data suggest that conduction through the atria travels preferentially through loosely connected bundles of atrial muscle called the anterior, middle, and posterior internodal pathways. A division of the anterior internodal pathway, the Bachman's bundle, connects the left and right atria. However, the functional importance of these pathways in providing specialized tracts for conduction is unsettled. Most experts agree that these pathways are *not* analogous to the specialized conducting pathways in the ventricles, e.g., the bundle branches and Purkinje fibers, which are discrete histologically identifiable tracts of tissue. However, preferential internodal conduction (more rapid conduction velocity between nodes in some parts of atrium compared with other parts) probably does exist and may be caused by fiber orientation, size, geometry or other factors, rather than by specialized tracts located between the SA and AV nodes.

The speed at which the impulse travels (conduction velocity) becomes reduced as the impulse traverses the AV node but once again accelerates through the His bundle, bundle branches, and Purkinje fibers. The Purkinje fibers distribute the impulse rapidly and uniformly over the ventricular endocardium, finally depolarizing the ventricular myocardium (Fig. 5-1). It is important to remember that the surface ECG records only ventricular muscle depolarization (QRS) and repolarization (T wave), atrial depolarization (P wave), and sometimes repolarization (Ta wave). Activity from the SA and AV nodes, His bundle, bundle branches, and Purkinje fibers is not recorded in the ECG. Special intracardiac electrodes can be employed to record activity from some of these structures and are discussed briefly later in this chapter.

It has been postulated that the bundle branches are really composed of three divisions, called fascicles,[2] that are formed by the right bundle branch and two divisions of the left bundle branch, the anterosuperior division, and the posteroinferior division. The term *hemiblock* has been used to describe block in one of these fascicles.[2] A more accurate term is *fascicular block*. Although a number of careful anatomic and pathologic studies of human hearts have failed to substantiate the anatomic separation of the left bundle branch into two distinct and specific divisions, the fascicular block concept has been useful to explain observed electrocardiographic and clinical entities (see discussion of bundle branch block) (Fig. 5-2).

The electric pattern of a typical cardiac cycle is displayed in Fig. 5-3 and is discussed in Table 5-1 (see also Chapter 4).

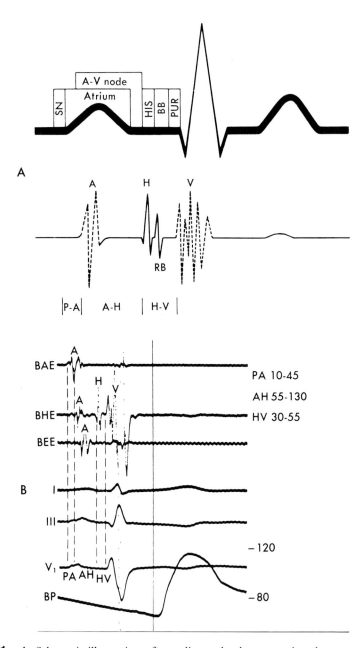

**Fig. 5-1** **A,** Schematic illustration of a cardiac cycle, demonstrating the normal ECG *(top)* and an intracardiac recording *(bottom)*. The diagram illustrates the approximate time of activation of various structures in the specialized conduction system. It is important to emphasize that conduction has already reached the Purkinje fibers just before the onset of the QRS complex. *SN,* sinus node; *HIS,* bundle of His; *BB,* bundle branches; *PUR,* Purkinje fibers; *A,* low right atrial deflection; *H,* His bundle deflection; *RB,* right bundle branch deflection; *V,* ventricular septal muscle depolarization; *P-A,* interval from the onset of the P wave in the surface tracing to the onset of the low right atrial deflection, serving as a measure of intraatrial conduction; *A-H,* measurement of conduction across the AV node; *H-V* measurement of conduction through the His bundle distal to the recording electrode, the bundle branches, and the Purkinje system up to the point of ventricular activation. (Top panel modified from Hoffman BF and Singer DH: Prog Cardiovasc Dis 7:226, 1964.) **B,** Electrophysiologic and blood pressure recordings during one cardiac cycle. *BAE,* Bipolar high right atrial electrogram; *BHE,* bipolar His electrogram; *BEE,* bipolar esphageal electrogram. Normal intervals in milliseconds to the right.

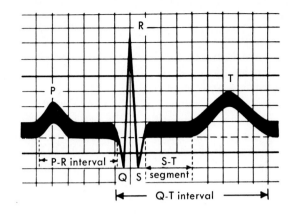

**Fig. 5-2**    Electric pattern of cardiac cycle (refer to Table 5-1).

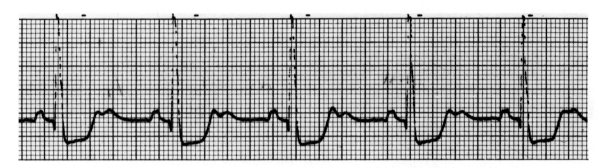

**Fig. 5-3    Calculation of atrial and ventricular rates.** Heart rate is almost 60 beats/min, determined by dividing time interval between consecutive P waves and/or consecutive R waves by 1 second; by dividing 5 large squares into 300 or 25 small squares into 1500; or by 5 multiplying the number of complexes occurring in a 6-second strip by 10. See Table 5-2.

---

**TABLE 5-1**    Definition and significance of ECG intervals*

| Description | Duration | Significance of Disturbance |
|---|---|---|
| PR interval: from beginning of P wave to beginning of QRS complex; represents time taken for impulse to spread through the atria, AV node and His bundle, the bundle branches and Purkinje fibers, to a point immediately preceding ventricular activation | 0.12 to 0.20 second | Disturbance in conduction usually in AV node, His bundle, or bundle branches but can be in atria as well |
| QRS interval: from beginning to end of QRS complex; represents time taken for depolarization of both ventricles | 0.06 to 0.10 second | Disturbance in conduction in bundle branches and/or in ventricles |
| QT interval: from beginning of QRS to end of T wave; represents time taken for entire electric depolarization and repolarization of the ventricles | 0.36 to 0.44 second | Disturbances usually affecting repolarization more than depolarization such as drug effects, electrolyte disturbances, and rate changes |

*Heart rate influences the duration of these intervals, especially that of the PR and QT intervals.

## DETERMINATION OF HEART RATE

Several methods are available for determining the heart rate from an ECG recording. When the atrial and ventricular rates are different, as in third-degree AV Block, both atrial and ventricular rates should be determined separately.

Five possible methods for determining heart rate follow:

1. **6-Second Interval Method** (Figs. 5-3 and 5-4): This method is the easiest and most practical. It is accurate for both regular and irregular rhythms.
   a. Count the cardiac waves (i.e., "P" and/or "QRS") in a 6-second interval and multiply by 10.
   b. The ECG paper is marked at the top into 3-second intervals. If these marks are absent, there are 15 large ECG squares in a 3-second interval.

2. **1500 Small Squares Method** (see Fig. 5-3): At the standard ECG paper speed of 25 mm/sec, 1500 mm (or 1500 small squares) will run under the ECG stylus in 1 minute. This method is accurate only with regular rhythms. For irregular rhythms, calculate the lowest and highest rates.
   a. Count the number of small squares between the cardiac waves (i.e., "P" and/or "QRS").
   b. Divide 1500 by the number of small squares between the cardiac waves.
   c. The result gives the rate of occurrence of the wave per minute.

3. **300 Large Squares Method** (see Fig. 5-3): At the standard ECG paper speed of 25 mm/sec, 300 mm (or 300 large squares) will run under the ECG stylus in 1 minute. This method is accurate only with regular rhythms. For irregular rhythms, calculate the lowest and highest rates.
   a. Count the number of large squares between the cardiac waves (i.e., "P" and/or "QRS").
   b. Divide 300 by the number of large squares between the cardiac waves.
   c. The result gives the rate of occurrence of the wave per minute.

4. **Quick Glance Method** (see Fig. 5-5): This method illustrates a simple way of approximating heart rate. Although not exact, it permits a quick method of determining rate if the rate is over 100 but less than 150.
   a. Determine the number of large squares between waves. (For convenience, select a wave that coincides with a heavy line.)
      1. If 1 large square, the rate = 300. (300 ÷ 1)
      2. If 2 large squares, the rate = 150. (300 ÷ 2)
      3. If 3 large squares, the rate = 100. (300 ÷ 3)
      4. If 4 large squares, the rate = 75. (300 ÷ 4)
      5. If 5 large squares, the rate = 60. (300 ÷ 5)
      6. If 6 large squares, the rate = 50. (300 ÷ 6)
      7. If 7 large squares, the rate = 42. (300 ÷ 7)
      8. If 8 large squares, the rate = 38. (300 ÷ 8)
   b. Memorize the resulting mnemonic: "300, 150, 100, 75, 60, 50, 42, 38."
   c. Using mnemonic, select wave and go to next occurrence of wave. ("guesstimate" rate.) (Fig. 5-5)

5. **Precalculated Table Method** (Table 5-2): This method is most accurate for regular rhythms. For irregular rhythms calculate the highest and lowest rates.
   a. Count the number of small squares between cardiac waves.
   b. Find this number on the table.
   c. Read rate from column to the right of this number in the table.

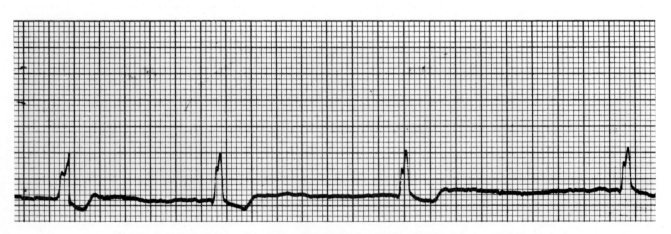

**Fig. 5-4** **Calculation of the rate of an irregular rhythm.** Heart rate is 40 beats/min, determined by multiplying 4 (the number of R waves occuring in 6 second strip) by 10.

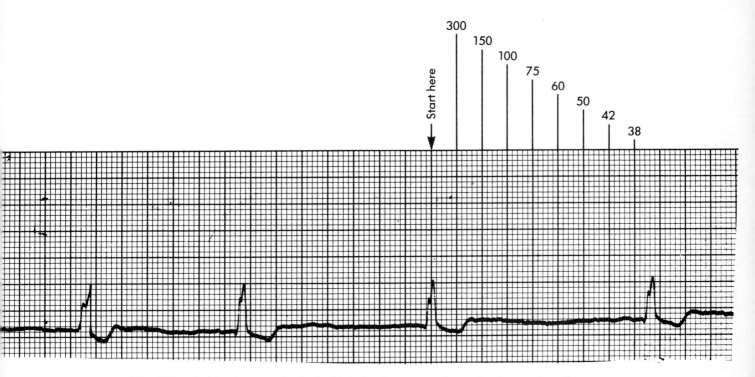

**Fig. 5-5**  **Quick glance method of calculating heart rate.** Determine the number of large squares between waves. (For convenience, select a wave that coincides with a heavy line.) Count the number of large squares between waves. If 1 large square, the rate is 300. If 2 large squares, the rate is 150. If 3 large squares, the rate is 100. If 4 large squares, the rate is 75. If 5 large squares, the rate is 60. If 6 large squares, the rate is 50. If 7 large squares, the rate is 42. If 8 large squares, the rate is 38. Memorize the resulting mnemonic: "300, 150, 100, 75, 60, 50, 42, 38."

| TABLE 5-2 | Determination of heart rate from the ECG | | | | |
|---|---|---|---|---|---|
| Time (Second) | No. of Small Squares | Rate (Beats/Min) | Time (Second) | No. of Small Squares | Rate (Beats/Min) |
| 0.10 | 2.5 | 600 | 0.60 | 15.00 | 100 |
| 0.12 | 3.0 | 500 | 0.64 | 16.00 | 94 |
| 0.15 | 3.75 | 400 | 0.70 | 17.50 | 86 |
| 0.16 | 4.0 | 375 | 0.72 | 18.00 | 83 |
| 0.20 | 5.0 | 300 | 0.76 | 19.00 | 79 |
| 0.24 | 6.0 | 250 | 0.80 | 20.00 | 75 |
| 0.26 | 6.5 | 230 | 0.84 | 21.00 | 71 |
| 0.28 | 7.0 | 214 | 0.88 | 22.00 | 68 |
| 0.30 | 7.5 | 200 | 0.92 | 23.00 | 65 |
| 0.32 | 8.0 | 188 | 0.96 | 24.00 | 63 |
| 0.34 | 8.5 | 176 | 1.00 | 25.00 | 60 |
| 0.36 | 9.0 | 167 | 1.08 | 27.00 | 56 |
| 0.38 | 9.5 | 158 | 1.14 | 28.50 | 53 |
| 0.40 | 10.0 | 150 | 1.20 | 30.00 | 50 |
| 0.42 | 10.5 | 143 | 1.40 | 35.00 | 43 |
| 0.44 | 11.0 | 136 | 1.50 | 37.50 | 40 |
| 0.46 | 11.5 | 130 | 1.60 | 40.00 | 38 |
| 0.48 | 12.0 | 125 | 1.80 | 45.00 | 33 |
| 0.50 | 12.5 | 120 | 2.00 | 50.00 | 30 |
| 0.52 | 13.0 | 115 | 2.50 | 62.50 | 25 |
| 0.56 | 14.0 | 107 | 3.00 | 75.00 | 20 |

## ELECTROPHYSIOLOGIC PRINCIPLES

Certain specialized cells, such as those in the sinus node, some parts of the atria, AV node, and His-Purkinje system, are able to discharge spontaneously; they do not require an external or propagated stimulus to fire. This property, known as *automaticity* (also called diastolic depolarization), creates the potential for these cells to depolarize the rest of the heart. Normally the sinus node rules as the pacemaker, since it spontaneously discharges at a rate of 60 to 100 times/min, which is faster than these other latent pacemakers.

Should a latent pacemaker possessing the property of automaticity discharge more rapidly than the sinus node, it may depolarize atria, ventricles, or both. This may occur in two ways. If the SA node discharges more slowly than the discharge rate of the latent pacemaker (see Fig. 5-13), or if the sinus impulse is blocked before reaching the latent pacemaker site (see Fig. 5-13), the latent pacemaker may passively *escape* sinus domination and discharge automatically at its own intrinsic rate. Such escape beats are slower than normal, since the AV junction and bundle branch–Purkinje system (two probable escape focus sites) generally beat at 40 to 60 times/min and 30 to 40 times/min, respectively. However, should a latent pacemaker abnormally accelerate its discharge rate and actively *usurp* control of the heartbeat from the sinus node, a premature beat results. This may happen in the atria, ventricles, or AV junction. A series of these premature beats in a row produces a tachycardia. A shift in the normal manner of atrial or ventricular activation, such as might be produced by a shift in pacemaker focus, is reflected by a change in P or QRS contour.

Automatic discharge of a pacemaker focus is not sufficient to depolarize a cardiac chamber; the impulse must also be conducted from its site of origin to surrounding myocardium. The heart possesses the property of *excitability,* which is a characteristic enabling it to be depolarized by a stimulus; this is an integral part of the propagation or conduction of the impulse from one fiber to the next. Many factors may influence the level of excitability but the most important, in the normal state, is how long after depolarization the heart is restimulated. Cardiac tissue requires a recovery period following depolarization. If a stimulus occurs too early, the heart has had insufficient time to recover, and it will not respond to the stimulus no matter how intense it is (absolute refractory period, excitability zero). A slightly later stimulus allows more time for recovery (relative refractory period, excitability improving), and a still later stimulus finds the heart completely recovered (no longer refractory, full excitability).

If conduction becomes unevenly depressed, with block in some areas and not in others, some regions of the myocardium (unblocked areas) must necessarily be activated (and recover) earlier than others. Under appropriate circumstances, when the block is in only one direction (unidirectional), this uneven conduction may allow the initial impulse to *reenter* areas previously inexcitable but that have now recovered. Should the reentering impulse then be able to depolarize the entire atria and/or ventricles, a corresponding premature extrasystole results; maintenance of the *reentrant excitation* establishes a tachycardia. A special form of reentry may produce echo or reciprocal beats (see Fig. 5-54, *D*).

Thus disorders of impulse *formation* (automaticity) or *conduction* (unidirectional block and reentry) or, at times, combinations of both may initiate dysrhythmias.

Only indirect evidence exists to enable a clinical classification of dysrhythmias according to electrophysiologic mechanisms. In addition, a dysrhythmia may be initiated and perpetuated by different mechanisms. For example, spontaneous diastolic depolarization (automaticity) may trigger a premature atrial or ventricular systole that initiates a dysrhythmia caused by reentry. Also, studies on parasystole,[3] a type of automaticity, and reflection,[4] a form of reentry, is causing us to rethink many of our clinical definitions (Table 5-3). Thus the clinical classification of dys-

---

**TABLE 5-3** Probable electrophysiologic mechanism responsible for various cardiac dysrhythmias

| Automaticity | Reentry | Automaticity or Reentry |
|---|---|---|
| Escape beats—atrial, junctional, or ventricular | AV nodal reentry | Premature systoles—atrial, junctional, or ventricular |
| Atrial rhythm | AV reciprocating tachycardia using an accessory (WPW) pathway | Flutter and fibrillation |
| Atrial tachyardia with or without AV block | Atrial flutter | Ventricular tachycardia |
| Junctional rhythm | Artrial fibrillation | |
| Nonparoxysmal AV junctional tachycardia | Ventricular tachycardia | |
| Accelerated idioventricular rhythm | Ventricular flutter | |
| Parasystole | Ventricular fibrillation | |

rhythmias according to mechanism remains speculative. Antidysrhythmic agents specifically indicated to treat one mechanism or the other do not yet exist.[5]

Depolarization of cells in the atria, ventricles, and His-Purkinje system depends on a rapid movement of sodium into the cell. Such an event is called the *fast response*. In the sinus and AV nodes depolarization depends primarily on intracellular movement of calcium and is called the *slow response*.[6] The slow response may play a role in the genesis of certain cardiac dysrhythmias and is affected by a specific class of drugs called calcium entry blockers such as verapamil, diltiazem and nifedipine.[7]

## DYSRHYTHMIA ANALYSIS (Table 5-4)

For proper analysis, each dysrhythmia must be approached in a systematic manner. A suggested guide follows:

1. What is the rate? Is it too fast or too slow? Are P waves present? Are atrial and ventricular rates the same?
2. Are the PP and RR intervals regular or irregular? If irregular, is it a consistent, repeating irregularity?
3. Is there a P wave (and therefore atrial activity) related to each ventricular complex? Does the P wave precede or follow the QRS complex? Is the PR or RP interval constant?
4. Are all P waves and QRS complexes identical and normal in contour? To determine the significance of changes in P or QRS contour or amplitude, one must know the lead being recorded.
5. Are the PR, QRS, and QT intervals normal?
6. Are premature complexes present? If so, are they atrial, junctional, or ventricular? Is there a constant coupling interval between the premature complex and the normal complex? Is there a constant interval between premature complexes?
7. Are escape beats present? If so, are they atrial, junctional, or ventricular in origin?
8. What is the dominant rhythm?
9. Considering the clinical setting, what is the significance of the dysrhythmia?
10. How should the dysrhythmia be treated?

**TABLE 5-4** Classification of normal and abnormal cardiac rhythms

| | |
|---|---|
| *Rhythms originating in the sinus node* | *Rhythms originating in the ventricles* |
| Sinus rhythm | Ventricular escape complexes |
| Sinus tachycardia | Premature ventricular complex |
| Sinus bradycardia | Ventricular tachycardia |
| Sinus dysrhythmia | Idioventricular tachycardia (accelerated idioventricular rhythm) |
| Sinus arrest | |
| Sinus exit block | |
| Sinus nodal reentry | Ventricular flutter |
| *Rhythms originating in the atria* | Ventricular fibrillation |
| Wandering pacemaker between sinus node and atrium or AV junction | *AV block* |
| | First-degree |
| | Second-degree |
| Premature atrial complex | Type I (Wenckebach) |
| | Type II |
| Intraatrial reentry | Third-degree (complete) |
| Atrial flutter | *Bundle branch block* |
| Atrial fibrillation | Right |
| Atrial tachycardia (with or without block) | Left |
| | Fascicular blocks (hemiblocks) |
| Multifocal atrial tachycardia | *Parasystole* |
| *Rhythms originating in the AV junction (AV node—His bundle)* | Atrial |
| | Junctional |
| | Ventricular |
| Premature AV junctional complex | |
| AV junctional escape complexes | |
| AV junctional rhythm | |
| AV nodal reentry | |
| AV reciprocating tachycardia using an accessory (WPW) pathway | |

From reference 8.

## THERAPY OF DYSRHYTHMIAS (Table 5-5)
### General Therapeutic Concepts[9,10,11]

Initial assessment. The therapeutic approach to a patient who has a cardiac dysrhythmia begins with an accurate electrocardiographic *interpretation* of the dysrhythmia and continues with determination of the *cause* of the dysrhythmia (if possible), the nature of the underlying *heart disease* (if any), and the *consequences* of the dysrhythmia for the individual patient. Thus one cannot treat dysrhythmias as isolated events without having knowledge of the clinical situation; *patients* who have dysrhythmias, not dysrhythmias themselves, are treated.

Electrophysiologic and hemodynamic consequences. The ventricular rate and duration of a dysrhythmia, its site of origin, and the cardiovascular status of the patient primarily determine the electrophysiologic and hemodynamic consequences of a particular rhythm disturbance. Electrophysiologic consequences, often influenced by the presence of underlying heart disease such as acute myocardial infarction, include the development of serious dysrhythmias as a result of rapid (and slow) rates, initiation of sustained dysrhythmias by premature complexes, or the degeneration of rhythms like ventricular tachycardia into ventricular fibrillation. Hemodynamic performance of the heart and circulation may be altered by extremes of heart rate or by loss of atrial contribution to ventricular filling. Rapid rates greatly shorten the diastolic filling time, and, particularly in diseased hearts, the increased heart rate may fail to compensate for the reduced stroke output; blood pressure, along with cardiac output, declines. Dysrhythmias such as nonparoxysmal AV junctional tachycardia (see Fig. 5-51) that prevent sequential AV contraction mitigate the hemodynamic benefits of the atrial booster pump, whereas atrial fibrillation causes complete loss of atrial contraction and may reduce cardiac output.

Slowing the ventricular rate. When a patient develops a tachydysrhythmia, slowing the ventricular rate is the initial and frequently the most important therapeutic maneuver. Because medical therapy frequently involves a time-consuming and potentially dangerous biologic titration of drugs such as digitalis or quinidine, electric direct current (DC) cardioversion may be preferable, depending on the clinical situation. Therapy may differ radically for the very same dysrhythmia in two different patients because the consequences of the tachycardia on the individual patients differ. For example, a supraventricular tachycardia at 200

### TABLE 5-5  Cardiac dysrhythmias*

| Type of Dysrhythmia | P Waves | | | QRS Complexes | | |
|---|---|---|---|---|---|---|
| | Rate | Rhythm | Contour | Rate | Rhythm | Contour |
| Sinus rhythm | 60 to 100 | Regular† | Normal | 60 to 100 | Regular | Normal |
| Sinus bradycardia | <60 | Regular | Normal | <60 | Regular | Normal |
| Sinus tachycardia | 100 to 180 | Regular | May be peaked | 100 to 180 | Regular | Normal |
| AV nodal reentry | 150 to 250 | Very regular except at onset and termination | Retrograde; difficult to see; lost in QRS complex | 150 to 250 | Very regular except at onset and termination | Normal |
| Atrial flutter | 250 to 350 | Regular | Sawtooth | 75 to 175 | Generally regular in absence of drugs or disease | Normal |
| Atrial fibrillation | 400 to 600 | Grossly irregular | Baseline undulations; no P waves | 100 to 160 | Grossly irregular | Normal |

*In an effort to summarize these dysrhythmias in a tabular form, generalizations have to be made, especially under therapy. Particularly, acute therapy to terminate a tachycardia may be different from chronic therapy to prevent a recurrence. Some of the exceptions are indicated by the footnotes, but the reader is referred to the text for a complete discussion.
†P waves initiated by sinus node discharge may not be precisely regular because of sinus dysrhythmia.
‡Often, carotid sinus massage fails to slow a sinus tachycardia.

beats/min may produce little or no symptoms in a healthy young adult and therefore require little or no therapy; the very same dysrhythmia may precipitate pulmonary edema in a patient with mitral stenosis, syncope in a patient with aortic stenosis, shock in a patient with an acute myocardial infarction, or hemiparesis in a patient with cerebrovascular disease. In these situations the tachycardia requires prompt electric conversion.

Etiology. The etiology of the dysrhythmia may influence therapy markedly. Electrolyte imbalance (potassium, magnesium, calcium), acidosis or alkalosis, hypoxemia, and many drugs may produce dryrhythmias. Because heart failure may cause dysrhythmias, digitalis may effectively suppress dysrhythmias during heart failure when all other agents are unsuccessful or prevent more severe dysrhythmias by reversing early congestive heart failure. Similarly, a dysrhythmia secondary to hypotension may respond to leg elevation or vasopressor therapy. Mild sedation or reassurance may be successful in treating some dysrhythmias related to emotional stress. Precipitating or contributing disease states such as infection, hypovolemia, anemia, and thyroid disorders should be sought and treated. Aggressive management of premature atrial or ventricular complexes that often presage or precipitate the occurrence of sustained tachydysrhythmias may prevent later occurrence of more serious tachydysrhythmias.

Risks of therapy. Since therapy always involves some risk, one must decide, particularly as the therapeutic regimen escalates, if the risks of not treating the dysrhythmia continue to outweigh the risks of the therapy. The antidysrhythmic agents[7,10,12] lidocaine, procainamide, quinidine, propranolol, disopyramide, and phenytoin exert negative inotropic effects on the myocardium, and when given parenterally, they may produce hypotension. Antidysrhythmic agents may slow conduction velocity, depress the activity of normal (sinus) as well as abnormal (ectopic) pacemaker sites, and cause dysrhythmias. It should be remembered that doses of all drugs may need to be adjusted according to the size of the patient, routes of excretion or degradation, presence of impaired organ function (heart, liver, kidney), degree of absorption (if given orally), adverse side effects, interaction with other drugs, electrolyte imbalance, hypoxemia, and the like.

The remainder of this chapter will be devoted to a discussion of cardiac dysrhythmias (see Tables 5-4 and 5-5). The systematic approach, previously discussed under dysrhythmia analysis will be used.

| Ventricular Response to Carotid Sinus Massage | Physical Examination | | | Treatment |
|---|---|---|---|---|
| | Intensity of S₁ | Splitting of S₂ | A Waves | |
| Gradual slowing and return to former rate | Constant | Normal | Normal | None |
| Gradual slowing and return to former rate | Constant | Normal | Normal | None, unless symptomatic; atropine, isoproterenol |
| Gradual slowing‡ and return to former rate | Constant | Normal | Normal | None, unless symptomatic; treat underlying disease |
| Abrupt slowing caused by termination of tachycardia, or no effect | Constant | Normal | Constant cannon A waves | Vagal stimulation, verapamil, digitalis, propranolol, DC shock, pacing |
| Abrupt slowing and return to former rate; flutter remains | Constant; variable if AV block changing | Normal | Flutter waves | DC shock, digitalis, quinidine, propranolol, verapamil, pacing |
| Slowing; gross irregularity remains | Variable | Normal | No A waves | Digitalis, quinidine, DC shock, verapamil, propranolol |

§Any independent atrial dysrhythmia may exist or the atria may be captured retrogradely.
‖Constant if atria captured retrogradely.
¶Atrial rhythm and rate may vary, depending on whether sinus bradycardia or tachycardia, atrial tachycardia, or something else is the atrial mechanism.
**Regular or constant if block is unchanging.

*Continued.*

TABLE 5-5  Cardiac dysrhythmias—cont'd

| Type of Dysrhythmia | P Waves | | | QRS Complexes | | |
|---|---|---|---|---|---|---|
| | Rate | Rhythm | Contour | Rate | Rhythm | Contour |
| Atrial tachycardia with block | 150 to 250 | Regular; may be irregular | Abnormal | 75 to 200 | Generally regular in absence of drugs or disease | Normal |
| AV junctional rhythm | 40 to 100§ | Regular | Normal | 40 to 60 | Fairly regular | Normal |
| Reciprocating tachycardia using an accessory (WPW) pathway | 150 to 250 | Very regular except at onset and termination | Retrograde; difficult to see; follows the QRS complex | 150 to 250 | Very regular except at onset and termination | Normal |
| Nonparoxysmal AV junctional tachycardia | 60 to 100§ | Regular | Normal | 70 to 130 | Fairly regular | Normal |
| Ventricular tachycardia | 60 to 100§ | Regular | Normal | 110 to 250 | Fairly regular; may be irregular | Abnormal, >0.12 second |
| Accelerated idioventricular rhythm | 60 to 100§ | Regular | Normal | 50 to 110 | Fairly regular; may be irregular | Abnormal, >0.12 second |
| Ventricular flutter | 60 to 100§ | Regular | Normal; difficult to see | 150 to 300 | Regular | Sine wave |
| Ventricular fibrillation | 60 to 100§ | Regular | Normal; difficult to see | 400 to 600 | Grossly irregular | Baseline undulations; no QRS complexes |
| First-degree AV block | 60 to 100¶ | Regular | Normal | 60 to 100 | Regular | Normal |
| Type I second-degree AV block | 60 to 100¶ | Regular | Normal | 30 to 100 | Irregular** | Normal |
| Type II-second-degree AV block | 60 to 100¶ | Regular | Normal | 30 to 100 | Irregular** | Abnormal, >0.12 second |
| Complete AV block | 60 to 100§ | Regular | Normal | <40 | Fairly regular | Abnormal, >0.12 second |
| Right bundle branch block | 60 to 100 | Regular | Normal | 60 to 100 | Regular | Abnormal, >0.12 second |
| Left bundle branch block | 60 to 100 | Regular | Normal | 60 to 100 | Regular | Abnormal, >0.12 second |

| Ventricular Response to Carotid Sinus Massage | Physical Examination | | | Treatment |
|---|---|---|---|---|
| | Intensity of $S_1$ | Splitting of $S_2$ | A Waves | |
| Abrupt slowing and return to former rate; tachycardia remains | Constant; variable if AV block changing | Normal | More A waves than CV waves | Stop digitalis if toxic; digitalis, if not toxic; possibly verapamil, quinidine |
| None; may be slight slowing | Variable‖ | Normal | Intermittent cannon waves‖ | None, unless symptomatic; atropine |
| Abrupt slowing caused by termination of tachycardia, or no effect | Constant but decreased | Normal | Constant cannon waves | See paroxysmal supraventricular tachycardia above |
| None; may be slight slowing | Variable‖ | Normal | Intermittent cannon waves‖ | None, unless symptomatic; stop digitalis if toxic |
| None | Variable‖ | Abnormal | Intermittent cannon waves‖ | Lidocaine, procainamide, DC shock, quinidine |
| None | Variable‖ | Abnormal | Intermittent cannon waves‖ | None, unless symptomatic; lidocaine, atropine |
| None | None | None | Cannon waves | DC shock |
| None | None | None | Cannon waves | DC shock |
| Gradual slowing caused by sinus slowing | Constant, diminished | Normal | Normal | None |
| Slowing caused by sinus slowing and an increase in AV block | Cyclic decrease and then increase after pause | Normal | Normal; increasing AC interval; A waves without C waves | None, unless symptomatic; atropine |
| Gradual slowing caused by sinus slowing | Constant | Abnormal | Normal; constant AC interval; A waves without C waves | Pacemaker |
| None | Variable‖ | Abnormal | Intermittent cannon waves‖ | Pacemaker |
| Gradual slowing and return to former rate | Constant | Wide | Normal | None |
| Gradual slowing and return to former rate | Constant | Paradoxical | Normal | None |

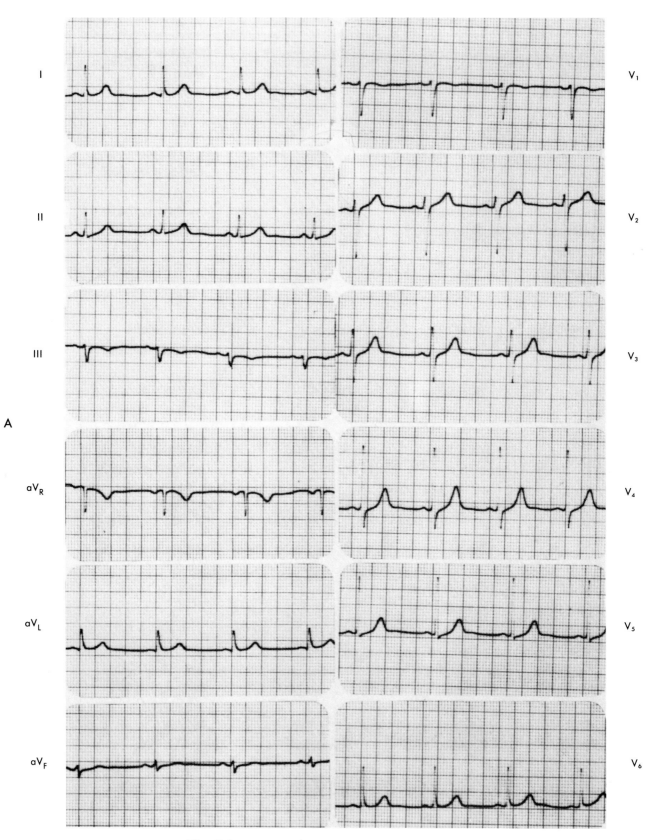

**Fig. 5-6** **A,** Normal sinus rhythm. The ECG is normal.

## NORMAL SINUS RHYTHM (Fig. 5-6)

Normal sinus rhythm, in adults, is arbitrarily limited to rates of 60 to 100 beats/min. The P wave is upright in leads I and II and negative in lead $aV_R$ with a vector in the frontal plane between 0 and +90 degrees. In the horizontal plane the P vector is directed anteriorly and slightly leftward and may therefore be negative in $V_1$ and $V_2$ but is positive in $V_3$. The PP interval characteristically varies slightly but by less than 0.16 second per cycle. The PR interval is between 0.12 and 2.0 seconds and may vary slightly with rate. The QRS duration is 0.06 to 0.20 second, and the QT duration is 0.36 to 0.44 second. The sinus node responds readily to autonomic stimuli; parasympathetic (cholinergic) stimuli slow and sympathetic (adrenergic) stimuli speed the rate of discharge. The resulting rate depends on the net effect of these two opposing forces.

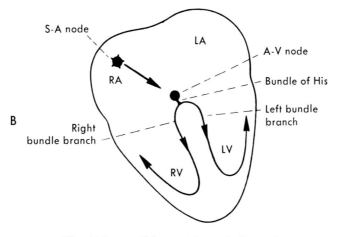
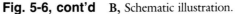

**Fig. 5-6, cont'd**    B, Schematic illustration.

## SINUS TACHYCARDIA (Figs. 5-7 and 5-8)

The conduction pathway in sinus tachycardia is the same as that in normal sinus rhythm, but, because of enhanced discharge of the sinus node from vagal inhibition or sympathetic stimulation (or both), the sinus rate is between 100 and 180 beats/min. It may be higher with extreme exertion and in infants. It has a gradual onset and termination, and the PP interval may vary slightly from cycle to cycle. P waves have a normal contour but may develop a larger amplitude and become peaked. Carotid sinus massage and Valsalva or other vagal maneuvers gradually slow a sinus tachycardia, which then accelerates to its previous rate. More rapid sinus rates may fail to slow in response to a vagal maneuver.

Significance. Sinus tachycardia is the normal physiologic response to such stressors as fever, hypotension, thyrotoxicosis, anemia, anxiety, exertion, hypovolemia, pulmonary emboli, myocardial ischemia, congestive heart failure, or shock. Inflammation such as pericarditis may produce sinus tachycardia. Sinus tachycardia is usually of no physiologic significance; however, in patients with organic myocardial disease, reduced cardiac output, congestive heart failure, or dysrhythmias may result. Since heart rate is a major determinant of oxygen requirements, angina or perhaps an increase in the size of an infarction may accompany persistent sinus tachycardia in patients with coronary artery disease.

Treatment. Therapy should be directed toward correcting the underlying disease state that caused the sinus tachycardia. Elimination of tobacco, alcohol, coffee, tea, or other stimulants (for example, sympathomimetic vasoconstrictors in nose drops) may be helpful. If sinus tachycardia is not secondary to a correctable physiologic stress, treatment with sedatives, reserpine, or clonidine is occasionally useful. The only currently available medication that consistently slows a sinus tachycardia directly is propranolol, administered orally, 10 to 60 mg, four times daily. Drugs that block the slow inward current, such as verapamil, may also slow the rate of sinus node discharge.

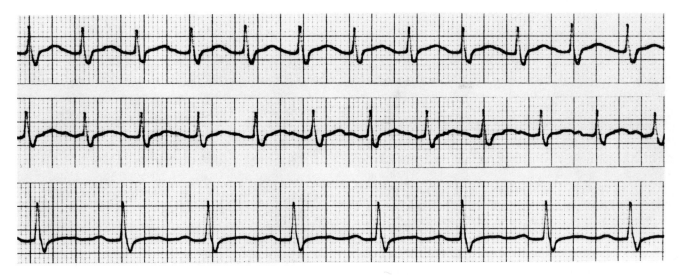

**Fig. 5-7    Sinus tachycardia.** Sinus tachycardia gradually slows to reveal clearer P waves in the bottom tracing, which is a sinus rhythm with a first degree AV block. Monitor lead.

| | |
|---|---|
| **Rate:** | Top, 125 beats/min; middle, 122 beats/min; bottom, 82 beats/min. |
| **Rhythm:** | Regular. |
| **P waves:** | Difficult to see in top strip. Precede each QRS complex at a regular interval with unchanging contour in middle and bottom strip. |
| **PR interval:** | Top, cannot measure; middle, 0.20 second; bottom, 0.24 second. |
| **QRS:** | 0.09 second. |

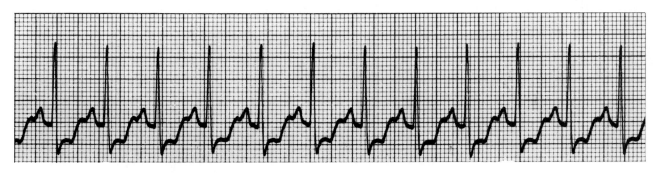

**Fig. 5-8    Sinus tachycardia.** Patient complained of chest pain and was noted to have sinus tachycardia with ST segment depression, consistent with anginal episode. Lead II.

| | |
|---|---|
| **Rate:** | 125 beats/min. |
| **Rhythm:** | Regular. |
| **P waves:** | Normal; precede each QRS complex with regular contour at fixed interval. |
| **PR interval:** | 0.16 second. |
| **QRS:** | Normal, 0.08 second. ST segments are depressed. |

## SINUS BRADYCARDIA (Figs. 5-9 and 5-10)

In sinus bradycardia, impulses travel down the same pathway as in sinus rhythm, but the sinus node discharges at a rate less than 60 beats/min. P waves have a normal contour and occur before each QRS complex with a constant PR interval exceeding 0.12 second. Sinus dysrhythmia is frequently present.

Significance. Sinus bradycardia results from excessive vagal or decreased sympathetic tone or both. Eye surgery, meningitis, intracranial tumors, cervical and mediastinal tumors, and certain disease states such as myocardial infarction, myxedema, obstructive jaundice, and cardiac fibrosis may produce sinus bradycardia. In most instances, sinus bradycardia is a benign dysrhythmia and may actually be beneficial by producing a longer period of diastole and increased ventricular filling. It occurs commonly in well-trained athletes, during sleep, vomiting, or vasovagal syncope and may be produced by carotid sinus stimulation or by the administration of parasympathomimetic drugs. Sinus bradycardia occurring in patients who have myocardial infarction, more commonly diaphragmatic or posterior, may compromise optimum myocardial function and predispose to premature systoles and sustained tachydysrhythmias. Sinus bradycardia may be beneficial in some patients who have acute myocardial infarction because it reduces oxygen demands, may help to minimize the size of the infarction, and may lessen the frequency of some dysrhythmias. Patients with acute myocardial infarction who have sinus bradycardia generally have lower mortality than patients who have sinus tachycardia.

Treatment. Treatment of sinus bradycardia is needed only when such symptoms as chest pain, dyspnea, light-headedness, hypotension, or ventricular ectopy occur. If the patient with an acute myocardial infarction is asymptomatic, it is probably best not to try to speed the sinus rate. If the cardiac output is inadequate, or if dysrhythmias are associated with the slow rate, atropine (0.5 mg IV as an initial dose, repeated if necessary) to a total dosage of 2.0 mg or isoproterenol (2 to 10 μg/minute IV) is usually effective.[13] These drugs should be used cautiously, with care taken not to produce too rapid a rate. In patients who have symptoms as a result of chronic sinus bradycardia, electric pacing may be needed, since few, if any, drugs successfully speed sinus node discharge chronically without producing side effects. Theophylline drugs or dermally applied scopolamine may be tried, although they are not approved for the treatment of sinus bradycardia.

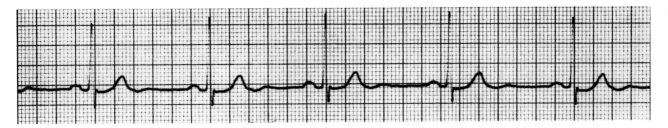

**Fig. 5-9    Sinus bradycardia.** Sinus bradycardia is present in this patient because of administration of propranolol. Lead II.

**Rate:**          46 beats/minute.
**Rhythm:**        Regular.
**P waves:**       Precede each QRS with a normal contour.
**PR interval:**   0.19 second.
**QRS:**           0.09 second.

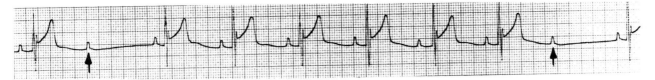

**Fig. 5-10    Sinus bradycardia in a young patient.** Type I (Wenckebach) AV block is also present and probably represents excessive vagal tone that may be normal in young individuals. Monitor lead. ST elevation is early repolarization.

**Rate:**          Atrial, 55 beats/minute.
**Rhythm:**        Atrial, regular; ventricular, irregular because of nonconducted P waves *(arrows)*.
**PR interval:**   Increasing slightly from 0.18 second to 2.2 seconds.
**QRS:**           0.09 second.

### SINUS DYSRHYTHMIA (Figs. 5-11 to 5-13)

Sinus dysrhythmia is characterized by a phasic variation in cycle length exceeding 0.16 second during sinus rhythm. It is the most frequent form of dysrhythmia and occurs as a normal phenomenon. The P waves do not vary in morphology, and the PR interval exceeds 0.12 second and remains unchanged, since the focus of discharge is fixed within the sinus node. Occasionally the pacemaker focus may wander within the sinus node, producing P waves of slightly different contour (but not retrograde) and a changing PR interval (but not less than 0.12 second). Sinus dysrhythmia commonly occurs in the young or aged, especially with slower heart rates or following enhanced vagal tone from digitalis or morphine administration. Sinus dysrhythmia appears in two basic forms. In the respiratory form the PP interval cyclically shortens during inspiration as a result of reflex inhibition of vagal tone or enhancement of sympathetic tone or both. Breath-holding eliminates the cycle length variation. Nonrespiratory sinus dysrhythmia is characterized by a phasic variation unrelated to the respiratory cycle. In both forms, impulses are generated in the sinus node and travel over the normal pathway to the AV node.

**Significance.** Sinus dysrhythmia commonly occurs in the young or aged especially with slower heart rates or from enhanced vagal tone after morphine or digitalis administration. Symptoms produced by sinus dysrhythmias are rare, but on occasion, if the pauses between beats are excessively long, palpitations or dizziness may be experienced. Marked sinus dysrhythmia can produce a sinus pause sufficiently prolonged to induce syncope if not accompanied by an escape rhythm.

**Treatment.** Treatment is usually not necessary. Increasing the heart rate by exercise or drugs will abolish sinus dysrhythmia. Symptomatic individuals may experience relief from feelings of palpitations through the use of sedatives, tranquilizers, atropine, ephedrine, or isoproterenol administration, as in the treatment of sinus bradycardia.

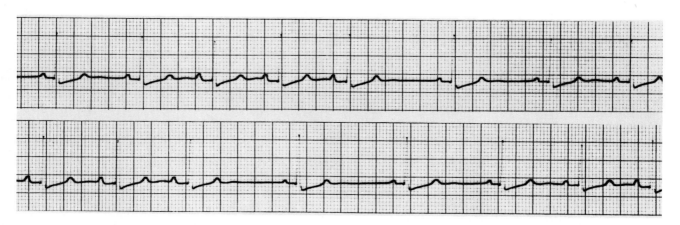
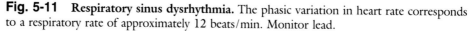

**Fig. 5-11** **Respiratory sinus dysrhythmia.** The phasic variation in heart rate corresponds to a respiratory rate of approximately 12 beats/min. Monitor lead.

| | |
|---|---|
| **Rate:** | Sinus rate increases with inspiration and decreases with expiration at a rate of 53 to 80 beats/min. |
| **Rhythm:** | Irregular with repetitive phase variation in cycle length according to respiratory cycles. Cycle lengths vary by more than 0.16 second. Breath-holding eliminates the rate variations (not shown). |
| **P waves:** | Precede each QRS complex with a normal, fairly constant contour. |
| **PR interval:** | Normal, constant, 0.18 second. |
| **QRS:** | Normal, 0.08 second. |

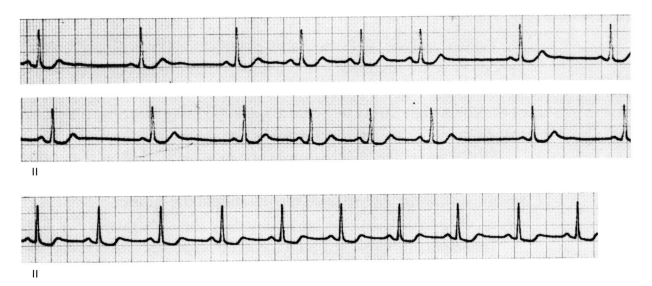

**Fig. 5-12** **Nonrespiratory sinus dysrhythmia.** In this instance if was caused by digitalis toxicity **(A).** One week following discontinuation of digitalis the nonrespiratory sinus dysrhythmia disappeared **(B).**

**Rate:**       Rate increases and decreases independently of respiration in **A** (47 to 80 beats/min). Rate constant (78 beats/min) in **B.**

**Rhythm:**       **A,** Irregular with a repetitive phasic variation in cycle length that continues during breath-holding. **B,** Regular.

**P waves:**       Precede each QRS with a normal, fairly constant contour.

**PR interval:**       0.12 second.

**QRS:**       Normal, 0.06 second.

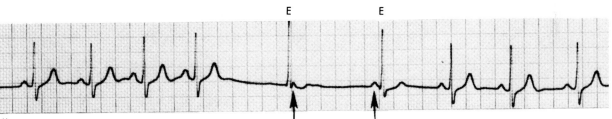

**Fig. 5-13** **Respiratory sinus dysrhythmia.** The first four P waves are fairly regular; the PR interval is 0.16 second and constant. Then the sinus node slows and the next two P waves occur much later *(arrows)*. The marked sinus slowing allows a latent pacemaker—possibly located in the His bundle or high in the fascicles—to escape sinus domination, depolarize automatically, and discharge the ventricles *(E, junctional escapes)*. A slight change in QRS contour is apparent in these beats. The sinus node then speeds up to resume control. This slightly complex dysrhythmia is completely normal in an otherwise healthy person.

**Rate:**       Rate increases with inspiration and decreases with expiration (55 to 80 beats/min).

**Rhythm:**       Irregular with a repetitive phasic variation in cycle length.

**P waves:**       Normal, fairly constant contour

**PR interval:**       0.16 second during sinus-conducted beats.

**QRS:**       Normal, 0.08 second during sinus-conducted beats.

## SINUS ARREST (Figs. 5-14 and 5-15)

Failure of sinus node discharge results in absence of atrial depolarization and periods of ventricular asystole if escape beats produced by latent pacemakers do not discharge. Sinus arrest may be produced by involvement of the sinus node or the sinus node artery by acute myocardial infarction, digitalis toxicity, excessive vagal tone, or degenerative forms of fibrosis. It may occur as a side effect of therapy with certain drugs such as amiodarone.

Significance. Transient sinus arrest may have no clinical significance by itself if latent pacemakers promptly escape to prevent ventricular asystole (Fig. 5-14). Prolonged ventricular asystole results should the latent pacemakers fail to escape. Other dysrhythmias may be precipitated by the slow rates (Fig. 5-15).

Treatment. Atropine (0.5 mg IV initially, repeated if necessary to total dosage of 2.0 mg) or isoproterenol (2 to 10 μg/min IV) may be tried as the first therapeutic approach.[13] If these drugs are unsuccessful, atrial or ventricular pacing may be required. In patients who have a chronic form of sinus node disease characterized by marked sinus bradycardia or sinus arrest (sick sinus syndrome), permanent pacing is often necessary. Some of these patients experience sinus bradycardia alternating with periods of supraventricular tachycardia (bradycardia-tachycardia syndrome). These patients are best treated by a combination of drugs (to slow the ventricular rate during the supraventricular tachycardia) and implantation of a permanent demand pacemaker (to prevent the slow rate when the tachycardia terminates).

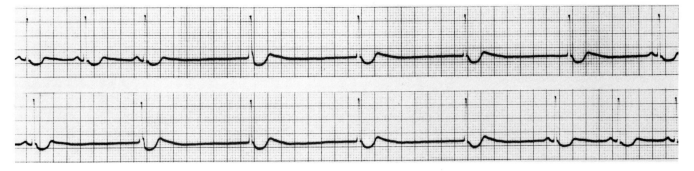

**Fig. 5-14** **Sinus arrest.** After three sinus beats in the top strip, sinus arrest occurs followed by junctional escape beats. The sinus rhythm returns at the end of the strip and once again restores sinus rhythm. A similar event happens in the lower recording. Monitor lead.

| | |
|---|---|
| **Rate:** | Varying: junctional escape rate, 38 beats/min; sinus rate, 70 beats/min. |
| **Rhythm:** | Irregular |
| **P waves:** | Normal contour, intermittently precedes QRS complexes. |
| **PR interval:** | Constant when P waves precede QRS contour. 0.18 second. |
| **QRS:** | Normal, 0.09 second. |

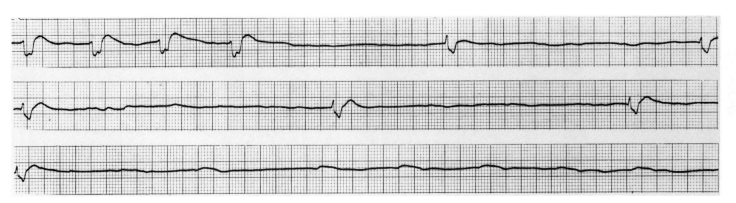

**Fig. 5-15.** **Sinus arrest with asystole.** These monitor lead tracings were recorded during a resuscitation procedure in a patient with recurrent syncope. No atrial activity is apparent, and the slight undulations in the baseline represent chest compression during resuscitation. The patient has intermittent junctional or most probably ventricular escapes and then develops complete atrial and ventricular asystole.

| | |
|---|---|
| **Rate:** | Varying. |
| **Rhythm:** | Irregular. |
| **P waves:** | Not seen. |
| **PR interval:** | Not measurable. |
| **QRS:** | 0.16 second. |

## SINUS EXIT BLOCK (Figs. 5-16 and 5-17)

Sinus exit block is a conduction disturbance during which an impulse formed within the sinus node is blocked from depolarizing the atria. Sinus exit block is indicated on the ECG by the absence of the normally expected P wave(s). The length of the pause between P waves is a multiple of the basic PP interval, approximately two, less commonly three or four times the normal PP interval (type II exit block). Type I (Wenckebach) sinus exit block may also occur, in which case the PP interval progressively shortens prior to the pause, and the duration of the pause is less than two PP cycles.

Significance. Sinus exit block may be caused by excessive vagal stimulation, by acute infections such as diphtheria or rheumatic carditis, by atherosclerosis involving the sinus nodal artery, or by fibrosis involving the atrium. Occlusion of the sinus nodal artery owing to acute myocardial infarction may result in an atrial infarction and produce sinus exit block. Medications such as quinidine, procainamide, amiodarone, and digitalis may lead to sinus exit block. Sinus exit block is usually transient and often of no clinical importance except to prompt a search for the underlying cause. Syncope may result if the sinus exit block is prolonged and unaccompanied by an AV junctional or ventricular escape rhythm. Digitalis produces type II sinus exit block (but not type I AV block).

Treatment. Therapy for symptomatic sinus exit block is directed toward increasing sympathetic tone and decreasing parasympathetic tone. Thus atropine and isoproterenol are useful, as described under sinus bradycardia. If the clinical situation demands therapy and pharmacologic measures are not effective, atrial or ventricular pacing may be indicated.

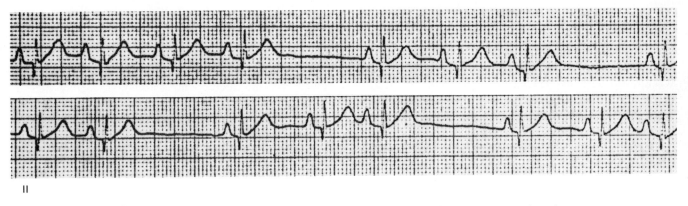

II

**Fig. 5-16 Sinus exit block (type III).** The longer PP intervals are approximately twice the shorter PP intervals, indicating an intermittent 2:1 sinus exit block of the type II variety.

**Rate:** Varying, slow (43 to 68 beats/min).
**Rhythm:** Irregular; pauses are twice as long as the shorter intervals.
**P waves:** Contour normal, precede each QRS complex; intermittent loss of P wave.
**PR interval:** 0.16 second.
**QRS:** Normal, 0.08 second.

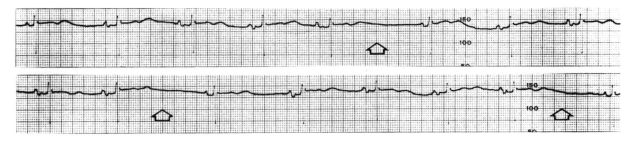

**Fig. 5-17 Sinus exit block, type I (Wenckebach block).** The following characteristics of this tracing suggest the diagnosis of a Wenckebach exit block from a sinus node. *1,* The PP intervals progressively shorten until *(2)* a pause in atrial activity occurs as depicted by the arrows. *3,* The duration of the pause is less than twice the shortest PP interval. *4,* The PP interval after the pause exceeds the PP interval preceding the pause, which is the shortest PP interval. Monitor lead.

**Rate:** Varying from 33 to 50 beats/min.
**Rhythm:** The four features mentioned above.
**P waves:** Biphasic, but fairly constant contour; intermittent loss of P wave, producing a pause *(arrows)*.
**PR interval:** 0.24 second.
**QRS:** 0.07 second.

## WANDERING PACEMAKER (Figs. 5-18 and 5-19)

Wandering pacemaker, a variant of sinus dysrhythmia, involves the passive transfer of the dominant pacemaker focus from the sinus node to latent pacemakers with the next highest degree of automaticity, in other atrial sites or in the AV junctional tissue. Thus only one pacemaker is operative at a time. As with other forms of sinus dysrhythmia, the change occurs in a gradual fashion over the duration of several beats. The ECG displays a cyclic increase of the RR interval, a PR interval that gradually shortens and may become less than 0.12 second, and a change in P wave configuration until it becomes negative in lead I or II or becomes buried in the QRS complex. A slight change in QRS configuration may occur owing to aberrant conduction. Generally these changes occur in reverse as the pacemaker shifts back to the sinus node. Rarely a wandering pacemaker may appear without changes in rate.

**Significance.** Wandering pacemaker is a normal phenomenon that is often seen in the very young or in the aged, and particularly in athletes. Persistence of an AV junctional rhythm for long periods of time, however, usually indicates underlying heart disease.

**Treatment.** Treatment of a wandering pacemaker usually is not indicated. Sympathomimetic agents such as ephedrine or isoproterenol or parasympatholytic agents such as atropine can be used if necessary (see discussion of sinus bradycardia).

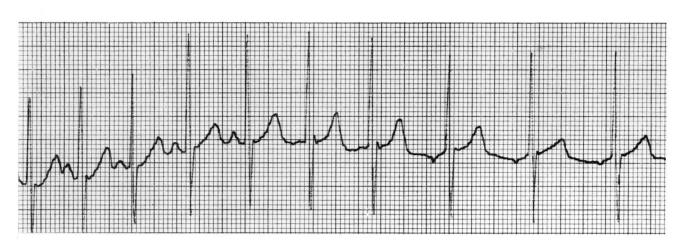

**Fig. 5-18   Wandering atrial pacemaker.** When the heart rate is fast, the P wave is upright and gradually becomes inverted as the heart rate slows and the site of impulse formation shifts. Monitor lead.

**Rate:**          Varying, 80 to 135 beats/min.
**Rhythm:**        Irregular with a repetitive phasic variation in cycle length, as in sinus dysrhythmia.
**P waves:**       Varying contour, indicating shift in pacemaker site or change in activation sequence.
**PR interval:**   Constant, 0.13 second.
**QRS:**           0.10 second.

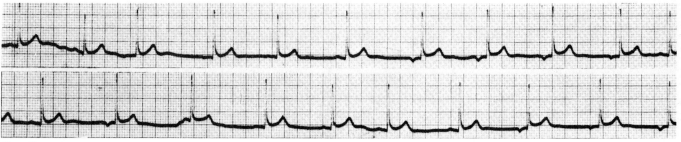

II-continuous

**Fig. 5-19   Wandering atrial pacemaker.** As the heart rate slows, the P waves become inverted and then gradually revert toward normal as the heart rate speeds. The PR interval shortens to 0.14 second with the inverted P wave and is 0.16 second with the upright P wave.

**Rate:**          Varying, slow (52 to 72 beats/min).
**Rhythm:**        Irregular with a repetitive phasic variation in cycle length as in sinus dysrhythmia.
**P waves:**       Varying contour, indicating shift in pacemaker site. Become negative in lead II.
**PR interval:**   Varies, 0.14, 0.16 second.
**QRS:**           Normal, 0.08 second.

## PREMATURE ATRIAL COMPLEXES
(Figs. 5-20 to 5-24)

Premature complexes are the most common cause of an intermittent pulse. They may originate in any area of the heart, most frequently in the ventricles, less often in the atria and the AV junctional region, and rarely in the sinus node. Although premature complexes arise in normal hearts, they are more often associated with organic disease, particularly in older patients.

The diagnosis of premature atrial complexes is indicated by a premature P wave and a PR interval greater than 0.12 second. Although the contour of the premature P wave may resemble the normal sinus P wave, it generally is different. Variations in the basic sinus rate at times may make the diagnosis of prematurity difficult, but differences in the contour of the P wave are usually quite apparent and indicate a different focus of orgin. When a premature atrial complex occurs early in diastole, conduction may not be completely normal. The AV junction may still be refractory from the preceding beat and will prevent propagation of the impulse (blocked premature atrial complex) or cause conduction to be slowed in the AV junction (prolonged PR interval) or ventricle (functional bundle branch block). As a general rule, a short RP interval produced by an early premature atrial complex close to the preceding QRS complex is followed by a long PR interval. On occasion, when the AV junction has sufficiently repolarized to conduct normally, the supraventricular QRS complex may be aberrant in configuration because the ventricle has not completely repolarized (see discussion of supraventricular dysrhythmias with abnormal QRS complexes, Figs. 5-23 and 5-24).

The length of the pause following any premature beat or series of premature beats is determined by the interaction of several factors. If the premature atrial complex occurs when the sinus node is not refractory, the impulse may conduct to the sinus node, discharge it prematurely, and cause the next sinus cycle to begin from that point. The interval between the two normal beats flanking a premature atrial complex that has reset the timing of the basic sinus rhythm is less than twice the normal cycle, and the pause after the premature atrial complex is said to be "noncompensatory." The interval following the premature atrial complex is generally slightly longer than one sinus cycle, however. Less commonly the premature atrial complex may find the sinus node refractory, in which case the timing of the basic sinus rhythm is not altered, and the interval between the two normal beats flanking the premature atrial complex is twice the normal PP cycle. The interval following this premature atrial discharge is therefore said to be a "full compensatory pause." A *compensatory pause* is one of sufficient duration to make the interval between the two normal beats on each side of the premature beat equal to twice the basic cycle length. However, sinus dysrhythmia may lengthen or shorten this pause.

Significance. Premature atrial complexes may occur in a variety of situations: for example, during infection, inflammation, or myocardial ischemia, or they may be provoked by a variety of medications, by tension states, or by tobacco and caffeine. Premature atrial complexes may precipitate or presage the occurrence of a sustained supraventricular tachycardia.

Treatment. In the absence of organic heart disease, treatment may not be necessary, unless the patient complains of symptoms such as palpitations or has recurrent tachycardias or an excessive number of premature atrial complexes. If treatment is indicated, for example, in a patient with acute myocardial infarction, initial therapy should probably be with digitalis, combined with quinidine or procainamide if digitalis alone is not successful. Sedation and/or omission of alcohol, cafffeine, smoking or other stimulants (e.g., amphetamines, cocaine) may be helpful in some patients.

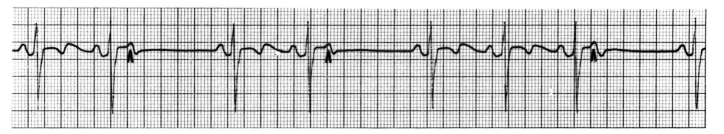

**Fig. 5-20** **Premature atrial complexes, blocked and hidden in the T wave.** The deformed T waves *(arrows)* indicate a nonconducted premature atrial complex that blocks within the AV node or His bundle. The premature atrial complex discharges the sinus node and delays its return so that the PP interval from the premature atrial complex to the next sinus P wave exceeds the normal sinus PP interval. A noncompensatory pulse follows the blocked PACs. Monitor lead.

**Rate:** 67 beats/min during sinus rhythm.
**Rhythm:** Varying because of premature atrial complexes.
**P waves:** Premature atrial complexes are hidden within and deform the T waves.
**PR interval:** Of normal sinus beats, 0.18 second.
**QRS:** 0.10 second.

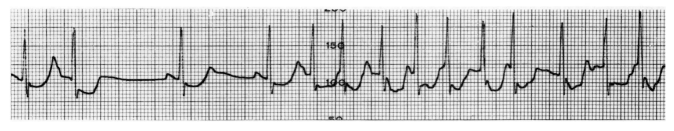

**Fig. 5-21** **Premature atrial complex precipitating atrial flutter-fibrillation.** A premature atrial complex is hidden within the T wave of the first QRS complex and occurs again in the T wave of the fourth QRS complex. This premature atrial complex precipitates atrial flutter fibrillation. Monitor lead.

**Rate:** Varying.
**Rhythm:** Varying because of premature atrial complexes and atrial flutter-fibrillation.
**P waves:** Premature atrial complexes hidden in the T waves.
**PR interval:** Of normally conducted beats, 0.14 second.
**QRS:** 0.08 second.

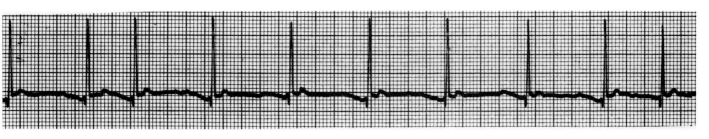

**Fig. 5-22** **Premature atrial complexes.** Third and tenth complexes represent premature atrial complexes. Monitor lead.

**Rate:** 68 beats/min during sinus rhythm.
**Rhythm:** Varying because of premature atrial complexes.
**P waves:** Precede each QRS complex.
**QRS interval:** 0.06 second.

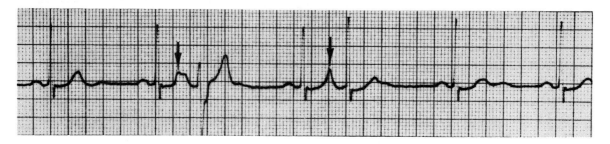

**Fig. 5-23** **Premature atrial complexes with and without aberrancy.** The first premature atrial complex *(arrow)* occurs at a shorter RP interval than does the second premature atrial complex *(arrows)* and conducts with a bundle branch block contour (probably right bundle branch block in this monitor lead). The first premature atrial complex conducts with aberrancy while the second does not because the first reaches the bundle branch system before complete recovery of repolarization.

| | |
|---|---|
| **Rate:** | 50 beats/min during the normally conducted complexes. |
| **Rhythm:** | Irregular because of the premature atrial complexes. |
| **P waves:** | Normal for the normally conducted sinus beats. Premature atrial complexes deform the T waves. |
| **PR interval:** | Of premature atrial complexes, prolonged because the AV node and/or His bundle has incompletely recovered. PR interval of first premature atrial complex is approximately 0.26 second and that of the second premature atrial complex approximately 0.22 second. The PR interval of normally conducted sinus beats is 0.19 second. |
| **QRS:** | Of normally conducted beats, 0.07 second; of aberrantly conducted QRS complex, 0.12 second. |

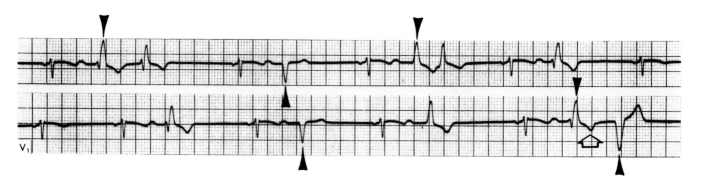

**Fig. 5-24** **Premature atrial complexes that produce functional right and functional left bundle branch block.** Upright arrowheads point to QRS complexes that conduct with complete or incomplete functional left bundle branch block while inverted arrowheads point to some of the QRS complexes that conduct with functional right bundle branch block. Note that the latter have both a monophasic and triphasic contour. The deformed T waves *(open arrow* at the end of the last strip) indicate a premature atrial complex. They occur singly and in pairs.

| | |
|---|---|
| **Rate:** | Varying because of premature atrial complexes. |
| **Rhythm:** | Irregular because of premature atrial complexes. |
| **P waves:** | During sinus rhythm, normal; P waves of premature atrial complexes are hard to discern because they occur in the preceding T wave. |
| **PR interval:** | Of normal sinus beats, 0.12 second; of premature atrial complexes, prolonged and of differing durations because of differencecs in RP intervals. |

## AV NODAL REENTRY (Figs. 5-25 to 5-28)

The tachycardias formerly called paroxysmal atrial (PAT) and junctional (PJT) tachycardias are caused most commonly by AV nodal reentry or reentry over an accessory pathway. They are often called, nonspecifically, paroxysmal supraventricular tachycardia (PSVT) when the mechanism responsible for the tachycardia cannot be determined with certainty (Figs. 5-25 to 5-28). In this section AV nodal reentry is examined. Reentry over an accessory pathway is dealt with in the section on Wolff-Parkinson-White syndrome.

AV nodal reentry is characterized by a rapid, regular tachycardia of sudden onset and termination, occurring at rates generally between 150 and 250 beats/min. Uncommonly the rate may exceed 250 beats/min. Unless aberrant ventricular conduction exists, the QRS complex is normal in contour and duration. The retrograde P wave is usually lost within the QRS complex. AV nodal reentry is most commonly caused by reentry within the AV node, anterogradely over a slowly conducting pathway and retrogradely over a more rapidly conducting pathway (Fig. 5-28).

AV nodal reentry recorded at the onset begins abruptly, usually following a premature atrial complex that conducts with a prolonged PR interval; the abrupt termination is sometimes followed by a brief period of asystole, which results in part from tachycardia-induced depression of sinus nodal automaticity. The RR interval may shorten during the course of the first few beats at the onset or lengthen during the course of the last few beats preceding termination of the tachycardia. Variation in cycle length is usually caused by variation in AV nodal conduction time. The mechanism of the tachycardia is reentry within the AV node (see Fig. 5-91).

**Significance.** AV nodal reentry may occur at any age and is often unassociated with underlying heart disease. The dysrhythmia may be related to specific inciting causes such as overexertion, emotional stimuli, and coffee and smoking, although this is often difficult to prove it may follow a specific pattern, or its onset may be unrelated to any particular event.

Symptoms frequently accompany the attack and range from feelings of palpitations, nervousness, or anxiety to angina, frank heart failure, or shock, depending on the duration and rate of the AV nodal reentry and the presence of organic heart disease. The AV nodal reentry may cause syncope because of the rapid ventricular rate, reduced cardiac output, and cerebral circulation or because of asystole when the AV nodal reentry terminates. The prognosis for patients without heart disease is usually quite good.

**Treatment.** Treatment of the acute attack depends on the clinical situation, how well the AV nodal reentry is tolerated, the natural history of the attacks in the individual patient, and the presence of associated disease. For some patients, rest, reassurance, and sedation may be all that are required to abort an attack.

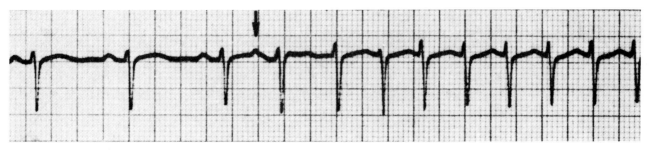

V₁

**Fig. 5-25** **Paroxysmal supraventricular tachycardia.** Three sinus beats are interrupted by a premature atrial complex *(arrow)*, which conducts with PR prolongation and initiates the supraventricular tachycardia.

| | |
|---|---|
| **Rate:** | Sinus rhythm, 83 beats/min; paroxysmal supaventricular tachycardia, 190 beats/min. |
| **Rhythm:** | Regular during sinus rhythm and during paroxysmal supraventricular tachycardia. |
| **P waves:** | Seen in first four beats but not afterward. |
| **PR interval:** | Normal during sinus beats, 0.16 second; slightly prolonged (0.20 second) during premature atrial complex. |
| **QRS:** | Normal, 0.08 second. |
| **Dysrhythmia:** | Sudden initiation of paroxysmal supraventricular tachycardia by a premature atrial complex that conducts with PR prolongation. In the absence of a recognizable P wave (probably buried in the QRS complex). The tachycardia is most likely AV nodal reentry. |

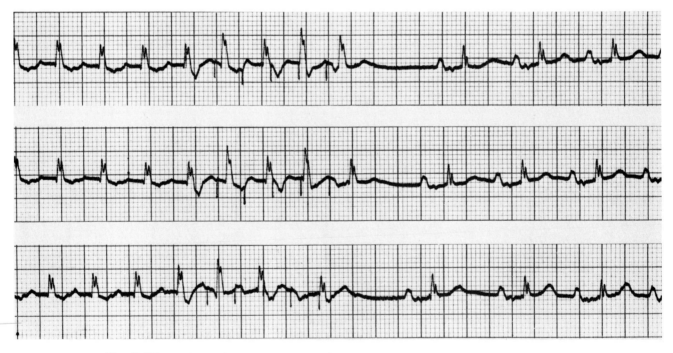

**Fig. 5-26** Initiation of paroxysmal supraventricular tachycardia (PSVT) following a **premature ventricular complex and spontaneous termination of PSVT.** In the top panel, PSVT begins after the fifth QRS complex, which is a premature ventricular complex (PVC). Two interpretations are possible. The first possibility is that the normally conducted sinus complex occurs in the T wave of the PVC and conducts with a prolonged PR interval (i.e., the PVC is interpolated) and initiates PSVT. The second possibility is that the PVC conducts retrogradely to the atrium and initiates the PSVT in that manner. In the bottom strip, the PSVT terminates spontaneously with a slight pause. Monitor lead.

| | |
|---|---|
| **Rate:** | During PSVT, 120 beats/min. |
| **Rhythm:** | Fairly regular during PSVT. |
| **P waves:** | Cannot be seen during PSVT. |
| **PR interval:** | Cannot determine during PSVT. |
| **QRS:** | Normal, 0.07 second. |
| **Dysrhythmia:** | Probably AV nodal reentry. |

**Fig. 5-27** **Pacing-induced termination of PSVT.** The patient had recurrent episodes of PSVT that were easily terminated by rapid atrial pacing. Pacing stimuli can be seen before the onset of sinus rhythm in the midportion of each monitor lead tracing.

| | |
|---|---|
| **Rate:** | During PSVT, 150 beats/min. |
| **Rhythm:** | During PSVT, regular. |
| **P waves:** | Not seen during PSVT. P waves during sinus rhythm are abnormal with a low-amplitude biphasic component following an initial positive component. |
| **PR interval:** | During sinus rhythm, 0.24 second; during PSVT, cannot be discerned. |
| **QRS:** | 0.08 second. |
| **Dysrhythmia:** | AV nodal reentry (documented by invasive electrophysiologic study). |

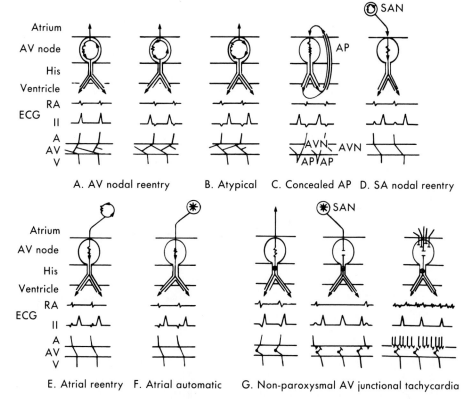

A. AV nodal reentry    B. Atypical   C. Concealed AP   D. SA nodal reentry

E. Atrial reentry   F. Atrial automatic   G. Non-paroxysmal AV junctional tachycardia

**Fig. 5-28**   **Diagrammatic representation of various tachycardias.** In the top portion of
each example is a schematic representation of the presumed anatomic pathways. In the lower
portion the ECG presentation in the explanatory ladder diagram is depicted. **A,** AV nodal
reentry. *Left,* reentrant excitation is confined to the AV node with retrograde atrial activity
occurring simultaneously with ventricular activity, owing to anterograde conduction over
the slow AV nodal pathway and retrograde conduction over the fast AV nodal pathway.
*Right,* atrial activity occurs slightly later than ventricular activity, owing to retrograde conduction delay. **B,** Atypical AV nodal reentry as a result of anterograde conduction over a
fast AV nodal pathway and retrograde conduction over a slow AV nodal pathway. **C,** Concealed accessory pathway (AP). Reciprocating tachycardia is caused by anterograde conduction over the AV node and retrograde conduction over the accessory pathway. Retrograde P
waves occur after the QRS complex. **D,** Sinus nodal reentry. The tachycardia occurs as a
result of reentry within the sinus node, which then conducts to the rest of the heart.
**E,** Atrial reentry. Tachycardia is caused by reentry with the atrium, which then conducts to
the rest of the heart. **F,** Automatic atrial tachycardia. Tachycardia is result of automatic discharge in the atrium, which then conducts to the rest of the heart. It is difficult to distinguish this tachycardia from tachycardia caused by atrial reentry. **G,** Nonparoxysmal AV
junctional tachycardia. Various presentations of this tachycardia are depicted with retrograde
atrial capture, AV dissociation with the sinus node in control of the atria, and AV dissociation with atrial fibrillation. (From Zipes DP: Specific arrhythmias: diagnosis and treatment.
In Braunwald E, editor: Heart disease: textbook of cardiovascular medicine, ed 3, Philadelphia, 1988, WB Saunders Co.)

1. For stable patients, simple vagal maneuvers, including carotid sinus massage, Valsalva, gagging, or activation of the "diving reflex" by ice water facial immersion (in the absence of ischemic heart disease), serve as the first line of therapy and either terminate AV nodal reentry by prolonging AV nodal refractoriness or leave it unaffected (actually, slight slowing may occur during vagal stimulation). These maneuvers should be retried after *each* pharmacologic approach.

2. Verapamil, a calcium antagonist, at a dose of 5 to 10 mg IV, terminates AV nodal reentry successfully in about 2 minutes in over 90% of instances. A second injection may be administered in 15 to 20 minutes if necessary. It has become the preferred treatment if the simple vagal maneuvers fail.[13-15]

3. If signs or symptoms of cardiac decompensation (such as chest pain, dyspnea, hypotension, or congestive heart failure) occur, synchronized cardioversion is the treatment of choice. DC shock, synchronized to the QRS complex to avoid precipitating ventricular fibrillation, successfully terminates AV nodal reentry with energies in the range of 10 to 50 watt-seconds; higher energies may be required in some instances. Short-acting barbiturates like sodium methohexital (Brevital), 50 to 120 mg given IV at a rate of 50 mg/30 seconds, may be used to provide anesthesia, or diazepam (Valium), 5 to 15 mg given IV at a rate of 5 mg/min, may be used to provide sedation and amnesia. Doses must be individualized and in general should be reduced for patients who have heart failure, hypotension, or liver disease. During DC cardioversion a physician skilled in airway management should be in attendance, an IV route established, and all equipment and drugs necessary for emergency resuscitation immediately accessible. One hundred percent oxygen is administered throughout the procedure, employing manually assisted ventilation if necessary. If DC shock becomes necessary in patients who have received large amounts of digitalis, one should begin with 1 to 5 watt-seconds and gradually increase the energy level in increments of approximately 25 to 50 watt-seconds as long as premature ventricular systoles do not result. If premature ventricular systoles occur but can be suppressed with lidocaine or phenytoin, the next higher energy level may be tried.

4. Cholinergic drugs, particularly edrophonium chloride (Tensilon), a short-acting cholinesterase inhibitor, may terminate AV nodal reentry when administered initially at a dose of 3 to 5 mg IV and, if unsuccessful, repeated at a dose of 10 mg IV. Its action is rapid in onset and short in duration, with minimal side effects. Edrophonium chloride should be used cautiously or not at all in patients who are hypotensive or who have lung disease, especially asthmatics.

5. Pressor drugs may terminate AV nodal reentry by inducing reflex vagal stimulation mediated via baroreceptors in the carotid sinus and aorta when the systolic blood pressure is acutely elevated to levels of about 180 mm Hg. One of the following drugs, diluted in 5 to 10 ml of 5% dextrose and water, may be given over a period of 1 to 3 minutes; phenylephrine hydrochloride (Neo-Synephrine), 0.5 to 1.0 mg; methoxamine hydrochloride (Vasoxyl), 3 to 5 mg; or metaraminol (Aramine), 0.5 to 2.0 mg. Pressor drugs should be used cautiously or not at all in the elderly or in patients with organic heart disease, significant hypertension, hyperthyroidism, or acute myocardial infarction. This potentially dangerous and almost always uncomfortable procedure is rarely needed any longer, unless the patient is also hypotensive. Other, safer procedures are preferred.

6. If these approaches are unsuccessful, IV digitalis administration may be attempted next, using one the following short-acting digitalis preparations: ouabain, 0.25 to 0.50 mg IV, followed by 0.1 mg every 30 to 60 minutes if needed, keeping the total dosage less than 1.0 mg within a 24-hour period; digoxin (Lanoxin), 0.5 to 1.0 mg IV, followed by 0.25 mg every 2 to 4 hours, with a total dosage less than 1.5 mg within a 24-hour period; or deslanoside (Cedilanid-D), 0.8 mg IV, followed by 0.4 mg every 2 to 4 hours, restricting the total dosage to less than 2.0 mg within a 24-hour period. Oral digitalis administration to terminate an acute attack is generally not indicated. Vagal maneuvers, previously ineffective, may terminate AV nodal reentry following digitalis administration and therefore should be repeated.

7. Propranolol (Inderal) given IV at a rate of 0.5 to 1 mg/min for a total dose of 1 to 3 mg may be tried if digitalis administration is unsuccessful. Propranolol must be used cautiously, if at all, in patients who have heart failure or chronic lung disease because its adrenergic beta-receptor blocking action depresses myocardial contractility and may produce bronchospasm.

Prior to administering digitalis or propranolol, it is advisable to reassess the clinical status of the patient and consider whether DC cardioversion may be advisable at this stage. DC shock, administered to patients who have received excessive amounts of digitalis, may be dangerous and result in serious postshock ventricular dysrhythmias.

8. In the event that digitalis has been given in large doses and DC shock is contraindicated, right atrial pacing may restore sinus rhythm, presumably by prematurely depolarizing one of the pathways required for continued reentry (Fig. 5-27). In some patients, right atrial pacing may precipitate atrial fibrillation;

however, because the latter is generally accompanied by a slower ventricular rate, the patient's clinical status improves.

9. Procainamide (Pronestyl), quinidine, or disopyramide (Norpace) may be required to terminte AV nodal reentry in some patients. Unless contraindicated, DC cardioversion should be employed prior to using these agents, which are more often administered to prevent recurrences.

Prevention of recurrences is often more difficult than terminating the acute episode. Smoking, alcohol, or excessive fatigue, if identified as precipitating factors, should be avoided. Initially, one must decide whether the frequency and severity of the attacks warrant drug prophylaxis. For example, an attempt should probably not be made to suppress AV nodal reentry occurring twice yearly in an otherwise healthy patient.

1. If drug prophylaxis is indicated, digitalis is the initial drug of choice. The speed at which digitalization is achieved is determined by the clinical situation. Using digoxin, rapid oral digitalization can be accomplished in 24 to 36 hours with an initial dose of 1.0 to 1.5 mg, followed by 0.25 to 0.5 mg every 6 hours for a total dose of 2.0 to 3.0 mg. A less rapid oral regimen digitalizes in 2 to 3 days with an initial dose of 0.75 to 1.0 mg, followed by 0.25 to 0.5 mg every 12 hours for a total dose of 2.0 to 3.0 mg. Alternatively, digoxin administered as a maintenance dose of 0.125 to 0.5 mg achieves digitalization in about 1 week. Because of its shorter half-life, digoxin may provide more effective control when administered twice daily. Digitoxin, which has a longer duration of action, may be used instead of digoxin. Oral digitalization with digitoxin may be accomplished in 24 to 36 hours with an initial dose of 0.5 to 0.8 mg, followed by 0.2 mg every 6 to 8 hours until reaching a total dose of 1.2 mg. A slower approach involves administering 0.2 mg three times daily for 2 to 3 days. Complete digitalization can also be accomplished in about 1 month by simply giving a maintenance dose of 0.05 to 0.2 mg daily.

2. If digitalis alone is unsuccessful, one can then add quinidine, 200 to 400 mg every 6 hours, or propranolol (Inderal), 10 to 40 mg every 6 hours. Verapamil (80 to 120 mg every 6 to 8 hours) combined with digitalis may be very effective treatment.

3. If a combination of digitalis and quinidine or digitalis and propranolol is unsuccessful, concomitant administration of all three drugs, that is, digitalis, quinidine, and propranolol, may be tried. If this regimen also fails, empiric trials with other antidysrhythmic agents such as procainamide or disopyramide may be warranted. Flecainide or amiodarone often is effective in patients with supraventricular tachycardia but is investigational for that purpose.

4. For many patients, pacemaker implantation is an acceptable treatment. Rapid atrial pacing promptly terminates AV nodal reentry, restoring sinus rhythm immediately or sometimes after a transient episode of atrial fibrillation. Some pacemaker units need to be activated by the patient when AV nodal reentry occurs; other units discharge automatically when they detect the onset of AV nodal reentry. Such pacing devices can be combined with drug therapy.

5. Ablation of the AV node—His bundle area by catheter or surgical techniques may be indicated on occasion to eliminate episodes of the tachycardia. Such an approach may make the patient pacemaker-dependent if complete AV heart block results.

## PREEXCITATION (WOLFF-PARKINSON-WHITE) SYNDROME (Figs. 5-29 to 5-38)

Ventricular preexcitation[1,8,16] exists when the atrial impulse activates the whole or some part of ventricular muscle earlier than would be expected if the atrial impulse reached the ventricles by way of the normal specialized conduction system only. Four basic features typify the usual ECG of a patient with the preexcitation (Wolff-Parkinson-White [WPW]) syndrome: (1) PR interval less than 0.12 second during sinus rhythm, (2) QRS complex duration greater than 0.12 second with a slurred, slow-rising onset of the R wave upstroke in some leads (delta wave) and usually normal terminal QRS portion, (3) secondary ST-T wave changes that are usually directed opposite the major delta and QRS vectors, and (4) paroxysmal tachydysrhythmias in many patients (the exact percentage varies widely, from 4% to 80%, and depends on the patient population studied). The explanation for those ECG findings is the presence of a rapidly-conducting muscular accessory pathway connection that bypasses the AV node by communicating directly from atrium to ventricle. Other patients may possess variants of the preexcitation syndrome that are explained by the presence of bypass tracts between the AV node and ventricle (nodoventricular) or between the fascicles and ventricle (fasciculoventricular). The group of patients who have a short PR interval (less than 0.12 second) and a normal QRS complex with supraventricular tachycardias most often do not have a bypass tract from atrium to His bundle (so-called Lown-Ganong-Levine syndrome). These patients may simply possess an AV node that conducts rapidly and also have episodes of supraventricular tachycardia (Fig. 5-29).

The site of the accessory pathway can be determined by a careful analysis of the spatial direction of the delta wave in maximally preexcited QRS complexes (Fig. 5-34), as well as from electric recordings made directly on the heart using catheters during an electrophysiologic study or at the time of open heart surgery. Once identified, the accessory pathway can be interrupted surgically or by other ablation techniques.

Because of the accessory pathway, two parallel routes of AV conduction are possible, one subject to physiologic delay over the AV node and the other passing directly without delay over the accessory pathway from atrium to ventricle. This produces the typical QRS complex that is a fusion beat caused by depolarization of the ventricle in part by the wavefront traveling over the accessory pathway and in part by the wavefront traveling over the normal AV node-His bundle route. The delta wave represents ventricular activation from input over the accessory pathway. The extent of contribution to ventricular depolarization by the wavefront over each route depends on the relative activation time of each wavefront.

The usual tachycardia is characterized by anterograde conduction over the normal pathway and retrograde con-

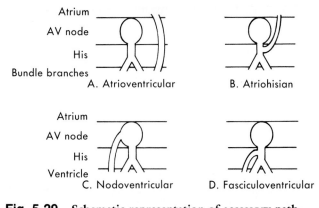

**Fig. 5-29** Schematic representation of accessory pathways. **A,** The usual atrioventricular connection often called a Kent bundle. **B,** Atriohisian bypass tract in which the connection is from the atrium to the His bundle, thus bypassing the AV node. **C,** Nodoventricular connection from the AV node to the ventricle. **D,** Fasciculoventricular connection from the His bundle or bundle branches to the ventricle. (From Zipes DP: Specific arrhythmias: diagnosis and treatment. In Braunwald E, editor: Heart disease: a textbook of cardiovascular medicine, Philadelphia, ed 3, 1988, WB Saunders Co.)

duction over the accessory pathway, which results in a normal QRS complex at rates of 150 to 250/min. Because the reentrant loop involves atria and ventricles, the tachycardia is called an atrioventricular reciprocating tachycardia (AVRT). In contrast to most patients who have AV nodal reentry, the retrograde P wave during AVRT occurs in the ST segment.

The rhythm of AVRT may change spontaneously into atrial flutter or atrial fibrillation, and patients with Wolff-Parkinson-White syndrome may have other types of tachycardia as well. Patients who have atrial fibrillation almost always have AVRT that can be induced during electrophysiologic study. Atrial fibrillation presents a potentially serious risk because of the possibility for rapid conduction over the accessory pathway and rapid ventricular rates. On occasion, ventricular fibrillation may result.

**Significance.** The reported incidence of the preexcitation syndrome averages about 1.5 in 1000 persons, although the actual incidence is unknown. It occurs in all age groups and more often (60% to 70%) in males. Two thirds of patients with the short PR interval and normal QRS complex are female. Patients may seek help because of recurrent supraventricular tachycardia, atrial fibrillation with a rapid ventricular response, heart failure, syncope, or symptoms related to associated cardiac anomalies; or the symptoms may be discovered during examintion for noncardiac-related reasons. Of adults with preexcitation syndrome, 60% to 70% have normal hearts; a higher proportion of children have heart disease. A variety of acquired and congenital cardiac defects have been reported in patients with the preexcitation syndrome, including Eb-

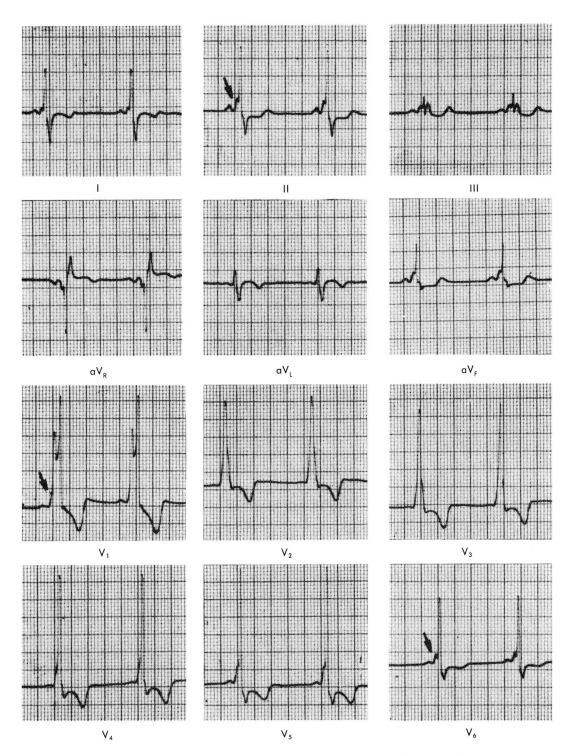

**Fig. 5-30** **Twelve-lead ECG illustrating preexcitation (Wolff-Parkinson-White) syndrome.** Arrows indicate delta waves. The short PR interval is apparent. The vector of the delta wave suggests that the accessory pathway is in a left anterior (position 9) or left anterior paraseptal (position 10) position. See Fig. 5-34 for position.

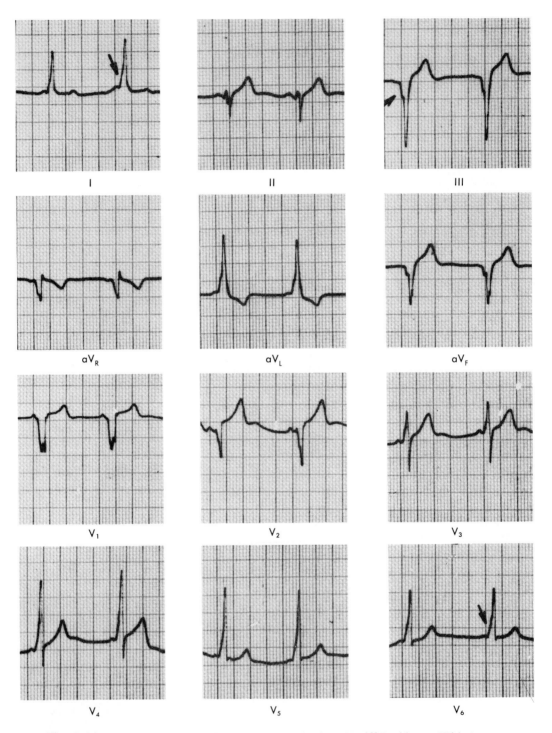

**Fig. 5-31**   **Twelve-lead ECG illustrating preexcitation (Wolff-Parkinson-White) syndrome.** Arrows indicate delta waves. The short PR interval is apparent. The vector of the delta wave suggests accessory pathway is located in a right lateral (area 3) position (see Fig. 5-34).

stein's anomaly, cardiomyopathies, and mitral valve prolapse.

Of patients with the preexcitation syndrome who have recurrent tachydysrhythmias, 80% have AVRT, 15% to 30% have atrial fibrillation, and 5% have atrial flutter. Ventricular tachycardia rarely occurs, and most reports have misdiagnosed as ventricular tachycardia the aberrant QRS complexes caused by anomalous conduction. Recognition of the preexcitation syndrome is clinically important, since the tachydysrhythmias at times do not respond to conventional therapy and may be associated with very rapid ventricular rates. For example, digitalis may accelerate the ventricular rate in some patients who have atrial fibrillation and the WPW syndrome. The anomalous complexes may mask or mimic myocardial infarction, bundle branch block, or ventricular hypertrophy, and the presence of the preexcitation syndrome may call attention to an associated cardiac defect.

The prognosis is excellent in patients without tachycardia or associated cardiac anomaly. In most patients with recurrent tachycardia the prognosis is good, but sudden unexpected death can occur, especially when the ventricular rate during atrial fibrillation is rapid or associated congenital defects are present. Ventricular fibrillation has been documented in humans and in dogs with WPW syndrome and is probably caused by extremely rapid ventricular rates, permitted by the bypass during atrial flutter or fibrillation that exceed the ability of the ventricle to follow in an organized fashion. Consequently, fragmented, disorga-nized ventricular activation results and leads to ventricular fibrillation. Alternatively, supraventricular discharge, by-passing the AV nodal delay, may activate the ventricle during the vulnerable period of the antecedent T wave and precipitate ventricular fibrillation.

**Treatment.**[7,9,16] Patients with ventricular preexcitation who have none or only occasional episodes of tachydys-rhythmias unassociated with significant symptoms do not require electrophysiologic evaluation or therapy. However, if the patient has frequent episodes of tachydysrhythmia and/or the dysrhythmias cause significant symptoms, therapy should be instituted.

Drugs that increase the refractory period, slow conduction, or cause block in one of the reentrant pathways may suppress reciprocating tachycardia. Verapamil, propranolol, and digitalis prolong conduction time and refractoriness in the AV node. Verapamil and propranolol do not directly affect conduction in the accessory pathway, whereas digitalis has variable effects. However, because digitalis has been reported to shorten refractoriness in the accessory pathway and speed the ventricular response in some patients with atrial fibrillation, it is advisable not to use digitalis as a single drug in patients with the WPW syndrome who have or may develop atrial flutter or atrial fibrillation. Since many patients may develop atrial flutter or fibrillation during the reciprocating tachycardia, the caveat about digitalis probably applies to all patients who have tachycardia and the WPW syndrome.

*Text continued on p. 146.*

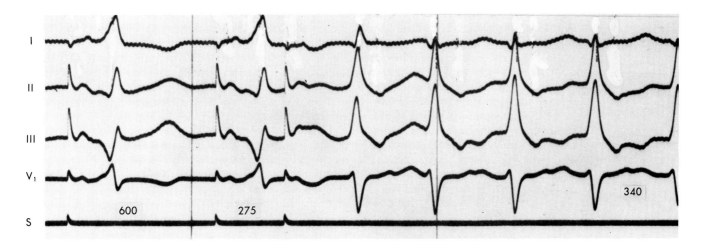

**Fig. 5-32**   **Onset of reciprocating tachycardia in a patient with preexcitation (WPW) syndrome.** The first two beats are paced from the right atrium (cycle length 600 msec) and conduct over the accessory pathway. The third beat is premature (275 msec) and conducts over the normal AV node—His bundle (note loss of delta wave). Following this a recipro-cating tachycardia in a patient with Wolff-Parkinson-White syndrome. *S,* Stimulus.

Reciprocating tachycardias

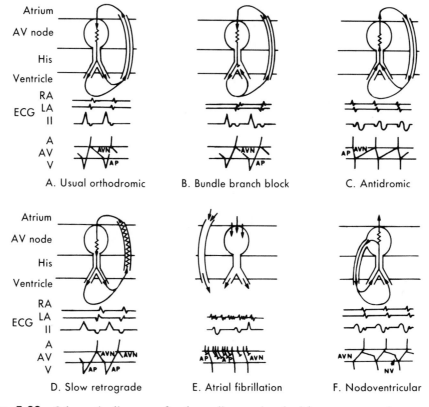

**Fig. 5-33** **Schematic diagram of tachycardia associated with accessory pathways.** **A,** Usual (orthodromic) form of tachycardia with anterograde conduction over the AV node—His bundle route and retrograde conduction over the accessory pathway (left-sided as depicted here by left atrial activation preceding right atrial activation). **B,** Usual (orthodromic) form of tachycardia and functional bundle branch block on the same side as the accessory pathway. **C,** Unusual (antidromic) form of tachycardia with anterograde conduction over the accessory pathway and retrograde conduction over the AV node—His bundle route. **D,** Orthodromic tachycardia with a slowly conducting accessory pathway. **E,** Atrial fibrillation conducting over the accessory pathway and the AV node. **F,** Nodoventricular tachycardia with anterograde conduction over a portion of the AV node and a nodoventricular pathway and retrograde conduction over the AV node. (From Zipes DP: Specific arrhythmias: diagnosis and treatment. In Braunwald E, editor: Heart disease: a textbook of cardiovascular medicine, ed 3, Philadelphia, 1988, WB Saunders Co.)

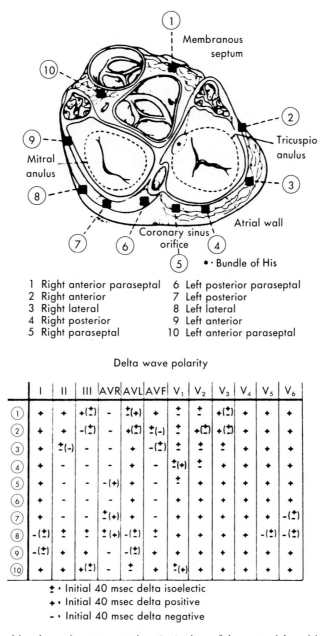

1 Right anterior paraseptal   6 Left posterior paraseptal
2 Right anterior              7 Left posterior
3 Right lateral               8 Left lateral
4 Right posterior             9 Left anterior
5 Right paraseptal           10 Left anterior paraseptal

Delta wave polarity

|    | I | II | III | AVR | AVL | AVF | V$_1$ | V$_2$ | V$_3$ | V$_4$ | V$_5$ | V$_6$ |
|----|---|----|-----|-----|-----|-----|----|----|----|----|----|----|
| 1  | + | + | +(±) | − | ±(+) | + | ± | ± | +(±) | + | + | + |
| 2  | + | + | −(±) | − | +(±) | ±(−) | ± | +(±) | +(±) | + | + | + |
| 3  | + | ±(−) | − | − | + | −(±) | ± | ± | ± | + | + | + |
| 4  | + | − | − | − | + | − | ±(+) | ± | + | + | + | + |
| 5  | + | − | − | −(+) | + | − | ± | + | + | + | + | + |
| 6  | + | − | − | + | + | − | + | + | + | + | + | + |
| 7  | + | − | − | ±(+) | + | − | + | + | + | + | + | −(±) |
| 8  | −(±) | ± | ± | ±(+) | −(±) | ± | + | + | + | + | −(±) | −(±) |
| 9  | −(±) | + | + | −(±) | + | + | + | + | + | + | + | + |
| 10 | + | + | +(±) | − | ± | + | ±(+) | + | + | + | + | + |

± · Initial 40 msec delta isoelectic
+ · Initial 40 msec delta positive
− · Initial 40 msec delta negative

**Fig. 5-34**   In this schematic representation *(top),* sites of the potential position of the accessory pathways are indicated by filled boxes numbered 1 through 10. Delta wave polarity in the 12-lead ECG for each of the 10 sites is depicted in the table at the bottom. (From Gallagher JJ and others: Prog Cardiovasc Dis 20:285, 1978.)

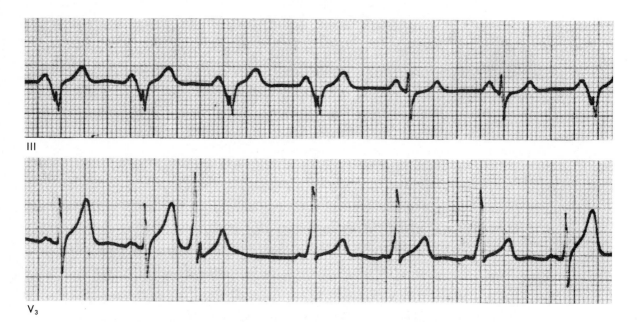

III

V₃

**Fig. 5-35** **Preexcitation (Wolff-Parkinson-White) syndrome.** Spontaneous onset and termination of preexcitation conduction account for the variable QRS conduction in lead III and V₃. The fifth and sixth QRS complexes in III and the first, second, and last QRS complexes in V₃ are normally conducted. In lead V₃ the onset of anomalous conduction follows a premature atrial complex (third QRS) with a Wolff-Parkinson-White pattern. This patient was erroneously admitted to the coronary care unit because of the Q waves in lead III, which were misinterpreted as indicating an inferior myocardial infarction.

| | |
|---|---|
| **Rate:** | 78 beats/min. |
| **Rhythm:** | Regular. |
| **P waves:** | Normal. |
| **PR interval:** | Varies between 0.10 and 0.13 second. |
| **QRS:** | Normal (0.08 second) during conduction over the AV node with a normal PR interval; abnormal (0.12 second) during conduction over the bypass tract with a short PR interval. |

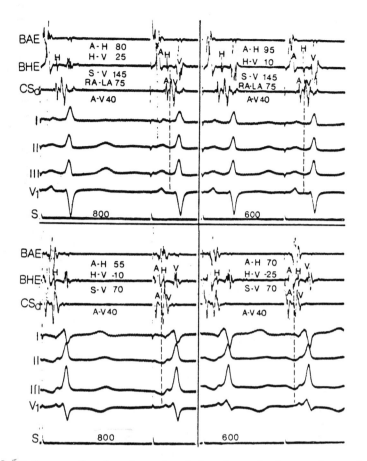

**Fig. 5-36** Influence of pacing site and cycle length on the degree of preexcitation. In this patient with a left anterolateral accessory pathway (site 9 in Fig. 5-34), pacing the high right atrium at a cycle length of 800 msec *(top left panel)* produced an A-H interval of 80 msec and an H-V interval of 25 msec. The interval from the stimulus to the onset of ventricular activity *(S-V)* was 145 msec and the right-to-left atrial activation time was 75 msec. The interrupted line indicates the onset of the delta wave. Little preexcitation is seen in the ECG because the fairly rapid AV conduction time over the normal pathway allows much of the ventricle to be activated normally before the impulse traveling from right to left atrium and then over the accessory pathway can depolarize the ventricles. Shortening the pacing cycle length to 600 msec *(top right panel)* without changing the pacing site lengthened the A-H interval by 15 msec and shortened the H-V interval by 10 msec. The other intervals remained the same and the QRS complex changed very slightly. The coronary sinus is paced at a cycle length of 800 msec *(bottom left panel)*. Even though the A-H interval shortens to 55 msec because of coronary sinus pacing, the S-V shortens to 70 msec, His bundle activation follows the onset of ventricular depolarization by 10 msec, and the QRS complex becomes more aberrant. By pacing at a site near the atrial insertion of the accessory pathway, conduction rapidly reaches the ventricle over the accessory pathway to activate more of the ventricle than when pacing the right atrium at the same cycle length. Shortening the pacing cycle length to 600 msec *(bottom right panel)* lengthens the A-H interval 15 msec, and His bundle activation begins 25 msec after the onset of QRS complex. S-V and A-V intervals remain unchanged and the QRS complex becomes even more aberrant. (From Zipes DP: Specific arrhythmias: diagnosis and treatment. In Braunwald E, editor: Heart disease: a textbook of cardiovascular medicine, ed 3, Philadelphia, 1988, WB Saunders Co.)

Drugs, such as quinidine (see the box on p. 147), that prolong the refractory period in the accessory pathway should be used to treat patients with atrial flutter or fibrillation. Lidocaine does not prolong refractoriness of the accessory pathway in patients whose effective refractory period is less than 300 msec. Verapamil and lidocaine given intravenously may increase the ventricular rate during atrial fibrillation in patients with the WPW syndrome.

Termination of the acute episode of AVRT, suspected electrocardiographically by a normal QRS complex, regular RR intervals at rate of about 200 beats/min, and a P wave in the ST segment, should be approached as for AV nodal reentry. For atrial flutter or fibrillation, drugs that prolong refractoriness in the accessory pathway—often coupled with drugs that prolong AV nodal refractoriness (for example, quinidine and propranolol) or a drug that affects both pathways (for example, encainide or amiodarone)—must be used. In some patients, particularly those with a very rapid ventricular response during atrial fibrillation, electric cardioversion should be the initial treatment of choice.

For long-term therapy to prevent a recurrence, drugs are selected on the basis of their effects on the AV node or accessory pathway. Invasive electrophysiologic studies are often necessary.

Some patients may require surgical ablation of the accessory pathway, particularly when symptomatic tachydysrhythmias are recurrent or incompletely controlled by

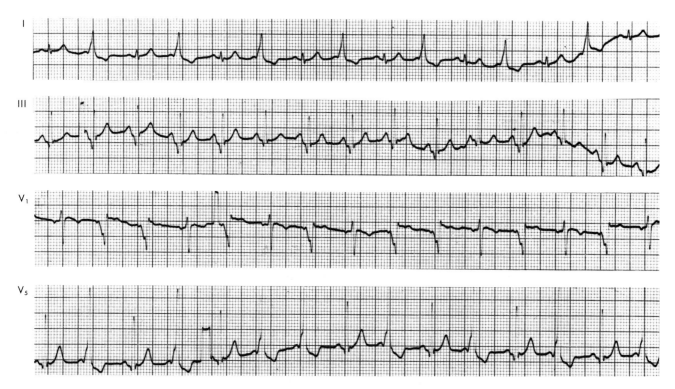

**Fig. 5-37** **Alternating conduction over the accessory pathway in preexcitation (Wolff-Parkinson-White) syndrome during normal sinus rhythm.** Almost throughout the recording, the QRS complexes alternate between conduction over the accessory pathway and conduction over the normal pathway. Occasionally two consecutive beats conduct over the accessory pathway. Conduction over the accessory pathway is characterized by a short PR interval, delta wave, prolonged QRS duration, and secondary T wave changes. Such intermittent conduction over an accessory pathway suggests that its refractory period is prolonged and implies that extremely rapid rates during atrial flutter or atrial fibrillation, as seen in Fig. 5-38, would not occur.

| | |
|---|---|
| **Rate:** | 105 beats/min. |
| **Rhythm:** | Regular. |
| **P waves:** | Normal. |
| **PR interval:** | Alternating between 0.08 and 0.12 second. |
| **QRS:** | Normal, 0.06 second during conduction over the AV node abnormal, 0.12 second, during conduction over the accessory pathway. |

drugs or are associated with rapid ventricular rates. Improved surgical techniques now permit surgery as a logical therapy for a young person who would otherwise face many years of drug management.

For patients who are symptomatic because of drug-refractory, recurrent tachycardia, surgery to interrupt the accessory pathway has been extremely useful.[7]

It is now known that some patients who have supraventricular tachycardia without any overt evidence of WPW may have an accessory pathway that only conducts retrogradely (concealed WPW).[16] The surface ECG during AVRT may provide some clues about the presence of a concealed accessory pathway by demonstrating the retrograde P wave to be in the ST segment (rather than simultaneous with the QRS, as in AV nodal reentry) and, if the accessory pathway is left-sided, a negative P wave in lead I. Naturally, the short PR interval, delta wave, and prolonged QRS duration during sinus rhythm are not present.

## DRUG THERAPY IN WPW SYNDROME

| AFFECTS AV NODE | AFFECTS ACCESSORY PATHWAY | AFFECTS BOTH |
|---|---|---|
| Digitalis | Quinidine | Flecainide |
| Propranolol | Procainamide | Encainide |
| Verapamil | Disopyramide | Amiodarone |
| Vagal stimulation | | |

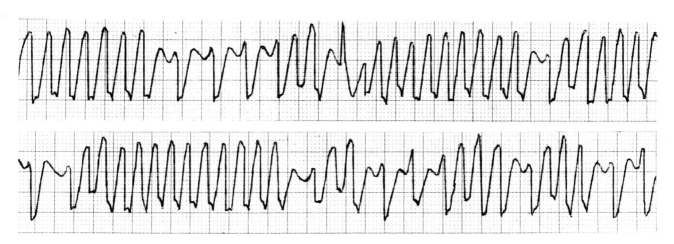

**Fig. 5-38** **Atrial fibrillation with an extremely rapid ventricular response in a patient who has preexcitation (Wolff-Parkinson-White) syndrome.** In this monitor lead the extremely rapid ventricular rates and gross irregularity of the RR intervals (remember, ventricular tachycardia can be irregular also; see Fig. 5-57) suggest the diagnosis of atrial fibrillation in a patient who has Wolff-Parkinson-White syndrome. The atrial fibrillatory impulses conduct to the ventricle over the accessory pathway, bypassing the AV node.

| | |
|---|---|
| **Rate:** | Atrial, indeterminant; ventricular, 150 to 350 beats/min. |
| **Rhythm:** | Irregular. |
| **P waves:** | Cannot be seen. |
| **PR interval:** | Cannot be determined. |
| **QRS:** | Difficult to determine, but approximately 0.12 to 0.14 second. |

## ATRIAL FLUTTER (Figs. 5-39 to 5-42)

Atrial flutter is an atrial tachydysrhythmia characterized electrocardiographically by identically recurring, regular, sawtooth-shaped flutter waves and evidence of continual electric activity (lack of an isoelectric interval between flutter waves), often best visualized in leads II, III, $aV_F$, or $V_1$. Commonly the flutter waves appear inverted in these leads. Less commonly the flutter waves are upright (positive) in these leads. In most instances, reentry in the atria causes atrial flutter. If the AV conduction ratio remains constant, the ventricular rhythm will be regular; if the ratio of conducted beats varies (usually the result of a Wenckebach AV block), the ventricular rhythm will be irregular. Impure flutter (flutter-fibrillation), occurring at a faster rate than pure flutter, shows variability in the contour and spacing of the flutter waves and may represent dissimilar atrial rhythms, that is, fibrillation in one atrium or part of the atrium and a slower, more regular rhythm in the opposite atrium.

The atrial rate during atrial flutter is usually 250 to 350 beats/min; antidysrhythmic drugs such as quinidine or procainamide may reduce the rate to 200 beats/min. In patients who have untreated atrial flutter the ventricular rate is usually half the atrial rate, that is, 150 beats/min. A significantly slower ventricular rate (in the absence of drugs) suggests abnormal AV conduction. Atrial flutter in children, in patients who have the preexcitation syndrome or hyperthyroidism, and occasionally in otherwise normal adults may conduct to the ventricle in a 1:1 fashion, producing a ventricular rate of 300 beats/min. In patients whose atrial flutter rate has been slowed by drugs, 1:1 conduction to the ventricle may also occur.

**Significance.** Atrial flutter is a less common tachydysrhythmia than is atrial fibrillation. Although paroxysmal atrial flutter usually indicates the presence of cardiac disease, it may occur in normal hearts. Chronic (persistent) atrial flutter rarely occurs in the absence of underlying heart disease. Atrial flutter usually responds to carotid sinus massage with a decrease in ventricular rate in stepwise multiples, reversing to the former ventricular rate at the termination of carotid massage. The ratio of conducted atrial impulses to ventricular responses is most often of an even number, for example, 2:1 or 4:1. Very rarely will sinus rhythm follow carotid sinus massage. Exercise, by enhancing sympathetic tone, lessening parasympathetic tone, or both, may reduce the AV conduction delay and produce an increase in the ventricular rate.

**Treatment.** Treatment for atrial flutter, aimed at slowing the ventricular rate, is as follows:

1. Synchronous DC cardioversion is commonly the preferred initial treatment for atrial flutter, since it promptly and effectively restores sinus rhythm with initial energy of 25 watt-seconds. If DC shock results in atrial fibrillation, a second shock of 100 watt-seconds may be used to restore sinus rhythm, or,

depending on the clinical circumstance, the atrial fibrillation may be left untreated. The untreated fibrillation will usually revert to atrial flutter or sinus rhythm.

2. If the patient cannot be cardioverted or the DC cardioversion is contraindicated (for example, after administering large amounts of digitalis), rapid atrial pacing can effectively terminate atrial flutter in many patients.

3. If the patient cannot be cardioverted or if the atrial flutter recurs at frequent intervals, therapy with a short-acting digitalis preparation, such as digoxin should be prescribed. The dose of digitalis necessary to slow the ventricular response varies and at times may result in toxic levels because it is often difficult to slow the ventricular rate during atrial flutter. Frequently, atrial fibrillation develops after digitalization, and it may revert to normal sinus rhythm on withdrawal of digitalis; occasionally, normal sinus rhythm may occur without intervening atrial fibrillation.

4. Verapamil, in an initial bolus of 5 mg IV with a repeat dose of 10 mg IV in 15 to 20 minutes followed by a constant infusion at a rate of 0.005 mg/kg/min, may be used to slow the ventricular response. Peak therapeutic effects occur within 3 to 5 minutes of bolus injection.[13] Verapamil less commonly restores sinus rhythm in patients who have atrial flutter.

5. If the atrial flutter persists after digitalization, quinidine, 200 to 400 mg orally every 6 hours, is used to restore sinus rhythm. Large doses of quinidine, formerly used to terminate atrial flutter prior to the development of DC cardioversion, are no longer warranted. If atrial flutter persists after digitalis and quinidine adminstration, termination may be attempted with DC cardioversion and the patient may be maintained on both digitalis and quinidine following reversion to sinus rhythm. Sometimes, treatment of the specific, underlying disorder, for example, thyrotoxicosis, is necessary to effect conversion to sinus rhythm.

6. In certain instances atrial flutter may continue, and if the ventricular rate can be controlled with digitalis, conversion may not be indicated. Quinidine maintenance therapy should be discontinued if flutter remains. It is important to remember that quinidine and procainamide should *not* be used unless the patient is fully digitalized. Both drugs have a vagolytic action and also directly slow the atrial rate. These two effects may facilitate AV conduction sufficiently to result in a 1:1 ventricular response to the atrial flutter, unless digitalis has been administered previously.

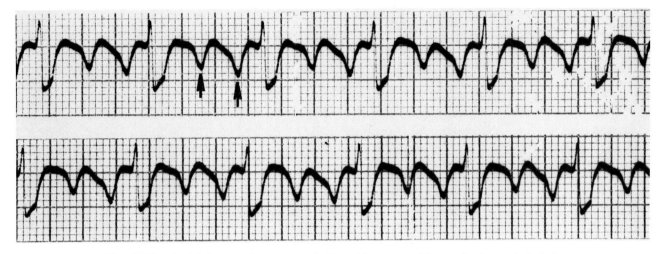

**Fig. 5-39   Atrial flutter.** Flutter waves indicated by arrows. The conduction ratio is 3:1, that is, three flutter waves to one QRS complex and is a less common conduction ration than is 2:1 or 4:1. Monitor lead.

**Rate:**         Atrial, 270 beats/min; ventricular, 90 beats/min.
**Rhythm:**       Atrial, regular; ventricular, regular.
**P waves:**      Flutter waves with regular oscillations resembling a sawtooth pattern are apparent.
**PR interval:**  Flutter-R interval is constant. Assuming that the flutter wave immediately preceding
                  the QRS complex conducts to the ventricle, the flutter-R interval is approximately
                  0.18 second.
**QRS:**          0.12 second.

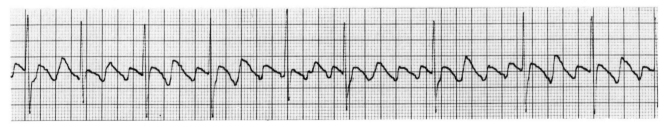

**Fig. 5-40   Atrial flutter rate slowed by an antidysrhythmic agent.** The atrial flutter in this patient had a rate of 300 beats/min before therapy but was slowed by an experimental antidysrhythmic agent, amiodarone. Monitor lead.

**Rate:**         Atrial, 220 beats/min; ventricular, 52 to 86 beats/min.
**Rhythm:**       Atrial, regular; ventricular, irregular.
**P waves:**      Flutter waves are apparent.
**PR interval:**  The flutter-R interval varies as the conduction ratio varies.
**QRS:**          Normal, 0.08 second.

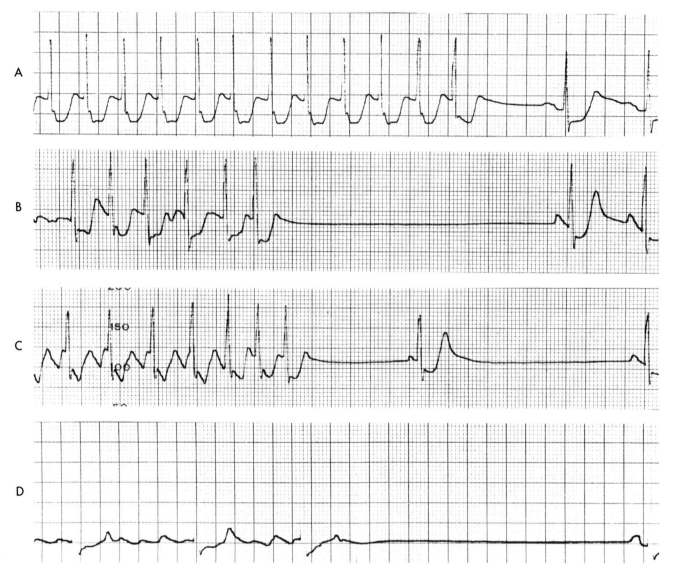

**Fig. 5-41** **Termination of multiple supraventricular tachycardias.** In panel *A*, paroxysmal supraventricular tachycardia abruptly terminates with only a short pause before restoration of sinus rhythm. In panels *B* and *C*, atrial flutter-fibrillation and pure atrial flutter, respectively, terminate on separate occasions in the same patient. In panel *B*, a fairly long period of asystole results before restoration of the first sinus beat while the lengthy pause is interrupted by an escape beat in panel *C*. In panel *D*, termination of atrial flutter-fibrillation in another patient results in a long period of asystole before the first sinus beat occurs. The long pauses in *B*, *C*, and *D* are consistent with sick sinus syndrome and episodes of bradycardia-tachycardia. Monitor leads.

| | |
|---|---|
| **Rate:** | 158 beats/min in panel *A*; varying ventricular rate, approximately 150 beats/min in panel *B*; 136 beats/min in panel *C*; 48 beats/min in panel *D*. |
| **Rhythm:** | Atrial and ventricular rhythm regular in panel *A*; atrial and ventricular rhythm irregular in panel *B*; atrial rhythm regular and ventricular rhythm irregular in panel *C*; atrial rhythm and ventricular rhythm irregular in panel *D*. |
| **PR interval:** | Not measurable. |
| **QRS:** | Normal in all panels. |

7. Propranolol effectively diminishes the ventricular response to atrial flutter and may be used together with digitalis in patients in whom the ventricular rate is not decreased after digitalization. Propranolol does not appear to affect the atrial rate during atrial flutter.

8. Uncommonly, atrial flutter may be resistant to cardioversion as well as to the AV blocking effects of digitalis. Rapid atrial pacing, on a temporary or permanent basis, may be used to convert flutter to fibrillation with a decrease in the ventricular rate.

9. Rarely, neostigmine (Prostigmin), 0.25 to 0.5 mg subcutaneously, or edrophonium (Tensilon), 0.25 to 2.0 mg/min in an IV solution, may be administered over a few days to control the ventricular rate.

Prevention of recurrent atrial flutter is often difficult to achieve but should be approached as outlined for the prevention of PSVT caused by AV nodal reentry. If recurrences cannot be prevented, the aim of therapy is directed toward a controlled ventricular rate when the flutter does recur, with digitalis alone or combined with propranolol, or with oral verapamil.

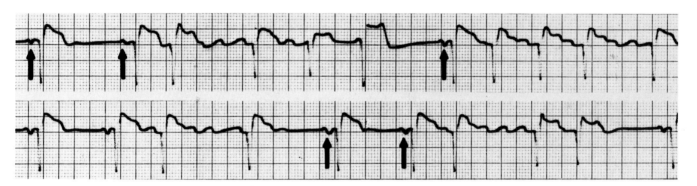

**Fig. 5-42  Intermittent atrial flutter.** Atrial flutter starts and stops intermittently throughout this continuous recording. Monitor lead.

| | |
|---|---|
| **Rate and Rhythm:** | Both atrial and ventricular rate and rhythm vary. |
| **P waves:** | Precede same QRS complexes. Atrial flutter waves precede other QRS complexes. Several P waves indicated by arrows. |
| **PR interval:** | 0.14 second when it can be measured. |
| **QRS:** | 0.08 second. |

## ATRIAL FIBRILLATION (Figs. 5-43 and 5-44)

Atrial fibrillation is characterized by a total disorganization of atrial activity without effective atrial contraction. The ECG reveals small deflections appearing for the most part as irregular baseline undulations of variable amplitude and contour at a rate of 305 to 600/min. The ventricular response is totally irregular, and if the patient is untreated, the rate is usually between 100 and 160 beats/min. Carotid sinus massage slows the ventricular rate, but the ventricular rhythm remains completely irregular. The conversion of atrial flutter to atrial fibrillation is usually accompanied by a *slowing* of the ventricular rate because more atrial impulses become blocked at the AV node. As a result, it is generally easier to slow the ventricular rate with digitalis during atrial fibrillation than during atrial flutter. When the ventricular rhythm becomes regular in patients with atrial fibrillation, four explanations are possible: conversion to sinus rhythm, conversion to atrial flutter, development of atrial tachycardia, or development of an independent junctional or ventricular rhythm (or tachycardia) controlling the ventricles and giving rise to AV dissociation. In the last two instances, digitalis intoxication must be suspected. If after a period of regularization the ventricular rhythm becomes irregular again in a patient who has been given an excessive amount of digitalis, it may be caused by an exit block, generally of the Wenckebach type from the junctional or ventricular focus.

Because irregular ventricular cycle lengths cause changes in ventricular refractoriness (long cycles lengthening refractoriness and short cycles shortening refractoriness), when a short ventricular cycle follows a long ventricular cycle, aberrant ventricular conduction may occur, generally of right bundle branch block configuration. This is called the Ashman phenomenon (see Figs. 5-103 and 5-109).

**Significance.** Similar to other tachydysrhythmias, atrial fibrillation may be chronic or intermittent; the former is almost always associated with underlying heart disease, whereas the latter may occur in clinically normal patients. Underlying heart disease is more frequent in patients who have atrial fibrillation than in patients who have atrial flutter. The dysrhythmia is commonly seen in patients who have rheumatic mitral stenosis, thyrotoxicosis, cardiomyopathy, hypertensive heart disease, pericarditis, and coronary heart disease.

Approximately 30% of all patients who have atrial fibrillation have systemic or pulmonary emboli. Such a catastrophe is most common in patients who have rheumatic mitral valvular disease. Of the emboli that occur in patients with mitral stenosis, 90% occur in patients who have atrial fibrillation.

**Treatment.** It is of paramount importance in treating the patient who has atrial fibrillation for the first time to search for a precipitating cause. Thyrotoxicosis, mitral stenosis, acute myocardial infarction, pericarditis, and other known associated causes should be considered.

1. Initial therapy is determined by the patient's clinical status. The primary therapeutic objective is to slow the ventricular rate and, secondarily, to restore atrial systole. DC cardioversion may accomplish both of these objectives. If the sudden onset of atrial fibrillation with a rapid ventricular rate results in acute cardiovascular decompensation, DC cardioversion is the preferred treatment, beginning with 100 watt-seconds.

2. In the absence of hemodynamic decompensation the patient may be given digitalis to maintain a resting apical rate of 60 to 80 beats/min, which does not exceed 100 beats/min after slight exercise. The speed, route, dosage, and type of digitalis preparation administered are determined by the degree of cardiovascular compensation (see the discussion of the treatment of AV nodal reentry). The ventricular rate cannot be slowed sufficiently by digitalis administration in some patients, and digitalis toxicity may result before slowing the ventricular rate. In such cases, complicating factors such as pulmonary emboli, atelectasis, myocarditis, infection, congestive heart failure, and hyperthyroidism should be excluded and treated if found. In some instances[11] verapamil may be useful (see atrial flutter).

3. The combined use of digitalis and propranolol or digitalis and verapamil may be used to slow the ventricular rate when digitalis alone fails. Occasionally, conversion of atrial fibrillation to normal sinus rhythm may result from this combination or following the administration of digitalis alone.

4. Most often the use of quinidine to maintain a controlled ventricular rate, together with digitalis administration[1] is necessary to convert the atrial fibrillation to sinus rhythm medically. Because of the availability and safety of the electric cardioverter, it is preferable not to administer the large doses of quinidine that were used formerly to produce drug reversion to normal sinus rhythm. Rather, maintenance doses in the range of 1.2 to 2.4 g/day should be administered for a few days prior to the planned DC cardioversion. During this time, 10% to 15% of patients establish a normal sinus rhythm. If sinus rhythm does not occur, DC cardioversion is carried out. Experience suggests that digitalis may not have to be discontinued prior to cardioversion if the patient has not received an excessive amount of digitalis. Pretreatment with quinidine establishes an effective tissue concentration, determines whether the drug will be tolerated, improves chances of maintaining normal sinus rhythm after cardioversion, and reduces the number of shocks and level of energy required to restore normal sinus rhythm. Successful establishment of normal sinus rhythm by electric DC cardioversion occurs in over 90% of patients; with

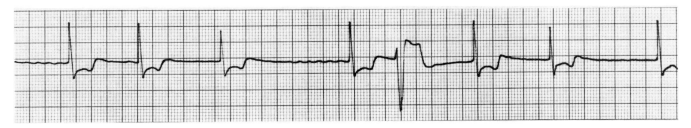

**Fig. 5-43  Atrial fibrillation.** Atrial activity is present as the undulating wavy baseline seen in the midportion of the ECG strip. Note that the premature ventricular complex follows the longest RR cycle. This conforms to a phenomenon known as the *rule of bigeminy,* that is, ventricular ectopy during atrial fibrillation more commonly follows the long RR cycles. The premature ventricular complex would have to be differentiated from aberrant supraventricular conduction. Monitor lead.

| | |
|---|---|
| **Rate:** | Atrial, cannot be determined accurately; ventricular, 36 to 105 beats/min. |
| **Rhythm:** | Atrial and ventricular are both irregularly irregular. |
| **P waves:** | Only the fibrillatory (*F*) waves of atrial fibrillation can be seen. |
| **PR interval:** | Not measurable. |
| **QRS:** | 0.08 second. |

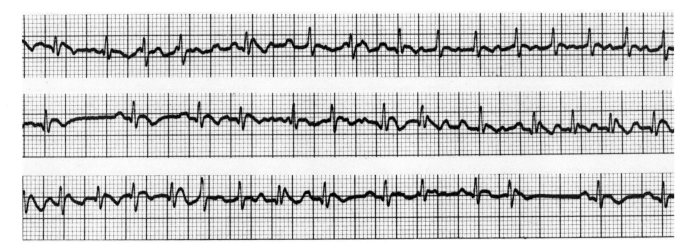

**Fig. 5-44  Intermittent, "coarse" atrial flutter-fibrillation.** Throughout this recording sinus beats are interrupted by premature atrial complexes that initiate episodes of atrial flutter-fibrillation. The fibrillatory waves appear more coarse than usual, and the flutter waves are irregularly spaced and of varying amplitude. Such atrial rhythms are often called *coarse atrial flutter* and are probably caused by portions of the atria that are fibrillating and other portions that are fluttering. A more appropriate term might be *flitter.* monitor lead.

| | |
|---|---|
| **Rate:** | Atrial, varying; ventricular, 69 to 150 beats/min. |
| **P waves:** | Appear before the sinus beats; otherwise the undulating baseline indicates flutter-fibrillation. |
| **PR interval:** | 0.16 second for the sinus beats. |
| **QRS:** | 0.08 second. |

maintenance quinidine therapy approximately 30% to 50% continue to have normal sinus rhythm for 12 months. In patients who do not tolerate quinidine, disopyramide or procainamide may be tried. Amiodarone is very effective in maintaining sinus rhythm but is investigational for that purpose.

Certain patients should *not* be considered for cardioversion. These include patients who have (1) known sensitivity or intolerance to quinidine or other antidysrhythmic agents (according to some studies, the recurrence rate of atrial fibrillation is higher in the absence of prophylactic quinidine administration), (2) repetitive paroxysmal atrial fibrillation that cannot be prevented by drugs, (3) digitalis intoxication, (4) numerous conversion procedures without clinical improvement or preservation of sinus rhythm, (5) difficult-to-control atrial tachydysrhythmias that finally eventuate into atrial fibrillation with clinical improvement and stability of dysrhythmia, (6) cardiac surgery planned in the near future, (7) a high degree of partial or complete AV block and thus a slow ventricular response, and (8) sick sinus syndrome (Fig. 5-41).

Many elderly patients in the last two groups tolerate the atrial fibrillation well because the ventricular rate is slow, and they often do not require treatment with digitalis, unless the ventricular rate increases or congestive heart failure develops. These patients may demonstrate serious supraventricular and ventricular dysrhythmias after cardioversion because concomitant sinus node disease becomes manifest. A related group of patients may have supraventricular tachycardias that alternate with bradycardias; these patients represent a subgroup of the sick sinus syndrome called "bradycardia-tachycardia syndrome." Usually, these patients are best treated with a ventricular pacemaker (to correct the slow rates) and digitalis (to control the ventricular rates during the supraventricular tachycardia).[17]

In general, all other patients in whom improved circulatory hemodynamics are desirable may be considered candidates for electric cardioversion. Failure to maintain normal sinus rhythm after electric reversion is related to the duration of atrial fibrillation, the functional classification of the patient, and the cause of the underlying heart disease. The likelihood of establishing and maintaining sinus rhythm should be weighed against the risks of cardioversion or other forms of therapy. The presence of multiple factors that adversely affect maintenance of sinus rhythm militates against cardioversion attempts.

Anticoagulation before cardioversion is indicated in patients with a high risk of emboli, that is, those who have mitral stenosis, recent onset of atrial fibrillation, recent or recurrent emboli, or enlarged heart.[18,19] The incidence of embolization during conversion to normal sinus rhythm is 1% to 3%. Some experts suggest anticoagulation for patients for 2 weeks before elective cardioversion of atrial fibrillation present for more than 1 to 2 weeks, if no contraindications to anticoagulation exist, and continuing anticoagulation for 2 additional weeks. However, few controlled studies exist to establish that approach definitively.

## ATRIAL TACHYCARDIA WITH AND WITHOUT AV BLOCK (Figs. 5-45 and 5-46)

The atrial rate is usually between 150 and 200 beats/min, with a range similar to AV nodal reentry, 150 to 250 beats/min. When caused by digitalis excess, the atrial rate is generally less than 200 beats/min and may be noted to increase gradually as the digitalis is continued. The PR interval also may gradually lengthen until Wenckebach second-degree AV block develops. On occasion the degree of AV block may be more advanced. Frequently other manifestations of digitalis excess, such as premature ventricular complexes coexist. In nearly 50% of cases of atrial tachycardia with block the atrial rate is irregular, whereas in AV nodal reentry the atrial rate is generally exceedingly regular. Characteristic isoelectric intervals between P waves, in contrast to atrial flutter, are usually present in all leads. However, at rapid atrial rates the distinction between atrial tachycardia with block and atrial flutter may be quite difficult. As in atrial flutter, carotid sinus massage slows the ventricular rate by increasing the degree of AV block but does not terminate the tachycardia.

**Significance.** Atrial tachycardia with block occurs most commonly in patients who have significant organic heart disease such as coronary artery disease or cor pulmonale. It is associated with digitalis excess in 50% to 75% of such patients.

A different type of atrial tachycardia, multifocal atrial tachycardia, is characterized by atrial rates of 100 to 250 beats/min and marked variation in P wave morphology and in the PP interval, it is associated with a high mortality, and it is rarely produced by digitalis. Verapamil may be effective therapy.

**Treatment.** If the ventricular rate is within a normal range and the patient is asymptomatic, often no therapy at all is necessary.

1. Very slow ventricular rates may respond to atropine (0.5 mg IV, repeated as needed to a total dose of 2.0 mg[13]) or, rarely, they may require ventricular pacing.
2. Atrial tachycardia with block in a patient who is not taking digitalis may be treated with digitalis to slow the ventricular rate.

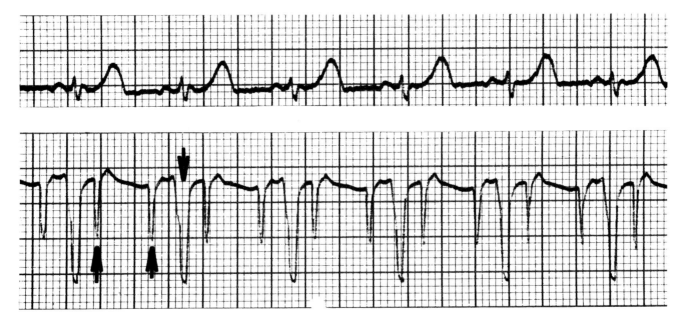

**Fig. 5-45**  Atrial tachycardia with 2:1 block. In the top tracing (lead II) alternate P waves cannot be seen because they are lost within the ST segment and the ECG appears to be sinus rhythm at a rate of 95 beats/min. The extra deflection in the terminal portion of the T wave suggests the presence of a second P wave, which is revealed in the esophageal recording *(bottom tracing)*. The atrial rate actually is 190 beats/min with 2:1 conduction to the ventricle. Upright arrows indicate P waves, inverted arrow indicates QRS complex. Monitor lead.

| | |
|---|---|
| **Rate:** | Atrial, 190 beats/min; ventricular, 95 beats/min. |
| **Rhythm:** | Atrial and ventricular, regular. |
| **P waves:** | Seen with clarity in the esophageal recording. |
| **PR interval:** | 0.14 second fro the conducted beats. |
| **QRS:** | 0.07 second. |

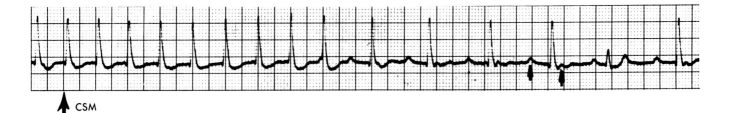

CSM

**Fig. 5-46**  Atrial tachycardia with 1:1 conduction becoming 2:1 conduction during carotid sinus massage. At the left portion of the ECG, P waves can be seen to conduct to each QRS complex. Carotid sinus massage (CSM) performed at the large arrow, precipitates 2:1 conduction. Clear atrial activity can be seen *(arrows)* as 2:1 conduction occurs. Monitor lead.

| | |
|---|---|
| **Rate:** | Atrial, 150 beats/min; ventricular, 150 beats/min in left portion and 75 beats/min in right portion. |
| **Rhythm:** | Atrial, regular; ventricular, regular. |
| **P waves:** | Can be seen in the ST segment in the left portion of the tracing and are quite clear in the right portion of the tracing. |
| **PR interval:** | Difficult to measure in the left portion of the tracing, but P waves conduct with a PR interval of 0.25 second in the right poriton of the tracing. |
| **QRS:** | 0.09 seconds. |

3. If atrial tachycardia with block remains after digitalization, oral quinidine, disopyramide, or procainamide may be added. Amiodarone or flecainide may be tried, but they are investigational for this purpose.

4. The rhythm in some patients may resist termination by pharmacologic means, and, if digitalis excess is not the cause, DC cardioversion may be tried.

5. If atrial tachycardia with (or without) block appears in a patient receiving digitalis, it should be assumed initially that the digitalis is responsible for the dysrhythmia, especially if the patient recently has received diuretics, the serum potassium level is low, the digitalis dose has been increased, quinidine has been added to the therapeutic regimen, or multiple premature ventricular complexes are also present. In such patients, initial therapy includes omission of digitalis and potassium-depleting diuretics (discontinuation of quinidine if it has been started recently) and the administration of potassium chloride, orally (30 to 45 mEq initially, repeated if necessary in 1 hour) or intravenously (0.5 mEq/min in 5% dextrose and water during constant electrocardiographic monitoring, for a total of 30 to 60 mEq initially). A gradual slowing of the atrial rate with a decrease in AV block usually occurs if the dysrhythmia is caused by digitalis. In the presence of advanced AV block, potassium, as well as other antidysrhythmic agents, must be given with great caution and under constant electrocardiographic monitoring. It should be remembered that renal dysfunction, acidosis, and excess digitalis predispose to the development of hyperkalemia, and therefore potassium must be administered cautiously, along with frequent ECG, serum potassium, and blood urea nitrogen (BUN) checks.

6. Verapamil 5 mg IV may be given; then verapamil 10 mg IV, repeated in 15 to 20 minutes if needed.[13]

7. Propranolol, 0.5 to 1 mg/min IV for a total dose of 0.5 to 3 mg, or phenytoin, 50 to 100 mg IV every 5 minutes until the tachycardia terminates, the patient develops signs of toxicity such as nystagmus, vertigo, or nausea, or a total dose of 1 g is given, may be quite useful for digitalis-induced dysrhythmias, including atrial tachycardia with block. The latter agent, since it does not appear to slow AV conduction, may be particularly useful.

8. If these agents are not effective, further short-acting digitalis preparations may be given cautiously, assuming that the development of atrial tachycardia with block was not caused by digitalis.

## PREMATURE AV JUNCTIONAL COMPLEXES
(Fig. 5-47)

Rhythms formerly called nodal, coronary nodal, and coronary sinus are now termed AV *junctional*. This term, which includes the AV nodal—His bundle area, is preferred to terms that imply a more exact site of impulse origin because the exact location at which the impulse originates often cannot be determined from the surface ECG. A premature AV junctional complex arises in the AV junction and spreads in an anterograde and retrograde fashion. If unimpeded in its course, the impulse discharges the atrium to produce a premature retrograde P wave and a QRS complex with a supraventricular contour. Retrograde atrial activation generally results in a negative P wave in leads II, III, $aV_F$, and $V_6$, with positive P waves in leads I, $aV_L$, $aV_R$, and $V_1$. The retrograde P wave may occur before, be buried in, or (less commonly) follow the QRS complex. The site at which the impulse originates, as well as the relative speeds of anterograde and retrograde conduction, determines the relationship of the P wave to the QRS complex. A compensatory pause commonly follows a premature AV junctional complex, but if the atrium and sinus node are discharged retrogradely, a noncompensatory pause results.

Significance and treatment. Premature AV junctional complexes usually do not cause symptoms and are rarely of any consequence. If symptoms occur, this dysrhythmia has the same significance and treatment as premature atrial contractions (PACs).

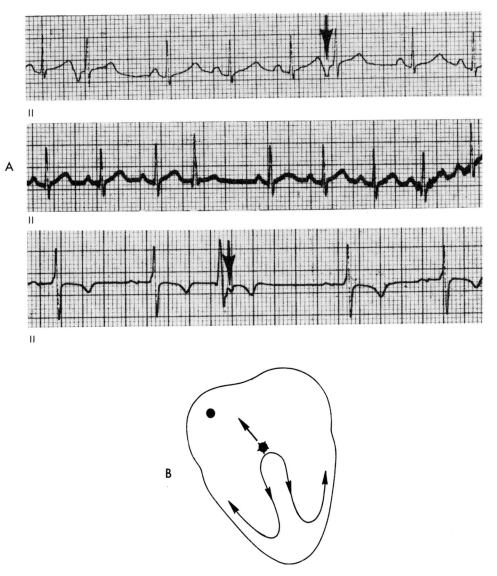

**Fig. 5-47** **A,** Premature AV junctional complexes. Premature junctional complexes seen in the top, middle, and bottom tracings were formerly called upper, middle, and lower nodal premature complexes, respectively, because the regrograde P wave was inscribed before, during, and after the QRS complex. Since not only the site of origin, but also the relative speeds of anterograde and retrograde conduction determine the P-QRS complex relationships during a premature AV junctional complex, it is best to use the nonspecific term *premature AV junctional complex* for all three types. Note that the QRS complex maintains an almost identical contour to the normally conducted beats. Slight QRS aberration occurs in the middle recording. Monitor lead from three different patients; arrows indicate P waves. In **B,** schematic illustration is presented.

| | |
|---|---|
| **Rate:** | Determined by basic rate and number of premature complexes. |
| **Rhythm:** | Irregular because of premature complexes; may be a regular irregularity, as in bigeminy or trigeminy. |
| **P waves** | Atria discharged in a retrograde direction, producing negative (inverted) P waves in lead II. P waves occur before (*top tracing*), during (*middle tracing*), and after (*bottom tracing*) the QRS complex, depending on the site of origin of the premature complex and the status of anterograde and retrograde conduction. |
| **PV interval:** | Less than 0.12 second. |
| **RP interval:** | If P wave follows QRS, less than 0.20 second. |
| **QRS:** | Normal, 0.08 second, reflecting normal anterograde conduction to the ventricles. Contour may differ slightly from normal. |

## AV JUNCTIONAL RHYTHMS (Figs. 5-48 to 5-50)

An AV junctional escape beat occurs when the rate of impulse formation of the primary pacemaker (usually sinus node) becomes less than that of the AV junctional pacemaker, or when impulses from the primary pacemaker do not penetrate to the region of the escape focus (AV block). The interval from the last normally conducted beat to the escape beat therefore exceeds the normal RR interval and is a measure of the initial rate of discharge of the AV junctional focus. The inherent discharge rate of the AV junctional escape focus (usually 40 to 60 per minute) determines when the junctional escape beat occurs. A continued series of AV junctional escape beats is called an AV junctional rhythm. An AV junctional escape rhythm is usually fairly regular. Intervals between subsequent escape beats after the initial escape beat may gradually shorten as the rate of discharge of the escape focus increases (rhythm of development). The configuration of the QRS complex may differ from the normal sinus-initiated QRS complex; usually, it maintains the same contour as the normally conducted QRS.

The atria may be under retrograde control of the AV junctional pacemaker, or the atria may discharge independently (see discussion of AV dissociation).

**Significance.** An AV junctional escape beat(s) or rhythm may be a normal phenomenon owing to the effects of vagal tone on higher pacemakers, or it may occur during pathologic slow sinus discharge and heart block. The escape beat or rhythm serves as a safety mechanism that assumes control of the cardiac rhythm owing to *default* of the primary pacemaker, so as to prevent the occurrence of complete ventricular asystole.

**Treatment.** Treatment, if indicated, lies in increasing the discharge rate of higher pacemakers or improving conduction with atropine or isoproterenol. Rarely, pacing may be needed. AV junctional escape beat(s) should not be suppressed.

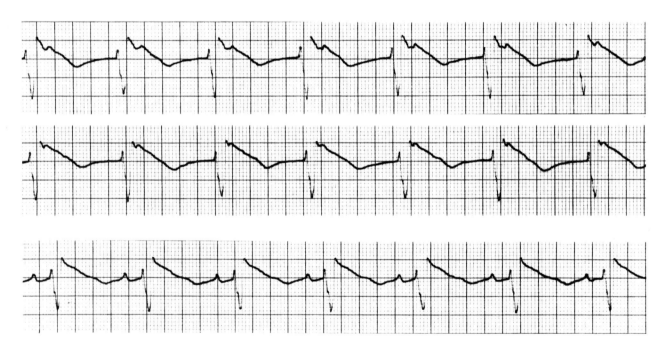

**Fig. 5-48 AV junctional rhythm.** The top tracings are a continuous recording, whereas the bottom tracing is recorded some time later. In the top two tracings, isorhythmic AV dissociation is present. P waves are in the ST segment and gradually move into the QRS complex (compare the QRS-P relationship in the first complex in the top strip with the last complex in the second strip). In the top strip, sinus slowing initially allowed the escape of the junctional rhythm (not shown). Monitor lead.

| | |
|---|---|
| **Rate:** | Top two strips, atrial is 60 beats/min and ventricular is 58 beats/min; bottom strip, atrial and ventricular rate 57 beats/min. |
| **Rhythm:** | Atrial, regular; ventricular, regular. |
| **P waves:** | Normal. |
| **PR interval:** | Varying in the top two strips; regular (0.22 second) in the bottom strip. |
| **QRS:** | 0.10 second (appears prolonged in this monitor lead but was normal by 12-lead ECG). |

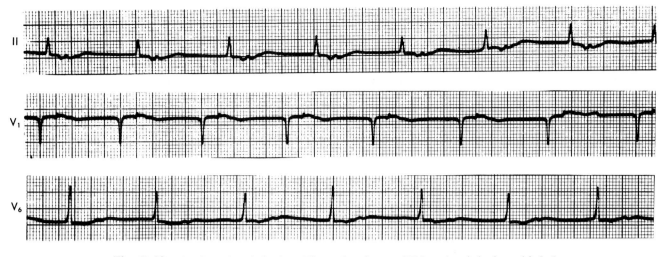

**Fig. 5-49  AV junctional rhythm.** The patient has an AV junctional rhythm with 1:1 retrograde capture. Thus AV dissociation is not present.

| | |
|---|---|
| **Rate:** | Atrial and ventricular, 55 beats/min. |
| **Rhythm:** | Regular. |
| **P waves:** | Retrograde. |
| **RP interval:** | 0.18 second. |
| **QRS:** | 0.06 second. |

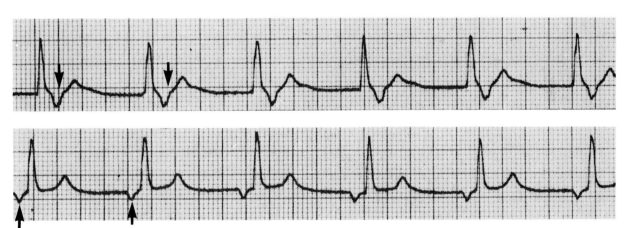

**Fig. 5-50  AV junctional rhythm with a changing P-QRS relationship.** In the top tracing, retrograde atrial activity ( ↓ ) follows the QRS complex. In the bottom tracing, retrograde atrial activity ( ↑ ) precedes the QRS complex. Thus with the same AV junctional rhythm in the same patient, atrial activity first followed and then preceded the QRS complex.

| | |
|---|---|
| **Rate:** | Atrial, 65 beats/min; ventricular, 65 beats/min. |
| **Rhythm:** | Regular. |
| **P waves:** | Inverted; follow QRS in top tracing; precede QRS in bottom tracing. |
| **PR interval:** | 0.12 second, bottom. |
| **RP interval:** | 0.12 second, top. |
| **QRS:** | Generally normal, 0.08 second. |

## NONPAROXYSMAL AV JUNCTIONAL TACHYCARDIA (Figs. 5-51 and 5-52)

Accepted terminology confers the label of tachycardia to rhythms that exceed 100 beats/min. However, since rates greater than 60 to 70 beats/min represent, in effect, a tachycardia for the AV junctional tissue, the term *nonparoxysmal AV junctional tachycardia* (NPJT), although not entirely correct, has been generally accepted when the rate of junctional discharge exceeds 60 to 70 beats/min.[16] NPJT usually has a more gradual onset and termination than does AV nodal reentry, with a ventricular rate commonly between 70 and 130 beats/min. The rate sometimes may be slowed by vagal maneuvers, as in sinus tachycardia, and the rhythm may not always be entirely regular. Although retrograde atrial activation may occur, more commonly the atria are controlled by an independent sinus or atrial focus resulting in AV dissociation.

**Significance.** The distinction between NPJT and AV nodal reentry is etiologically and therapeutically quite important. NPJT occurs most commonly in patients who have underlying heart disease, such as inferior wall infarction and acute rheumatic myocarditis, and following open-heart surgery. Probably the most important cause is excessive digitalis, which only rarely produces AV nodal reentry. It is especially important to recognize slowing and regularization of the ventricular rhythm caused by NPJT as an early sign of digitalis intoxication in a patient who has atrial fibrillation.

**Treatment.** The treatment for NPJT is as follows:

1. If the ventricular rate is rapid, the cardiovascular status compromised, and the patient is not taking digitalis, digitalization should be the first measure.
2. Uncommonly in an emergency situation or if the dysrhythmia does not respond to digitalization and is *clearly not induced by digitalis*, electric DC cardioversion may be employed with initial energies of 75 to 100 watt-seconds.
3. However, if the patient tolerates the dysrhythmia well, careful monitoring and attention to the underlying heart disease is usually all that is needed. The dysrhythmia will usually abate spontaneously.
4. If digitalis toxicity is the causative factor, the drug must be immediately stopped. Potassium may be given (see discussion of treatment of atrial tachycardia with block). The ECG should be monitored, since the blocking effects of potassium administration and digitalis are additive in the AV junctional tissue, and advanced AV heart block may result. The rate of potassium administration is important, since a rapid infusion of the potassium, especially in a potassium-depleted patient, may result in transient cardiac arrest or depression of AV conduction.
5. Lidocaine, propranolol, phenytoin, or verapamil also may be tried.

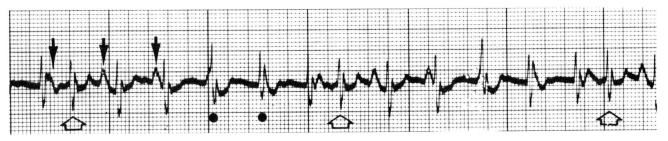

Lead II

**Fig. 5-51    Nonparoxysmal AV junctional tachycardia.** Atrial activity *(inverted dark arrows)* intermittently capture the ventricles *(upright arrow outlines)* to produce incomplete AV dissociation. The junctional tachycardia fails to capture the atria retrogradely, but the sinus tachycardia intermittently captures the ventricles. Unidirectional block (i.e., retrograde) is present. Incomplete AV dissociation occurs because of the accelerated AV junctional discharge. Two uninterrupted junctional cycles indicated by filled circles.

| | |
|---|---|
| **Rate:** | Atrial, 111 beats/min; ventricular, 125 beats/min. |
| **Rhythm:** | Atrial, regular; ventricular, fairly regular with intermittent speeding because of sinus captures. |
| **P waves:** | Normal and can be "marched out." P waves are not influenced by ventricular activity. |
| **PR interval:** | Difficult to measure but prolonged before the captures. |
| **QRS:** | 0.06 second. |

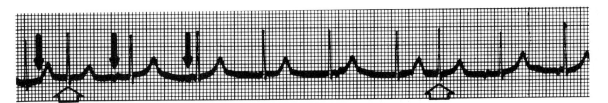

Lead I

**Fig. 5-52    Nonparoxysmal AV junctional tachycardia.** Atrial activity *(inverted dark arrows)* can be seen as small inverted P waves that occur regularly throughout the QRS complex, uninfluenced by ventricular activity. The ventricular rhythm is regular except for intermittent atrial captures indicated by the unfilled upright arrows. The rhythm is explained as in Fig. 5-51 except that an ectopic pacemaker, rather than a sinus pacemaker, controls the atria. This ectopic pacemaker could be an atrial focus or an upper junctional focus. Incomplete AV dissociation is present with unidirectional conduction from atria to ventricles but retrograde block (the ventricular rhythm does not capture the atria retrogradely).

| | |
|---|---|
| **Rate:** | Atrial, 72 beats/min; ventricular, 79 beats/min. |
| **Rhythm:** | Atrial, regular; ventricular irregular because of intermittent atrial captures. |
| **P waves:** | Abnormal. |
| **PR intervals:** | Prolonged during ventricular captures. |
| **QRS:** | 0.06 second. |

## VENTRICULAR ESCAPE BEATS (Fig. 5-53)

A ventricular escape beat results when the rate of impulse formation of supraventricular pacemakers (sinus node and AV junctional) becomes less than that of potential ventricular pacemakers or when supraventricular impulses do not penetrate to the region of the escape focus because of SA or AV block. The inherent rate of discharge of ventricular escape pacemakers is usually 20 to 40 per minute. A continued series of ventricular escape beats is called a ventricular escape rhythm. The ventricular rhythm is usually fairly regular, although the rhythm may accelerate for a few complexes shortly after its onset (rhythm of development). The duration of the QRS complexes is prolonged to greater than 0.12 second because the origin of ventricular discharge is located in the ventricles. Sometimes the escape focus may shift from one to another portion of ventricle and may generate QRS complexes with a different contour and rate.

**Significance.** The presence of ventricular escape beats indicates significant slowing of supraventricular pacemakers or a fairly high degree of SA or AV block and would, therefore, generally be considered abnormal.

**Treatment.** Depending on the cause, atropine, isoproterenol, or pacing generally represent the therapeutic approach.

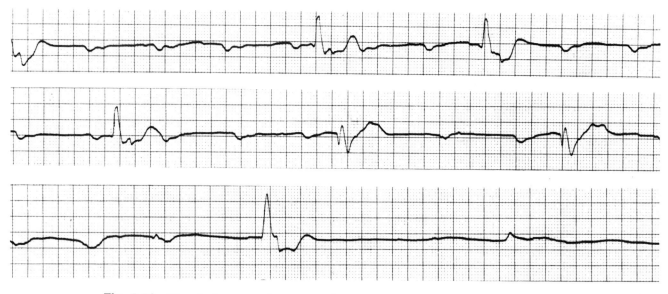

**Fig. 5-53  Ventricular escape beats occurring in a dying patient.** Ventricular escape beats occur with changing contour and at irregular intervals in this ECG from a dying patient. AV block is also present, since the P waves do not appear to conduct to the ventricles. The changing QRS contour may be caused by shifting pacemakers or changing activation sequence.

| | |
|---|---|
| **Rate:** | Varying. |
| **Rhythm:** | Atrial and ventricular rhythms are varying. |
| **P waves:** | Can be seen in the top strip and then more intermittently in the second and third strips. |
| **PR interval:** | Varying. |
| **QRS:** | Varying but approximately 0.16 second. |

# PREMATURE VENTRICULAR COMPLEXES
(Figs. 5-54 to 5-56)

A premature ventricular complex is characterized by the premature occurrence of a QRS complex, initiated in the ventricle, that has a contour different from the normal supraventricular complex and a duration usually greater than 0.12 second. The T wave is generally large and opposite in direction to the major deflection of the QRS. The QRS complex generally is not preceded by a premature P wave but may be preceded by a sinus P wave occurring at its expected time. However, these criteria may be met by a supraventricular complex or rhythm that conducts aberrantly through the ventricle; in fact, aberrant supraventricular conduction may mimic all the manifestations of ventricular dysrhythmia except ventricular fibrillation.

Retrograde transmission to the atria from premature ventricular complex occurs more frequently than has often been affirmed but still probably does not occur commonly. The retrograde P wave produced in this fashion is often obscured by the distorted QRS complex. Usually a fully compensatory pause follows a premature ventricular complex. If the retrograde impulse discharges the sinus node prematurely and resets the basic timing, it may produce a pause that is not fully compensatory. A compensatory pause results when the premature complex does not alter the discharge rate or rhythm of the sinus node, so that a P wave occurs at its normal time. The P wave does not reach the ventricle, since the AV node is refractory because of (concealed) retrograde penetration into the AV node by the premature junctional or ventricular complex. Therefore the RR interval produced by the two QRS complexes on either side of the premature complex equals twice the normally conducted RR interval. A compensatory pause occurs more commonly with ventricular and AV junctional premature complex, but the presence of a compensatory pause is not invariably diagnostic of the site of origin of the premature complex.

The normal sinus P wave following a premature ventricular complex may conduct to the ventricles with a long PR interval, in which case a pause does not follow the premature ventricular complex, and the premature complex is said to be *interpolated*. *A ventricular fusion beat* (the simultaneous activation of one chamber by two foci) represents a blend of the characteristics of the normally conducted beat and the beat originating in the ventricles, indicating that the ventricle has been depolarized from both atrial and ventricular directions. *Atrial fusion beats* may occur during ectopic atrial discharge and represent a blend of the characteristics of the sinus-initiated and ectopic atrial P waves. Whether a compensatory or noncompensatory pause, a retrograde atrial excitation, an interpolated complex, a fusion complex, or an echo beat (see Fig. 5-54) occurs in merely a function of how well the AV junction conducts and the timing of the events taking place.

The term *bigeminy* refers to pairs of beats or two complexes and may be used to indicate couplets of normal and ectopic ventricular complex. Premature ventricular complexes may have differing contours and often are called multifocal. More properly they should be called multiform, since it is not known from a surface ECG recording that there are multiple foci discharging.

**Significance.** The frequency of premature ventricular complexes increases with age. The presence of premature complexes may be manifested by symptoms of palpitations or discomfort in the chest or neck; this is caused by the greater than normal contractile force of the postectopic beats or the feeling that the heart has stopped during the long pause after the premature complexes. Long runs of premature complexes in patients who have heart disease may produce angina or hypotension. Frequent interpolated premature complexes actually represent a doubling of the heart rate and may compromise the patient's hemodynamic status. In the absence of underlying heart disease the presence of premature complexes may have no significance and not require suppression. Premature ventricular complexes and complex ventricular dysrhythmias occurring in asymptomatic healthy subjects portends no increased risk of death and their long term prognosis is similar to that of the healthy U.S. population. Ventricular ectopy recorded after myocardial infarction represents an independent risk factor for subsequent death. However, it has not been demonstrated that the premature ventricular complexes or complex ventricular dysrhythmias play a *precipitating* role in the genesis of sudden death; they may be simply a marker of heart disease. Nor has it been shown unequivocally that antidysrhythmic therapy given to suppress the premature ventricular complexes or complex ventricular dysrhythmias reduces the incidence of sudden death in these patients.

Most of the drugs used to suppress premature complexes also may produce them on certain occasions. This is especially true of the digitalis preparations. On the other hand, digitalis may be effective in controlling premature atrial and ventricular complexes, especially those related to the presence of congestive heart failure. In patients suffering from acute myocardial infarction, it has been commonly held that so-called warning dysrhythmias (premature ventricular complexes occurring close to the preceding T wave, greater than five or six per minute, bigeminal, multiform, or occurring in salvos of two, three, or more) may presage or precipitate ventricular tachycardia or fibrillation. However, it has been demonstrated that about half of the patients who develop ventricular fibrillation have no warning dysrhythmias, and half of those who do have warning dysrhythmias do not develop ventricular fibrillation.

**Treatment.** In the hospitalized patient with or without an acute myocardial infarction, lidocaine IV is the initial drug of choice when suppression of premature ventricular complexes is deemed necessary.

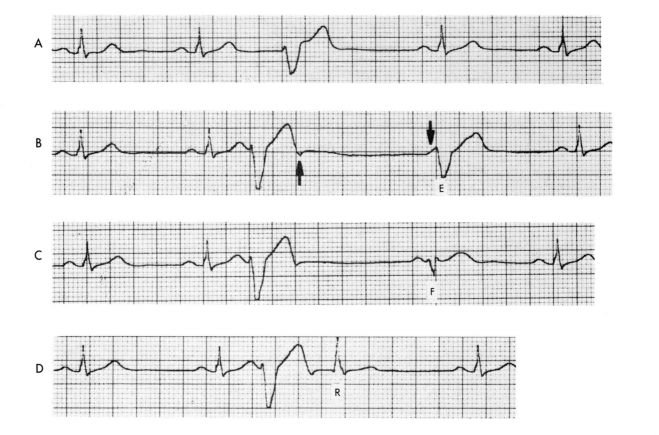

**Fig. 5-54** **Premature ventricular complexes.** All four tracings were recorded from the same patient. In **A** a relatively late premature ventricular complex is followed by a full compensatory pause. Sinus slowing makes the pause after the ventricular complex slightly greater than compensatory, but its characteristics are essentially the same, that is, the interval between the two normal QRS complexes flanking the premature ventricle complex is twice the basic RR interval. In **B** an earlier premature ventricular complex in the same patient retrogradely discharges the atrial ( ↑ ). This resets the sinus node and a ventricular escape beat *(E)* escapes before the next P wave ( ↓ ) can conduct to the ventricles. In strip **C** the sequence is the same as in **B**, except that the atrial rate is faster. This permits the P wave, following the premature ventricular complex and retrograde P wave, to partially depolarize the ventricles at the same time the ventricular escape beat occurs, resulting in a fusion beat *(F)*. In **D**, the sequence is the same as in **C**, except that after the impulse from the ventricle retrogradely discharges the atria, it returns to the ventricles to produce a ventricular echo, or reciprocal beat *(R)*. In **E**, a schematic illustration is presented.

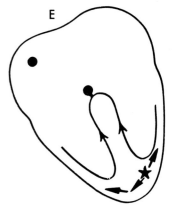

| | |
|---|---|
| **Rate:** | Determined by basic rate and number of ventricular complexes. |
| **Rhythm:** | Irregular because of premature complexes. |
| **P waves:** | Generally normal; may be captured retrogradely; often lost in QRS or T wave of premature ventricular complex. |
| **PR interval:** | Determined by whether P wave is blocked, conducted with a prolonged PR interval, or retrogradely activated. |
| **QRS:** | 0.14 second. |

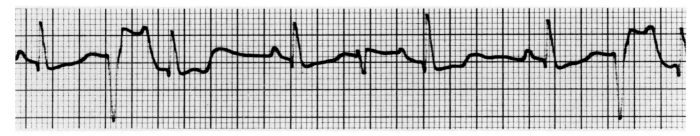

**Fig. 5-55** **Interpolated premature ventricular complexes.** The second, fifth, and eighth QRS complexes are premature ventricular complexes. The sinus P wave that follows those premature ventricular complexes conducts to the ventricle with a long PR interval. Thus the normally expected compensatory pause is not present. The premature ventricular complex does not replace a normally conducted complex (see Fig. 5-54, *A*) but occurs in addition to the normally conducted complex. The PR interval following the premature ventricular complex is prolonged because of incomplete recovery of the AV node because of partial retrograde penetration by the interpolated premature ventricular complex. Monitor lead.

| | |
|---|---|
| **Rate and Rhythm:** | Varying because of the premature ventricular complexes. |
| **P waves:** | Normal. |
| **PR interval:** | 0.16 second for the normally conducted beats and 0.20 to 0.25 second after the interpolated premature ventricular complexes. |
| **QRS:** | 0.09 second for the normal beats and 0.12 second for the premature ventricular complexes. |

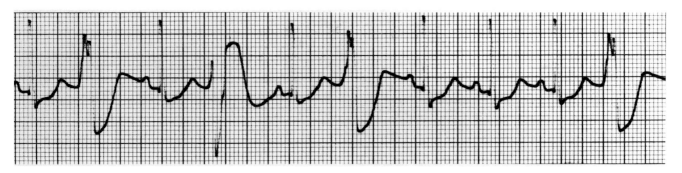

**Fig. 5-56** **Multiform premature ventricular complexes.** Each sinus beat is followed by premature ventricular complexes that have two contours, one predominantly upright and the other predominantly negative. These premature ventricular complexes of different contours are more properly called multiform rather than multifocal, since one cannot be certain if more than one focus is active or if different activation sequences are emerging from the same focus. Monitor lead.

| | |
|---|---|
| **Rate:** | 100 beats/min but varying. |
| **Rhythm:** | Varying because of premature ventricular complexes. |
| **P waves:** | Normal preceding the normally conducted beats. |
| **PR interval:** | 0.14 second preceding the normally conducted beats. |
| **QRS:** | 0.09 second for the normally conducted beats and 0.16 second for the premature ventricular complexes. |

### Immediate suppression[13]

1. Lidocaine 1 mg/kg is given as an IV bolus. If ectopy is not suppressed, repeat lidocaine 0.5 mg/kg every 2 to 5 minutes until there is no ectopy or up to 3 mg/kg is given.

   Lidocaine produces less hypotension and negative inotropic effects than procainamide or quinidine in doses having equivalent antidysrhythmic effects. It is ideal for use in patients who have renal disease, since less than 10% is excreted unaltered in the kidney and the rest is metabolized by the liver. In patients exhibiting allergic reactions to quinidine or procainamide, lidocaine is useful, since there appears to be no cross-sensitivity.

2. If maximum doses of lidocaine are unsuccessful, then procainamide is administered IV 20 mg/min until there is no ectopy or up to 1 g is given. Toxic effects include hypotension and QRS widening. If successful, procainamide may then be given as a continuous IV infusion of 1 to 4 mg/min.[13]

3. If ectopy is still unsuppressed and if it is not contraindicated, Bretylium IV 5 to 10 mg/kg over 8 to 10 minutes may be tried.[13]

4. If ectopy is still unsuppressed, overdrive pacing may be considered.

### Maintenance[13]

Once ectopy is suppressed, maintain as follows:

1. If the lidocaine bolus is successful, start a lidocaine drip:

| Bolus dose | Drip rate |
| --- | --- |
| 1 mg/kg | 2 mg/min |
| 2 mg/kg | 3 mg/min |
| 3 mg/kg | 4 mg/min |

2. After using a procainamide bolus, start a procainamide drip at 1 to 4 mg/min. Check blood level.

3. After the bretylium bolus, start a bretylium drip at 2 mg/min.

### Long-term suppression

1. Oral maintenance therapy can be achieved with procainamide, 375 to 500 mg every 3 to 4 hours to produce therapeutic blood levels of 4 to 8 mg/L, or with quinidine sulfate, 200 to 400 mg every 6 hours to produce serum levels of 3 to 6 mg/L. A long-acting procainamide preparation can be given at a dose of 750 to 1000 mg every 6 hours.

2. Disopyramide (Norpace), 100 to 250 mg every 6 hours, may be useful at serum concentrations of 2 to 5 $\mu$g/ml.

3. Tocainide (Tonocard) 400 to 600 mg every 8 to 12 hours achieving serum concentrations of 4 to 10 $\mu$g/ml may be effective, particularly if lidocaine has successfully suppressed the dysrhythmia.

4. Flecainide (Tambocor) is given in doses of 100 to 200 mg every 12 hours to produce serum concentrations in the range of 0.6 $\mu$g/ml and may be useful.

5. Amiodarone (Cordarone) is generally given in a loading dose of 800 to 1600 mg/day for 1 to 2 weeks and then at maintenance doses of 400 to 800 mg/day (or less), titrating the dose to the lowest effective amount. Therapeutic serum concentrations range between 1 and 3.5 $\mu$g/ml.

6. Mexiletine (Mexitel) may be tried in doses of 250 to 400 mg every 8 hours to achieve plasma concentrations of 1 to 2 $\mu$g/ml.

7. Propranolol or phenytoin may be tried if the above drugs fail (see discussion of treatment of ventricular tachycardia.

# VENTRICULAR TACHYCARDIA
(Figs. 5-57 to 5-59)

Ventricular tachycardia is usually an ominous finding, indicating the presence of significant underlying cardiac disease. In many instances the responsible electrophysiologic mechanism is probably reentry.[1] Although ventricular tachycardia occurs most commonly in patients who have acute myocardial infarction and coronary artery disease, this dysrhythmia also occurs in patients who have a variety of cardiac diseases, including cardiomyopathy, mitral valve prolapse, prolonged QT syndrome, and other problems. It has been reported in patients who have no evidence of structural heart disease.

The electrocardiographic diagnosis of ventricular tachycardia is suggested when a series of three or more bizarre, premature ventricular complexes occur that have a duration exceeding 0.12 second, with the ST-T vector pointing opposite to the major QRS deflection. The ventricular rate is between 110 and 250 beats/min, and the RR interval may be exceedingly regular, or it may vary. Atrial activity may be independent of ventricular activity (AV dissociation) or the atria may be depolarized by the ventricles in a retrograde fashion (in which case AV dissociation is *not* present). Ventricular tachycardia may be sustained (defined in the electrophysiology laboratory as lasting longer than 30 seconds or requiring termination because of hemodynamic deterioration) or nonsustained (lasting less than 30 seconds), and the patient's prognosis as well as the electrophysiologic mechanism may differ for the two forms. One type of nonsustained ventricular tachycardia is characterized by repetitive bursts of premature ventricular complexes separated by a series of sinus beats. Another type of ventricular tachycardia that may be sustained or nonsustained is called *torsades de pointes* and is characterized by a QRS contour that gradually changes its polarity from negative to positive or vice versa over a series of beats. It often occurs in a setting of QT prolongation.[8]

The distinction between supraventricular and ventricular tachycardia may be difficult at times because the features of both dysrhythmias frequently overlap, and under certain circumstances a supraventricular tachycardia can mimic the criteria established for ventricular tachycardia. Ventricular complexes with abnormal configurations indicate only that conduction through the ventricle is not normal; they do not necessarily indicate the origin of impulse formation or the reason for the abnormal conduction (see discussion of supraventricular dysrhythmia with abnormal QRS complex).

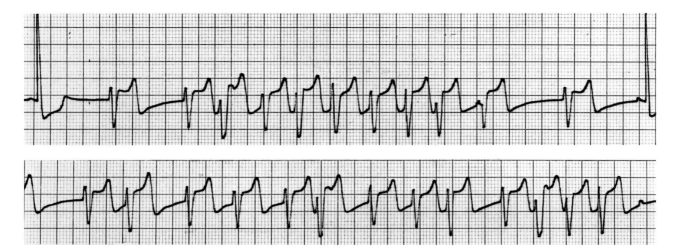

**Fig. 5-57 Ventricular tachycardia.** Ventricular tachycardia may be irregular at times, as exemplified in this ECG. The origin of the ventricular tachycardia was documented by electrophysiologic study. The interectopic intervals do not conveniently fit a diagnosis of exit block. Monitor lead.

| | |
|---|---|
| **Rate:** | Atrial, cannot be determined; ventricular, varying. |
| **Rhythm:** | Atrial, cannot be determined; ventricular, irregular. |
| **P waves:** | Can be seen occasionally and precede the first and next to last QRS complexes in the top strip, which are the only normally conducted QRS complexes. The nonconducted P wave at the terminal portion of the bottom strip probably results from incomplete AV nodal recovery of refractoriness caused by retrograde penetration from the last beat in the ventricular tachycardia. |
| **PR interval:** | 0.12 second for the normally conducted beats. |
| **QRS:** | 0.08 second for the normally conducted beat and 0.11 second for the ventricular tachycardia. |

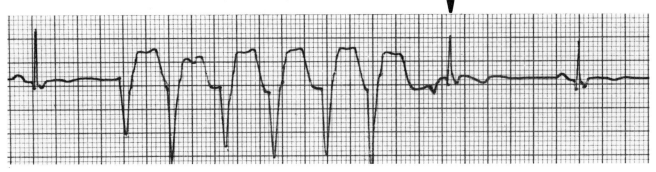

II

**Fig. 5-58  Ventricular tachycardia ending with a ventricular echo.** Six beats of ventricular tachycardia occur following the first sinus beat. The last ventricular tachycardia beat conducts retrogradely to the atrium (note the small negative P wave in lead II), which then returns to reexcite the ventricle (ventricular echo, *arrow*).

| | |
|---|---|
| **Rate:** | Atrial, 55 to 75 beats/min; ventricular, approximately 150 beats/min. |
| **Rhythm:** | Atrial, cannot be determined during ventricular tachycardia; regular during sinus rhythm. Ventricular, slightly irregular during ventricular tachycardia. |
| **P waves:** | Normal during sinus-conducted beats; retrograde P wave following the last ventricular tachycardia beat. |
| **PR interval:** | 0.16 second during sinus rhythm. RP interval following the last ventricular tachycardia beat, 0.52 second. |
| **QRS:** | 0.08 second during sinus rhythm and 0.10 second during ventricular tachycardia. |

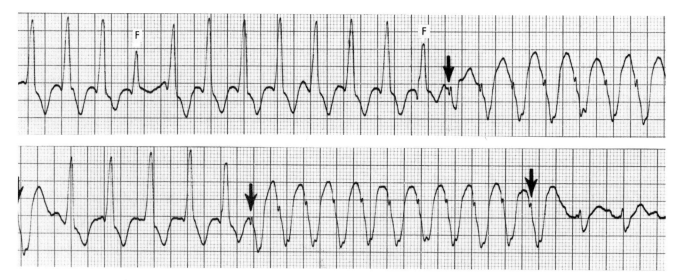

**Fig. 5-59  Termination of ventricular tachycardia by rapid ventricular pacing.** Intermittent fusion beats *(F)* in the top strip support the diagnosis of ventricular tachycardia. Between the first and second arrows, competitive ventricular pacing is performed at a rate of 166 beats/min, but the ventricular tachycardia continues. Between the third and fourth arrows, competitive ventricular pacing is performed at a rate of 176 beats/min, and following cessation of pacing, sinus rhythm occurs. Monitor lead.

| | |
|---|---|
| **Rate:** | Atrial, cannot be determined; ventricular 136 beats/min. |
| **Rhythm:** | Atrial, cannot be determined; ventricular, fairly regular. |
| **P waves:** | Cannot be seen. |
| **PR interval:** | Cannot be determined. |
| **QRS:** | 0.13 second. |

The presence of *fusion* and *capture* beats provides evidence in favor of ventricular tachycardia. Fusion beats indicate simultaneous activation of the ventricles by two separate impulses (suggesting that one of the impulses arose in the ventricles), whereas the capture beats signal supraventricular control of the ventricles, generally at a rate faster than the ventricular tachycardia. This proves that normal ventricular conduction can occur at cycle lengths equal to or shorter than the tachycardia in question, again implying that the origin of the wide QRS complexes lies in the ventricles rather than in aberrant supraventricular conduction.

**Significance.** Symptoms occurring during ventricular tachycardia depend on the ventricular rate, the duration of the tachydysrhythmia; and the severity of the underlying heart disease. The location of impulse formation and, therefore, the way in which the depolarization wave spreads across the myocardium also may be important because it influences the ventricle's contraction. The immediate significance of ventricular tachycardia to the patient relates to the hemodynamic dysfunction it produces and the possible development of ventricular fibrillation.

A premature ventricular (rarely, atrial) complex can initiate ventricular tachycardia or ventricular fibrillation when the premature complex occurs during the vulnerable period of the antecedent T wave. The vulnerable period represents an interval of 20 to 40 msec located near the apex of the T wave during which the heart, when stimulated, is prone to develop ventricular tachycardia or fibrillation (see discussion of ventricular fibrillation). The stimulus may be from an intrinsic source such as a spontaneous premature complex or from an extrinsic source such as a pacemaker or DC shock. During the interval of the vulnerable period, maximum electric nonuniformity in the ventricular muscle is present; that is, ventricular muscle fibers are at varying stages of recovery of excitability. Some fibers may have completely repolarized, others may have only partially repolarized, and still others may be completely refractory. Therefore stimulation during this period establishes nonuniform conduction with some areas of slowed conduction or actual block and sets the stage for repetitive ventricular discharge possibly caused by reentrant excitation. Equally important, however, is that ventricular tachycardia or fibrillation may begin without preexisting or precipitating premature ventricular complexes or may be ushered in by a *late* premature ventricular complex. In fact, the majority of recorded episodes of ventricular tachycardia begin with a late premature ventricular complex that occurs after the vulnerable period has ended.

**Treatment.** The treatment for ventricular tachycardia is as follows:

1. Striking the patient's chest, sometimes called "*thumpversion,*" may terminate ventricular tachycardia by mechanically inducing a premature ventricular complex that presumably interrupts the reentrant pathway necessary to support the ventricular tachycardia. It is a simple treatment to try initially. Stimulation at the time of the vulnerable period during ventricular tachycardia may provoke ventricular fibrillation.

2. Acute termination of ventricular tachycardia that does not cause any hemodynamic decompensation may be achieved medically, by administering lidocaine IV in an initial bolus of 1 mg/kg body weight. Lidocaine may be given in doses of 0.5 mg/kg every 8 minutes until VT resolves, up to 3 mg/kg.[13] The dosage should be reduced in patients who have liver disease, heart failure, or shock. If lidocaine abolishes the ventricular tachycardia, then a continuous IV infusion of 1 to 4 mg/min can be given to the patient. Other infusion schedules also are effective.[7]

3. If maximum doses of lidocaine are unsuccessful, procainamide administered IV (at 20 mg/min until termination of the tachycardia occurs, toxic effects such as QRS widening or significant hypotension result, or up to 1000 mg is administered) may be tried. If successful, procainamide may then be given as a continuous IV infusion (1 to 4 mg/min, titrated to patient's response).[13]

4. When first-line antidysrhythmic agents such as lidocaine or procainamide have failed, IV bretylium at a dose of 5 mg/kg is given over several minutes and may be increased to 10 mg/kg 15 to 30 minutes later. Doses may be repeated at 15- to 30-minute intervals, not to exceed a total of 40 mg/kg. A continuous infusion at 1 to 2 mg/min can be initiated.

5. If the dysrhythmia does not respond to medical therapy, electric DC cardioversion may be used. Ventricular tachycardia that precipitates hypotension, shock, angina, or congestive heart failure should be treated promptly with DC cardioversion. Start cardioversion with 50 watt-seconds. If unsuccessful, increase watt-seconds progressively to 100, 200, up to 360 watt-seconds. If the dysrhythmia is recurrent, give lidocaine and cardiovert again, starting at the energy level previously successful. Then use procainamide or bretylium IV infusions.[13] Digitalis-induced ventricular tachycardia is best treated medically. After reversion of the dysrhythmia to a normal rhythm, it is essential to institute measures to prevent a recurrence.

6. In patients who have recurrent ventricular tachycardia, a pacing catheter can be inserted into the right ventricle, and single, double, or multiple stimuli can be introduced competitively to terminate the ventricular tachycardia (Fig. 5-59). This procedure incurs the risk of accelerating the ventricular tachycardia to ventricular flutter or ventricular fibrillation. A catheter electrode is available through which synchronized cardioversion can be performed. In the

awake, conscious patient shocks of 0.25 watt-seconds that successfully terminate ventricular tachycardia can be delivered through this catheter electrode.[20]

7. A search for reversible conditions contributing to the initiation and maintenance of ventricular tachydysrhythmias should be made and the conditions corrected if possible. For example, ventricular dysrhythmia related to hypotension or hypokalemia at times may be terminated by vasopressors or potassium, respectively. Slow ventricular rates that are caused by sinus bradycardia or AV block may permit the occurrence of premature ventricular complexes and ventricular tachydysrhythmias that can be corrected by administering atropine, 0.5 to 1.0 mg IV, temporary isoproterenol administration (1 to 2 μg/min in an IV drip), or temporary transvenous pacing.

8. Intermittent ventricular tachycardia, interrupted by one or more supraventricular beats, generally is best treated medically. Lidocaine or procainamide should be tried. If they prove unsuccessful, then quinidine, disopyramide (IV administration is approved for investigational use only), propranolol, or drugs such as flecainide and amiodarone (IV administration investigational) may be tried.

Prevention of recurrences may be difficult at times.

1. Initial preventive drug therapy for recurrent ventricular dysrhythmias in the ambulatory patient should be with quinidine, procainamide, disopyramide, flecainide, or tocainide. Amiodarone is reserved for the patient in whom these other drugs fail to work or for those who cannot tolerate them. Procainamide is given as a loading dose of 0.5 to 1 g orally, followed by 375 to 500 mg three to six times daily. Because procainamide has a shorter duration of action than quinidine, the long-acting preparation must be used when giving procainamide at 6-hour intervals to provide therapeutic blood levels (4 to 8 mg/L) for the entire 6-hour period. Hard-to-control dysrhythmias may reflect poor absorption of the drug or nontherapeutic blood levels between two widely spaced doses.

2. Alternatively, quinidine may be used, administered at a dosage of 200 to 400 mg four times daily, to achieve therapeutic blood levels of 3 to 6 mg/L.

3. If quinidine is unsuccessful, disopyramide, 100 to 250 mg every 6 hours, flecainide, 50 to 300 mg every 12 hours, or tocainide, 400 to 600 mg every 8 to 12 hours, may be tried. Amiodarone, after a loading dose of 800 to 1600 mg/day for 1 to 2 weeks, is given at a maintenance dose of 400 to 800 mg/day working down to the lowest effective dose daily.

4. Following an initial approach with the above drugs,

phenytoin or propranolol may be tried; these two drugs are often not very effective in preventing recurrences of ventricular tachydysrhythmias.

5. Combinations of drugs with different mechanisms of action may be successful and allow one to use low doses of both agents rather than high or toxic doses of one drug. For example, propranolol, 40 mg daily, combined with average doses of quinidine or procainamide may be efficacious. Similarly, procainamide or quinidine might be effectively combined with amiodarone.

6. Administration of potassium to maintain serum potassium levels in the 5+ range, in addition to antidysrhythmic agents, may be helpful on occasion.

7. A trial of ventricular or atrial pacing, combined with antidysrhythmic agents if necessary, may be tried empirically; if successful, permanent pacing may be instituted. Generally, unless the initiation of the ventricular tachycardia is related to significant bradycardia, such as ventricular rates in the 30s caused by complete AV block, attempts at rapid "overdrive" pacing are often ineffective in the long term.

8. Surgery may be used in selected patients to treat ventricular tachycardia. Multiple surgical techniques are available and include a single ventriculotomy in some patients, cryosurgery, and encircling endocardial ventriculotomy to isolate the arrhythmogenic area or endocardial resection to remove the arrhythmogenic area (preferably directed by electrophysiologic mapping techniques) in patients who have ventricular tachycardia related to coronary artery disease (Fig. 5-60). If the surgery alone fails to eliminate recurrences of the dysrhythmias, it may make previously ineffective drug regimens efficacious. Coronary bypass surgery alone, without electrophysiologic mapping and myocardial resection, in patients who do not have ventricular tachycardia definitely associated with ischemia, for example, ventricular tachycardia induced by stress testing, has not been very successful.

9. A number of new antidysrhythmic agents offer promise to control recurrent, life-threatening ventricular tachydysrhythmias.[22]

10. Implantable electric devices that competitively pace, synchronously cardiovert or defibrillate may be very effective in some patients.

**Evaluation of therapy.** Evaluating the adequacy of drug therapy in patients who have widely spaced episodes of ventricular tachycardia is a difficult problem because there exists no adequate end point to judge therapy until the patient has another spontaneous recurrence. Because of this, many groups have taken a more aggressive approach. The patient undergoes a control electrophysiologic study, during which the ventricular tachycardia is initiated and a variety of electrophysiologic and hemodynamic parameters are assessed. Then the patient is treated with a drug and the electrophysiologic study is repeated. If the drug prevents reinduction of the ventricular tachycardia, there is a high likelihood that the drug will also prevent spontaneous recurrences. If the drug fails to prevent reinitiation of the tachycardia, in many instances the drug may still be successful clinically by slowing the rate of the ventricular tachycardia, converting a sustained form to a nonsustained episode, or preventing a recurrence.[23]

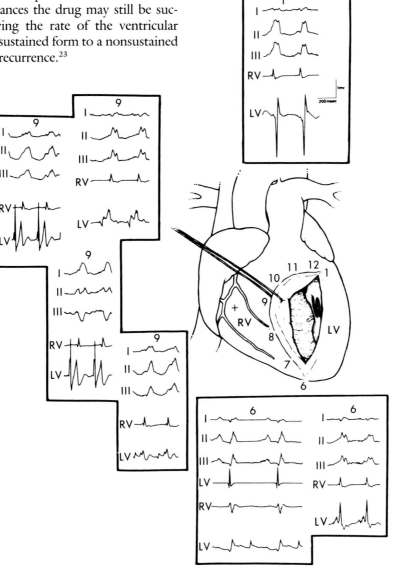

**Fig. 5-60**   **Partial activation map during ventricular tachycardia;** tracings have been redrawn for clarity. Left ventricular aneurysm is opened and numbered in a clockwise fashion. Left ventricular endocardial recordings *(LV)* from a handheld exploring electrode are shown in the inserts for sites 1, 6, and 9. A stationary right ventricular epicardial electrode *(RV)* was sewn in place (+ on right ventricle). Ventricular tachycardia with four different contours (see surface leads, insert 9) was initiated. Left ventricular endocardial recordings at site 9 showed earliest activation during each ventricular tachycardia *(arrows)*. Left ventricular recordings at site 6 (right portion of insert 6) show activation starting later than the left ventricular recordings at site 9 but before the left ventricular recording at site 1, which is relatively normal and late in the QRS complex. However, during sinus rhythm (left portion of insert 6), recording at site 6 shows a split, late potential *(arrow)*. Endocardial resection was carried out between sites 6 and 9 with elimination of ventricular tachycardia. (From Braunwald E, editor: Heart disease: a textbook of cardiovascular medicine, Philadelphia, ed 3, 1988, WB Saunders Co.)

## Torsades de Pointes

The term *torsades de pointes* refers to a ventricular tachycardia characterized by QRS complexes of changing amplitude and morphology that appear to twist around the isoelectric line and occur at rates of 200 to 250 beats/min (Fig. 5-61). The peaks of the QRS complexes appear successively on one side and then the other of the isoelectric baseline, giving the typical twisting appearance with continuous and progressive changes in QRS contour and amplitude. Torsades de pointes connotes a *syndrome* characterized by prolonged ventricular repolarization with corrected QT intervals generally exceeding 500 msec. The U wave also may be prominent but its role in this syndrome and in the long QT syndrome is not clear. Patients experience recurrent episodes of ventricular tachycardia often precipitated by a late premature complex. Tachycardia may terminate with progressive prolongation of cycle lengths and larger and more distinctly formed QRS complexes.

Rarely ventricular fibrillation supervenes. Of interest is the fact that cycle length changes that occur immediately before the onset of torsades de pointes often show a long-short RR cycle sequence: a pause in the supraventricular rhythm, caused by sinus bradycardia or the compensatory pause following a premature ventricular complex, is followed by the next sinus beat that has a premature ventricular complex in its T wave. The premature ventricular complex appears to initiate torsades de pointes.

**Significance.** Conditions that can prolong the QT interval may be associated with torsades de pointes. These include bradycardia; SA block; cardiac drug therapy (especially quinidine, procainamide, disopyramide, and amiodarone); electrolyte imbalances (especially hypokalemia and hypomagnesemia); myocardial infarction, angina, and other ischemic heart conditions; subarachnoid hemorrhage; tricyclic antidepressants and phenothiazines; vagal response; and congenital QT prolongation.

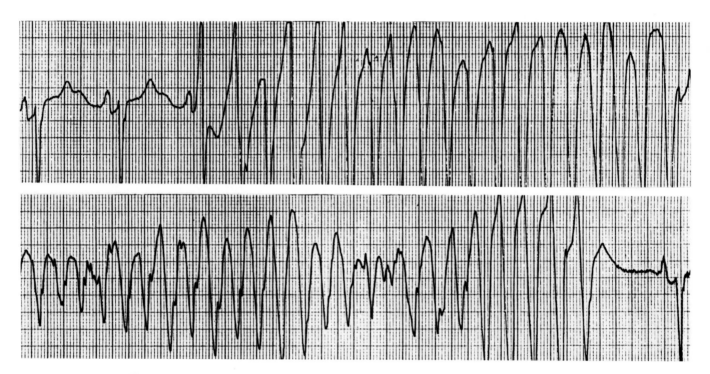

**Fig. 5-61** **Long QT interval and torsades de pointes.** Congenital long QTU interval (approximately 680 msec, uncorrected) in a 16-year-old with recurrent syncope. Characteristic contour of torsades de pointes is present in the lower recording just before termination of the ventricular tachycardia.

| | |
|---|---|
| **Monitor lead:** | Continuous recording. |
| **Rate:** | Atrial 60 beats/min. Ventricular irregular. |
| **Rhythm:** | Atrial regular. Ventricular irregular. |
| **P waves:** | Normal when visible. |
| **PR interval:** | 0.18 second during sinus rhythm. |
| **QRS:** | Normal during sinus rhythm. QT interval prolonged. |
| **Dysrhythmia:** | Torsades de pointes. |

Treatment. Treatment of ventricular tachycardia that has a polymorphic pattern depends on whether or not the QT interval is prolonged. Thus it is important to restrict the definition of torsades de pointes to the typical electrocardiographic morphology described above that occurs in the setting of a long QT and/or long Q-T U wave. In patients with torsades de pointes, administration of antidysrhythmic agents such as quinidine, disopyramide and procainamide tends to increase the abnormal QT interval and worsen the dysrhythmia.

1. Temporary ventricular or atrial pacing should be instituted. Pacing at rapid rates suppresses the ventricular tachycardia, which often does not recur after cessation of pacing. Isoproterenol can be tried until pacing is instituted.
2. Magnesium sulfate given intravenously has been reported to suppress torsades de pointes in a small number of patients. The dosage is 2 g IV push over 1 to 2 minutes with an IV infusion of 1 to 2 g/hour for 4 to 6 hours.
3. The cause of the long QT interval and torsades de pointes should be determined and corrected if possible.
4. Antidysrhythmic drugs that do not prolong the QT interval, such as lidocaine, mexiletine, or tocainide, may be tried.

## Long QT Syndrome

Long QT syndrome exists when an abnormally prolonged QT interval is present that exceeds 0.44 seconds after correction for rate, or when the Q-T U pattern appears abnormal in configuration. The nature of the U wave and its relationship to the long QT syndrome are not clear. Notched, bifid and sinusoidal T waves may occur.

Significance. Repolarization abnormalities can be divided into two groups: (1) a primary or idiopathic group that includes a congenital, often familial disorder sometimes, but not always, associated with deafness, and (2) an acquired group caused by various drugs like quinidine, disopyramide and procainamide, phenothiazines and tricyclic antidepressants, metabolic abnormalities such as hypokalemia, central nervous system lesions, autonomic nervous system dysfunction, coronary artery disease with myocardial infarction, and other problems. Symptomatic patients with the long QT syndrome develop a type of ventricular tachycardia, torsade de pointes. Since sudden death may occur in this group of patients, it is obvious that, in some, the ventricular dysrhythmia becomes sustained and probably results in ventricular fibrillation. Patients with congenital long QT syndrome who are at increased risks for developing sudden cardiac death include those who have family members who died suddenly at an early age and those who have experienced syncope.

Treatment. (1) For patients who do not have syncope, complex ventricular dysrhythmias or a family history of sudden cardiac death, no therapy is recommended; (2) in asymptomatic patients with complex ventricular dysrhythmias or a family history of premature sudden cardiac death, beta blockers at maximally tolerated doses are recommended; (3) in patients with syncope, beta blockers at maximally tolerated doses, at times combined with phenytoin and phenobarbital, are suggested; (4) in patients who continue to have syncope despite triple drug therapy, left-sided cervicothoracic sympathetic ganglionectomy that interrupts the stellate ganglion and the first three or four thoracic ganglia has been proposed; (5) finally, implantable automatic defibrillators may be needed in the symptomatic patient who has not responded to other therapy.

## ACCELERATED IDIOVENTRICULAR RHYTHM
(Figs. 5-62 and 5-63)

The ventricular rate, commonly between 50 and 110 beats/min, usually hovers within 10 beats of the sinus rate so that control of the cardiac rhythm may be passed back and forth between these two competing pacemaker sites. Consequently, long runs of fusion beats often appear at the onset and termination of the dysrhythmia as the pacemakers vie for control of ventricular discharge. Because of the slow rates, capture beats are common. The onset of this dysrhythmia is generally gradual (nonparoxysmal) and occurs when the rate of ectopic ventricular discharge exceeds the sinus rate because of sinus slowing, or SA or AV block. The ectopic mechanism may also begin following a premature ventricular complex or the ectopic ventricular rate may simply accelerate sufficiently to overtake the sinus focus. The slow rate and nonparoxysmal onset usually avoid the problems initiated by excitation during the vulnerable period, and consequently, precipitation of more rapid ventricular dysrhythmias is rarely seen. Termination of the rhythm generally occurs gradually as the dominant sinus rhythm accelerates or the ectopic ventricular rhythm decelerates. Occasionally, an accelerated idioventricular rhythm may be present in a patient who also has a more rapid ventricular tachycardia at other times.

Significance. The dysrhythmia occurs as a rule in patients with heart disease such as in a setting of acute myocardial infarction or as an expression of digitalis toxicity. Generally it is transient and intermittent, with episodes lasting a few seconds to a minute, and does not appear to seriously affect the course or prognosis of the disease. Suppressive therapy is usually unnecessary because the ventricular rate is commonly less than 100 beats/min. Basically, five conditions exist during which therapy may be considered: (1) when AV dissociation results in loss of sequential AV contraction and, with it, the hemodynamic benefits of atrial contraction; (2) when accelerated idioventricular rhythm occurs together with more rapid forms of ventricular tachycardia; (3) when accelerated idioventricular rhythm begins with a premature ventricular complex that initiates more rapid ventricular tachycardia; (4) when the ventricular rate is too rapid and produces symp-

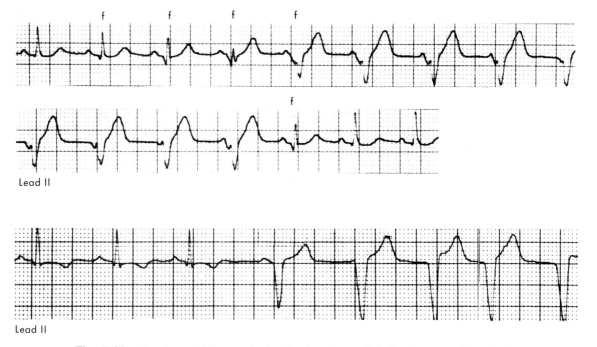

**Fig. 5-62   Accelerated idioventricular rhythm.** In panel **A** the sinus rate slows slightly and allows the escape of an idioventricular rhythm. A series of fusion beats *(F)* result, In panel **B** the sinus rate speeds slightly and once again regains control of the ventricular rhythm. A similar sequence occurs in panel **C**.

| | |
|---|---|
| **Rate:** | In panels **A** and **B** the atrial rate is 94 beats/min but slows and speeds; ventricular is 90 beats/min. In panel **C** the atrial rate is 75 beats/min but slows and speeds; ventricular rate is 75 beats/min but speeds to 86 beats/min. |
| **Rhythm:** | Fairly regular. |
| **P waves:** | Normal P waves preceding each normally conducted QRS complex. |
| **PR interval:** | 0.14 second for the normally conducted beats. |
| **QRS:** | 0.06 second for the normally conducted beats and 0.14 second for the accelerated idioventricular beats. |

toms; and (5) if ventricular fibrillation develops. The latter appears only rarely.

Treatment. Treatment for accelerated idioventricular rhythm is as follows:

1. The best initial therapeutic approach would appear to be close observation, rhythm monitoring, and care for the underlying heart disease.
2. Digitalis administration should be discontinued if the drug is implicated in the genesis of the dysrhythmia.
3. Atropine, 0.5 mg IV initially, repeated if necessary, may be used to speed the sinus rate and capture the ventricles. Rarely, pacing may be considered to speed the basic heart rate and suppress the accelerated idioventricular rhythm.
4. Lidocaine or other antidysrhythmic drugs may be given to suppress the ectopic ventricular focus.

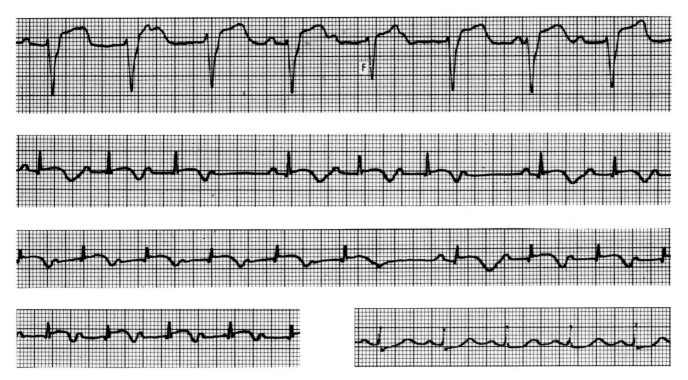

**Fig. 5-63  Accelerated idioventricular rhythm and second-degree AV block.** This series of tracings was recorded over a period of several days in a patient who had an acute inferior myocardial infarction. In panel **A** an accelerated idioventricular rhythm occurs at a rate of 70 beats/min. Note the fusion QRS complex (*F*) in the midportion of the strip preceded by a long PR interval. The long PR interval suggests the presence of an AV conduction disturbance, but its exact degree cannot be determined from his ECG. Thus incomplete AV dissociation is present, caused by a combination of accelerated idioventricular rhythm and AV block. In panel **B** the accelerated idioventricular rhythm has stopped, but Wenckebach second-degree AV block is still present with a conduction ratio of 4 : 3. In panel **C** the Wenckebach second-degree AV block is still present, but the conduction ratio has increased significantly. On the following day (**D**) the second-degree AV block has disappeared and is now replaced by first-degree AV block. Finally, after several days the first-degree AV block is barely present (**E**). **A.** Monitor lead. **B-E,** Lead II.

| | |
|---|---|
| **Rate:** | Panel **A**: atrial, 88 beats/min; ventricular, 70 beats/min. Panel **B**: atrial, 87 beats/min; ventricular, varying. Panel **C**: atrial, 86 beats/min; ventricular, varying. Panel **D**: atrial and ventricular, 88 beats/min. Panel **E**: atrial and ventricular, 88 beats/min. |
| **Rhythm:** | Panel **A**:, atrial and ventricular, regular. Panel **B**: atrial, regular; ventricular, irregular. Panel **C**: atrial, regular; ventricular, irregular. Panel **D**: atrial and ventricular, regular. Panel **E**: atrial and ventricular, regular. |
| **P waves:** | Normal in all traces. |
| **PR interval:** | Not measurable in panel **A**, progressively increasing in panels **B** and **C**, regular at 0.3 second in panel **D**, and regular at 0.20 second in panel **E**. |
| **QRS:** | 0.12 second in panel **A**, and 0.06 second in panels **B** to **E**. |

## VENTRICULAR FLUTTER AND VENTRICULAR FIBRILLATION (Figs. 5-64 to 5-66)

Ventricular flutter and ventricular fibrillation represent severe derangements of the heartbeat that usually terminate fatally within 3 to 5 minutes unless they are promptly stopped. Ventricular flutter resembles a sine wave in appearance, with regular, large oscillations occurring at a rate between 150 and 300 beats/min, usually exceeding 200 beats/min. Ventricular fibrillation is recognized by the presence of irregular undulations of varying contour and amplitude. Distinct QRS complexes, ST segment, and T waves are absent. The difference between rapid ventricular tachycardia and ventricular flutter may be difficult to discern and is usually of academic interest only.

Significance. Ventricular fibrillation occurs in a variety of clinical situations but is most commonly associated with coronary heart disease, acute myocardial infarction, and cardiomyopathy. The dysrhythmia occurs frequently as the terminal event in a variety of diseases. It also may be seen during cardiac pacing, cardiac catheterization, operation, anesthesia, drug toxicity (for example, antidysrhythmic drugs), and hypoxia. It may occur after electric shock administered during cardioversion or accidentally by improperly grounded equipment. Premature stimulation during the vulnerable period (R-on-T phenomenon; see discussion of ventricular tachycardia) may precipitate ventricular tachycardia, flutter, or fibrillation, particularly when the electric stability of the heart has been altered by the ischemia of an acute myocardial infarction, for example. In many patients, sustained ventricular tachycardia may precede ventricular fibrillation.[23] However, ventricular fibrillation may occur without antecedent or precipitating ventricular tachycardia or premature ventricular complexes. Experimentally, it may occur when a previously occluded coronary artery undergoes sudden restoration of flow. Clinically, this condition may be replicated by streptokinase infusion or percutaneous transluminal and angioplasty (PTCA) that restores flow to an occluded coronary artery, or possibly when coronary spasm relaxes. Conceivably, the latter event could result in ventricular fibrillation without myocardial infarction.

Ventricular flutter or fibrillation results in faintness followed by loss of consciousness, seizures, apnea, and, if the rhythm continues untreated, death. The blood pressure is unobtainable, and heart sounds are usually absent. The atria may continue to beat at an independent rhythm or be retrogradely captured for a time. Eventually, electric activity of the heart is completely absent.

Many patients who suffer ventricular fibrillation out of hospital have been resuscitated. It is interesting that only 20% to 30% of them develop a myocardial infarction, and those that do have a myocardial infarction experience a 2% to 3% recurrence rate of ventricular fibrillation in the first year. However, those patients who are resuscitated from out-of-hospital ventricular fibrillation but do not develop a myocardial infarction have a 1-year recurrence rate of almost 25%.

Treatment. Ventricular flutter and ventricular fibrillation are totally unphysiologic life-threatening dysrhythmias for which immediate electric (nonsynchronized) DC cardioversion, using 200 to 400 watt-seconds, is the only reliable treatment. When ventricular tachycardia produces

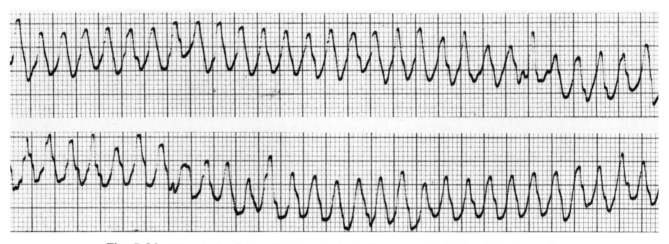

**Fig. 5-64   Ventricular flutter.** During ventricular flutter, ventricular depolarization and repolarization appear as a sine wave with regular oscillations. The QRS complex cannot be distinguished from the ST segment or T wave. Monitor lead is continuous recording.

| | |
|---|---|
| **Rate:** | Ventricular, 300 beats/min. |
| **Rhythm:** | P waves cannot be seen; ventricular, fairly regular. |
| **PR interval:** | Not measurable. |
| **QRS:** | 0.18 second. |

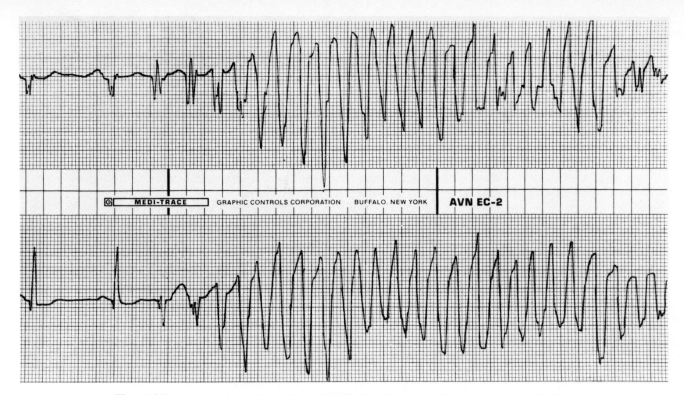

**Fig. 5-65   Ventricular tachycardia to fibrillation.** During a 24-hour ambulatory ECG recording the patient experienced sudden death. The ECG demonstrated the development of a rapid ventricular tachycardia that progressed promptly to ventricular fibrillation. Ventricular fibrillation at its onset may appear fairly regular. Dual tracing records simultaneously.

| | |
|---|---|
| **Rate:** | During sinus rhythm, 65 beats/min; ventricular rate during the rapid ventricular tachycardia is approximately 300 beats/min. |
| **Rhythm:** | During sinus rhythm, regular; during rapid ventricular tachycardia, grossly irregular. |
| **P waves:** | Normal during sinus rhythm. Cannot be seen during ventricular tachycardia-fibrillation. |
| **PR interval:** | 0.16 second during sinus rhythm. |
| **QRS:** | 0.08 second during sinus rhythm. Cannot be measured accurately during the ventricular tachycardia-fibrillation. |

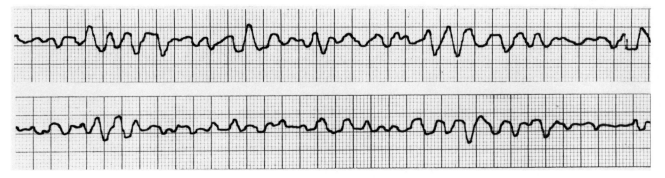

**Fig. 5-66   Ventricular fibrillation.** In this monitor lead the irregular, undulating baseline without any electric evidence of organized ventricular activity is characteristic of ventricular fibrillation. The rhythm in Fig. 5-65 proceeded to degenerate and resemble the rhythm in 5-66.

| | |
|---|---|
| **Rate:** | Cannot be determined. |
| **Rhythm:** | Grossly irregular. |
| **P waves:** | Cannot be seen. |
| **PR interval:** | Cannot be determined. |
| **QRS:** | Cannot be measured. |

the same hemodynamic response as ventricular flutter or fibrillation, it also must be terminated immediately by DC shock. A sharp blow to the chest may terminate some forms of ventricular tachydysrhythmias ("thumpversion"), but it should only be used in a witnessed arrest.

Termination of ventricular flutter or fibrillation within 30 to 60 seconds prevents the biochemical derangements accompanying ventricular fibrillation, eliminates the need for endotracheal intubation, and significantly increases the success rate of such procedures.

In an unwitnessed arrest, CPR should be initiated until a defibrillator is available. Start defibrillation at 200 watt-seconds. If unsuccessful, increase watt-seconds progressively to 300, then 360. If still unsuccessful, resume CPR and establish IV access. Administer epinephrine 1:10,000, 0.5 to 1 mg IV push. Intubate if possible. Defibrillate with up to 360 watt-seconds. If ventricular fibrillation is still present, give lidocaine 1 mg/kg IV push. Defibrillate with up to 360 watt-seconds. If ventricular fibrillation continues, consider bretylium 5 mg/kg IV push. Also consider administration of bicarbonate. (Ideally, bicarbonate is given according to blood gases.) Defibrillate up to 360 watt-seconds. Repeat bretylium 10 mg/kg IV push. Defibrillate up to 360 watt-seconds. Repeat lidocaine or bretylium; defibrillate up to 360 watt-seconds.[13]

The DC shock may cause the asystolic heart to begin discharging, as well as terminate ventricular fibrillation if the latter is present. Following a successful cardioversion, measures must be taken to prevent a second episode of ventricular fibrillation, including monitoring of the cardiac rhythm, administration of lidocaine, procainamide, or bretylium, and so forth.

## ATRIOVENTRICULAR BLOCK[24]

The conduction of an impulse may be slowed or completely blocked at sites along the conduction pathway. If the site of conduction impairment is in the AV node, His bundle or surrounding tissue, the resultant conduction abnormality is called an AV block. AV blocks are further described as first degree, second degree (Type I and Type II), or third degree based on the following criteria.

### FIRST-DEGREE AV BLOCK (Figs. 5-67 and 5-68)

During first-degree heart block, every atrial impulse is conducted to the ventricles producing a regular ventricular rhythm. However, the duration of AV conduction is abnormally prolonged, and this is manifested by a PR interval exceeding 0.20 second in the adult. PR intervals as long as 1.0 second have been recorded.

**Significance.** First-degree AV block is a common conduction disturbance that may occur in healthy or diseased hearts. It is common in elderly individuals without clinical evidence of heart disease. It may be a precursor to more advanced degrees of block. Acute first degree block is commonly caused by digitalis toxicity, acute myocardial infarction (inferior), or myocarditis.

#### Treatment

**First-degree AV block.** Generally no therapy is required. If digitalis, quinidine, or procainamide is implicated, the offending drug must be stopped or its dosage reduced.

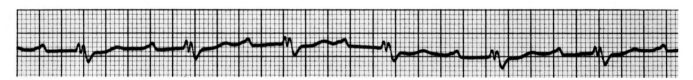

**Fig. 5-67  First-degree heart block.** In this monitor lead one cannot be certain of the type of intraventricular conduction delay. The prolonged AV conduction time may be caused by conduction delay within the AV node and/or His-Purkinje system (see His bundle section).

| | |
|---|---|
| **Rate:** | 60 to 70 beats/min. |
| **Rhythm:** | Regular. |
| **P waves:** | Normal contour and precede each QRS complex. |
| **PR interval:** | Prolonged 0.36 to 0.40 second. |

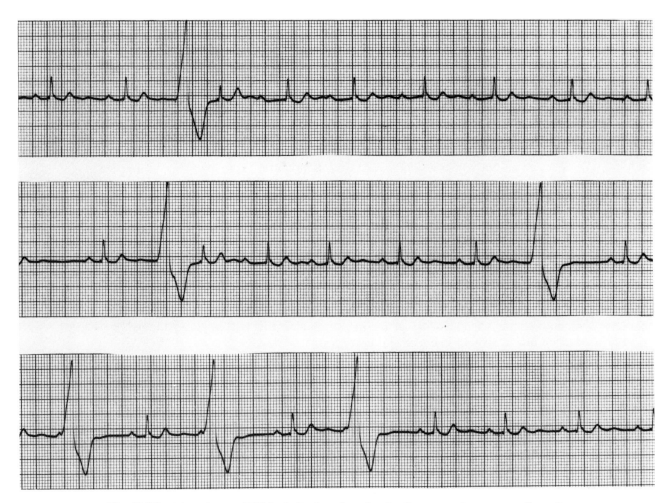

**Fig. 5-68** **First-degree AV block.** In the selected strips from a continuous recording of lead 1, premature ventricular complexes occur and are either interpolated (PVC in the first strip and first PVC in the second strip) or result in a compensatory pause. The PR interval of the QRS complexes preceding the PVC is slightly prolonged. However, following the interpolated PVC the PR interval prolongs further and remains prolonged for a series of beats, finally returning to the resting PR interval duration. When the premature ventricular complex produces a compensatory pause, additional PR prolongation does not occur. Monitor lead.

| | |
|---|---|
| **Rate:** | 63 beats/min. |
| **Rhythm:** | Regular for the most part; irregularities caused by premature ventricular complexes. |
| **P waves:** | Normal. |
| **PR interval:** | 0.22 to 0.24 second prior to the interpolated premature ventricular complexes, lengthening to 0.4 second immediately following the interpolated premature ventricular complex. |
| **QRS:** | 0.07 second for the normally conducted beats and 0.16 second for the PVC. |

## SECOND-DEGREE AV BLOCK (Figs. 5-69 to 5-73)

Failure of some atrial impulses to conduct to the ventricles at a time when physiologic interference would not be expected constitutes second-degree AV block. The nonconducted P wave may be intermittent, frequent, or infrequent, occur at regular or irregular intervals, and may be preceded by fixed or lengthening PR intervals. A distinguishing feature is that conducted P waves relate to a QRS complex with recurring PR intervals, that is, the association of P with QRS is not random. The two types of second-degree AV block can be distinguished with an acceptable degree of accuracy by analysis of the PR intervals.

### Second-Degree AV Block Mobitz Type I (Wenckebach)(Figs. 5-69 to 5-70)

In a classic type I (Wenckebach) second-degree AV block a gradual lengthening of the PR interval occurs because of lengthening AV conduction time, until an atrial impulse is nonconducted, so a P wave is not followed by a QRS. Then the sequence begins again. The blocked P wave may occur occasionally or frequently; regularly or irregularly. The ratio of atrial impulses to ventricular responses is frequently 5:4, 4:3, 3:2, or 3:1. The duration of the QRS complex may be normal or prolonged. Type I AV block occurs most commonly in the AV node. Because the increment in conduction time is greatest in the second beat of the Wenckebach group and then *decreases* progressively over succeeding cycles, (1) the interval between successive RR cycles prior to the nonconducted P wave progressively *decreases*, (2) the duration of the pause produced by the nonconducted P wave is less than twice the shortest cycle, (3) the duration of the RR cycle following the pause exceeds the RR cycle preceding the pause.

In atypical Wenckebach (which occurs commonly) the increment in AV conduction time may increase in the last beat so that the last RR cycle preceding the blocked P wave lengthens rather than shortens.

**Significance.** Of the second-degree blocks, type I is the most common, is usually transitory, and rarely progresses to complete heart block. It produces little or no clinical symptoms.

**Treatment.** Generally no therapy is required. Treatment may be necessary for patients who are symptomatic with very slow ventricular rates. This may be more common in elderly patients who develop type I AV block. Atropine, in 0.5 mg increments IV, or isoproterenol, 1 or 2 µg/min, may be tried initially, with care taken not to produce a sinus tachycardia in patients who have an acute myocardial infarction. If there is no response or if the block remains for prolonged periods, pacemaker therapy may be used. Digitalis, if implicated, must be stopped.

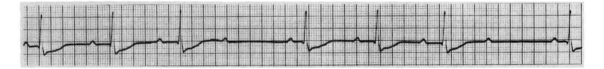

**Fig. 5-69 Second-degree AV heart block (type I, Wenckebach).** In this monitor lead classic AV Mobitz I Wenckebach heart block is characterized by four features in the surface electrodiogram: (1) progressive PR prolongation preceding the nonconducted P wave; (2) progressive shortening of the RR interval because the increment in PR interval decreases in succeeding cycles; (3) the duration of the pause (generated by the blocked P wave) is less than twice the duration of the shortest cycle, which is the cycle that precedes the nonconducted P wave; and (4) the duration of the RR cycle following the pause exceeds the duration of the RR cycle preceding the pause. The increment in PR interval is greatest in the second cycle following the pause. Wenckelbach AV block often may be "atypical"; the increment in PR interval does not decrease but rather increases, so that the last RR interval preceding the nonconducted P wave lengthens rather than shortens. In the setting of a normal QRS complex, Wenckebach AV heart block almost always occurs at the level of the AV node.

| | |
|---|---|
| **Rate:** | Atrial, 54 beats/min; ventricular, varying. |
| **Rhythm:** | Atrial, regular; ventricular, varying. |
| **P waves:** | More numerous than QRS complexes but are related to ventricular beats in a consistent repetitive fashion. |
| **PR interval:** | Progressive PR prolongation preceding the nonconducted P wave. Finally, one P wave is blocked, and the cycle then repeats. |
| **QRS:** | Prolonged, 0.14 second. Therefore in this tracing one cannot be certain that the level of block is at the AV node but indeed could occur distal to the His bundle recording site (see His bundle section). |

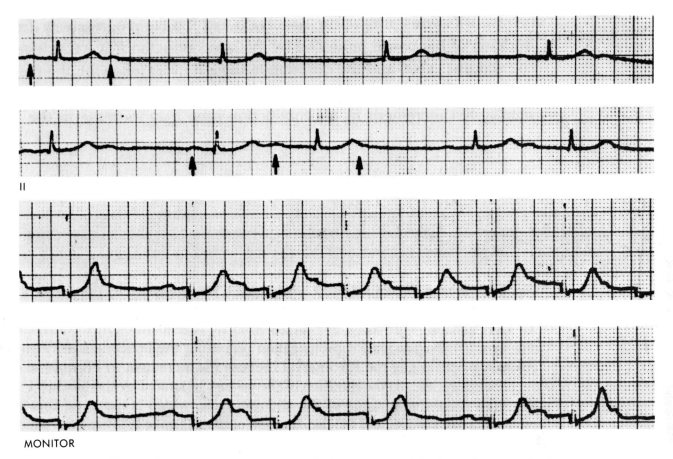

II

MONITOR

**Fig. 5-70  Second-degree AV heart block (type I Wenckebach).** In A, 2:1 conduction occurs (arrows indicate P waves). Since 2:1 conduction can occur with either type I and type II second-degree heart block, sometimes the two cannot be readily differentiated. However, the presence of a normal QRS complex is an indicator of type I second-degree AV heart block. In **B** the 2:1 AV heart block becomes 3:2 and PR prolongation for the second conducted P wave *(second arrow)* establishes the diagnosis of type I second-degree AV heart block. **C** (continuous recording) illustrates the response of Wenckebach AV block to intravenous atropine. Both the atrial rate and the conduction ratio increase.

| | |
|---|---|
| **Rate:** | Atrial: in **A** and **B**, 72 beats/min; in **C**, 79 beats/min; ventricular: in **A**, 36 beats/min; in **B**, varying; in **C**, varying but increased. |
| **Rhythm:** | Atrial, regular; ventricular, varying, depending on the degree of AV block. |
| **P waves:** | Normal. |
| **PR interval:** | Progressive increase in PR interval until one P wave fails to conduct. |
| **QRS:** | Normal, 0.07 second. |

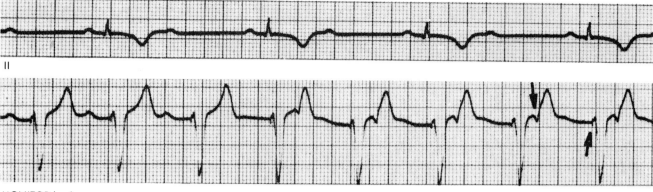

II

MONITOR lead

**Fig. 5-71    2:1 anterograde AV block 1:1 retrograde VA conduction.** In the top tracing alternate P waves conduct to the ventricles. In the lower tracing (same patient) ventricular pacing (upright arrow indicates pacemaker artifact) establishes 1:1 retrograde atrial conduction beginning with the fourth paced QRS complex. Inverted arrow indicates retrograde atrial activation.

| | |
|---|---|
| **Rate:** | Atrial, top tracing, 68 beats/min; bottom tracing, 70 beats/min; ventricular; top tracing, 34 beats/min; bottom tracing, 70 beats/min. |
| **Rhythm:** | Atrial, regular; ventricular, regular. |
| **P waves:** | Top tracing, normal; bottom tracing, normal and retrograde. |
| **PR interval:** | Top tracing, 0.20 second; conduction of alternate P waves. |
| **RP interval:** | Bottom tracing, 0.16 second. |
| **QRS:** | Top tracing. 0.08 second; bottom tracing, 0.14 second. |

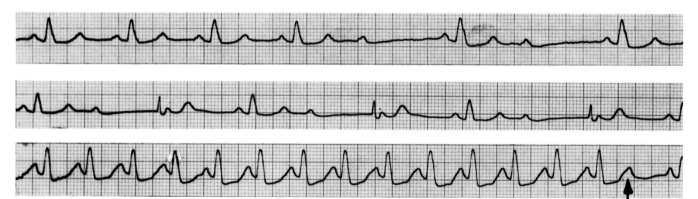

Isoproterenol

**Fig. 5-72    Second-degree AV heart block, type II.** Left bundle branch block is present in this recording of lead I. Sudden failure of AV conduction results without antecedent PR prolongation. In the second strip the escape beats interrupt the pause produced by the blocked P wave. In the bottom strip isoproterenol infusion has increased the atrial rate and also increased the conduction ratio significantly. Only one nonconducted P wave occurs *(arrow)*.

| | |
|---|---|
| **Rate:** | Atrial, 62 beats/min in the top strip. 71 beats/min in the middle strip, and 122 beats/min in the bottom strip; ventricular, varying. |
| **Rhythm:** | Atrial, regular; ventricular, varying, depending on the degree of AV block. |
| **P waves:** | Normal. |
| **PR interval:** | Normal and constant at 0.19 second in the top and middle strips and difficult to measure in the bottom strip. |
| **QRS:** | Prolonged to 0.12 second with a left bundle branch block contour. |

## Second-Degree AV Block Mobitz Type II
### (Figs. 5-72 and 5-73)

In type II second-degree AV block a P wave is blocked without progressive antecedent PR prolongation and occurs almost always in a setting of bundle branch block. The PR interval of the conducted atrial impulses may be prolonged or normal, but it usually remains fairly constant. The pause caused by the nonconducted P wave is equal to or may be slightly less than twice the normal RR interval. Sinus dysrhythmia, premature beats, AV junctional escape beats, or changes in neurogenic influences may disturb the timing of the expected pauses. Type II AV block almost always occurs in the His-Purkinje system.

**Significance.** Type II second-degree block is less common and frequently progresses to complete heart block. Clinical symptoms such as dizziness or faintness may occur with frequent nonconducted P waves.

**Treatment..** If type II block develops in the setting of an acute myocardial infarction, temporary transvenous pacing is necessary because this form of block often precedes the occurrence of sudden complete AV block with ventricular asystole and Adams-Stokes syncope. Prior to pacemaker insertion, isoproterenol (IV, 2 to 10 μg/min titrated to patient response) may be used temporarily. Atropine (IV 0.5 to 1 mg) by increasing the atrial rate without decreasing the AV block, may cause more P waves to block and reduce the ventricular rate. Symptomatic (for instance, with syncope, or presyncope) patients who do not have an acute myocardial infarction should receive a permanent pacemaker. For asymptomatic patients, many physicians recommend permanent pacemaker implantation prophylactically, since the natural history of type II AV block is to progress to complete AV block.

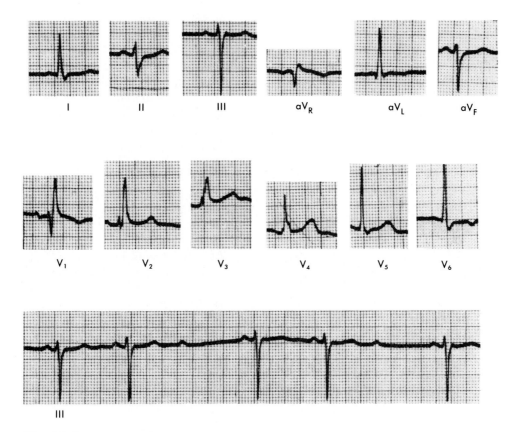

**Fig. 5-73  Second-degree AV heart block, type II.** The 12-lead ECG indicates the presence of left anterior fascicular block and right bundle branch block. In the rhythm recording (lead III) sudden failure of AV conduction results without antecedent PR prolongation.

| | |
|---|---|
| **Rate:** | 62 beats/min. |
| **Rhythm:** | Atrial, regular; ventricular, varying, depending on the degree of AV block. |
| **P waves:** | Normal. |
| **PR interval:** | Normal, constant (0.14 second) or may be prolonged, constant; sudden failure of conduction. |
| **QRS:** | Prolonged, 0.12 second. |

## COMPLETE AV BLOCK (Figs. 5-74 to 5-76)

Complete AV block occurs when no P waves are conducted to the ventricles. The atria and ventricles are controlled by independent pacemakers, and, as such, complete AV block constitutes one form of complete AV dissociation. The atrial pacemaker may be of sinus, ectopic atrial or (uncommonly) junctional origin (tachycardia, flutter, or fibrillation). The ventricular focus may be above or below the His bundle bifurcation, depending on the site of the block. In congenital complete AV block, the block is usually at the level of the AV node, proximal to the His bundle. The escape focus is supraventricular and, as such, is more stable and faster than that which occurs with distal His block. The rhythm, usually regular, may vary because of premature ventricular beats, a shift in pacemaker site, or an irregularly discharging pacemaker focus. The QRS is normal, and Adams-Stokes syncope occurs less often. In acquired complete AV block, the ventricular rate is 30 to 40 beats/min because the site of block is distal to the His bundle and consequently the escape focus is in the bundle branch—Purkinje system (Fig. 5-62). Less commonly, block within the bundle of His may occur (Fig. 5-76).

Significance. In the adult, drug toxicity (predominantly digitalis, but other drugs as well) and degenerative heart disease are the most common causes of acquired AV heart block. The degenerative process produces partial or complete anatomic or electric disruption within the AV nodal region, the His bundle, or both bundle branches. Multiple factors may contribute to this degenerative process. They include fibrosclerosis of the cardiac skeleton, fibrosis of the conduction system, coronary artery disease, myocarditis, and cardiomyopathies. Cardiac surgery has become an infrequent but still important cause of heart block. Less commonly, electrolyte disturbances, endocarditis, myocarditis, tumors, Chagas' disease, syphilitic gummas, rheumatoid nodules, myxedema, infiltrative processes such as amyloidosis, sarcoidosis, or scleroderma, and other systemic illnesses may lead to AV heart block. Calcium deposition in the region of the aortic and mitral valves may extend to involve the conduction pathways. Digitalis excess produces type I, not type II, second-degree AV block.

AV heart block occurring during a myocardial infarction may be divided into two groups: that which occurs during an anterior or anteroseptal infarction and that which occurs during a diaphragmatic (inferior) infarction. When an anterior wall infarction produces AV block, it is usually the result of extensive necrosis of the summit of the interventricular septum, which spares the AV node and His bundle but inflicts severe damage to the bundle branches. Consequently, the block is apt to be distal to the His bundle (type II) and associated with right bundle branch block and a form of fascicular block. Complete AV block may develop, during which the ventricular rate is less than 40 beats/min, asystole and syncope occur more commonly,

and mortality is 75% or higher. Death results from pump failure or shock, owing to the large size of the infarction.

When AV block results from diaphragmatic infarction, the block, type I, usually occurs in the region of the AV node, owing to inflammation or edema that results from ischemia or infarction of neighboring myocardium. The ventricular pacemaker is faster and more stable, located in the region of the AV node or His bundle, and the block is usually transient, without residua. Advanced block and syncope are uncommon, and the mortality in patients without associated heart failure does not appear to be increased. Some overlap occurs between these two divisions.

Atropine, isoproterenol, and exercise normally shorten the PR interval as the atrial rate increases; when the atrial rate is increased by atrial pacing, the PR interval lengthens. Steroids and thyroid hormones tend to improve AV conduction, which may lengthen during adrenal insufficiency or myxedema. In patients with type II AV block occurring in the His-Purkinje system, an increase in the atrial rate following atropine, isoproterenol, or exercise may not concomitantly improve AV conduction and result in a greater number of blocked P waves.

Symptoms during second-degree AV block are infrequent unless periods of complete AV block occur. The slow ventricular rate during complete heart block may not maintain circulation effectively and may result in angina, congestive heart failure, or syncope. Ventricular asystole may occur or the slow rate may initiate premature ventricular systoles or tachydysrhythmias.

### Treatment

**Third-degree (complete) AV block.** If third-degree (complete) AV block develops in a setting of an acute myocardial infarction, temporary transvenous pacing is necessary.

Atropine 0.5 mg IV push may be used and repeated as needed to a total dose of 2.0 mg prior to insertion of the pacemaker. Pacemaker insertion is preferable to repeated doses of atropine.[13]

Asymptomatic patients with chronic stable complete AV block may need no specific therapy, although many physicians recommend prophylactic pacemaker implantation for them, to prevent an Adams-Stokes attack. For those patients with symptoms of congestive heart failure or Adams-Stokes syncope caused by ventricular asystole, severe ventricular bradycardia, or ventricular tachydysrhythmias occurring as a result of the AV block, long-term drug therapy is generally unreliable, and permanent pacemaker implantation is indicated. It has been suggested that patients who develop transient high-degree AV block during myocardial infarction and survive should receive prophylactic permanent pacemaker implantation even though the block resolves.[25] This conclusion needs to be supported by other studies.

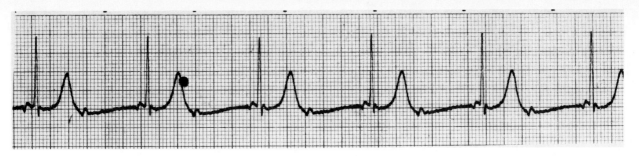

**Fig. 5-74  Congenital complete AV block in a 7-year-old.**

| | |
|---|---|
| **Rate:** | Atrial: 95 beats/min. |
| **Ventricular:** | 48 beats/min. |
| **Rhythm:** | Atrial: Slightly irregular, possibly caused by ventriculophasic sinus dysrhythmia. |
| **P waves:** | Vary in contour. |
| **PR interval:** | There is no consistent PR interval indicating that the atrial and ventricular impulses are not related. |
| **QRS:** | Normal; 0.06 second. |
| **Dysrhythmia:** | Third degree AV block. |

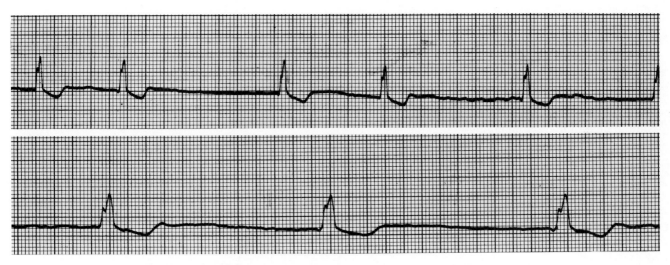

**Fig. 5-75  Atrial fibrillation in an elderly male with complete AV block.**

| | |
|---|---|
| **Rate:** | 20 to 70 beats/min. |
| **Rhythm:** | Irregular. |
| **P waves:** | Irregular baseline indicated atrial fibrillation. |
| **PR interval:** | Not measurable. |
| **QRS interval:** | 0.10 second in top strip to 0.14 second in bottom strip. |
| **Dysrhythmia:** | The underlying atrial rhythm is atrial fibrillation. In the bottom strip there is complete AV dissociation (as a result of complete AV block) manifested by ventricular escape beats while the atrial continued to fibrillate. |

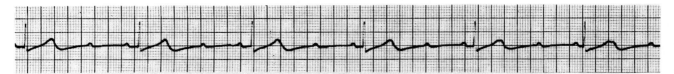

**Fig. 5-76  Third-degree (complete) AV heart block.** This tracing was recorded from an 80-year-old man who had recurrent syncope caused by an acquired complete AV block. The ECG is uncommon, since the QRS complexes are normal in this monitor lead and suggest that the site of block is AV nodal or, more likely, intrahisian. Congenital complete AV block has this appearance, although with a faster ventricular rate. His bundle recording would be necessary to establish site of block.

| | |
|---|---|
| **Rate:** | Atrial, 107 beats/min; ventricular, 36 beats/min. |
| **Rhythm:** | Atrial, regular; ventricular, regular. |
| **P waves:** | Normal. |
| **PR interval:** | Totally variable. |
| **QRS:** | Normal, 0.6 second. |

## BUNDLE BRANCH BLOCK (Figs. 5-77 and 5-78)

Anatomic or functional discontinuity in one of the bundle branches may prevent or slow conduction so that the ventricle on the affected side becomes activated late, because this ventricle, normally supplied by the blocked bundle branch, must be activated by impulses traveling through the ventricular wall and interventricular septum from the unaffected side. Conduction along this circuitous route proceeds more slowly, and therefore the QRS complex becomes widened to 0.10 to 0.12 second (incomplete) or more than 0.12 second (complete right or left bundle branch block). Transient bundle branch block may occur as a result of tachycardia, bradycardia, pulmonary embolism, anemia, infection, myocardial ischemia or infarction, congestive heart failure, metabolic derangements, hypoxia, and other causes.

The following criteria are helpful in diagnosing bundle branch block:

1. QRS 0.12 seconds
2. Supraventricular rhythm
3. PR interval 0.12 seconds
4. Wide QRS complex with "M" shape or rSR' pattern (When "M" is in $V_1$ consider RBBB; when "M" is in $V_6$ consider LBBB.)

## LEFT BUNDLE BRANCH BLOCK (Fig. 5-77)

In complete left bundle branch block (LBBB) the QRS complex becomes prolonged more than 0.12 second, with the major slowing occurring in the middle and terminal forces. The initial forces are deformed and prevent the development of the normal septal Q wave in I or $V_6$. Initial R waves in $V_1$ to $V_3$ are small or absent, followed by deep, large, slurred S waves, and large, prolonged R waves in $V_5$ and $V_6$. Significant mean axis deviation is usually absent. The ST segment and T wave shift are characteristically 180 degrees opposite the major QRS deflection.

**Significance.** LBBB is often associated with serious heart disease such as coronary artery disease, valvular heart disease, and hypertension. Although both RBBB and LBBB can occur in patients without apparent heart disease, LBBB correlates significantly with cardiomegaly and suggests a more serious prognosis. The conduction defect caused by LBBB alters the initial QRS vector, often obscuring the normal ECG signs of an acute myocardial infarction.[24]

**Treatment.** The cause is treated and not LBBB response.

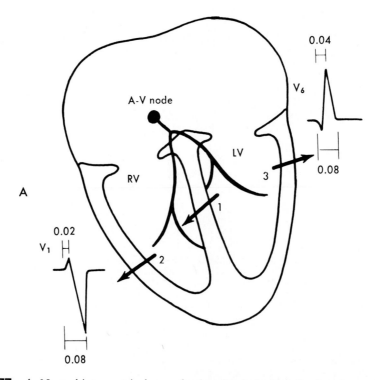

**Fig. 5-77** **A,** Normal intraventricular conduction. Intrinsicoid deflection (interval from onset of QRS complex to peak of R wave, upper brackets) is usually about 0.02 second in right precordial leads and 0.03 to 0.04 second in left precordial leads. The intrinsicoid deflection prolongs during bundle branch block.

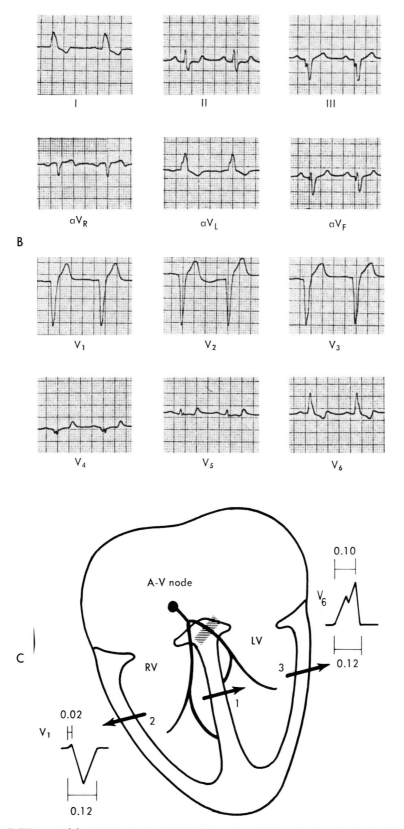

**Fig. 5-77, cont'd    B,** Twelve-lead ECG illustrating left bundle branch block. The axis is −30 degrees. **C,** Schematic illustration is presented.

## RIGHT BUNDLE BRANCH BLOCK (Fig. 5-78)

In uncomplicated complete right bundle branch block (RBBB) the QRS complex is 0.11 second or wider. The initial and middle forces of the vector loop are in a normal direction, and the terminal force is directed to the right and anteriorly. These changes produce large S waves in I, II, $V_5$ and $V_6$, often a terminal R wave in III, and R' in $V_1$ and $V_2$. Incomplete RBBB is associated with the same electrocardiographic pattern, but the QRS complex is 0.10 second or less.

Significance. In a young individual, right ventricular hypertrophy may produce RBBB; in an older patient, coronary artery disease is a more likely cause. Early supraventricular complexes that are conducted aberrantly through the ventricle are more likely to develop RBBB than LBBB, presumably because the right bundle branch takes longer to repolarize than does the left bundle branch. The initial forces in RBBB are not altered, and therefore the ECG signs of myocardial infarction are not obscured.

Treatment. There is no treatment for RBBB itself, but the cause is treated.

According to electrocardiographic concepts, the left bundle branch divides into two subdivisions or fascicles:

1. The anterior (superior), which traverses the base of the anterior papillary muscle of the left ventricle
2. The posterior (inferior), which traverses the posterior papillary muscle

When the two subdivisions are intact, the impulse is transmitted simultaneously down both fascicles and gives a resultant force *(3)* of its vectors *(1)* and *(2)*. (Fig. 5-79). The term *hemiblock* is used when one of the subdivisions is blocked.

*Left anterior hemiblock* occurs if the anterior (superior) division is blocked. The vector *(1)* is no longer present and the left ventricle is activated by the posterior division, vector *(2)*. The ECG manifestations include left axis deviation; a small q in I and a small r in III; and a normal QRS when not accompanied by RBBB (Fig. 5-79, B and D).

*Left posterior hemiblock* occurs if the posterior (inferior) division is blocked. The vector *[2]* is no longer present and the left ventricle is activated by the anterior division, vector *(1)*. The ECG manifestations include right axis deviation: a small r in lead I and a small q in lead III; normal QRS duration; and no evidence of right ventricular hypertrophy (Figs. 5-79, C, and 5-80.

*Significance:* left anterior hemiblock is more common than left posterior hemiblock because the posterior branch is shorter and thicker and less influenced by the stresses of the outflow tract. The posterior branch also has a double blood supply. Chronic hemiblock may be seen in the elderly without demonstrable heart disease. Acute hemiblock is nearly always caused by an anterior myocardial infarction. Less common causes include cardiomyopathies, a calcified aorta, and hypercalemia. Two large groups of patients develop ventricular conduction disorders because of either a sclerodegenerative process limited to the conduction system (Lenegre's disease) or fibrosclerosis of structures adjacent to the conduction system (Lev's disease). Patients with Lenegre's disease appear to be younger and more prone to developing AV block than those with Lev's disease.

*Bifascicular block* occurs when two fascicles are blocked simultaneously: RBBB and left anterior hemiblock (LAH) occur most commonly. Right bundle branch block RBBB and left posterior hemiblock (LPH) occur less commonly.

*Significance:* chronic bifascicular block is often asymptomatic. If symptoms occur they may include dizziness, syncope, hypotension, or congestive heart failure because of a slow heart rate and decreased cardiac output. Acute bifascicular block may occur in the presence of an acute myocardial infarction, especially anterior infarction, and may precede more advanced forms of heart block.

*Treatment:* chronic bifascicular block that is asymptomatic may not require any treatment. Pacemaker implantation is the treatment of choice if the patient becomes symptomatic. In acute bifascicular block, the patient should be paced regardless of symptoms because complete AV Block is likely to occur.

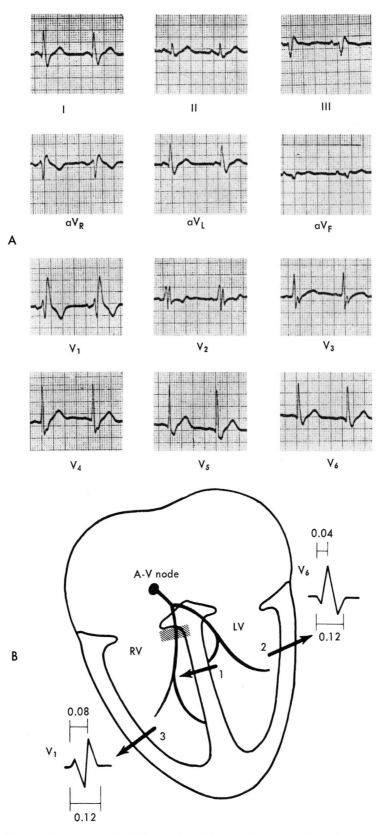

**Fig. 5-78** **A,** Twelve-lead ECG illustrating right bundle branch block. **B,** Schematic illustration is presented.

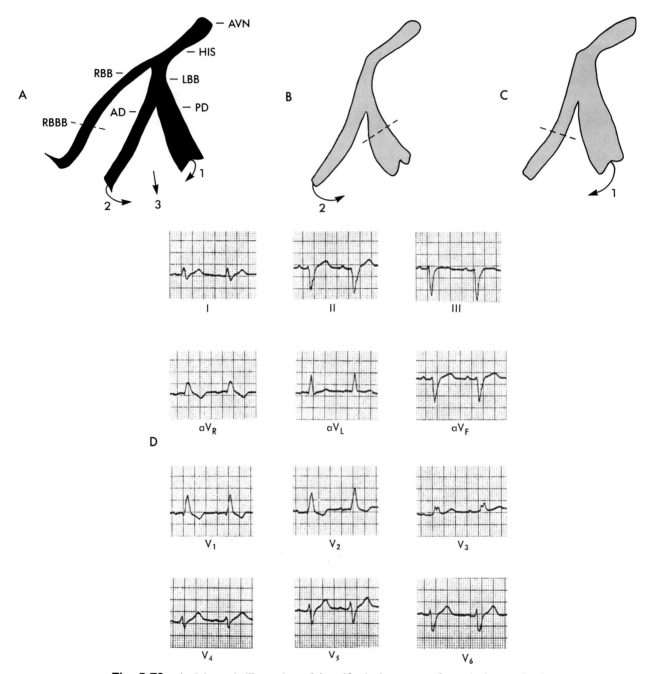

**Fig. 5-79** **A,** Schematic illustration of the trifascicular nature of ventricular conduction. *AVN,* Atrioventricular node; *HIS,* bundle of His; *RBB,* right bundle branch; *LBB,* main portion of left bundle branch; *AD,* anterior (superior) division (fascicle) of left bundle branch; *PD,* posterior (inferior) division (fascicle) of left bundle branch. When both divisions of the left bundle are activated simultaneously (vectors 1 and 2), the resultant force produces vector 3. **B,** When the anterior (superior) division is blocked, the impulse must travel through the intact posterior division. Left axis shift occurs. **C,** When the posterior (inferior) division is blocked, the impulse must travel through the intact anterior division. Right axis shift occurs. **D,** Twelve-lead ECG, illustrating right bundle branch block and left anterior hemiblock. See also Fig. 5-72.

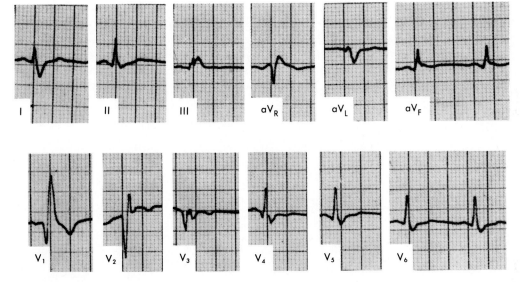

**Fig. 5-80**   Twelve-lead ECG illustrating right bundle branch block and left posterior fascicular block. The abnormal Q waves in leads $V_1$ to $V_4$ indicate the presence of an anteroseptal myocardial infarction.

## PARASYSTOLE (Fig. 5-81)

Premature complexes that lack a fixed relationship to the preceding complex (varying coupling intervals) may result from parasystole. As classically defined, a parasystolic focus is a protected pacemaker focus that discharges at a fixed rate. Parasystolic discharge becomes manifest when the area in which the parasystolic focus originates has recovered excitability. The parasystolic focus then may depolarize the atrium or ventricle to produce a premature complex. The resulting P wave or QRS complex has a configuration different from that of the dominant rhythm, depending on the site of origin. Although the dominant rhythm may be discharged by the parasystolic focus, the dominant rhythm does not depolarize the parasystolic focus because the latter is protected by unidirectional entrance block; that is, impulses may exit from the parasystolic focus to discharge the surrounding myocardium, but no impulse may enter the parasystolic focus and discharge it. For learning purposes, it can be thought of as a fixed-rate pacemaker that does not sense spontaneous complexes, is not reset by them but does cause depolarization of the rest of the heart. The manifest parasystolic rate may be much less than the actual rate because of exit block from the parasystolic focus.

That is, the parasystolic focus may discharge at more rapid rates than are apparent in the ECG because many of the discharges fail to exit and depolarize the surrounding myocardium. Exit block from the parasystolic focus may produce irregular spacing of the interectopic intervals. However, since the rate of discharge of the parasystolic focus is constant, the interectopic intervals between parasystolic impulses reduce to a common denominator. Premature complexes that are caused by a parasystolic focus ordinarily have no fixed relationship to the basic rhythm and often result in the production of fusion beats.

Parasystole should be suspected when the following criteria are met: (1) varying coupling intervals; (2) constant shortest interectopic intervals; and (3) frequent appearance of fusion beats.[26]

**Significance.** Atrial and junctional parasystole may occur in patients without clinical evidence of heart disease. Ventricular parasystole generally manifests in patients with heart disease; it is rarely, if ever, caused by digitalis excess.

**Treatment.** The therapeutic approach is basically the same as that discussed for premature atrial, junctional, and ventricular complexes. Parasystole is a benign rhythm disorder.

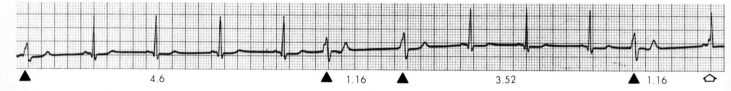

**Fig. 5-81   Ventricular parasystole.** The parasystolic ventricular beats are indicated by the solid triangles and the open arrow. The interval between parasystolic ventricular complexes is 1.16 seconds. The intervals of 4.6 and 3.52 seconds are 4 times and 3 times, respectively, the interectopic interval of 1.16 seconds. Note that the coupling interval varies and that a fusion beat (next to last QRS complex, indicated by open arrow) is also present. Ventricular refractoriness prevents emergence of the parasystolic ventricular rhythm during the long intervals in which it is absent. This tracing was recorded from an otherwise healthy 15-year-old boy.

| | |
|---|---|
| **Rate:** | 65 beats/min, with some variation; parasystolic rate, 63 beats/min. |
| **Rhythm:** | Atrial and ventricular rhythms during normally conducted beats, regular; parasystolic ventricular interval, regular. |
| **P waves:** | Normal. |
| **PR interval:** | 0.11 second during the normally conducted beats. |
| **QRS:** | Of normally conducted beats, 0.09 second; or parasystolic ventricular beats, 0.12 second. |

## AV DISSOCIATION

As the words imply, AV dissociation means that atria and ventricles are dissociated; they are controlled by separate pacemakers for one or more beats. The term used generically tells nothing about the nature of atrial or ventricular activity, except that these chambers are beating independently for a period of time. It is as if the term described a "symptom" without indicating what caused it. The atria may be fibrillating, fluttering, or responding to an ectopic tachycardia or sinus impulses; the ventricles may be controlled by AV junctional or ectopic ventricular beating. The only fact conveyed is that whatever controls one chamber does not also control the other during the period of AV dissociation.

AV dissociation is *never* a primary disturbance of rhythm but rather a consequence of a more basic disorder; for the term to be used properly, the cause(s) producing AV dissociation must also be described. Examples can be found throughout this chapter; some of them are as follows:

1. Slowing of the primary pacemaker to allow the escape of a subsidiary (latent) focus. In Fig. 5-13, sinus slowing allows two ventricular beats to escape under the control of a separate focus while the sinus node still controls the atria. During these two beats, AV dissociation exists.
2. Accelerated discharge of subsidiary focus. In Fig. 5-51, accelerated AV junctional discharge results in a nonparoxysmal AV junctional tachycardia without retrograde atrial capture. Since the atria remain under sinus domination, separate pacemakers control atria and ventricles, resulting in AV dissociation. Fig. 5-135 presents a similar example, called "isorhythmic" AV dissociation because atria and ventricles maintain similar rates and rhythms. AV dissociation may also occur during ventricular tachycardia if retrograde atrial capture does not ensue (see Figs. 5-57 to 5-62).
3. AV block. In Fig. 5-73, AV block reduces the number of effective (conducted) atrial impulses; this allows the escape of a subsidiary focus to produce AV dissociation. When AV block results in AV dissociation, the atrial rate generally exceeds the ventricular rate (see Fig. 5-162).
4. Combinations of 1, 2, or 3 may initiate AV dissociation, as, for example, when digitalis causes both first-degree (or Wenckebach) AV block and NPJT, or when acute myocardial infarction produces AV block and an accelerated idioventricular rhythm (Fig. 5-63).

In all these examples, but for diverse reasons, the ventricular rate either exceeds or becomes equal or nearly equal to the effective (conducted) atrial rate. It is this fact that allows AV dissociation to occur.

The preceding discussion makes it apparent that the presence or absence of AV dissociation depends on the rate and temporal relationships of the two pacemakers and the intactness of AV and VA conduction. Should the atrial pacemaker capture control of the ventricle, or vice versa, AV dissociation would be terminated during that period of capture (incomplete AV dissociation).

## SUPRAVENTRICULAR DYSRHYTHMIA WITH ABNORMAL QRS COMPLEXES
### (Figs. 5-82 to 5-85)

Wide, bizarre QRS complexes may occur during isolated supraventricular beats or sustained supraventricular rhythms. The term *aberrant ventricular conduction* is commonly applied to such complexes. Thus QRS contours that display prolonged abnormal configuration indicate that conduction through the ventricle is abnormal; they do not necessarily mean that the impulse *originated* in the ventricles.[28] The presence of fusion and capture complexes strongly supports the diagnosis of ventricular tachycardia or accelerated ventricular rhythm. However, the electrocardiographic manifestations of ventricular tachycardia, including the presence or absence of AV dissociation, and complexes that appear to represent capture or fusion beats, may be mimicked, under certain circumstances, by supraventricular dysrhythmias.

Intraventricular conduction defects, bundle branch blocks, and anomalous pathway conduction all may initiate abnormal ventricular depolarization with widened QRS complexes. Also, premature supraventricular stimulation may conduct to the ventricles before ventricular repolarization has been completed, causing the impulse to conduct aberrantly. The resulting widened QRS complex may display characteristic features that distinguish it from those beats arising in the ventricles during a true ventricular tachycardia. The following analysis may be helpful in distinguishing aberrant ventricular conduction initiated by a supraventricular impulse from ventricular tachycardia.

Identification of atrial activity. During sinus rhythm or an ectopic supraventricular rhythm, identification of distinct atrial activity initiating ventricular depolarization, regardless of how deformed the QRS complex may appear, establishes the diagnosis of supraventricular rhythm with QRS aberration. A casual relationship between the P and QRS complexes may be demonstrated in one or more of the following ways, depending on the nature of the supraventricular rhythms:

1. P waves with a normal contour precede and maintain a constant relationship to each QRS complex during sinus rhythm.
2. Interventions that alter the sinus rate, such as carotid sinus massage or exercise, secondarily alter the ventricular rate in exactly the same manner and maintain the same, or nearly the same, PR interval. This indicates that ventricular activation follows as a consequence of atrial discharge. Atrial pacing can be employed to alter the atrial rate during a tachycardia characterized by wide QRS complexes, and a diagnosis of ventricular tachycardia is considered likely when fusion and capture complexes result.
3. When atrial flutter, atrial fibrillation, or atrial tachycardia exists, carotid sinus massage, digitalis, verapamil, or edrophonium chloride (Tensilon) admin-

istration produces characteristic slowing of the ventricular response (at times also normalizing the QRS complex); during AV nodal reentry or AVRT the rhythm may remain unchanged or terminate and allow sinus rhythm to resume.

4. Atrial and ventricular rhythms may be so related as to suggest dependency of the latter on the former, during typical AV Wenckebach cycles, for example.
5. When atria and ventricles are dissociated, finding ventricular captures that have the same contour as the QRS of the tachydysrhythmia in question indicates a supraventricular rhythm.
6. Bursts of an intermittent tachycardia that are always initiated by a premature atrial complex provide indirect evidence supporting a supraventricular diagnosis. However, it is important to remember that, under certain circumstances, a premature atrial complex can initiate a ventricular tachycardia.
7. During retrograde atrial capture the RP interval is of too short a duration to be explained by retrograde conduction from a ventricular focus (about 0.10 second or less).
8. If the rate and rhythm of abnormal QRS complexes are the same as the rate and rhythm of a known supraventricular tachycardia, this provides some support in favor of aberration.
9. The presence of AV dissociation during a wide QRS tachycardia is much more consistent with ventricular than supraventricular tachycardias.

Analysis of QRS contours and intervals. The following clues suggest aberrant ventricular conduction initiated by a supraventricular impulse:

1. The contour of the QRS is a triphasic rsR' in $V_1$. RBBB patterns occur more frequently than LBBB patterns because, at a slower heart rate, the right bundle branch appears to require more time to repolarize than the left. Therefore premature discharge is more likely to encounter a refractory right bundle branch and produce RBBB.
2. Monophasic or diphasic complexes in $V_1$ or an LBBB pattern favor the diagnosis of ventricular tachycardia, as does a frontal QRS axis that is directed superiorly and to the right.
3. Faster rates speed repolarization, whereas slower rates retard it; the refractory period is proportional to the preceding cycle length. Therefore the heart takes longer to repolarize following a long cycle than it does after a short cycle. Because of this, when an early beat succeeds a long cycle, the early beat may encounter refractory tissue and conduct aberrantly. A comparison of such long-short cycle sequences aids in determining aberrant conduction.
4. During atrial flutter or fibrillation or a series of premature atrial complexes, aberrantly conducted beats persist in runs rather than maintain a bigem-

inal pattern and then lack a compensatory pause after their termination.

5. The initial vectors of aberrant and normal beats are similar during functional RBBB, since RBBB preserves the normal initial forces.

6. Aberrantly conducted supraventricular QRS complexes are not wildly bizarre or lengthened; most of the QRS prolongation occurs in the latter portion of the beat. QRS complexes with a duration exceeding 0.14 second are more likely to indicate ventricular tachycardia.

7. A fixed coupling interval between the normal and aberrant beats is absent during atrial flutter or atrial fibrillation. Conversely, fixed coupling during atrial

flutter or fibrillation favors ventricular ectopy.

8. The aberrant beats are not excessively premature.

9. During a narrow QRS supraventricular tachycardia (excluding atrial flutter and atrial fibrillation, the presence of alteration of QRS morphology favors the presence of a retrograde accessory pathway in the tachycardia circuit [i.e., AVRT associated with the WPW syndrome.]).[29]

10. The QRS configuration appears the same as that resulting from known supraventricular conduction at similar rates. Conversely, if the QRS contour is the same as that resulting from known ventricular conduction, the tachycardia is probably ventricular in origin.

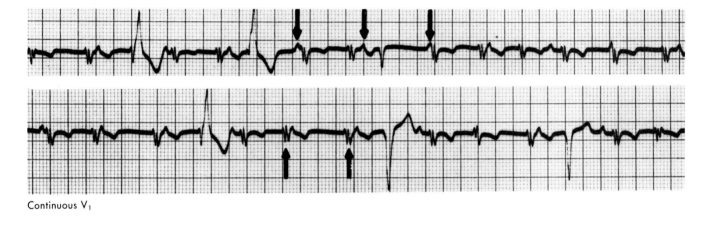

Continuous V₁

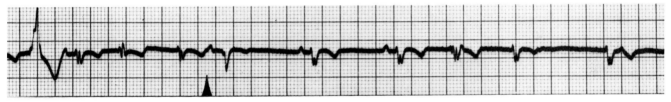

Carotid sinus massage V₁

**Fig. 5-82  Nonparoxysmal AV junctional tachycardia with intermittent atrial captures producing functional right and functional left bundle branch block.** The nonparoxysmal AV junctional tachycardia discharges at a slightly irregular rate and accounts for the W-shaped QRS complex, *(upright arrrows)*. intermittent sinus captures (p waves indicated by inverted arrows) shorten the cardiac cycle and result in either a normal, W-shaped QRS complex, functional right bundle branch block, or functional left bundle branch block. Carotid sinus massage (in the bottom tracing at the arrowhead) slows both the sinus and junctional discharge rates. This tracing was recorded from a 13-year-old boy with no heart disease other than the cardiac dysrhythmia. Therapy with digitalis slowed the junctional rate sufficiently so that the patient remained asymptomatic and had resting rates of 70 to 80 beats/min with a normal response to exercise.

| | |
|---|---|
| **Rate:** | Atrial, approximately 88 beats/min but varying; ventricular, approximately 88 beats/min but varying. |
| **Rhythm:** | Irregular; incomplete AV dissociation. |
| **P waves:** | Normal. |
| **PR interval:** | 0.14 second when premature capture does not occur. |
| **QRS:** | Normal, functional right and functional left bundle branch block with a duration of 0.12 second. |

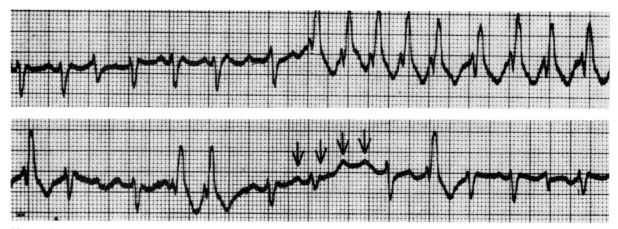

V₁—continuous

**Fig. 5-83  Functional right bundle branch block.** At first glance the tracing appears to be sinus rhythm interrupted by a burst of ventricular tachycardia and intermittent premature ventricular systoles. Closer inspection reveals flutter waves *(arrows)* when the ventricular rate slows slightly and suggests that the widened QRS complexes may be aberrantly conducted supraventricular beats. These beats conform in all respects to criteria established to differentiate supraventricular aberration from ventricular tachycardia. (See text.) The patient requires digitalis to slow the ventricular rate rather than lidocaine to suppress ectopic ventricular discharge.

| | |
|---|---|
| **Rate:** | Atrial, 280 beats/min; ventricular, 90 to 200 beats/min. |
| **Rhythm:** | Atrial, regular; ventricular, irregularly irregular. |
| **P waves:** | Flutter waves *(arrows)* can be seen when the ventricular rate slows and can be marched out with regularity. |
| **PR interval:** | Flutter-R interval varies. |
| **QRS:** | Varying contour between normal and functional right bundle branch block. |

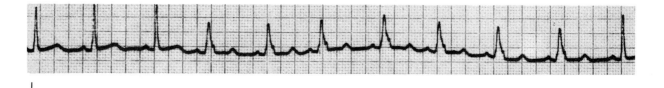

I

**Fig. 5-84  Rate-dependent aberrancy of the left bundle branch block type.** Gradual acceleration of the sinus rate results in a functional left bundle branch block that remains until the sinus rate slows sufficiently at the end of the tracing. This type of aberrancy is much more commonly of the left bundle rather than the right bundle branch block type and is more apt to be associated with cardiac disease than is functional right bundle branch block.

| | |
|---|---|
| **Rate:** | 60 to 78 beats/min. |
| **Rhythm:** | Slightly irregular. |
| **P waves:** | Normal. |
| **PR interval:** | Normal and constant, 0.14 second. |
| **QRS:** | Varies between normal and functional left bundle branch block. |

11. Vagal maneuvers remain a most important differentiating point, since vagal discharge does not usually affect ventricular tachycardia, whereas it slows the ventricular rate in most supraventricular mechanisms. However, ventricular tachycardia terminated by vagal discharge has been reported.

12. The presence of fusion and capture beats (see p. 163), as stated earlier, provides the most important evidence in favor of ventricular tachycardia.

None of the aforementioned features can be used to establish unequivocally the diagnosis of ventricular tachycardia, and in many instances invasive electrophysiologic studies must be performed.

### Esophageal Pill Electrode

When wide, bizarre QRS complexes are present, a 12-lead ECG recorded from an esophageal electrode facilitates differential diagnosis.[30] The esophageal pill electrode affords a simple and precise method for obtaining such an ECG. This electrode is a disposable bipolar electrode housed in a gelatin capsule. Two thin threadlike wires emerge from the electrode and facilitate its placement, attachment to the ECG, and ultimate retrieval. The capsule is easily swallowed by the patient. Optimum position within the esophagus is verified when maximum atrial voltage appears on the ECG. This simple device permits differentiation of supraventricular and ventricular dysrhythmias when a conclusive diagnosis cannot be made from the 12-lead ECG alone.

Moreover, the same electrode can also be used for therapeutic pacing after a definite diagnosis of a supraventricular tachydysrhythmia has been made. The pill electrode may be used for either atrial or ventricular pacing, although success with atrial pacing has been more uniform than that with ventricular pacing.[31,32]

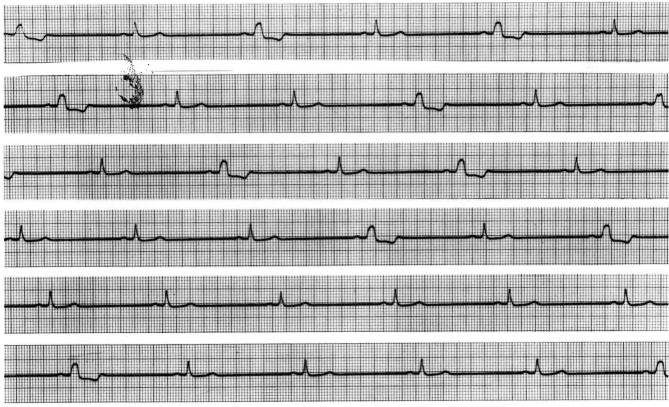

Continuous lead I

**Fig. 5-85** **Bradycardia-dependent left bundle branch block.** In this unusual tracing the patient has a sinus bradycardia. When the sinus cycle increases, the P wave conducts with a left bundle branch block. Shorter sinus cycles are ended with a normally conducted QRS complex. Very small changes in the sinus rate account for these differences.

| | |
|---|---|
| **Rate:** | 34 to 38 beats/min. |
| **Rhythm:** | Fairly regular. |
| **P waves:** | Normal and precede each QRS complex. |
| **PR interval:** | 0.19 second. |
| **QRS:** | Normal and left bundle branch block, 0.14 second. |

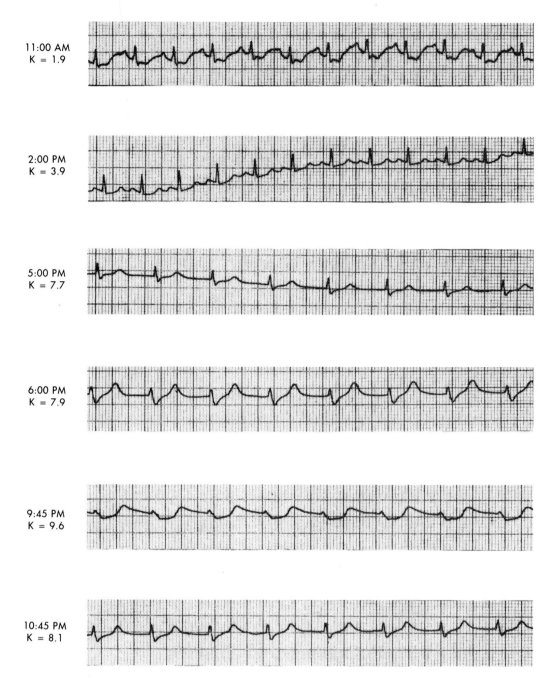

**Fig. 5-86   Serial ECG tracings in a patient with marked changes in serum potassium level.** In the 11:00 AM tracing the depressed ST segment and low amplitude T wave blending into a probable U wave (this cannot be seen with clarity because of the superimposed P waves) indicate the presence of hypokalemia. Following the administration of potassium the 2:00 PM tracing becomes relatively normal. Continued potassium administration results in hyperkalemia with the disappearance of atrial activity on the ECG and some prolongation of the QRS complex. By 7:00 PM the QRS complex is more prolonged, and by 9:45 PM the QRS complex is greatly prolonged Secondary ST-T wave changes are present. Improvement follows the administration of bicarbonate, glucose, and insulin at 10:45 PM with reduction in serum potassium level; improvement in the ECG results.

## ELECTROLYTE DISTURBANCES[33]
### Potassium (Figs. 5-86 and 5-87)

During induced hyperkalemia in animals, the ECG correlates closely with the potassium blood level. The T wave peaks when potassium concentration reaches about 5.5 mEq/L; the corrected QT interval is normal or shortens initially but may prolong as the QRS complex widens. The QRS complex may widen when the external potassium concentration exceeds 6.5 mEq/L; about 7.0 mEq/L, P wave amplitude diminishes, and P wave and PR interval duration are prolonged. About 8.0 to 9.0 mEq/L, the P wave frequently disappears. Sometimes ST segment deviation, both elevated and depressed, occurs and simulates an injury pattern. Clinically occurring potassium alterations do not correlate as well as during these experimental changes in animals, probably because the patient has multiple abnormalities that may influence the ECG differently. For example, in some studies less than 25% of patients with hyperkalemia developed the characteristic tall, narrow, peaked T waves. It is believed that extracellular potassium concentration accounts for the ECG patterns rather than changes in total body potassium or intracellular potassium concentration.

During hypokalemic states the ST segment becomes depressed, the U wave is exaggerated, and the T wave amplitude is decreased without changing the actual duration of QT interval (as long as it can be measured accurately). Actually, it is the QU interval that becomes prolonged. The P and QRS amplitude and duration may increase, and the PR interval may be prolonged. Clinical hypokalemia does not normally slow AV conduction significantly; however, isolated cases have been reported demonstrating varying degrees of PR prolongation. Intraven-

tricular conduction in adults seldom lengthens by more than 20 msec, but it may be more prolonged in children.

Spontaneous hyperkalemia rarely, if ever, produces more advanced AV block than simple PR prolongation; large doses of potassium administered rapidly may produce further advanced forms of AV block, however. Often the P wave disappears, which precludes the diagnosis of AV block. As the plasma potassium level continues to rise about 6.5 and 7.0 mEq/L, slowed intraventricular conduction results, manifested by uniform widening of the QRS complex. Areas of intraventricular block may occur and lead to ventricular fibrillation.

Potassium may potentiate the slowing effects of digitalis on AV conduction, particularly if the plasma potassium level rises rapidly. However, if AV conduction is also hampered by a rapid atrial rate, slowing the atrial rate with potassium actually may improve AV conduction and offset any direct depressing effects of potassium. Fortunately, administration of potassium to patients with digitalis-induced dysrhythmias suppresses ectopic discharge at a much lower blood potassium level than that which further depresses AV conduction.

Low blood potassium levels encourage spontaneous ectopic pacemaker discharge, presumably by enhancing automaticity and also possibly by slowing dominant pacemakers or producing conduction defects. Low potassium levels may initiate ventricular fibrillation in humans. Reduced potassium concentration may precipitate dysrhythmias in animals and humans receiving digitalis at plasma potassium levels that ordinarily do not produce ectopic beating in the absence of digitalis. Possibly the synergistic effects of digitalis and reduced potassium on automaticity and conduction make animals and humans receiving dig-

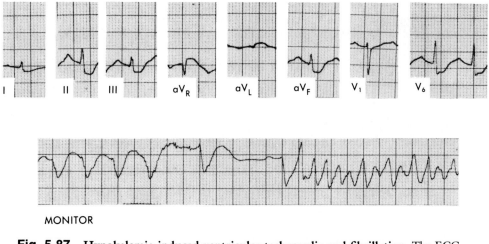

MONITOR

**Fig. 5-87** **Hypokalemia-induced ventricular tachycardia and fibrillation.** The ECG demonstrates the characteristic changes of hypokalemia: depressed ST segment, low-amplitude T wave, and large U wave, blending into the following P wave. In the monitor lead a ventricular tachycardia briefly stops and then degenerates into ventricular fibrillation that was reversed with DC shock.

italis particularly prone to dysrhythmias precipitated by hypokalemia.

The antidysrhythmic effects of potassium administration may suppress varied rhythms, regardless of cause and whether or not hypokalemia exists. Digitalis-induced ectopic discharge generally responds to potassium therapy at sufficiently low doses to avoid further AV conduction delay. Many believe that potassium remains the drug of choice for ectopic rhythms produced by excessive digitalis. Animals and humans with elevated potassium levels may tolerate large doses of digitalis without developing ectopic dysrhythmias, whereas reduced potassium level predisposes to ectopic activity in digitalized animals or patients. Also, a low level of potassium may worsen the depression of AV conduction produced by digitalis.

## Sodium

In general the magnitude of sodium change necessary to produce ECG alterations is not compatible with life, making clinical electrocardiographic manifestations of sodium derangements rarely seen, if ever.

## Calcium (Fig. 5-88)

In the ECG, low calcium level prolongs the duration of the ST segment and QT interval without prolonging the duration of the T wave, although the T wave may reverse polarity. Elevated calcium level shortens the ST segment and QT interval; the QRS duration may be prolonged during severe hypercalcemia, and AV block may develop. High calcium level opposes the effects of high potassium level, whereas low calcium level opposes the effects of low potassium. If the calcium level varies in a direction opposite that of potassium level, the effects of the latter are enhanced.

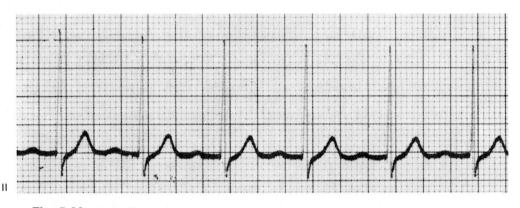

II

**Fig. 5-88** **The effects of hypercalcemia on the ECG.** Serum calcium level, 14.0/100 ml. The ST segment and QT interval are shortened, and the PR interval is slightly prolonged (0.22 second).

## INVASIVE ELECTROPHYSIOLOGIC STUDIES[23]
(Figs. 5-89 to 5-92)

Invasive electrophysiologic studies permit the direct study and manipulation of the electric activity of the heart by using electrodes placed inside the cardiac chambers.[34] The technique to record His bundle activation involves passing an electrode catheter that is introduced percutaneously into the femoral vein, in a cephalad direction up the inferior vena cava, and positioning the catheter tip near the septal leaflet of the tricuspid valve. The His bundle potential (H) appears as a well-defined, most often bipolar spike between the low right atrial (A) and ventricular (V) electrograms. The interval between the earliest onset of the surface P wave or a high right atrial deflection (P) and the low right atrial deflection (PA interval) is a measure of intraatrial conduction. The AH interval is a measurement of the conduction across the AV node and varies in duration from 55 to 130 msec, depending on the cycle length and autonomic influences. The interval from H to V (HV interval) is determined by the interval between the His bundle deflection and the earliest ventricular activity recorded in any lead. The HV interval is a measure of conduction through the His bundle distal to the recording electrode, the bundle branches, and the Purkinje system up to the point of ventricular activation. In contrast to a relatively wide range of values for the AH interval, the HV interval is fairly constant, measuring 30 to 55 msec, with an average value of 45 msec. In some patients, discharge of the right bundle branch may be recorded.

The ability to separate AV nodal and His-Purkinje conduction has enhanced our understanding of normal and abnormal AV conduction. Abnormal AV conduction may be caused by prolongation of P-A, A-H, or H-V intervals or all three. In addition, intra-His block has been demonstrated. During type I (Wenckebach) AV block in a patient with a normal QRS complex the conduction disturbance occurs at the AV node, proximal to the His bundle (Fig. 5-89). Type II AV block in a patient with a bundle branch block virtually always results distal to the His bundle (Fig. 5-90). Thus in type I AV block the blocked P wave is not followed by a His spike, whereas in type II AV block the blocked P wave is followed by a His spike.

Insertion of several electrode catheters (2 to 5) permits recording and stimulating from multiple atrial and ventricular sites and has been useful in differentiating ventricular tachycardia and aberrant ventricular conduction, in understanding the nature of many supraventricular and ventricular tachycardias and other dysrhythmias, in evaluating patients with the preexcitation syndrome or AV block, and in other areas as well, such as in initiating tachydysrhythmias in susceptible patients (Figs. 5-91 and 5-92). Significantly, adequacy of therapy can be judged by precipitating the patient's tachycardia in a control state and then attempting to restart it during therapy. Further, most recently catheters have been used for therapy (to ablate sites important for the genesis and/or maintenance of the dysrhythmia) as well as for diagnostic purposes. Although areas of application of these electrophysiologic studies are still evolving, fairly definitive indications can be stated.[35]

Further discussion is beyond the scope of this text and the reader is referred to other sources.

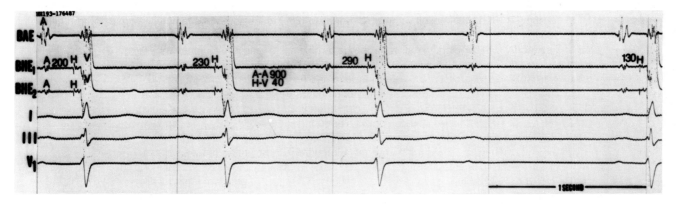

**Fig. 5-89   Type I (Wenckebach) AV nodal block.** Simultaneous recordings of electrograms from the high right atrium *(BAE)* and His bundle *(BHE₁, BHE₂)* and scalar leads I, III, and V₁ are displayed during normal sinus rhythm. The PR interval progressively lengthens until the fourth P wave fails to conduct. The conduction delay is caused by AH prolongation that increases from 200 msec in the first beat shown (not the first beat in this Wenckebach series) to 290 msec just before the block. The AH interval then shortens to 130 msec in the first beat of the next Wenckebach series. The nonconducted P wave blocks proximal to the His bundle.

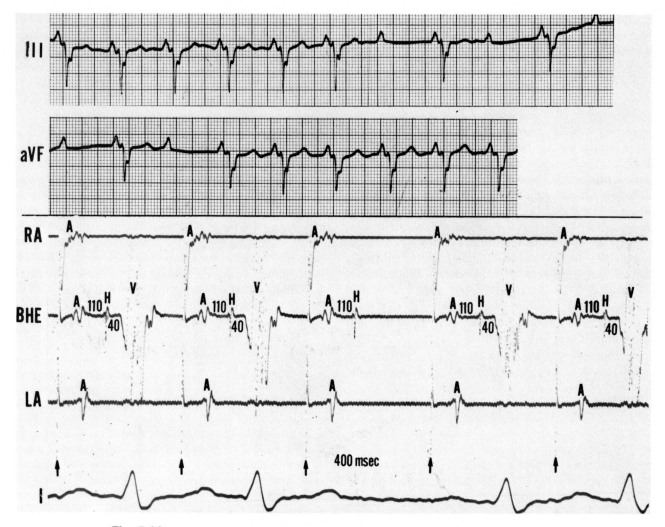

**Fig. 5-90** **Type II AV block.** The scalar recordings in the top portion of the figure (leads III and AV$_F$) demonstrate type II AV block characterized by a fixed PR interval preceding the nonconducted P wave. During the electrophysiologic study *(bottom)*, right atrial pacing at a cycle length of 400 msec resulted in a fixed AH interval of 110 msec and HV interval of 40 msec. The third P wave *(A)* blocked distal to the His bundle recording site, characteristic of type II AV block. *LA,* Left atrial electrogram. Arrows point to stimuli delivered to right atrium.

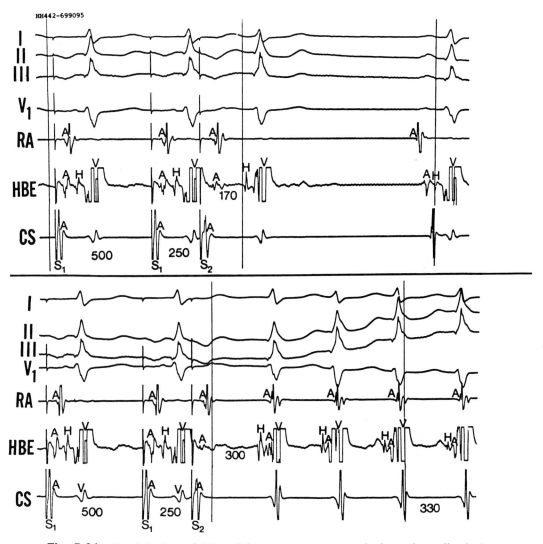

**Fig. 5-91** **Precipitation of AV nodal reentrant, supraventricular tachycardia. A,** Recordings were obtained simultaneously from scalar leads I, II, III, and $V_1$ and intracavitary recordings from the right atrium *(RA)*, His bundle area *(HBE)*, and coronary sinus *(CS)*. The coronary sinus was stimulated at a fixed cycle length of 500 msec ($S_1$ to $S_1$) and then stimulated prematurely ($S_2$) at a cycle length of 250 msec. The AH interval lengthened slightly to 170 msec, but tachycardia did not result. **B,** Premature stimulation at the same coupling interval produced an AH interval of 300 msec and precipitation of a supraventricular tachycardia caused by AV nodal reentry at a cycle length of 330 msec (rate: 182 beats/min). Findings are consistent with "dual AV nodal" pathways.

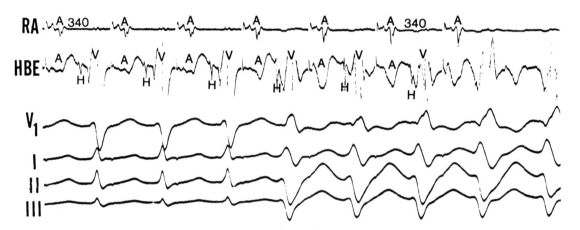

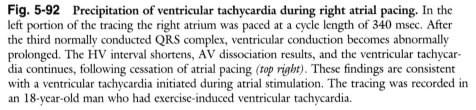

**Fig. 5-92** **Precipitation of ventricular tachycardia during right atrial pacing.** In the left portion of the tracing the right atrium was paced at a cycle length of 340 msec. After the third normally conducted QRS complex, ventricular conduction becomes abnormally prolonged. The HV interval shortens, AV dissociation results, and the ventricular tachycardia continues, following cessation of atrial pacing *(top right)*. These findings are consistent with a ventricular tachycardia initiated during atrial stimulation. The tracing was recorded in an 18-year-old man who had exercise-induced ventricular tachycardia.

## ARTIFACTS (Figs. 5-93 and 5-94)

Electronic instrumentation has provided vast dividends to the care of patients with heart disease. However, because we now rely so heavily on various types of monitoring devices, one must constantly be alert and recognize artifacts that mimic dysrhythmias. A tracing that resembles ventricular fibrillation *must* be artifactual if the patient is found sitting up in bed in no distress, reading a newspaper! The cardinal rule is to treat the patient and not the monitor.

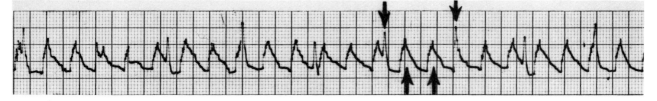

**Fig. 5-93  Toothbrush tachycardia.** This tracing was recorded from a patient brushing his teeth with an electric toothbrush at a rate of 188 brushes/min. Note the regularly occurring artifacts *(upright arrows)* that do not influence the QRS complexes *(inverted arrows)*.

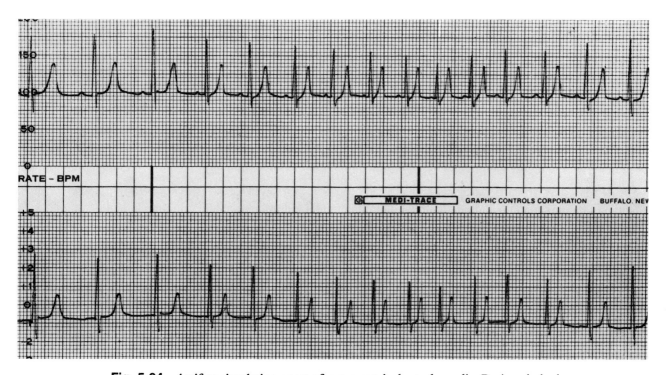

**Fig. 5-94  Artifact simulating onset of supraventricular tachycardia.** During playback of a tape-recorded ECG rhythm, the rate of revolutions per minute of the tape slowed and simulated the onset of a supraventricular tachycardia. The diagnosis of artifact is easily made, since, in addition to shortening of the RR interval, the PR, QRS, and QT intervals all decrease markedly. Both leads recorded simultaneously.

## Dysrhythmia Test Section

It is suggested that the reader use this section to test knowledge of dysrhythmias. Cover the interpretations in each legend, calculate intervals and irregularities as previously discussed, and determine the diagnosis. Consider also the significance of each dysrhythmia and what form of treatment would most likely be employed. There may be disagreements in interpretation of rhythm strips, but the essential point is to make your diagnosis by using the analytic method described in this chapter. This approach offers a justification for your interpretation.

*Text continued on p. 244.*

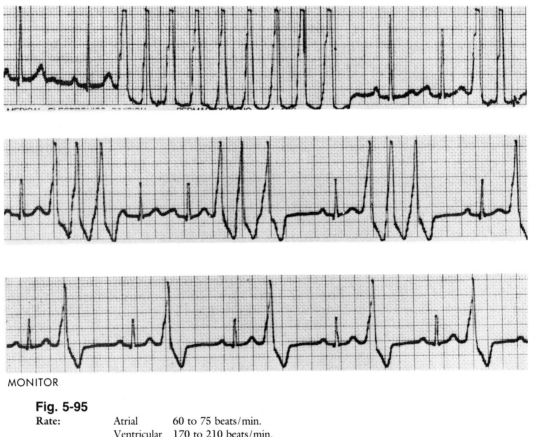

MONITOR

**Fig. 5-95**

| Rate: | Atrial | 60 to 75 beats/min. |
|---|---|---|
| | Ventricular | 170 to 210 beats/min. |
| **Rhythm:** | Atrial | Slightly irregular. |
| | Ventricular | Irregular because of bursts of ventricular ectopy. |
| **P waves:** | | Normal for the sinus-initiated QRS complexes. |
| **PR interval:** | | Normal for the sinus-initiated QRS complexes, 0.16 second. |
| **QRS:** | | Normal for the sinus-initiated complexes; wide, bizarre, prolonged (0.12 second) for the ventricular ectopy. |
| **Dysrhythmia:** | | Paroxysmal ventricular tachycardia gradually decreasing in frequency to bigeminy and then complete disappearance. This result followed administration of lidocaine, 50 mg IV in a patient with an acute myocardial infarction. |

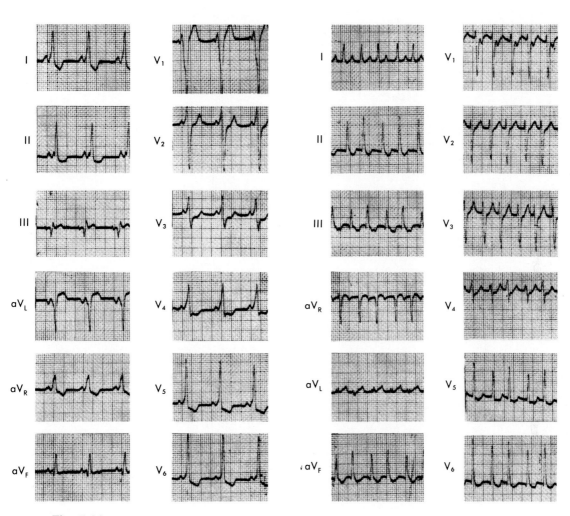

### Fig. 5-96

| | |
|---|---|
| **Rate:** | **A,** 82 beats/min; **B,** varying between 150 and 180 beats/min. |
| **Rhythm:** | **A,** Regular; **B,** slight variation in RR intervals with long cycles alternating with short cycles. |
| **P waves:** | **A,** Normal; **B,** retrograde; see $V_1$. |
| **PR interval:** | **A,** 0.08 second; **B,** RP interval 0.12 second. |
| **QRS:** | **A,** Prolonged, 0.12 second; **B,** normal, 0.08 second. |
| **Dysrhythmia:** | **A,** Normal sinus rhythm during preexcitation syndrome; **B,** AVRT in the same patient. |

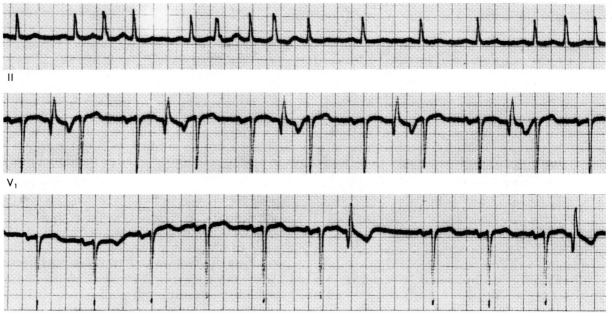

II

V₁

V₁

**Fig. 5-97**

| | |
|---|---|
| **Rate:** | 75 beats/min, with premature complexes. |
| **Rhythm:** | Irregular because of premature complexes. |
| **P waves:** | Normal and precede each of the normal QRS complexes. |
| **PR interval:** | Prolonged following the premature complexes. |
| **QRS:** | Normal for the sinus-initiated complexes; prolonged to almost 0.12 second for the premature complexes. |
| **Dysrhythmia:** | Interpolated premature ventricular complexes in the top and middle tracings. In the bottom tracing, premature ventricular complexes produce a compensatory pause and are therefore no longer interpolated. |

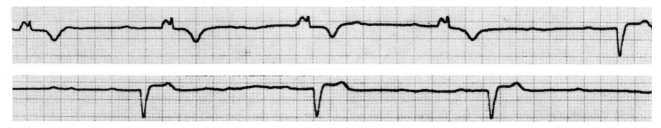

Continuous—MONITOR

**Fig. 5-98**

| | | |
|---|---|---|
| **Rate:** | Atrial | 86 beats/min. |
| | Ventricular | Upright complexes 38 beats/min; negative complexes 28 beats/min. |
| **Rhythm:** | Atrial | Regular. |
| | Ventricular | Fairly regular. |
| **P waves:** | | Normal and have no relationship to the QRS complexes. Clear P waves cannot be seen throughout the entire tracing. |
| **PR interval:** | | Not measurable. |
| **QRS:** | | Abnormal; upright complexes 0.14 second, negative complexes 0.12 second. |
| **Dysrhythmia:** | | Complete AV block with a ventricular escape rhythm. The simultaneous change in ventricular contour and rate probably indicates a shift in the ventricular escape focus site. |

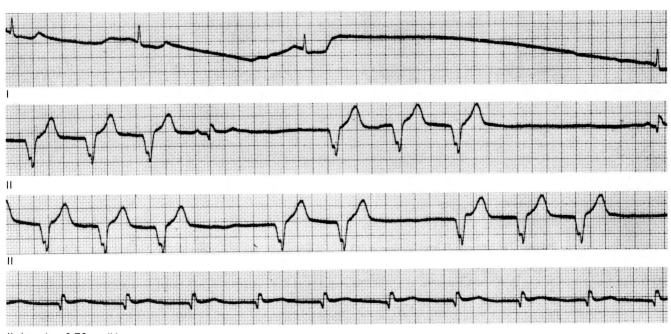

I

II

II

II Atropine, 0.75 mg IV

## Fig. 5-99

**Rate:** Top tracing, slow with periods of asystole. Middle two tracings, 75 beats/min with periods of asystole. Bottom tracing, 65 beats/min.

**Rhythm:** Top three tracings, irregular; bottom tracing, regular.

**P waves:** Normal contour, preceding the sinus-initiated QRS complexes in lead II but are hard to see in lead I.

**PR interval:** Normal for the sinus-initiated P waves, not present for the other QRS complexes. In the bottom tracing no P wave or PR interval is apparent.

**QRS:** Normal for the sinus-initiated QRS complexes, prolonged (0.13 second) for the ventricular ectopic beats.

**Dysrhythmia:** Various dysrhythmias recorded in a patient with an acute inferior myocardial infarction. Top tracing, marked sinus bradycardia and periods of sinus arrest.

Middle two tracings, an accelerated idioventricular rhythm, slightly irregular. The duration of the pauses in the third strip appears to be a multiple of the basic idioventricular cycle length, thus suggesting the possible presence of an intermittent exit block. Bottom tracing, a junctional rhythm following atropine administration suppresses the ventricular ectopy.

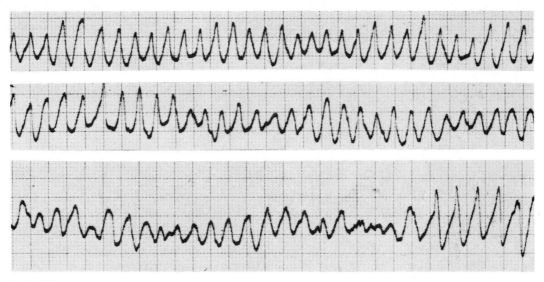

MONITOR

### Fig. 5-100

| | |
|---|---|
| **Rate:** | 300 to 500 beats/min. |
| **Rhythm:** | Grossly irregular. |
| **P waves:** | None seen. |
| **PR interval:** | Not measurable. |
| **QRS:** | Wide, bizarre, irregular. |
| **Dysrhythmia:** | Ventricular flutter that becomes ventricular fibrillation in the bottom tracing. The ventricular fibrillation then seems to organize and merge into ventricular flutter or possibly ventricular tachycardia in the terminal portion of the tracing. |

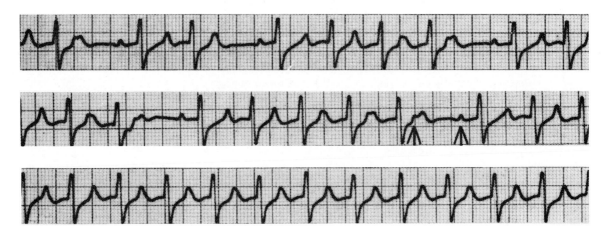

MONITOR

### Fig. 5-101

| | | |
|---|---|---|
| **Rate:** | Atrial | 115 beats/min. |
| | Ventricular | Varying, depending on the degree of block. |
| **Rhythm:** | Atrial | Regular. |
| | Ventricular | Irregular. |
| **P waves:** | | Precede each of the QRS complexes *(arrows)*. |
| **PR intervals:** | | Progressively lengthens until one P wave fails to conduct (Wenckeback AV block) |
| **QRS:** | | Normal (0.08 second). |
| **Dysrhythmia:** | | Atrial tachycardia with varying block. Note the varying T wave contour as P waves fall during portions of the antecedent T wave. In the bottom tracing 1 : 1 AV conduction occurs. |

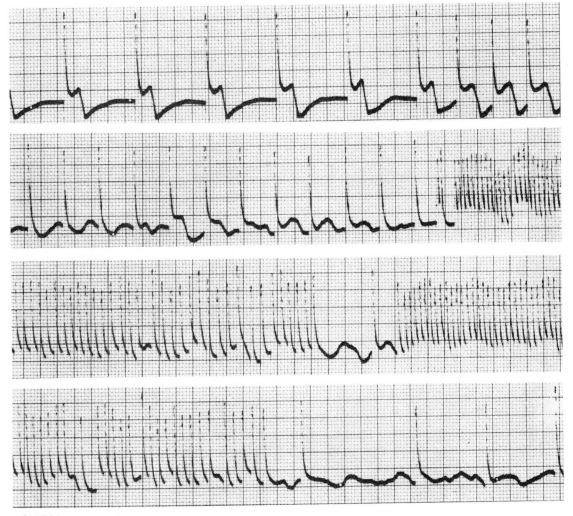

MONITOR

### Fig. 5-102

| | | |
|---|---|---|
| **Rate:** | Ventricular | 74 beats/min to very rapid rates. |
| **Rhythm:** | Ventricular | Periods of regularity replaced by gross irregularity. |
| **P waves:** | | None seen. |
| **PR interval:** | | Not measurable. |
| **QRS:** | | Wide, distorted, initiated by pacemaker spikes. |
| **Dysrhythmia:** | | Runaway pacemaker discharging at irregular and extremely rapid rates and finally initiating ventricular fibrillation. The pacemaker rate sped from 71 beats/min to approximately 145 beats/min and then greater than 1000 stimuli/min. |

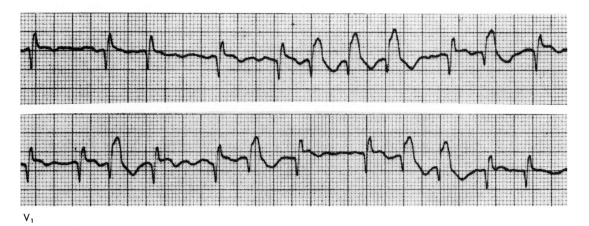

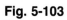

### Fig. 5-103

| | | |
|---|---|---|
| **Rate:** | Ventricular | 73 to 180 beats/min. |
| **Rhythm:** | Ventricular | Grossly irregular. |
| **P waves:** | | None seen. |
| **PR interval:** | | Not measurable. |
| **QRS:** | | Normal (0.08 second) and abnormal (0.12 second) with a right bundle branch block contour. |
| **Dysrhythmia:** | | Atrial fibrillation with a rapid ventricular response. QRS complexes, which demonstrate a right bundle branch block, terminate a short cycle (or a series of short cycles) that follows a long preceding cycle. The development of functional right bundle branch block caused by cycle length changes in this fashion is called the *Ashman phenomenon*. |

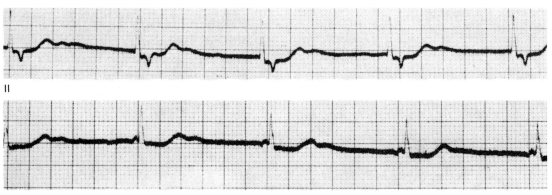

### Fig. 5-104

| | |
|---|---|
| **Rate:** | *Top, 52 beats/min.* |
| **Rhythm:** | Regular. |
| **P waves:** | Retrograde. |
| **PR interval:** | *Bottom,* 0.06 second. |
| **RP interval:** | *Top,* 0.08 second. |
| **QRS:** | Normal (0.06 second). |
| **Dysrhythmia:** | AV junctional rhythm recorded on two occasions in the same patient. In the top tracing, retrograde P waves followed the QRS complex; in the bottom tracing, retrograde) P waves preceded the QRS complex. |

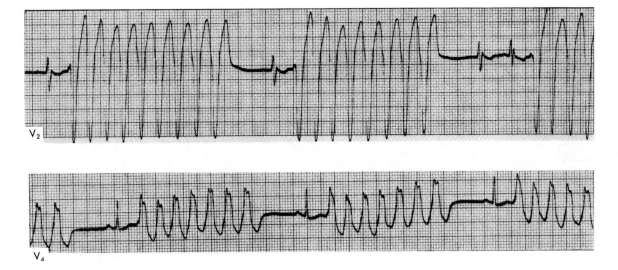

**Fig. 5-105**

| | | |
|---|---|---|
| **Rate:** | Ventricular | 250 beats/min. |
| **Rhythm:** | Ventricular | Regular in a recurrent paroxysmal fashion. |
| **P waves:** | | Precede the normally conducted QRS complexes. |
| **PR interval:** | | Normal for the normally conducted QRS complexes. |
| **QRS:** | | Normal for the sinus-initiated QRS complexes, QRS prolonged for the ventricular ectopic systoles (0.14 seconds). |
| **Dysrhythmia:** | | Repetitive monomorphic ventricular tachycardia. The lack of fusion or capture beats and precise determination of atrial activity during the tachycardia prevent an unequivocal diagnosis of ventricular tachycardia from this tracing, although the diagnosis is highly suggestive. |

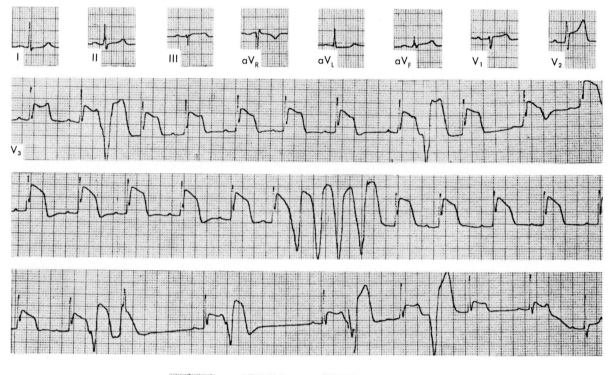

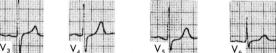

## Fig. 5-106

**Rate:**    During $V_3$, approximately 75 beats/min, interrupted by ventricular ectopy.

**Rhythm:**    Fairly regular except when interrupted by ventricular ectopy.

**P waves:**    Normal and precede each of the normally conducted QRS complexes.

**PR interval:**    Normal (0.16 second) and constant.

**QRS:**    Note abrupt ST segment elevation between $V_1$ and $V_2$ and during the $V_3$ rhythm strip. The $V_3$ at the bottom shows a normal ST segment. Abnormal complexes have a QRS duration greater than 0.12 second.

**Dysrhythmia:**    Atypical (Prinzmetal) angina pectoris characterized by ST segment *elevation* probably a result of coronary artery bypass. Premature ventricular complexes trigger a short run of ventricular tachycardia in the midportion of the tracing. ST segments return to the baseline as the chest pain abates and the ectopic ventricular activity ceases.

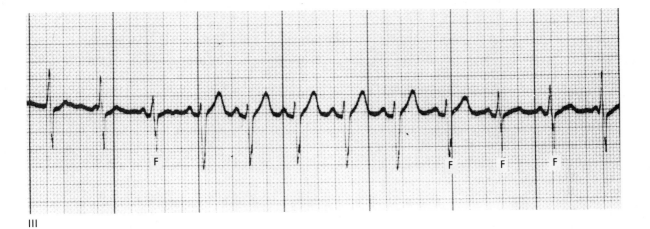

III

### Fig. 5-107

| | |
|---|---|
| **Rate:** | 107 beats/min. |
| **Rhythm:** | Regular. |
| **P waves:** | Normal and precede each of the QRS complexes in the midportion of the tracing. |
| **PR interval:** | Constant (0.16 second) for the QRS complexes in the midportion of the tracing. |
| **QRS:** | Normal duration (0.08 second) for both types of QRS complexes. Fusion QRS complexes indicated by *F*. |
| **Dysrhythmia:** | Ventricular tachycardia at beginning and end of tracing, which generates QRS complexes with a slightly different contour than during sinus tachycardia that occurs in the midportion of the tracing. The supraventricular origin of the tachycardia is suggested by the QRS duration (<0.12 second). However, recent data suggest that such a tachycardia actually may be ventricular, originating in the upper portions of the fascicular system and generating a QRS complex with a duration *less* than 0.12 second. The presence of fusion beats *(F)* supports this conclusion. In any event, during the tachycardia at the beginning and end of the ECG, QRS complexes are not related to atrial activity. Thus AV dissociation is present because of ventricular tachycardia. In the midportion of the tracing, slight acceleration of the sinus rate allows the sinus node to regain capture of the ventricles, suppress the tachycardia, and eliminate the periods of AV dissociation. |

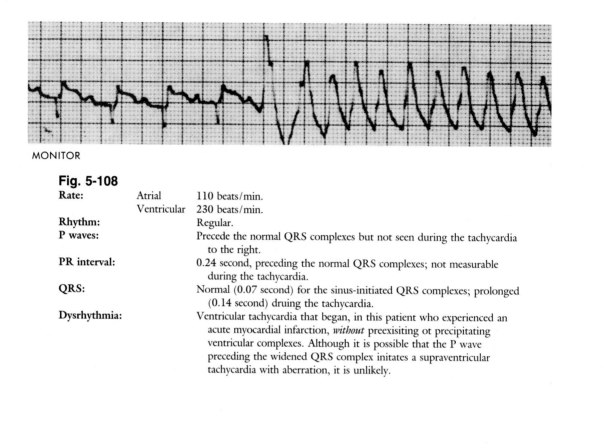

MONITOR

### Fig. 5-108

| | | |
|---|---|---|
| **Rate:** | Atrial | 110 beats/min. |
| | Ventricular | 230 beats/min. |
| **Rhythm:** | | Regular. |
| **P waves:** | | Precede the normal QRS complexes but not seen during the tachycardia to the right. |
| **PR interval:** | | 0.24 second, preceding the normal QRS complexes; not measurable during the tachycardia. |
| **QRS:** | | Normal (0.07 second) for the sinus-initiated QRS complexes; prolonged (0.14 second) druing the tachycardia. |
| **Dysrhythmia:** | | Ventricular tachycardia that began, in this patient who experienced an acute myocardial infarction, *without* preexisiting ot precipitating ventricular complexes. Although it is possible that the P wave preceding the widened QRS complex initates a supraventricular tachycardia with aberration, it is unlikely. |

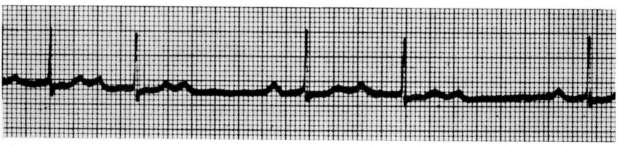

II

### Fig. 5-109

| | | |
|---|---|---|
| **Rate:** | Atrial | 75 beats/min. |
| | Ventricular | 3:2 conduction, average 50 beats/min. |
| **Rhythm:** | Atrial | Regular |
| | Ventricular | Irregular |
| **P waves:** | | Normal and precede each QRS complex. |
| **PR interval:** | | Progressively lengthens before the nonconducted P wave. |
| **QRS:** | | Normal (0.06 second). |
| **Dysrhythmia:** | | Second-degree AV block, type I (Wenckebach). |

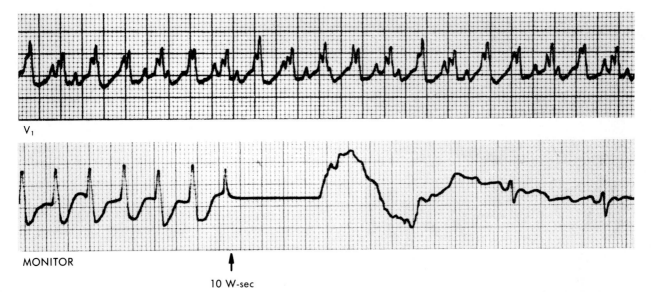

V₁

MONITOR

↑
10 W-sec

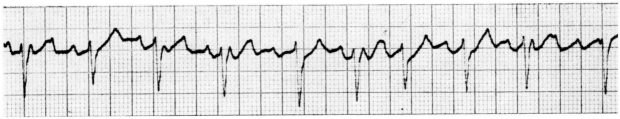

V₁

### Fig. 5-110

| | | |
|---|---|---|
| **Rate:** | Atrial | 300 beats/min (top panel). |
| | Ventricular | 200 beats/min (top panel). |
| **Rhythm:** | Atrial | Regular. |
| | Ventricular | Regular. |
| **P waves:** | | Atrial flutter. |
| **PR interval:** | | Completely variable. |
| **QRS:** | | Wide, prolonged (0.12 second) |
| **Dysrhythmia:** | | Atrial flutter and ventricular tachycardia in top tracing. Thus complete AV dissociation is present. In the monitor recording (middle tracing) the left portion reflects the same activity seen in V₁ above. However, the particular monitor lead fails to reveal the atrial flutter waves. Direct current cardioversion (*arrow,* 10 watt-seconds) terminates the ventricular tachycardia but allows the atrial flutter to persist, seen more clearly in V₁ below. The atrial flutter at this point is not as precisely regular as is was before the cardioversion. |

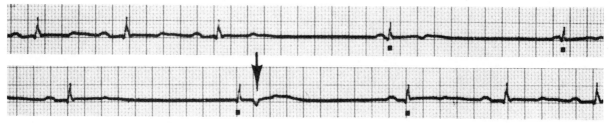

II

## Fig. 5-111

**Rate:**          30 to 50 beats/min.

**Rhythm:**     Fairly irregular.

**P waves:**     Precede and conduct to the QRS complexes that do not have dots beneath them. Those with dots beneath them are junctional escape beats.

**PR interval:**   Prolonged (0.26 second) and constant for the QRS complexes that do not have a dot beneath them.

**QRS:**         Normal duration and contour (0.08 second). Dots indicate AV junctional excape beats. The third AV junctional escape beat (lower tracing) retrogradely activates the atrium *(arrow)*.

**Dysrhythmia:**   Sinus bradycardia with intermittent sinus arrest and AV junctional escape beats, the "sick sinus syndrome."

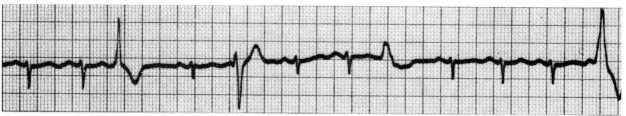

V₁

## Fig. 5-112

**Rate:**          98 beats/min.

**Rhythm:**     Irregular because of premature ventricular systoles.

**P waves:**     Normal and precede each sinus-initiated QRS complex.

**PR interval:**   Normal for the sinus-initiated QRS complexes (0.14 second).

**QRS:**         Normal for the sinus-initiated QRS complexes (0.08 second). Premature systoles are characterized by varied contour and a duration greater than 0.12 second.

**Dysrhythmia:**   Multiform premature ventricular complexes with four different contours.

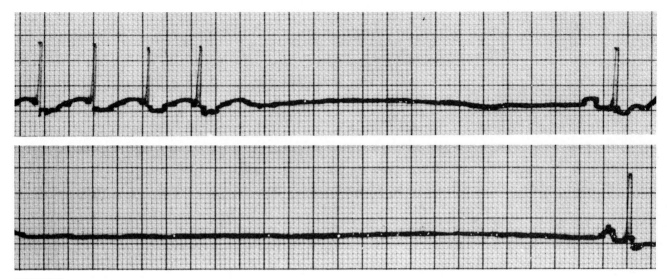

MONITOR

### Fig. 5-113

**Rate:** 140 beats/min, abruptly slowing following carotid sinus massage. Two periods of asystole are finally terminated by sinus rhythm.

**Rhythm:** Regular, followed by asystole, an atrial escape beat, and then sinus rhythm.

**P waves:** Can be seen when tachycardia terminates.

**P interval:** Normal (0.18 sec) in those beats preceded by P waves.

**QRS:** Normal.

**Dysrhythmia:** Abrupt termination of paroxysmal supraventricular tachycardia by carotid sinus massage (at beginning of recording). A lengthy period of asystole results when the tachycardia stops, before sinus rhythm resumes.

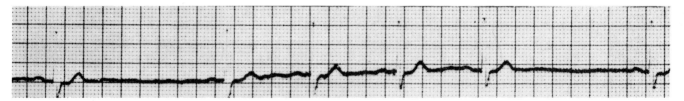

II

### Fig. 5-114

**Rate:** 33 to 66 beats/min.

**Rhythm:** Irregular.

**P waves:** Normal contour. Long PP cycles are exactly twice the short PP cycles.

**PR interval:** Normal (0.20 second).

**QRS:** Normal (0.08 second).

**Dysrhythmia:** 2:1 sinus exit block.

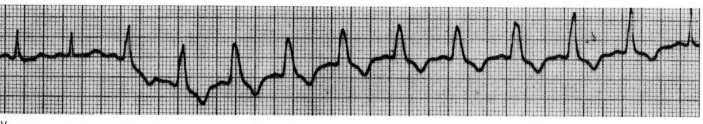

V₆

### Fig. 5-115

| | |
|---|---|
| **Rate:** | Gradually accelerates from 105 to 115 beats/min. |
| **Rhythm:** | Fairly regular. |
| **P waves:** | Normal and precede each QRS complex. |
| **PR interval:** | Normal (0.14 second) and constant. |
| **QRS:** | Normal at the slower rates; left bundle branch block (0.12 second) at the faster rates. |
| **Dysrhythmia:** | Rate-dependent aberration with functional left bundle branch block. |

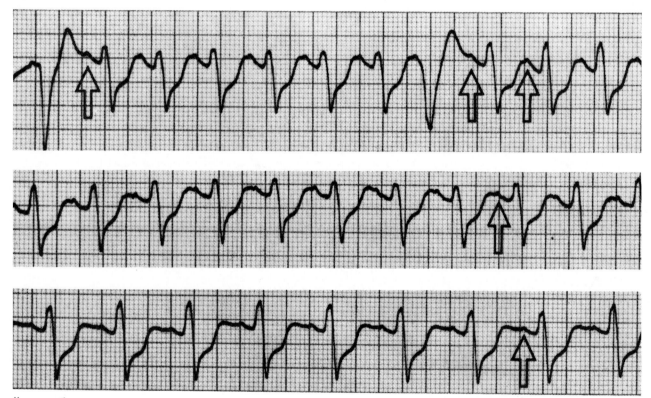

II—noncontinuous

### Fig. 5-116

| | |
|---|---|
| **Rate:** | 125 beats/min in top tracing; gradually slows to 100 beats/min in bottom tracing. |
| **Rhythm:** | Regular. |
| **P waves:** | Normal, but hidden by preceding T waves *(arrows)*. |
| **PR interval:** | 0.16 second. |
| **QRS:** | Abnormal, prolonged (0.14 second) because of the presence of a preexisting left bundle branch block. |
| **Dysrhythmia:** | Sinus tachycardia. Patient has a preexisting bundle branch clock. Clear P waves *(arrows)* can be seen in the pause that follows the two premature ventricular complexes (top tracing). The heart rate gradually slowed following edrophonium (Tensilon) adminstration (middle and bottom tracings). |

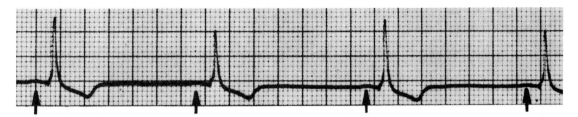

II

**Fig. 5-117**

| | |
|---|---|
| **Rate:** | 41 beats/min. |
| **Rhythm:** | Fairly regular. |
| **P waves:** | Precede each QRS with a normal contour. |
| **PR interval:** | 0.16 second. |
| **QRS:** | Borderline prolonged (0.11 second). |
| **Dysrhythmia:** | Sinus bradycardia. Patient is receiving methyldopa for hypertension. Normal rate was restored following discontinuation of methyldopa therapy. Low-amplitude P waves indicated by arrows. |

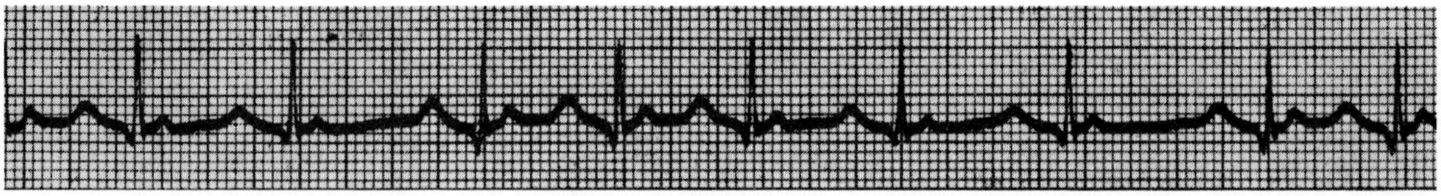

II

**Fig. 5-118**

| | |
|---|---|
| **Rate:** | Sinus rate increases with inspiration and decreases with expiration (70 to 110 beats/min). |
| **Rhythm:** | Irregular with a repetitive phasic variation in cycle length according to respiratory cycles. Cycle lengths vary by more than 0.16 second. Breath-holding eliminates the rate variations. |
| **P waves:** | Precede each QRS with a normal, fairly constant contour. |
| **PR interval:** | 0.12 second. |
| **QRS:** | Normal (0.08 second). |
| **Dysrhythmia:** | Respiratory sinus dysrhythmia. The phasic variation corresponds to a respiratory rate of approximately 18 breaths/min. |

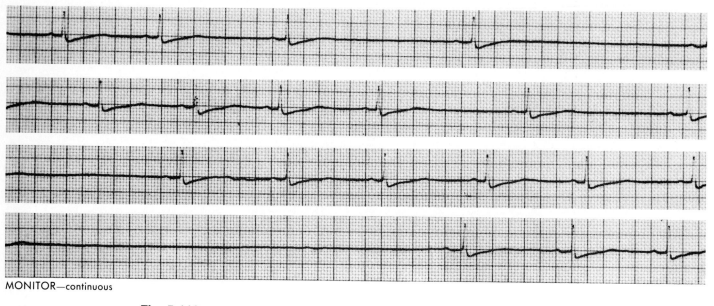

MONITOR—continuous

### Fig. 5-119

| | |
|---|---|
| **Rate:** | Varying, slow (maximum rate of 5 beats/min). |
| **Rhythm:** | Irregular; periods of asystole not a multiple of basic sinus cycle length. |
| **P waves:** | Precede each QRS with a normal contour; may be altered by escape beats. |
| **PR interval:** | Slightly prolonged (0.21 second). |
| **QRS:** | Normal (0.09 second). |
| **Dysrhythmia:** | Sinus arrest. Patient also has an acute inferior myocardial infarction. Asystolic intervals are not interrupted by escape beats. |

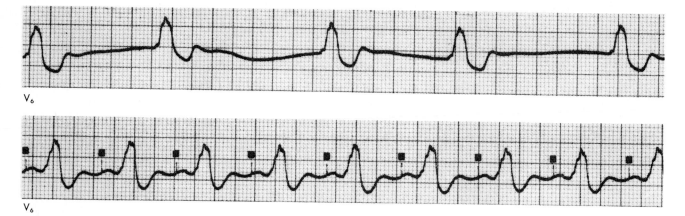

### Fig. 5-120

| | |
|---|---|
| **Rate:** | Varying, slow (36 to 50 beats/min) (*top*); normal (81 beats/min) (*bottom*). |
| **Rhythm:** | Irregular (*top*); regular (*bottom*). |
| **P waves:** | Not seen (*top*); follows pacemaker stimulus (*bottom*). |
| **PR interval:** | Not measurable (*top*); 0.16 second (*bottom*). |
| **QRS:** | Left bundle branch block (0.20 second). |
| **Dysrhythmia:** | Sinus arrest (*top*) and right atrial pacing (*bottom*). Patient also has a left bundle branch block. A supraventricular escape focus controls the rhythm in the top panel, but atrial activity is not apparent. Atrial pacing (stimuli indicated by filled squares, bottom tracing) results in atrial capture, producing a P wave and an unchanged QRS contour. |

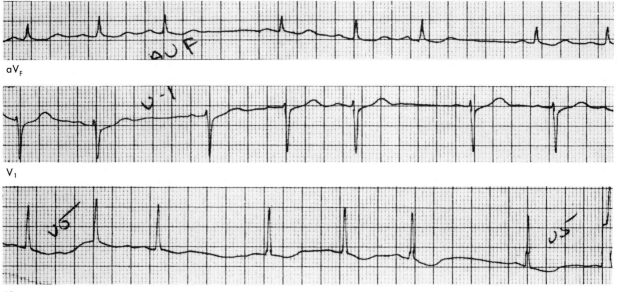

aVF

V₁

V₅

### Fig. 5-121

**Rate:** Varying, slow (50 to 88 beats/min).

**Rhythm:** (1) A pause in atrial activity occurs. (2) The PP interval progressively shortens up until the pause. (3) The duration of the pause is less than twice the shortest PP interval. (4) The PP interval following the pause exceeds the PP interval preceding the pause.

**P waves:** Contour normal, precede each QRS complex; intermittent loss of P wave.

**PR interval:** Normal, constant (0.20 second).

**QRS:** Normal (0.08 second).

**Dysrhythmia:** Sinus exit block (type I or Wenckebach). The four characteristic rhythm changes of this tracing allow the diagnosis of a Wenckebach exit block from the sinus node.

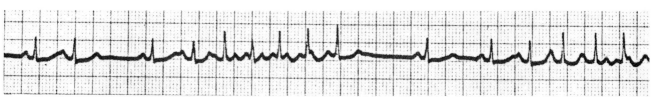

II

### Fig. 5-122

**Rate:** Varying.

**Rhythm:** Irregular because of premature atrial complexes.

**P waves:** Premature atrial complexes have different contour; some are buried in preceding T wave.

**PR interval (of atrial systole):** 0.14 second.

**QRS:** Generally normal; may be aberrantly conducted (normal, 0.08 second).

**Dysrhythmia:** Single and multiple premature atrial complexes can be seen hidden within preceding T waves and appear to initiate short bursts of anatrial tachydysrhythmia, probably atrial flutter-fibrillation.

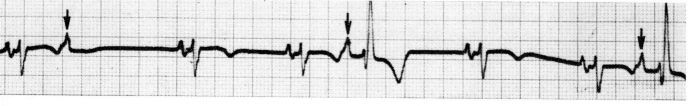

V₁

**Fig. 5-123**

| | |
|---|---|
| **Rate:** | Slow, because of nonconducted premature atrial complexes. |
| **Rhythm:** | Irregular. |
| **P waves:** | Premature atrial complexes have different contour and are buried in preceding T wave *(arrows)*. |
| **PR interval (of premature atrial systoles):** | First two premature atrial complexes are completely blocked; third and fourth premature atrial systoles conduct with a prolonged PR interval 0.21 second. |
| **QRS:** | Third and fourth premature atrial complexes initate aberrantly conducted QRS complex with a right bundle block pattern. |
| **Dysrhythmia:** | Nonconducted premature atrial complexes and premature atrial complexes initiating functional right bundle branch block. Sinus-initiated P waves are abnormal and suggest left atrial enlargement. Premature atrial complexes *(arrows)* can be seen hidden in the preceeding T waves. The first two premature atrial complexes are blocked and generate a pause in the ventricular rhythm. The second two premature atrial complexes conduct to the ventricle with a prolonged PR interval and initiate a functional right bundle branch block. |

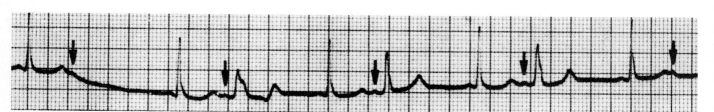

V₆

**Fig. 5-124**

| | |
|---|---|
| **Rate:** | Varying. |
| **Rhythm:** | Irregular because of premature atrial complexes. |
| **P waves:** | Premature atrial complexes have different contour and look like U waves *(arrows)*. |
| **PR interval (of premature atrial complexes):** | Later premature atrial complexes (second, third, and fourth) conduct whereas early premature atrial complexes (first, fifth, and sixth) fail to reach the ventricles. |
| **QRS:** | Second, third, and fourth premature atrial complexes produce varying degrees of left bundle branch block. |
| **Dysrhythmia:** | Nonconducted premature atrial complexes and premature atrial complexes that produce a functional left bundle branch block. Premature atrial complexes can be seen in the terminal portion of the preceding T waves and look like U wave *(arrows)*. Fairly early premature atrial complexes block whereas slightly later premature atrial complexes conduct to the ventricles with an increase in PR interval and varying degrees of left bundle branch block. |

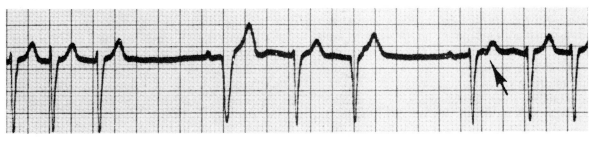

$V_1$

## Fig. 5-125

| | |
|---|---|
| **Rate:** | 150 beats/min. |
| **Rhythm:** | Varying. |
| **P waves:** | Not seen consistently. |
| **PR interval:** | Cannot determine. |
| **QRS:** | 0.08 second. |
| **Dysrhythmia:** | Paroxysmal supraventricular tachycardia. Paroxysmal sypraventricular tachycardia suddenly terminates, begins briefly, stops, and then restarts again following a premature atrial complex (*arriow*) that conducts with a prolong PR interval. |

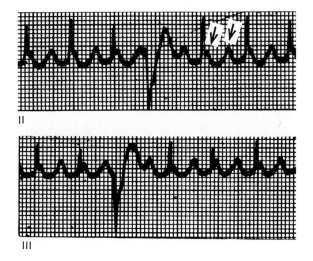

II

III

## Fig. 5-126

| | | |
|---|---|---|
| **Rate:** | Atrial | 280 beats/min. |
| | Ventricular | 140 beats/min. |
| **Rhythm:** | Atrial | Regular |
| | Ventricular | 2:1. |
| **P waves:** | | Flutter waves with regular oscillations resembling a sawtooth pattern. |
| **PR interval:** | | Flutter-R interval is constant. |
| **QRS:** | | Normal (0.08 second). |
| **Dysrhythmia:** | | Uncommon form of atrial flutter. Flutter waves indicated by arrows. A single premature ventricular complex occurs in each lead. The conduction ratio is 2:1; that is, flutter waves are conducted alternately to the ventricle. |

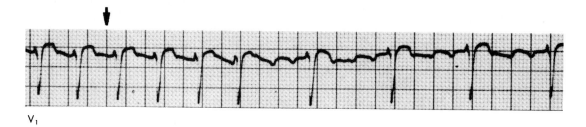

$V_1$

**Fig. 5-127**

| | | |
|---|---|---|
| **Rate:** | Atrial | 300 beats/min. |
| | Ventricular | 150 beats/min decreasing to 75 beats/min. |
| **Rhythm:** | Atrial | Regular. |
| | Ventricular | Regular. |
| **P waves:** | | Flutter waves clearly seen after carotid sinus massage *(arrows)* decreases the ventricular response. |
| **PR interval:** | | Flutter-R interval fairly constant. |
| **QRS:** | | Normal (0.08 second). |
| **Dysrhythmia:** | | Atrial flutter. Atrial flutter with a 2:1 ventricular response is present in the left portion of the tracing but cannot be clearly diagnosed from this lead. At the arrow, carotid sinus massage increases the degree of AV block to 4:1 and clearly exposes the atrial flutter waves. |

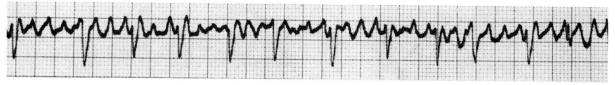

$V_1$

**Fig. 5-128**

| | | |
|---|---|---|
| **Rate:** | Atrial | 300 to 500 beats/min. |
| | Ventricular | 72 to 150 beats/min. |
| **Rhythm:** | Atrial | Irregular. |
| | Ventricular | Irregular. |
| **P waves:** | | Variability in the contour and spacing of the flutter-fibrillation waves. |
| **PR interval:** | | Nonmeasurable. |
| **QRS:** | | Normal (0.09 second). |
| **Dysrhythmia:** | | Impure atrial flutter (coarse atrial flutter or flutter-fibrillation). Impure atrail flutter is characterized by a faster atrial rate than pure atrial flutter, and more variability shows in the contour and spacing of the flutter waves. |

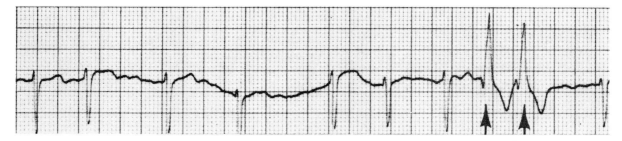

V₁

### Fig. 5-129

| | | |
|---|---|---|
| **Rate:** | Atrial | 350 to 600 beats/min. |
| | Ventricular | 65 to 160 beats/min. |
| **Rhythm:** | Atrial | Irregularly irregular. |
| | Ventricular | Irregularly irregular. |
| **P waves:** | | Irregular rapid baseline undulations indicate fibrillatory atrial activity. |
| **PR interval:** | | Not measurable. |
| **QRS:** | | 0.08 second; two complexes indicated by arrows are functional right bundle branch block QRS complexes with a duration of 0.13 second. |
| **Dysrhythmia:** | | Atrial fibrillation. A long ventricular pause followed by a short ventricular pause precedes the QRS complex with a right bundle branch block contour *(arrow)*; this QRS complex is followed after a short interval by a second QRS complex, also with right bundle branch block *(arrow)*. The aberrant QRS pattern indicates functional right bundle branch block (Ashman phenomenon). |

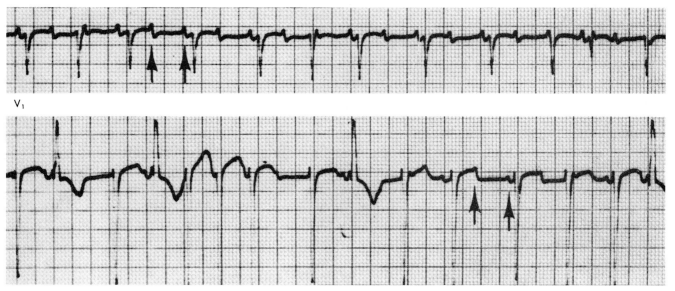

V₁

V₂

### Fig. 5-130

| | | |
|---|---|---|
| **Rate:** | Atrial | 167 beats/min. |
| | Ventricular | Varies according to the degree of AV block (83 to 120 beats/min). |
| **Rhythm:** | Atrial | Regular. |
| | Ventricular | Irregular (2:1, 3:2, and 4:3). |
| **P waves:** | | Contour differs from sinus-initiated P waves. |
| **PR interval:** | | Wenckebach cycles. |
| **QRS:** | | 0.08 second; functional right bundle branch block in lower tracing with a duration of 0.12 second. |
| **Dysrhythmia:** | | Atrial tachycardia with AV block. In the lower tracing, long-short QRS intervals, which follow longer intervals, set the stage for aberrant ventricular conduction that is manifest as a functional right bundle branch block. Arrows indicate P waves. |

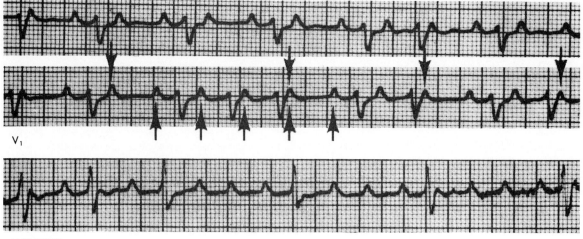

V₁

MONITOR

### Fig. 5-131

| | | |
|---|---|---|
| **Rate:** | Atrial | 150 beats/min, *top;* 193 beats/min, *bottom.* |
| | Ventricular | 83 to 125 beats/min, *top;* 50 to 94 beats/min, *bottom.* |
| **Rhythm:** | Atrial | Regular. |
| | Ventricular | Irregular (2:1, 3:1, 4:1, 4:3, etc.) |
| **P waves:** | | Contour differs from sinus-initiated P waves. |
| **PR interval:** | | Wenckebach cycles. |
| **QRS:** | | 0.09 second. |
| **Dysrhythmia:** | | Atrial tachycardia with AV block caused by digitalis toxicity. Top two tracings recorded on admission. In the bottom tracing, continued digitalis administration increased the atrial rate to 193 beats/min and increased the degree of AV block. Upright arrows indicate P waves; inverted arrows indicate nonconducted P waves. |

II

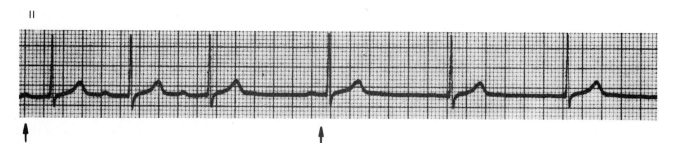

### Fig. 5-132

| | | |
|---|---|---|
| **Rate:** | Atrial | 75 beats/min initially; atrial activity not apparent during the junctional rhythm. |
| | Ventricular | 48 to 50 beats/min during the junctional rhythm. |
| **Rhythm:** | | Ventricular, generally regular. |
| **P waves and PR interval:** | | Relationship between P and QRS as explained under premature AV junctional complexes. (P waves not apparent.) PR interval not determinable during junctional rhythm. |
| **QRS:** | | Normal (0.08 second); may be conducted with slight aberration. |
| **Dysrhythmia:** | | AV junctional rhythm. Carotid sinus massage (*CSM,* between arrows) produces significant sinus slowing to allow the escape of an AV junctional rhythm (fifth QRS). Note unchanged QRS complexes. Atrial activity to the right of the last arrow is not apparent and may be caused by the AV junctional rhythm with retrograde capture of the P wave, lost within the QRS complex. |

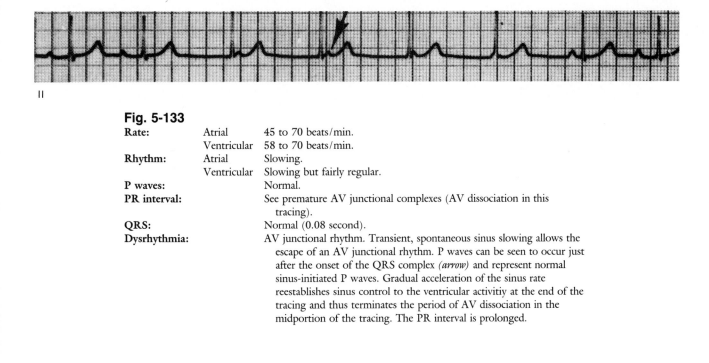

II

### Fig. 5-133

| | | |
|---|---|---|
| **Rate:** | Atrial | 45 to 70 beats/min. |
| | Ventricular | 58 to 70 beats/min. |
| **Rhythm:** | Atrial | Slowing. |
| | Ventricular | Slowing but fairly regular. |
| **P waves:** | | Normal. |
| **PR interval:** | | See premature AV junctional complexes (AV dissociation in this tracing). |
| **QRS:** | | Normal (0.08 second). |
| **Dysrhythmia:** | | AV junctional rhythm. Transient, spontaneous sinus slowing allows the escape of an AV junctional rhythm. P waves can be seen to occur just after the onset of the QRS complex *(arrow)* and represent normal sinus-initiated P waves. Gradual acceleration of the sinus rate reestablishes sinus control to the ventricular activitiy at the end of the tracing and thus terminates the period of AV dissociation in the midportion of the tracing. The PR interval is prolonged. |

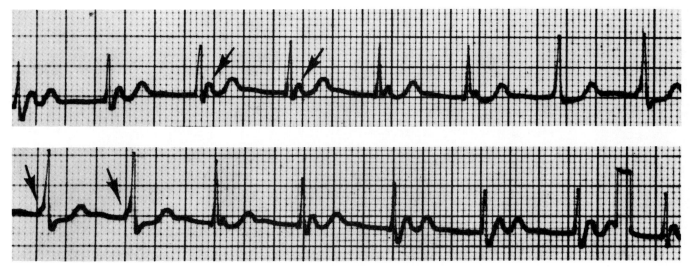

II

### Fig. 5-134

| | | |
|---|---|---|
| **Rate:** | Atrial | 100 beats/min. |
| | Ventricular | 100 beats/min. |
| **Rhythm:** | Atrial | Regular. |
| | Ventricular | Fairly regular. |
| **P waves:** | | Normal. |
| **PR interval:** | | Varying. |
| **QRS:** | | 0.08 second. |
| **Dysrhythmia:** | | Nonparoxysmal AV junctional tachycardia. Atrial activity *(arrows)* follows, then slightly precedes, and then once again follows the inscription of the QRS complex. Therefore AV dissociation is present because of the accelerated AV junctional discharge. This type of AV dissociation is called *isorhythmic*. |

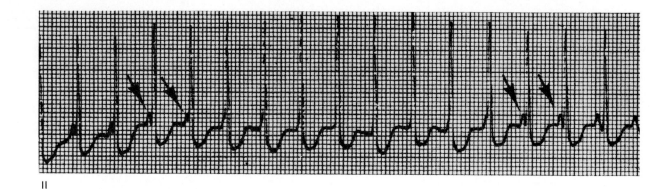

II

### Fig. 5-135

| Rate: | Atrial | 166 beats/min. |
|---|---|---|
| | Ventricular | 166 beats/min. |
| Rhythm: | Atrial | Regular. |
| | Ventricular | Regular. |
| P waves: | | Normal. |
| PR interval: | | Varying. |
| QRS: | | 0.06 second. |
| Dysrhythmia: | | Nonparoxysmal AV junctional tachycardia. Atrial activity *(arrows)* at a very similar rate and rhythm to the QRS can be seen to precede, then occur simultaneously with, and once again precede the onset of the QRS complex. This type of AV dissociation is called *isorhythmic*. |

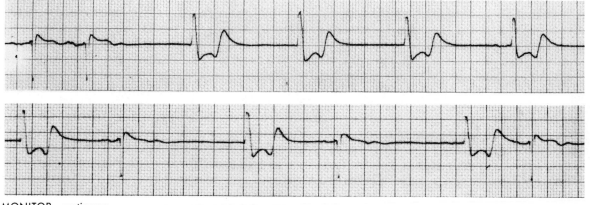

MONITOR—continuous

### Fig. 5-136

| Rate: | Atrial | Intermittent sinus arrest. |
|---|---|---|
| | Ventricular | 43 beats/min. |
| Rhythm: | Atrial | Irregular. |
| | Ventricular | Regular. |
| P waves: | | Normal. |
| PR interval: | | Varying. |
| QRS: of ventricular escape rhythm): | | 0.13 second. |
| Dysrhythmia: | | Ventricular escape beats. Intermittent sinus arrest produced periods of asystole terminated by ventricular escape beats that are characterized by a prolonged, abnormal QRS complex. Intermittent return of sinus node activity establishes periods of supraventricular capture. The reason why AV junctional escape beats did not terminate the asystolic periods is not known. |

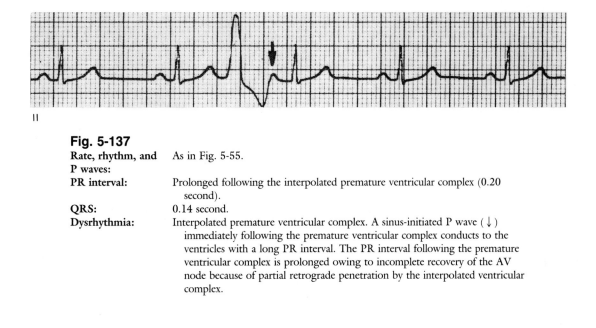

II

## Fig. 5-137

**Rate, rhythm, and**    As in Fig. 5-55.
**P waves:**

**PR interval:**    Prolonged following the interpolated premature ventricular complex (0.20
    second).

**QRS:**    0.14 second.

**Dysrhythmia:**    Interpolated premature ventricular complex. A sinus-initiated P wave ( ↓ )
    immediately following the premature ventricular complex conducts to the
    ventricles with a long PR interval. The PR interval following the premature
    ventricular complex is prolonged owing to incomplete recovery of the AV
    node because of partial retrograde penetration by the interpolated ventricular
    complex.

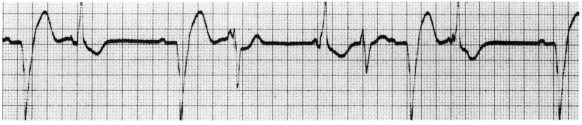

V₁

## Fig. 5-138

**Rate, rhythm, P waves,**    As in Fig. 5-54.
**and PR interval:**

**QRS:**    Wide, bizarre, greater than 0.12 second with varying contours and coupling
    intevals.

**Dysrhythmia:**    Multiform premature ventricular complexes. The normally conducted QRS
    complexes have a left bundle branch block morphology. The PR interval
    is slightly prolonged (0.24 second). Premature QRS complexes with
    varying contours and coupling intervals are present and called *multiform*
    *ventricular complexes.*

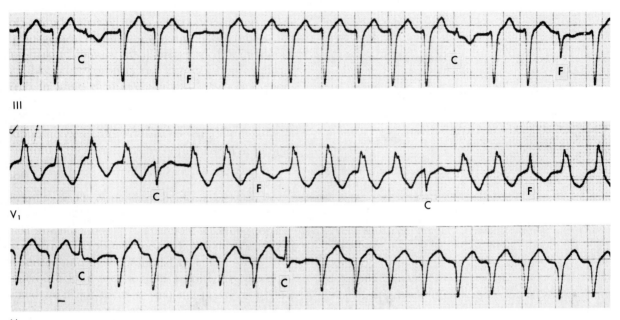

III

V₁

V₆

## Fig. 5-139

| | | |
|---|---|---|
| **Rate:** | Atrial | Clear P waves not seen. |
| | Ventricular | 150 beats/min. |
| **Rhythm:** | Atrial | Regular. |
| | Ventricular | Regular. |
| **P waves:** | | Atrial activity is probably under independent control of sinus node. |
| **PR interval:** | | Not measurable. |
| **QRS:** | | 0.14 second. |
| **Dysrhythmia:** | | Ventricular tachycardia. QRS complexes with a prolonged duration and a right bundle branch block morphology occur at a regular interval and are occasionally interrupted by QRS complexes with an intermediate contour (*C*, capture) or QRS complexes with a normal contour. (*F*, fusion). Atrial activity cannot be seen; most likely, the atria are discharging independently to produce intermittent QRS captures and fusion beats. Therefore the most reasonable diagnosis is a ventricular tachycardia with AV dissociation. |

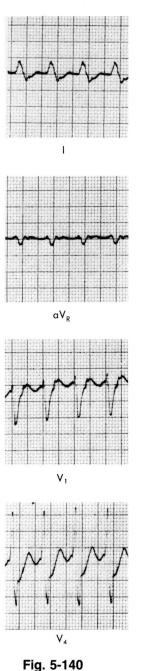
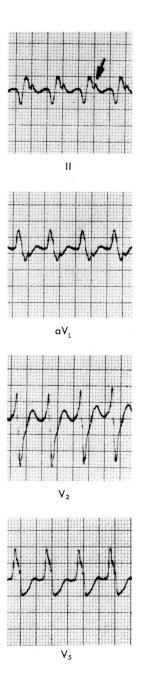
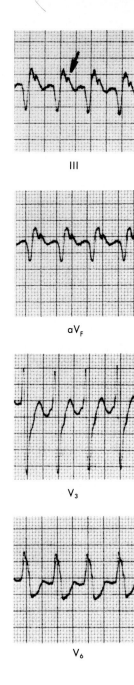

## Fig. 5-140

| Rate: | Atrial | 150 beats/min. |
|---|---|---|
| | Ventricular | 150 beats/min. |
| Rhythm: | Atrial | Regular. |
| | Ventricular | Regular. |
| P waves: | | Retrograde P waves inverted in 2, 3 *(arrows)*, and aVF. |
| RP interval: | | 0.16 second. |
| QRS: | | 0.12 second. |
| Dysrhythmia: | | Ventricular tachycardia with retrograde atrial capture. Ventricular tachycardia cannot be diagnosed with certainty from this surface ECG because all the features of this dysrhythmia can be mimicked by a supraventricular tachycardia with aberrant ventricular conduction of a left bundle branch block type. Electrophysiologic study proved that this was a ventricular tachycardia, however. The importance of the illustration lies in demonstrating 1:1 retrograde conduction to the atrium. Retrograde atrial activity is indicated by arrows. Thus AV dissociation is *not* present during this ventricular tachycardia. |

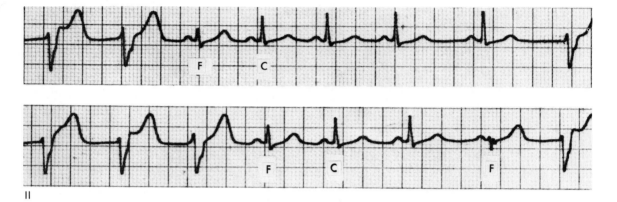

**Fig. 5-141**

| Rate: | Atrial | 70 to 90 beats/min. |
|---|---|---|
| | Ventricular | 72 beats/min. |
| **Rhythm:** | Atrial | Regular. |
| | Ventricular | Regular. |
| **P waves:** | | Independent. |
| **PR interval:** | | Not measurable during accelerated idioventricular rhythm. |
| **QRS:** | | 0.14 second; fusion beats and capture beats often present (labeled F and C). |

**Dysrhythmia:** Accelerated idioventricular rhythm. An accelerated idioventricular rhythm is present at the beginning and termination of the top and bottom strips. In the midportion of each tracing, slight sinus node acceleration reestablishes sinus node control by capturing the ventricles (C) and suppresses the accelerated idioventricular rhythm. When the sinus node shows, the accelerated idioventricular rhythm escapes. Fusion beats (F) may occur in the beginning and end of such dysrhythmias because sinus and ventricular foci have similar rates.

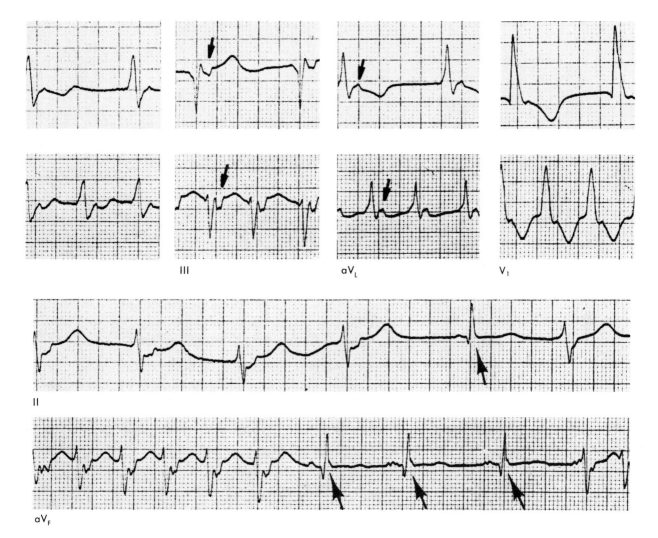

## Fig. 5-142

**Rate:** Accelerated idioventricular rhythm (60 beats/min). Ventricular tachycardia (varying slight, 150 beats/min.).

**Rhythm:** Accelerated idioventricular rhythm (regular). Ventricular tachycardia (regular).

**P waves:** Retrogradely captured.

**PR interval:** 0.14 second.

**QRS:** 0.14 second.

**Dysrhythmia:** Accelerated idioventricular rhythm and ventricular tachycardia. An accelerated idioventricular rhythm and a ventricular tachycardia occurred at different times in this patient. **A** illustrates leads, I, II, $aV_L$, $V_1$, and $V_6$ during the accelerated ventricular rhythm, whereas **C** (lead II) illustrates the onset of the accelerated idioventricular rhythm. **B** illustrates the ventricular tachycardia in leads I, II, $aV_L$, $V_1$, and $V_6$, whereas **D** ($aV_F$) illustrates the onset and termination of the ventricular tachycardia. Retrograde atrial capture ( ↓ ) occurred during both tachycardias. Normally conducted QRS complexes present in **C** and **D** ( ↑ ). Note identical QRS contours for both tachycardias ($aV_L$, $V_1$, and $V_6$ in **A** were recorded at different standardization), indicating that they arose at same or similar areas of the ventricle.

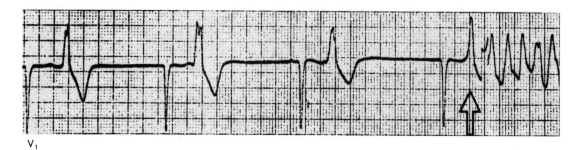

$V_1$

### Fig. 5-143

| | | |
|---|---|---|
| **Rate:** | Atrial | 60 to 100 beats/min; any independent atrial dysrhythmia may exist or the atria captured retrogradely. |
| | Ventricular | 400 to 600 beats/min. |
| **Rhythm:** | Atrial | Regular; may be irregular if the atria are retrogradely captured. |
| | Ventricular | Grossly irregular. |
| **P waves:** | | Generally cannot be seen. |
| **PR interval:** | | Generally not measurable. |
| **QRS:** | | Baseline undulations without distinct QRS contours. |
| **Dysrhythmia:** | | Ventricular fibrillation. Premature ventricular complexes occurred in a bigeminal pattern with a decreasing coupling interval. The fourth premature ventricular complex discharged during the vulnerable period of the antecedent T wave and precipitated ventricular fibrillation *(arrow)*. |

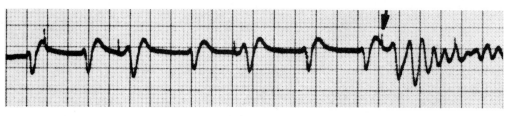

MONITOR

### Fig. 5-144

| | |
|---|---|
| **Rate, rhythm, and P waves, PR interval and QRS:** | As in Fig. 5-143. |
| **Dysrhythmia:** | Ventricular fibrillation. Pacemaker spikes *(arrow)* from a malfunctioning pacemaker fall randomly throughout the cardiac cycle at a slightly irregular interval. When the pacemaker spike discharged during the vulnerable period of the antecedent T wave *(arrow)*, it precipitated ventricular fibrillation. Ventricular rhythm preceding onset of ventricular fibrillation is probably slightly irregular, accelerated idioventricular rhythm. |

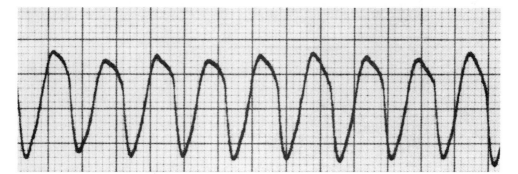

MONITOR

## Fig. 5-145

| Rate: | Atrial | P waves not seen. |
|---|---|---|
| | Ventricular | 195 beats/min. |
| **Rhythm:** | Ventricular | Regular. |
| **P waves:** | | Cannot be seen. |
| **PR interval:** | | Not measurable. |
| **QRS:** | | 0.16 second. |
| **Dysrhythmia:** | | Ventricular flutter. Sine wave with regular large oscillations. The QRS complex cannot be definitely distinguished from the ST segment or T wave. |

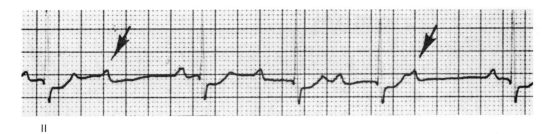

II

## Fig. 5-146

| Rate: | Atrial | Normal (83 beats/min). |
|---|---|---|
| | Ventricular | Depends on degree of AV block, which may vary between 2:1, 3:2, 4:3, 5:3, 5:3, etc. |
| **Rhythm:** | Atrial | Regular. |
| | Ventricular | Varying, depending on the degree of AV block. |
| **P waves:** | | More numerous than QRS complexes but are related to ventricular beats in a consistent, repetitive fashion. |
| **PR interval:** | | Progressive PR prolongation preceding the nonconducted P wave. Finaly, one P wave is blocked, and the cycle then repeats. |
| **QRS:** | | Normal; RR interval gradually shortens until the blocked P wave occurs; the cycle then repeats. |
| **Dysrhythmia:** | | Second-degree AV heart block (type I Wenckebach). AV Wenckebach is characterized by progressive PR prolongation preceding the nonconducted P wave. Wenckebach AV block, in the presence of a normal QRS complex, is virtually always at the level of the AV node. Conduction ratios (that is, the number of P waves to the number of QRS complexes) 2:1, 4:3, and 3:2 in this tracing. Because the increment in conduction time is greatest in the second cycle of the Wenckebach group and then decreases progressively over succeeding cycles, the following characteristics are also present: (1) the interval between successive RR cycles before the nonconducted P wave progressively decreases; (2) the duration of the pause produced by the nonconducted P wave is less than twice the shortest cycle, which is generally the cycle immediately preceding the pause; (3) the duration of the RR cycle following the pause exceeds the duration of the RR cycle preceding the pause. These features can be seen in the middle 4:3 grouping. Blocked P waves indicated by arrows. |

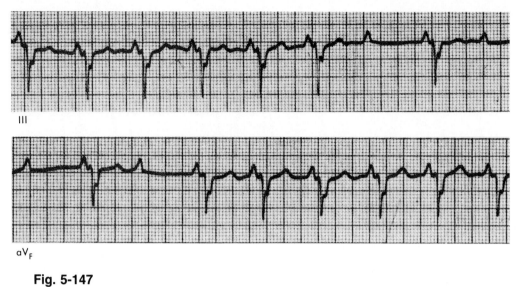

III

aV<sub>F</sub>

### Fig. 5-147

| | | |
|---|---|---|
| **Rate:** | | 86 beats/min. |
| **Rhythm:** | Atrial | Regular. |
| | Ventricular | Varying, dependent on the degree of AV block. |
| **P waves:** | | Normal. |
| **PR interval:** | | Normal, constant (0.12 second) with sudden failure of conduction. |
| **QRS:** | | Prolonged; right bundle branch block and left anterior hemiblock (0.12 second) |
| **Dysrhythmia:** | | Second-degree AV heart block, type II. Right bundle branch block (not readily apparent in leads III and aV<sub>F</sub>) along with left anterior fascicular block is present in this patient. Sudden failure of AV conduction results without antecedent PR prolongation. The PR interval for the conducted beats is normal, as it often is during type II second-degree AV heart block. |

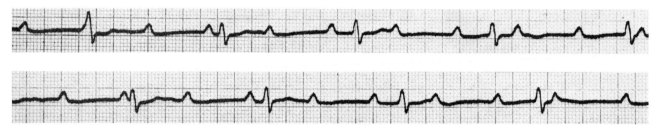

II

### Fig. 5-148

| | | |
|---|---|---|
| **Rate:** | Atrial | 85 beats/min. |
| | Ventricular | 38 beats/min. |
| **Rhythm:** | Atrial | Regular. |
| | Ventricular | Regular. |
| **P waves:** | | Normal. |
| **PR interval:** | | Completely variable. |
| **QRS:** | | Prolonged (0.12 second) |
| **Dysrhythmia:** | | Third-degree (complete) AV heart block. Complete AV dissociation is present *resulting from* complete heart block. The abnormal QRS complexes (prolonged duration) indicate a ventricular origin for the escape rhythm. |

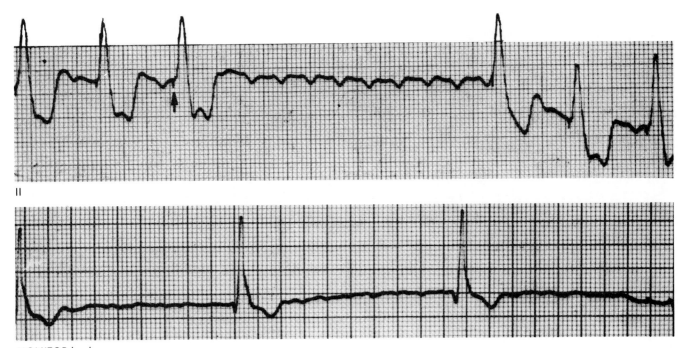

II

MONITOR lead

### Fig. 5-149

| | | |
|---|---|---|
| **Rate:** | Atrial | *Top*, 250 beats/min; *bottom*, 400 to 600 beats/min. |
| | Ventricular | *Top*, 100 beats/min; *bottom*, 32 beats/min. |
| **Rhythm:** | Atrial | *Top*, regular; *bottom*, irregular. |
| | Ventricular | *Top*, regular; *bottom*, regular. |
| **P waves:** | | *Top*, atrial flutter; *bottom*, atrial fibrillation. |
| **PR interval:** | | Totally variable or nonmeasurable. |
| **QRS:** | | *Top*, ventricular paced beats (0.16 second); *bottom*, 0.14 second. |
| **Dysrhythmia:** | | Complete (third-degree) AV heart block during atrial flutter and atrial fibrillation. In the top tracing a ventricular pacemaker controls ventricular activity (arrow indicates pacemaker artifact). In the midportion of the tracing the ventricular pacing was temporarily discontinued, and one can easily see the atrial flutter waves that fail to conduct to the ventricle. In the terminal portion of the tracing the ventricular pacemaker was turned on once again. In the bottom tracing the undulating baseline indicates the presence of atrial fibrillation. The regular ventricular rhythm establishes that none of the atrial fibrillatory impulses conduct to the ventricles; thus complete AV block is present during atrial fibrillation. |

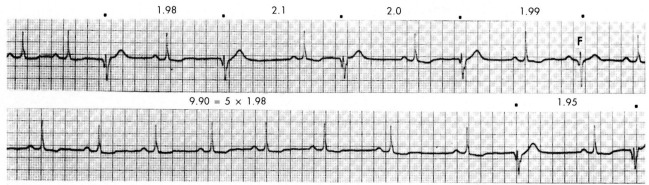

MONITOR—continuous

### Fig. 5-150

| | | |
|---|---|---|
| **Rate:** | Atrial | Approximately 60 beats/min. |
| | Ventricular parasystole | 30 beats/min. |
| **Rhythm:** | Atrial | Regular. |
| | Ventricular parasystole | Regular; interrupted by exit block or ventricular refractoriness. |
| **P waves:** | | Normal. |
| **PR interval:** | | During normally conducted beats, normal. |
| **QRS (of ventricular parasystole):** | | Prolonged (0.13 second) |
| **Dysrhythmia:** | | Ventricular parasystole. The interval between ectopic ventricular systoles ranges between 1.98 and 2.1 seconds. The coupling interval varies between the sinus-initiated QRS complex and the parasystole complex. A ventricular fusion beat is labeled *F*. Ventricular refractoriness prevents the emergence of the ventricular parasystole during the long interval in which it is absent. This interectopic interval equals 9.90 seconds and is 5 times the normal interectopic interval. The dark marks above the tracing indicate the parasystolic ventricular systoles. |

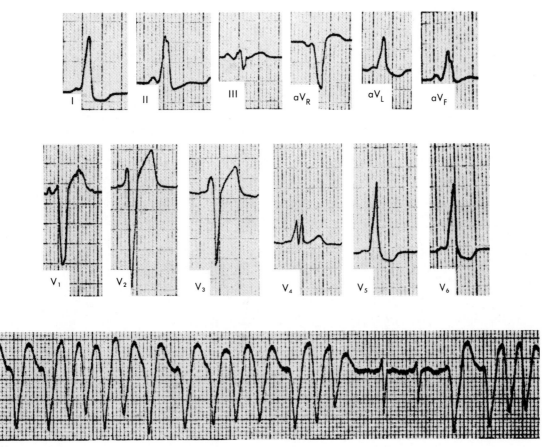

**Fig. 5-151**   Dysrhythmia: twelve-lead ECG illustrating the preexcitation (Wolff-Parkinson-White) syndrome with a right anterior or paraseptal pathway. The lower recording ($V_1$ half standard) demonstrates an extremely rapid ventricular rate during atrial fibrillation in this same patient. The grossly irregular ventricular rhythm, extremely rapid rate, and gradations in QRS contour from normal to prolonged (as conduction changes from the normal AV nodal pathway to the anomalous route) help distinguish this dysrhythmia from ventricular tachycardia. Bypass of the safety valve features provided by normal AV nodal delay accounts for the rapid ventricular rate that less commonly may actually cause the ventricles to fibrillate and result in sudden death.

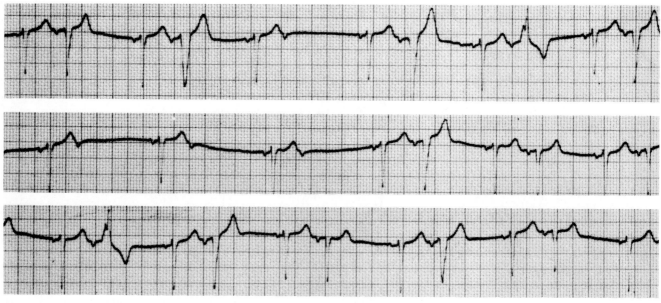

V₁—continuous

### Fig. 5-152

| | |
|---|---|
| **Rate:** | Determined by the number of premature atrial complexes. |
| **Rhythm:** | Irregular because of premature atrial complexes. |
| **P waves:** | Both sinus-initiated and premature atrial P waves are abnormal. |
| **PR interval:** | Normal (0.12 second) for the sinus-initiated P waves; prolonged following the premature atrial complexes. Some premature atrial complexes failed to conduct to the ventricle. |
| **QRS:** | Normal, following the sinus-initiated P waves; functional left bundle and functional right bundle branch block following the premature atrial complexes. |
| **Dysrhythmia:** | Functional right and left bundle branch block following atrial premature complexes. Premature atrial complexes occur at varying coupling intervals. When they occur with a very short PR interval, they fail to reach the ventricle and are therefore nonconducted atrial complexes. At slightly longer RP intervals, they conduct with both functional right and functional left bundle block. Differences in the duration of the preceding long cycle and in the duration of the short cycle account for whether functional right or left bundle branch block results. |

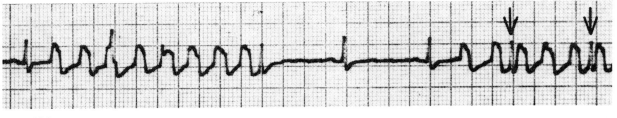

MONITOR

**Fig. 5-153   Artifact.** Regularly moving a loose electrode creates an artifact that mimics ventricular tachycardia. However, careful scrutiny uncovers the fairly regularly occurring normal QRS complexes *(arrows)*, each preceded by a P wave. The question of ventricular tachycardia may be eliminated and the diagnosis of artifact established by observing that the QRS complexes continue uninterrupted and unaffected by the apparent ventricular tachycardia.

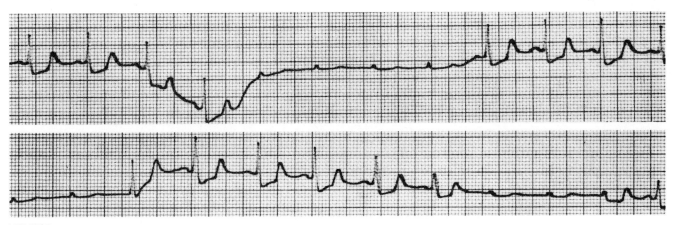

MONITOR

**Fig. 5-154   Artifact simulating AV block.** These tracings were recorded in a patient who presented with an acute anteroseptal myocardial infarction and 1 day later developed left anterior fascicular block. The monitored recording was interpreted as illustrating the development of advanced AV block with sequentially blocked P waves. Temporary transvenous pacemaker insertion was deemed immediately necessary. However, careful observation of the tracing reveals that the nonconducted P waves are artifactual in origin. In reality the "nonconducted P waves" are QRS complexes with a grossly diminished amplitude caused by intermittent poor ECG lead contact. The diagnosis is established by noting QRS complexes with intermediate amplitudes, by noting T waves that follow the diminutive QRS complexes, and by "matching out" the QRS complexes and finding that they occur at the same time as the apparent P waves.

## Electrocardiogram Test Section

The following section provides a series of ECG tracings of various conditions that have been discussed throughout this text. It is suggested that the reader cover the interpretations given at the end of each legend and attempt to identify the abnormal patterns that are found in each ECG.

*Text continued on p. 252.*

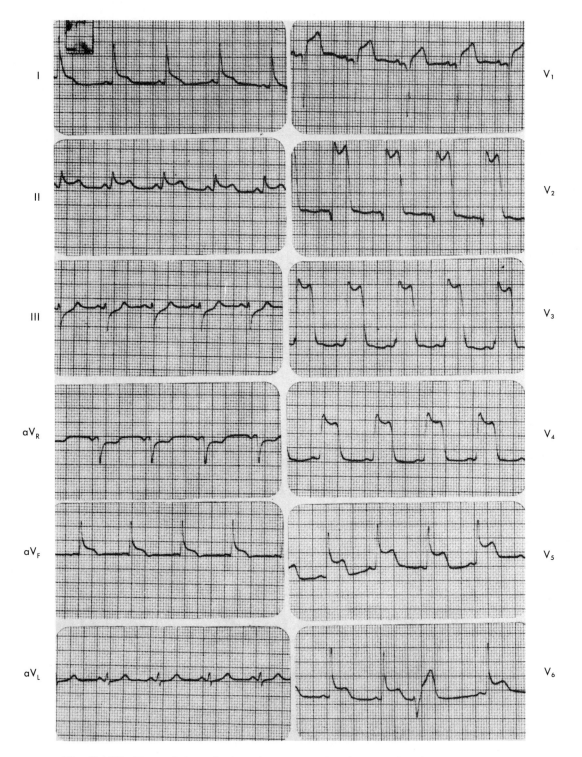

**Fig. 5-155** **Normal sinus rhythm, Q waves in $V^1$ and $V^2$.** Marked ST segment elevation in leads I, II, $aV_1$, and $V_1$ through $V_6$. T waves have not yet inverted.
ECG: *Hyperacute anterolateral, possibly apical, myocardial infarction.*

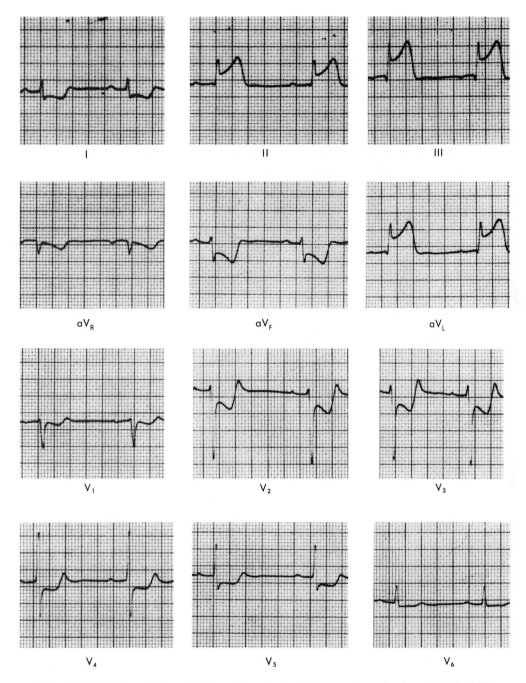

**Fig. 5-156   Normal sinus rhythm.** No pathologic Q waves have developed. Marked ST segment elevation in leads II, III, and aV_F, with reciprocal depression in leads I, aV_L and the anterior precordium. T waves are still upright.

ECG: *Hyperacute inferior (diaphragmatic) myocardial infarction.*

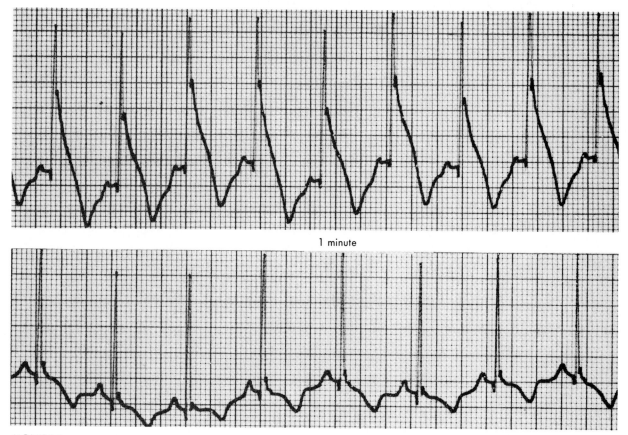

1 minute

MONITOR

**Fig. 5-157** Top tracing demonstrates marked ST segment elevation and T wave inversion. One minute later (bottom tracing) the ST segments have returned to baseline. The T waves are still inverted.
ECG: *The rapid ST changes from elevation to normal are characteristic of atypical (Prinzmetal) angina pectoris.*

9:30 AM                         11:45 AM

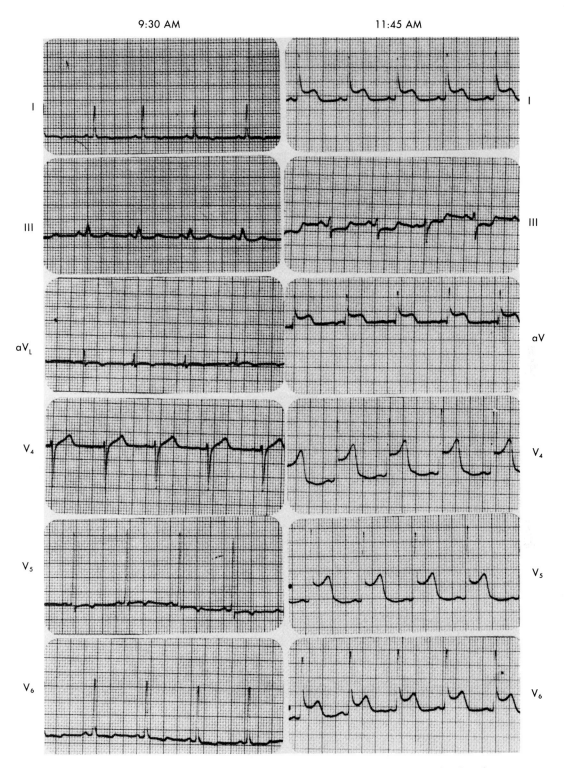

**Fig. 5-158    Normal sinus rhythm.** Tracing at 9:30 AM, (after the patient developed more chest pain) demonstrates ST segment elevation in leads I, aV₆ and V₄ through V₆. The T waves are still upright, and no pathologic Q waves have developed.
ECG: *Hyperacute lateral myocardial infarction.*

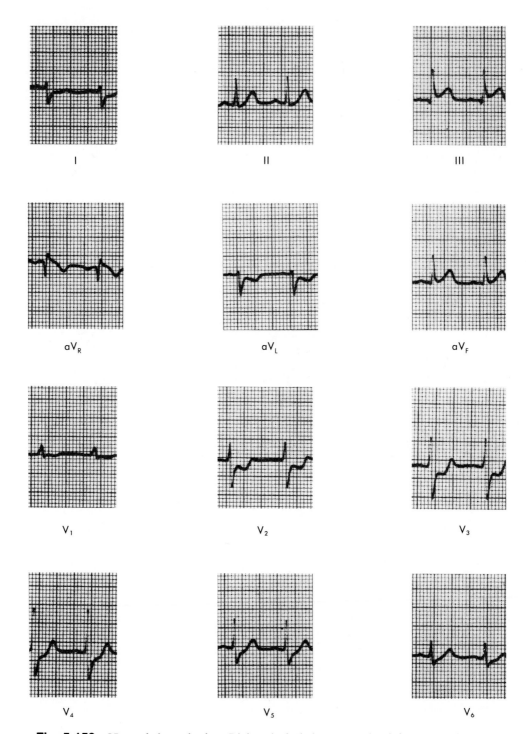

**Fig. 5-159    Normal sinus rhythm.** Right axis deviation suggesting left posterior hemi-block. ST segment elevation in lead III and slight ST segment elevation in lead aV$_F$ Large R wave in V$_1$, with slight ST segment depression in V$_1$, more marked in V$_2$ and V$_3$. T waves are still upright except for diphasic T waves in leads V$_1$ and V$_2$.
ECG: *Acute posteroinferior myocardial infarction.*

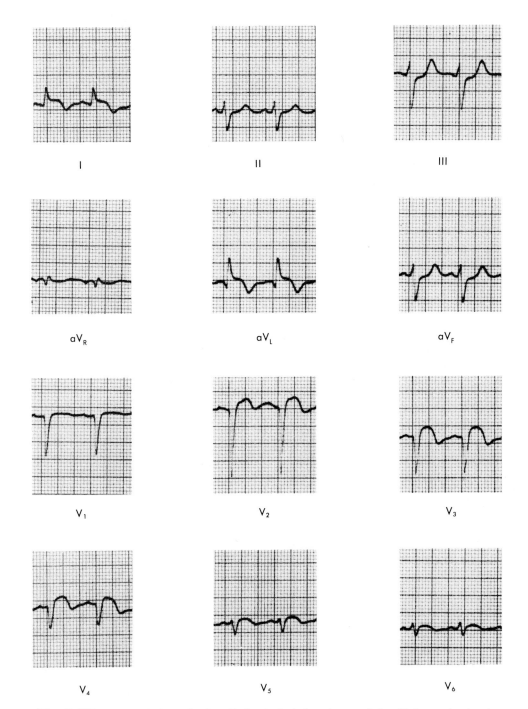

**Fig. 5-160   Normal sinus rhythm.** Left axis deviation characteristic of left anterior hemiblock. ST segment elevation in leads I, $aV_1$ and $V_2$ through $V_6$. Abnormal Q wave in $V_1$
through $V_4$, with small R waves in $V_5$ and $V_6$. T wave inversion in leads 1 and $aV_L$ and
terminal T wave inversion in $V_2$ through $V_5$.
Impression: *Acute anterolateral myocardial infarction and left anterior hemiblock.*

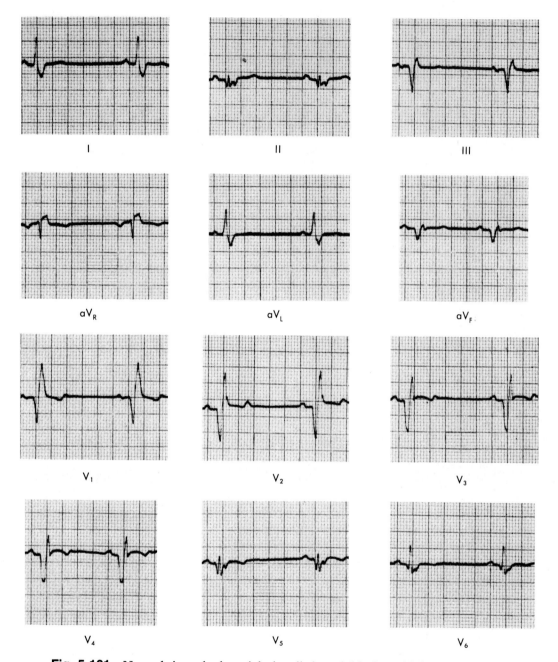

I

II

III

aV_R

aV_L

aV_F

V_1

V_2

V_3

V_4

V_5

V_6

**Fig. 5-161** **Normal sinus rhythm, right bundle branch block, and left axis deviation characteristic of left anterior hemiblock.** ST segments are normal. There are nonspecific T wave changes. A pathologic Q wave is present in leads II, III, aV_F, and V_1 through V_4 and makes the diagnosis of left anterior hemiblock difficult.

ECG: *Right bundle branch block, possible left anterior hemiblock, and anteroinferior myocardial infarction, probably old.*

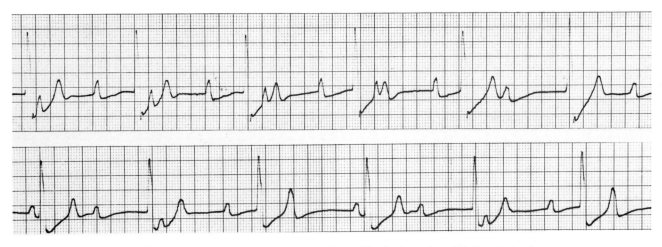

**Fig. 5-162    Third-degree (complete) AV heart block.** Complete AV dissociation is present caused by complete AV heart block. Atria and ventricles are under control of separate pacemakers, and the sinus node and an idioventricular escape rhythm, respectively. Monotor lead.

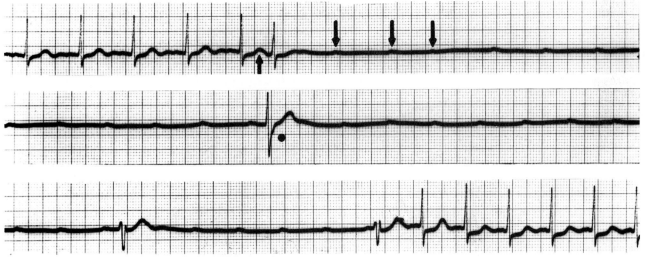

V₄ continuous

**Fig. 5-163    Paroxysmal AV block.** Periods of complete AV block interrupted only by an occasional escape beat occurred in this patient who had recurrent syncope. Each episode of AV block was always introduced by a premature atrial complex *(upright arrow),* which then resulted in a series of successive nonconducted P waves *(inverted arrows).* Finally, an escape beat occurred and restored conduction (bottom strip of this continuous recording of V₄). Electrophysiologic mechanism responsible for this form of paroxysmal AV block is not clear.

# REFERENCES

1. Zipes DP: Genesis of cardiac arrhythmias: electrophysiological considerations. In Braunwald E, editor: Heart disease: a textbook of cardiovascular medicine, ed 3, Philadelphia, 1984, WB Saunders Co.
2. Rosenbaum MB: The hemiblocks: diagnostic criteria and clinical significance, Mod Concepts Cardiovasc Dis 39:141, 1970.
3. Jalife J and Moe GK: A biologic model of parasystole, Am J Cardiol 43:761, 1979.
4. Anzelovitch V, Jalife J, and Moe GK: Characteristics of reflection as a mechanism of reentrant arrhythmias and its relationship to parasystole, Circulation 61:182, 1980.
5. Zipes DP: A consideration of antiarrhythmic therapy (editorial), Circulation 72:949, 1985.
6. Zipes DP, Bailey JC, and Elharrar V: The slow inward current and cardiac arrhythmias, The Hague, 1980, Martinus Nijhoff.
7. Zipes DP: Management of cardiac arrhythmias. In Braunwald E, editor: Heart disease: a textbook of cardiovascular medicine, Philadelphia, 1984, WB Saunders Co, p 648.
8. Zipes DP: Specific arrhythmias: diagnosis and treatment. In Braunwald E, editor: Heart disease: a textbook of cardiovascular medicine, Philadelphia, 1984, WB Saunders Co, p 683.
9. Prystowsky EN and Zipes DP: Treatment of tachycardia. In Rakel RE, editor: Conn's current therapy, Philadelphia, WB Saunders Co, p 188.
10. Zipes DP, editor: Symposium on cardiac arrhythmias, Cardiology Clinics, vol 1, 1983.
11. Zipes DP, editor: Symposium on cardiac arrhythmias, Med Clin North Am 68:793-1390, 1984.
12. Pick A and Langendorf R: Interpretation of complex arrhythmias, Philadelphia, 1979, Lea & Febiger.
13. Albarran-Sotelo R and others: Textbook of advanced cardiac life support, American Heart Association, Dallas, Tx, 1987.
14. Josephson ME and Seides SF: Clinical cardiac electrophysiology, Philadelphia, 1979, Lea & Febiger.
15. Nattel S and Zipes DP: Clinical pharmacology of old and new antiarrhythmic drugs, Cardiovasc Clin 11:221, 1980.
16. Rinkenberger RL and others: Effects of intravenous and chronic oral verapamil administration in patients with supraventricular tachyarrhythmias, Circulation 62:996, 1980.
17. Arcebal A and Lemberg L: Mechanisms of supraventricular tachycardia, Heart Lung 13:205, 1984.
18. Prystowsky EN and others: Preexcitation syndromes: mechanisms and management, Med Clin North Am 68:831, 1984.
19. Huerta B and Lemberg L: Anticoagulation in atrial fibrillation, Heart Lung 14:521, 1985.
20. Zipes DP and others: Development of the implantable transvenous cardioverter, Am J Cardiol 54:670, 1984.
21. Kienzle M and others: Antiarrhythmic drug therapy for sustained ventricular tachycardia, Heart Lung 13:614, 1984.
22. Markmann P and Chellemi J: Surgical management of ventricular tachycardia, Heart Lung 13:622, 1984.
23. Rahimtoola S and others: Consensus statement of the conference on the state of the art of electrophysiological testing in the diagnosis and treatment of patients with cardiac arrhythmias, Circulation 75:11, 1987.
24. Zipes DP: Second-degree atrioventricular block, Circulation 60:465, 1979.
25. Hindman MC and others: The clinical significance of bundle branch block complicating acute myocardial infarction, Circulation 58:689, 1978.
26. Chung EK: Electrocardiography: practical applications with vectorial principles; Norwalk, CT, 1985, Appleton-Century-Crofts, p 549.
27. Miles WM and others: Evaluation of the patient with wide QRS tachycardia, Med Clin North Am 68:1015, 1984.
28. Wellens HJJ, Barf WHM, and Lie KI: The value of the electrocardiogram in the differential diagnosis of a tachycardia with a widened QRS complex, Am J Med 64:27, 1978.
29. Green M and others: Value of QRS alternation in determining the site of origin of narrow QRS synaventricular tachycardia, Circulation 68:368, 1983.
30. Shaw M, Niemann JT, and Haskell RJ: Esophageal electrocardiography in acute cardiac care: efficacy and diagnostic value of a new technique, Am J Med 82:689–696, 1987.
31. Bense DW: Tranesophageal electrocardiography and cardiac pacing: state of the art, Circulation 75(III):86–92, 1987.
32. Gallager JJ and others: Esophageal pacing: a diagnostic and therapeutic tool, Circulation 65:336–341, 1982.
33. Commerford PJ and Lloyd EA: Arrhythmias in patients with drug toxicity, electrolyte and endocrine disturbances, Med Clin North Am 68:1051, 1984.
34. Vacek J, Smith W, and Phillips J: Cardiac electrophysiology: an overview, Practical Cardiol 10(13):83–97, 1984.
35. Akhtar M and others: NASPE Ad Hoc Committee on Guidelines for Cardiac Electrophysiological Studies, PACE 8:611, 1985.

# SUGGESTED READINGS

Chung EK: Electrocardiography: practical applications with vectorial principles, Norwalk, CT, 1985, Appleton-Century-Crofts.

Josephson ME and Wellens HJ, editors: Tachycardias: mechanisms, diagnosis, treatment, Philadelphia, 1984, Lea & Febiger.

Kennedy HL: Ambulatory electrocardiography, Philadelphia, 1981, Lea & Febiger.

Mandel WJ, editor: Cardiac arrhythmias, ed 2, Philadelphia, 1987, JB Lippincott Co.

Marriott HJL: Practical electrocardiography, ed 8, Baltimore, 1988, Williams & Wilkins.

Surawicz B, Reddy CP, and Prystowsky EN, editors: Tachycardias, Boston, 1984, Martinus Nijhoff.

Zipes DP and Jalife J, editors: Cardiac electophysiology and arrhythmias, Orlando, FL, 1985, Grune & Stratton, Inc.

# CHAPTER 6

# Coronary Artery Disease

Lynne T. Braun
Marcia Pencak Murphy
Elizabeth VanBeek Carlson

## INCIDENCE, PREVALENCE, MORBIDITY, AND MORTALITY

Despite the recent decline in age-adjusted death rates, cardiovascular disease remains the leading cause of death in the United States. In 1986 the American Heart Association (AHA) estimated that 4.94 million Americans had coronary artery disease. Among the nearly 66 million Americans with some form of cardiovascular disease, coronary artery disease (CAD) ranked second to hypertensive heart disease in prevalence. Of all heart attacks, 5% occur in people under the age of 40, and 45% occur in people under the age of 65. Sudden death is the first clinical manifestation in 20% to 25% of the first events, and 50% to 60% of all heart attack deaths occur during a first heart attack. Among the approximately 524,100 Americans who die annually from heart attacks, 25% are under the age of 65. Furthermore, two thirds of the deaths from heart attack occur outside the hospital and within the first 2 hours of an acute event.[1]

## PATHOGENESIS

*Arteriosclerosis* is a chronic disease of the arteries, characterized by abnormal thickening and hardening of the vessel walls that results in loss of elasticity. There are several possible causes of the arteriosclerotic process; its manifestations differ according to the type of vessel involved and the site and extent of the disease within the vessel. Arteriosclerosis may be categorized into the following types:

*Type I: Intimal atherosclerosis.* This form of arteriosclerosis affects the internal membranes (intima) of arteries and consists of irregular thickening and plaque formation. Plaques consist of lipid, proliferating smooth muscle cells, and variable amounts of collagen. Intimal atherosclerosis primarily affects the large vessels, may begin at a very young age, and to some degree is almost universally present in people over the age of 20.

*Type II: Medial sclerosis.* This process consists of calcification and hypertrophy of the muscular portion of the artery (media). It affects medium-sized blood vessels such as the brachial artery and the femoral artery, which become thickened, rigid, and tortuous. It is not necessarily associated with any reduction in the caliber of the involved vessel.

*Type III: Arteriolar sclerosis.* This type of the disease affects small blood vessels and is characterized by hypertrophy of the muscular media and thickening of the intima; it is usually seen in patients with long-standing hypertension. It often affects the small vessels in the fundus of the eye and in the kidney.

Although these three types of arteriosclerosis may exist separately, there is in fact considerable overlap. Type I, or intimal atheroclerosis, is the cause of most coronary artery disease but may be aggravated or accelerated by coexisting hypertension.

The natural history of CAD has three phases. The first phase begins with injury to the intimal endothelium, which may either heal or progress to a second phase. The second phase is the response to injury: blood platelets and other plasma constituents adhere to the site of injury, inducing proliferation of smooth muscle cells, and lipid accumulates abnormally in the arterial intima. At the earliest (and still reversible) part of this stage only a fatty streak may be produced. With more severe involvement, however, massive amounts of lipid, extensive smooth muscle proliferation, and the influx of cells, such as macrophages and collagen-producing fibroblasts, may combine to produce a full-blown atherosclerotic plaque. Although mature atherosclerotic lesions may occasionally regress, the usual course is a progressive encroachment on the lumen of the affected artery. The third phase in the natural history of CAD is the production of clinically manifest symptoms, either angina pectoris, myocardial infarction, or, all too frequently, sudden cardiac death.[2]

Different factors may contribute to the development of clinically evident heart disease during each of these three phases. For example, homocysteine, which accumulates in patients with congenital homocystinuria, a genetic disorder characterized by the early onset of severe and diffuse atherosclerosis, has been shown to produce diffuse sites of endothelial injury. Carbon monoxide inhaled during cigarette smoking may work through similar mechanisms. Elevated low-density lipoproteins in plasma produce accelerated atherosclerosis by increasing the accumulation of lipid at the sites of endothelial injury. Finally, other poorly identified factors must exist to explain the tremendous variations in longevity and clinical symptoms among subjects with equivalent amounts of coronary artery disease.

A number of pathologic events, either gradual or sudden, may affect the clinical course of coronary artery disease. Rose[3] and others have emphasized the dynamic interaction between platelets and vascular endothelium, and the participation of factors released from these cells, such as platelet-derived growth factor, thromboxane $A_2$, and prostacyclin, as determinants of both the acute and the gradual progression of atherosclerosis. Usually a plaque enlarges slowly as fat is deposited and scar tissue develops. Sometimes blood vessels that grow into the fibrous plaque rupture, producing small hemorrhages. Such subintimal hemorrhages increase the size of the plaque and are frequently followed by scarring and fibrosis, which further enlarge the lesion. Rupture of blood vessels within the plaque also may cause a sudden major obstruction of the lumen of the vessel. The intima covering a plaque may break, causing a clot to form on the surface, which adds to the building obstruction of the vessel's lumen. The clot or plaque also may embolize and occlude the vessel distally where the lumen becomes narrow. Evidence indicates that myocardial infarction is usually produced by an acute thrombotic event complicating preexisting atherosclerosis.[4,6] The discovery that acute coronary thrombosis is usually present in myocardial infarction has fostered attempts to restore coronary blood flow by chemical agents that dissolve blood clots (streptokinase or tissue plasminogen activator) or by mechanical disruption of the thrombus (balloon angioplasty) before the myocardium supplied by the occluded vessel is irreversibly damaged.

In addition to compromising blood supply by obstruction, the atherosclerotic process may cause weakening of the arterial wall and aneurysm formation. Thus obstruction and aneurysm may coexist in the same artery.

## GROSS PATHOLOGY AND PROGNOSIS

Atherosclerotic lesions usually form at branch points in the arterial tree. In the carotid and iliac arteries the disease is most prevalent at the bifurcation. Coronary arteries are particularly susceptible to atherosclerosis. Although it is unusual to have peripheral vascular disease without coronary artery involvement, coronary disease without involvement of peripheral arteries is not rare. In coronary circulation the atherosclerotic process is confined to the portions of the vessels that lie on the epicardial surface, sparing the smaller penetrating arteries. Such a pattern of distribution suggests that turbulence of flow at branch points and rhythmic torsion of untethered vessels may contribute to the genesis of the lesion.

In considering the natural history of coronary artery disease, it is important to distinguish factors that affect the underlying coronary artery disease per se, that is, the previously described accumulation of lipid, cellular material, and sometimes calcium within the vessel wall,[4] from factors that influence the occurrence of clinical complications such as sudden death, angina pectoris, or myocardial infarction. An additional discussion of pathophysiology will highlight the importance of this distinction.

Some degree of CAD is present in most individuals above the age of 30 in Western industrialized nations. However, such disease is almost always clinically silent until it progresses to occlude 75% of the diameter of a major coronary vessel. Even at this degree of obstruction, blood flow to the region of the myocardium supplied by the occluded vessel is usually normal at rest, and it becomes inadequate only when the oxygen requirements of the heart muscle are high, for example, during strenuous exercise. Only when the vessel lumen is narrowed to less than 5% of its normal vessel diameter is the blood flow insufficient to maintain a normal oxygen supply to the myocardium in the resting state. Furthermore, even with such severe stenosis, blood from other major coronary vessels may reach the muscle supplied by the severely narrowed vessel through alternative channels, termed *collaterals*, thereby maintaining normal blood flow, even during exercise.

The degree to which an individual patient's heart forms such collaterals is very unpredictable; therefore the relationship between the severity of the stenosis and the severity of symptoms is also unpredictable. Furthermore, some individuals may have serious limitations to myocardial blood flow, even developing myocardial infarction in the absence of chest pain, an occurrence that further complicates the clinical assessment of patients with coronary artery disease.

An additional anatomic feature of the coronary arteries that is clinically relevant is that they are not rigid pipes, but muscular structures capable of rapid variations in diameter under the influence of autonomic nerves that innervate them or vasoactive substances released in the vessel lumen by vascular endothelium, or by platelets.[7] The degree to which an atherosclerotic plaque present in a coronary vessel limits blood flow will depend not only on the severity of the plaque itself, but also on the muscular tone of the vessel around the plaque. Thus an insignificant 25% stenosis may rapidly become a critical 99% stenosis under the influence of a vasoconstrictive stimulus. This occurrence is termed *coronary spasm* and may be suspected clinically with observation of transient ST-segment elevation on the ECG, in the absence of the release of myocardial enzymes into blood that characterizes a myocardial infarction. To further complicate matters, such limitations in coronary blood flow, and even myocardial infarction, may occasionally occur in the absence of clinically demonstrable atherosclerosis.[8]

These pathophysiologic considerations, in addition to the marked variability in the rate of progression of the underlying atherosclerosis and also in the occurrence of sudden catastrophic events such as acute coronary thrombosis of ventricular fibrillation, account for the disconcerting unpredictability of the prognosis carried by an individual patient with coronary artery disease. These considerations also explain part of the difficulty in trying to detect coronary artery disease in its early stages. However, it is possible to use anatomic and physiologic data to yield probability estimates concerning prognosis. An important variable is the number of major coronary vessels with obstructions exceeding 75% of the vascular lumen. CAD occurs most frequently in the left anterior descending artery, less in the right coronary artery, and still less frequently (although not rarely) in the circumflex artery. Narrowing tends to be most severe in the proximal 2 to 3 cm of each artery, but distal involvement, particularly of the right coronary artery, is not uncommon. The site of vessel obstruction is clinically important, since proximal lesions are much more amenable to therapy by saphenous vein-grafting or by percutaneous transluminal coronary angioplasty with balloon-type catheters. In almost all pathologically examined cases of myocardial infarction, the vessel supplying the infarcted area demonstrates a lesion of 95% or greater. Thus significant disease of the right coronary artery is found in patients with inferior myocardial infarction, and disease of the left anterior descending artery is found in patients with anterior infarction.

A second factor with prognostic importance for the patient with CAD is the contractile function of the left ventricle, which is determined largely by the amount of muscle tissue damaged by previous myocardial infarction. Individuals with good ventricular function have a much better prognosis than those with impaired function, despite equivalent degrees of coronary obstruction. The increased mortality of patients with poor ventricular function is attributable largely to a higher incidence of sudden death, presumably caused by ventricular fibrillation, rather than to recurrent infarction or to inexorably progressive congestive heart failure. Sudden death also occurs in patients with coronary disease and normal ventricular function, although with a lower incidence, and, tragically, it can occur as the initial manifestation of coronary artery disease in previously asymptomatic persons. Frequent premature ventricular contractions or ventricular tachycardia in the postinfarction period also may identify persons at higher risk for sudden death.[9]

Although the number of diseased coronary vessels and left ventricular function are powerful predictors of both symptomatic improvement and prognosis in patients with CAD, exceptions to the general trends described above occur with some frequency. Patients with severe three-vessel CAD or markedly severe left ventricular dysfunction may be asymptomatic and may survive for more than a decade. Conversely, some patients with single-vessel disease may have disabling angina pectoris or may die unexpectantly as a result of myocardial infarction or ventricular dysrhythmia.

In summary, coronary atherosclerosis may be without symptoms for many years until the disease progresses to produce an obstruction that interferes with the arterial blood supply to the myocardium. If the obstruction progresses gradually over a period of years, intercoronary collateral circulation may develop, and clinical evidence of disease may be deferred or may never occur. Despite marked obstructive disease, the myocardial cells may receive adequate oxygen regardless of demands. On the other hand, when an artery is partially obstructed and sufficient collateral circulation has not yet developed, the obstruction may impair blood flow during conditions of increased demand, producing symptoms of intermittent vascular insufficiency.

## RISK FACTORS

Large-scale epidemiologic studies have identified certain cardiovascular risk factors that are associated with a higher incidence of CAD.[10] The 25% decline in mortality from cardiovascular disease in the last decade is partially attributable to increased public awareness of risk factors and subsequent lifestyle changes. The well-established major risk factors include hypertension, hypercholesterolemia, smoking, and diabetes mellitus. Other factors that may affect risk for CAD are obesity, sedentary lifestyle, and an aggressive response to stress. In this context risk is viewed as the probability of developing CAD, and that probability is determined by the number of risk factors in any individual, by the level of each factor (that is, the level of blood pressure or cholesterol), and by age. It is important to consider the cumulative nature of risk factors in the clinical evaluation of the patient. For example, a person who smokes and is hypertensive, has approximately twice the risk as one who smokes and is normotensive. Although the disease is more common when multiple risk factors are present, it can occur in the absence of any identifiable risk factors. Clearly, genetic or environmental variables can act independently of established risk factors and influence the clinical outcome. Nonetheless, identification and elimination of risk factors remain a priority to further lower the incidence of CAD.

### Age, Sex, and Race

Atherosclerosis is more prevalent in older people. In 1984, 611,416 deaths were caused by diseases of the heart, with 435,759 or 71.3% attributed to CAD. In addition, the death rate for persons with CAD rose steeply with age among the elderly. The death rate of men with CAD was higher than that of women in age groups 65 to 85. These differences were not found in individuals who were 85 years or older.[11] Men have a greater risk of heart attack than women,[1] but heart attacks remain the leading cause of death among women in the United States. The Framingham study[15] reported that after age 55, a woman's risk of CAD increases 10-fold and approaches, but does not reach, the risk of men.

Black men have similar or higher CAD death rates compared with white men age 65 and younger, but black men show lower death rates once they have reached 75 years of age. Black women have higher CAD death rates than white women until age 75, similar death rates from age 75 to 84, and lower death rates at 85 or more years of age.[1] Prevalence of self-reported CAD increased in the elderly between 1972 and 1984; this increase may be the result of improved care, which prevented deaths, or it may be the result of more complete self-reporting activities by the elderly.[11]

## Hypertension

Hypertension is the most common form of cardiovascular disease and is a major risk factor for CAD.

It was estimated in 1986 that over 60 million Americans age six and older had hypertension.[1] Essential hypertension refers to the 90% of cases in which the cause is unknown. Normal adult blood pressure is defined as a systolic blood pressure less than 140 mm Hg and a diastolic pressure less than 90 mm Hg. The Third Joint National Committee on Detection, Evaluation, and Treatment of High Blood Pressure recommended a specific classification scheme for hypertension (Table 6-1).[12] The risk for heart disease associated with essential hypertension is directly proportional to the level of elevated blood pressure, and either the systolic or the diastolic pressure may be used to predict risk. Diastolic hypertension is related to an increase in total peripheral resistance (arteriolar), and systolic hypertension reflects an elevated cardiac output or large vessel (arterial) stiffness. Young hypertensives may have an elevated systolic pressure as a result of an increased cardiac output, related to sympathetic nervous system overactivity. In middle-aged and older adults systolic hypertension is usually caused by atherosclerosis of the aorta and its major branches.[13] Systolic and diastolic hypertension may coexist however.

Data from the Framingham study[14,15] revealed that hypertensive persons (blood pressure greater than 160/95) have more than twice the risk for coronary heart disease compared with normotensive persons (blood pressure less than 140/90). Individuals with borderline hypertension have a 50% increase in risk. Systolic pressure exerts an even greater influence on coronary heart disease morbidity and mortality than diastolic pressure. A major focus of nursing is the identification of risk factors for hypertension, and assisting patients in reducing them. Congenital and environmental risk factors include: heredity, age, Black race, obesity, salt intake, alcohol, caffeine, smoking, oral contraceptives, socioeconomic factors, and stress.[16] Public education has produced considerable gains in the detection and treatment of hypertension.

**TABLE 6-1** Classification of blood pressure in adults aged 18 years or older[12]

| Range (mm Hg) | Category |
|---|---|
| **DIASTOLIC BLOOD PRESSURE** | |
| <85 | Normal blood pressure |
| 85-89 | High-normal blood pressure |
| 90-104 | Mild hypertension |
| 105-114 | Moderate hypertension |
| ≥115 | Severe hypertension |
| **SYSTOLIC BLOOD PRESSURE, WHEN DIASTOLIC BLOOD PRESSURE <90** | |
| <140 | Normal blood pressure |
| 140-159 | Borderline isolated systolic hypertension |
| ≥160 | Isolated systolic hypertension |

Joint National Committee: The 1988 report of the joint national committee on detection, evaluation, and treatment of high blood pressure, Arch Intern Med 148:1023, 1988.

There is evidence that some nonpharmacologic measures can assist in controlling blood pressure. In some individuals nonpharmacologic therapy, such as weight reduction, low sodium diet, and exercise, may be all that is required to normalize blood pressure. In most cases, however, these therapies alone are insufficient for achieving or maintaining a lower blood pressure. Nonpharmacologic approaches may not produce adequate blood pressure reduction or the individual may not comply with the necessary lifestyle changes.[13] However, because these measures may be effective either alone or in conjunction with drug therapy for certain individuals, health professionals must provide the appropriate counseling.

A strong association exists between obesity and elevated blood pressure.[17] Obesity may contribute to hypertension via an increase in blood volume, stroke volume, and cardiac output.[18] Weight reduction has been shown to reduce blood pressure in some individuals.[19]

The American diet contains excess sodium much beyond physiologic needs. A moderate restriction of dietary sodium, to about one half of the usual intake, lowers blood pressure 5 to 10 mm Hg below levels observed with higher sodium intake.[19] Elderly individuals with isolated systolic hypertension may respond to sodium restriction, because their hypertension usually is volume-dependent.[20] Dietary counseling encourages refraining from adding salt to foods, avoiding processed foods, and reading labels of purchased food items for sodium content.

A relationship between alcohol, caffeine, tobacco, and hypertension has been noted in some studies.[19,21] The prevalence of hypertension increases with the consumption of greater than 2 to 3 ounces of ethanol per day, which produces an acute pressor response and elevation of blood pressure. Caffeine ingestion and smoking may cause an acute rise in blood pressure by vasoconstriction, however, some studies have not shown a higher incidence of hypertension with chronic use. Smoking should be discouraged, however, since its combination with hypertension greatly potentiates the risk of CAD.

Isotonic or dynamic exercise, such as running, bicycling, and swimming, produces a progressive increase in systolic pressure, but little or no change in diastolic pressure in normotensive individuals.[22] Most studies have reported a greater increase in systolic and diastolic pressures with exercise in people with hypertension,[23] related to higher levels of total peripheral resistance. After exercise training, however, the rise in arterial pressure and heart rate is less marked. After an exercise session, blood pressure in hypertensive persons decreases to levels below resting, and remains there for variable amounts of time.[24] Similar to other forms of nonpharmacologic therapy, exercise training is not uniformly effective in lowering blood pressure. However, because it may be a useful adjunct to drug therapy, hypertensive individuals should be provided with an exercise program after a thorough medical evaluation. In addition, exercise contributes to weight reduction and stress management.

Recent studies on behavioral approaches to hypertension management have shown that various relaxation and biofeedback methods produce modest long-term reductions in blood pressure in selected groups.[25,26] The combination of biofeedback and relaxation techniques produces greater effects than either approach alone.[27] These approaches are primarily recommended for mild hypertension and may be used to reduce medication requirements. It is essential that blood pressure be closely monitored at rest and during daily activities in order to evaluate long-term effectiveness.

Most American physicians have adopted the philosophy of instituting early and aggressive drug therapy for patients with mild hypertension. In fact, treatment of hypertension is the major reason for office visits to physicians.[28] It has been shown that drug therapy is usually begun when diastolic pressure is between 90 and 94 mm Hg.[29]

Studies[30,31] indicate that reducing blood pressure with medications decreases cardiovascular morbidity and mortality in patients with diastolic pressures greater than 104 mm Hg. In patients with diastolic pressures between 90 and 104 mm Hg, drug therapy protects against stroke, congestive heart failure, progression to more severe levels of hypertension, and all-cause mortality. Clinical trials evaluating the effects of antihypertensive drug therapy show a trend toward reduced mortality from CAD.[32]

The Joint National Committee on Detection, Evaluation, and Treatment of High Blood Pressure recommends that drug therapy be instituted for individuals with a persistently elevated diastolic pressure greater than 94 mm Hg and for those with lesser elevations who have other CAD risk factors.[12] Lower risk individuals with diastolic pressures between 90 and 94 mm Hg should initially be treated with nonpharmacologic approaches.

Initial drug therapy may consist of thiazide diuretics, beta blockers, angiotension-converting enzyme inhibitors, or calcium channel blockers. Physiologic and biochemical measurements, such as resting heart rate, plasma renin activity, and urine sodium, assist the clinician in selecting the most appropriate medication.

## Hypercholesterolemia

Cholesterol is a lipid that is a primary component of cell membranes and a precursor of bile acids and steroid hormones. Cholesterol is transported through the circulation by lipoproteins, which are particles containing apolipoproteins and several lipids (including triglycerides, cholesterol, cholesteryl esters, and phospholipids). The apolipoproteins assist in maintaining the structural integrity and functional specificity of plasma lipoproteins.[33] Generally, the apolipoprotein B concentration in plasma is positively associated with CAD, and apolipoprotein A is negatively associated with CAD. Knowledge about both lipoproteins and apolipoproteins has increased dramatically in the last decade, providing the framework for understanding lipid metabolism in normal individuals and in those with lipid disorders. Lipoprotein metabolism is complex and beyond the scope of this chapter, but the reader is referred to current literature for more information.[33,34]

Three major classes of plasma lipoproteins can be measured in a fasting individual: very low-density lipoproteins (VLDL), low-density lipoproteins (LDL), and high-density lipoproteins (HDL). VLDL contain mostly triglycerides and 10% to 15% of the total serum cholesterol. LDL, derived from the metabolism of VLDL, contain 60% to 70% of the total serum cholesterol. The HDL are mostly protein and contain about 20% to 30% of the total cholesterol. Studies have demonstrated that HDL levels are inversely correlated and LDL levels are directly correlated with the risk of CAD.[35]

There are two common patterns of hyperlipidemia. In type IV, there are elevated levels of triglycerides with normal or only slightly elevated cholesterol, caused by increased VLDL. Type II includes elevated cholesterol with normal or only slightly elevated levels of triglycerides, caused by increased LDL.

Substantial evidence from epidemiologic, genetic, and animal studies supports a causal relationship between elevated serum cholesterol and CAD. Comparisons of world populations demonstrate the direct association between serum cholesterol levels and the incidence of CAD.[36] People who move to a country with a higher average serum cholesterol level eventually acquire the dietary habits, serum cholesterol levels, and CAD rate of their new country. Prospective epidemiologic studies have demonstrated that serum cholesterol levels predict future CAD morbidity and mortality, with risk increasing steadily as cholesterol levels rise above 200 mg/dl.[37]

In addition to the data that support the causal relationship between elevated serum cholesterol and CAD, several clinical trials have demonstrated that lowering LDLs by dietary or drug interventions can reduce the incidence of CAD. In the Lipid Research Clinics Coronary Primary Prevention Trial,[38] investigators compared the cholesterol lowering drug cholestyramine with a placebo and found that a 12.5% decrease in LDLs was associated with a 19% decrease in the incidence of acute myocardial infarction (AMI) and death in the cholestyramine treatment group.[38]

In the Helsinski Heart Study,[39,40] drug treatment that was associated with an 11% decrease in LDLs and an 11% increase in HDLs also was associated with a 34% decrease in the CAD endpoints of definite heart attack or death. In both studies the benefits of therapy were not evident until after 24 months. Data from the Coronary Drug Project[41] also evidenced a significant decrease in overall mortality in a 15-year follow-up in men after AMI who were treated with nicotinic acid, a cholesterol-lowering agent.

The pooled analysis of clinical findings suggest, therefore, that intervention is as effective in preventing recurrent MI and death in patients who have had an MI, as it is in primary prevention of CAD. The evidence is strongest in middle-aged men with initial high-cholesterol levels. Evidence suggests, however, that decreasing total cholesterol and LDL cholesterol also is likely to reduce CAD incidence in adults and in individuals with more moderate elevations of cholesterol.[42]

A recent review of the nine prospective studies that have examined the correlation between total cholesterol and CAD in women revealed that total cholesterol and possibly LDL are risk factors for CAD in women.[43] A high-triglyceride level is an independent risk factor for women and increased HDL is negatively associated with subsequent CAD.[44] Data indicate that women have much lower rates of CAD than men with similar cholesterol values.[43] Women, however, develop CAD an average of 10 years later than men.[44] Nevertheless, a recent study confirms the need for screening women for the risk of CAD because lifestyle changes can reduce the incidence of CAD morbidity and mortality.[45]

The Bogalusa Heart Study,[46] which included a 15-year span, established that cardiovascular risk can be predicted early in life and that the interrelationships of risk factors in children are similar to those observed in adults. Approximately 5% of 5- to 18-year-old American children have total plasma cholesterol levels exceeding 200 mg/dl.[47] In a recent study of 786 fourth-grade schoolchildren, 10% had blood cholesterol levels of 200 mg/dl or more and only one third had a family history of early CAD.[48]

In the past there has been some controversy among pediatric clinicians regarding the detection and treatment of hypercholesterolemia in children. Some of the objections that were made include the following: (1) normal values have not been established for identification of a child at "high risk"; (2) mass screening of blood cholesterol levels would be too expensive; and (3) modifying nutrition patterns in children would be very difficult.[48]

In the past couple of years, these objections have been addressed by long-term studies of children and their risk factors for CAD.[46] Based on current research, the American Heart Association recommends that all American children gradually decrease their intake of saturated fat.[47] Current AHA guidelines do not recommend mass routine screening of all children, but they do stress the importance of detection and treatment of children with inherited disorders of lipoprotein metabolism.[47] According to the AHA, a child with mild hypercholesterolemia should be treated initially with diet. The AHA recommends that cholesterol in the diets of children be restricted to 100 mg/1000 calories, not to exceed 300 mg/day; and that fat provide 30% of total calories, of which approximately 10% is saturated, up to 10% polyunsaturated, and 10% monosaturated.[47]

The strength of the association between LDL and CAD diminishes with age and there is little evidence that elderly patients benefit from intervention. The Expert Panel on the Detection, Evaluation, and Treatment of High Blood Cholesterol in Adults, or Adult Treatment Panel (ATP),[42] recommends, however, that lowering LDL through diet may be beneficial in the elderly based on the clinical trial evidence for effectiveness of intervention after MI. The ATP recommends that the value of dietary therapy for prevention of atheroscleratic disease in the elderly high-risk patient must be balanced with the possibility of inadequate nutrition, often a problem for the elderly.[49]

The ATP of the National Cholesterol Education Program recently developed guidelines for classification and treatment of individuals with high blood cholesterol.[42] It recommends that total serum cholesterol be measured in all adults 20 years of age and over once every 5 years. LDL is the primary atherogenic agent and because most of the cholesterol in the serum is found in LDL, it can be used initially in evaluating serum lipids. Serum cholesterol levels are categorized as desirable (<200 mg/dl), borderline (200 to 239 mg/dl), or high (>240 mg/dl).[42] In addition, assessments should include other risk factors such as hypertension, cigarette smoking, diabetes mellitus, severe obesity, male sex, peripheral vascular or cerebrovascular disease, HDL level below 35 mg/dl, and family or individual history of CAD.[50]

The Panel recommends that treatment decisions for hypercholesterolemia regarding diet or drugs be based on LDL values. LDL levels should be assessed in all individuals with high blood cholesterol levels and in those with borderline cholesterol levels who already have CAD or who have two other risk factors.[42]

Dietary therapy is recommended for individuals with LDL levels exceeding 160 mg/dl and for those with LDL levels of 130 mg/dl who already have CAD or two other risk factors. Treatment with medications is recommended when despite dietary changes, the LDL level remains above 190 mg/dl or 160 mg/dl in individuals with preexisting CAD or two other risk factors. The minimum treatment goal is an LDL level below 160 or below 130 for those with CAD or two other risk factors.[42]

Dietary measures are the first line of treatment for elevated LDL. The average American diet contains approximately 450 mg of cholesterol daily, 37% of calories as fat, and 14% of calories as saturated fat.[51] For patients with elevated LDL levels, a two-step approach is recommended. Initial efforts are to achieve ideal weight and to limit cholesterol intake to 300 mg/dl, fat intake to 30% of calories, and saturated fat intake to 10% of calories. Foods high in saturated fat include whole milk, cream, butter, cheeses, animal fats, organ meats, and palm and coconut oils. Reduction in cholesterol intake is best achieved by decreasing intake of egg yolks and fats of animal origin. For individuals whose LDL levels remain elevated despite the step I diet, the more rigorous step II diet is advised; in the step II diet cholesterol is limited to 200 mg a day and saturated fats are limited to 7% of calories.

The Panel recommends that dietary measures be undertaken for at least 6 months before the need for drug treatment is decided. Medications can be added earlier for patients with severe or familial hypercholesterolemia.[42]

The primary medications used for lowering LDL cholesterol include those that (1) stimulate the removal of LDL through receptor-mediated mechanisms (bile acid sequestrants); (2) decrease the rate of synthesis of VLDL, the precursor of LDL (nicotinic acid); (3) hasten the clearance of VLDL (fibric acid derivatives); and (4) stimulate the clearance of LDL via nonreceptor mechanisms (probucol). Because of their long-standing efficacy, niacin and bile acid sequestrants are the drugs of choice in lowering LDL.[51]

## Smoking

Cigarette smoking has been identified as a major health problem and the single most preventable cause of death in the United States.[52] During the last several decades, significant public health effort has been focused on decreasing the prevalence of smoking. Although these efforts have had a positive impact in reducing overall smoking prevalence, the rate of decline has been variable among population subgroups, such as women, blacks, and individuals with lower educational level and socioeconomic status.

According to the National Health Interview Surveys the estimated prevalence of smoking in men decreased from 43.4% in 1974 to 33.5% in 1985.[53] The decline was less for women with an estimated prevalence of 31.2% in 1974 to 27.6% in 1985. This slower decline in smoking prev-

alence for women is reflected in the changing epidemiology of lung cancer. In 1987, for the first time, breast cancer was replaced by lung cancer as the leading cause of cancer mortality in women.[53] A higher proportion of blacks than whites smoke, and lower socioeconomic status is associated with higher smoking rates.[54]

Smoking prevalence declined in all educational groups, but it declined 5 times faster among the more highly educated compared with the less educated. From 1974 to 1985 smoking prevalence declined to 34.2% among persons with less than a high-school diploma, whereas the prevalence declined to 18.4% for persons with 4 years or more of college.[53]

There also are important differences in smoking rates between age groups reported in the 1985 Health Interview Survey statistics. Smoking rates were fairly uniform between ages 20 and 55 years and dropped rapidly among older age groups, being 30.2% among those 55 to 64 years old, 21.5% among those 65 to 74 years old, and only 8.5% among those 75 years and older. Smoking among adolescents continues to be a problem. An estimated two million teenagers continue to smoke, and more than 100,000 children age 12 and under are habitual smokers.[53]

There has been a great deal of effort to reduce smoking in the work place, in public, and in the home. A significant trend is the negative attitude toward cigarette smoking reflected in numerous regulations separating smokers and nonsmokers in schools, restaurants, worksites, airplanes, and other public places. Nonsmokers have become outspoken in their demand for clean indoor air. By 1989, 43 states and the District of Columbia had restricted public smoking. The range was from simple laws, such as no smoking in school buses in operation, to comprehensive clean indoor air laws.[55]

Smoking is a major risk factor for coronary and peripheral vascular disease. Middle-aged men who smoke have 2 to 3 times the risk of developing a major manifestation of CAD as compared with nonsmokers. Continued smoking shortens life expectancy and increases the likelihood of recurrence among patients who have experienced an MI.[56]

Available data suggest that smoking cessation markedly decreases future CAD risk. One year after ceasing to smoke cigarettes, the risk of experiencing a cardiovascular event drops by 10%; in 10 years the risk approaches that of a lifelong nonsmoker.[56] Data indicate that smoking cessation is associated with a 20% to 50% decreased incidence of new infarction and sudden death in patients with myocardial infarction, a reduction in the risk of nonfatal reinfarction, and an extension of long-term benefits.[56,57] Even in the elderly aged 65 to 74 years, smoking cessation is associated with decreased cardiovascular risk, indicating that it is worthwhile to encourage patients of all ages to stop smoking.[58]

Smoking a cigarette causes an infusion of nicotine, which stimulates the sympathetic nervous system. In healthy people this results in an increased heart rate, blood pressure, stroke volume, cardiac output, and coronary blood flow. The peripheral vascular changes include cutaneous vasoconstriction associated with decreased skin temperature, systemic vasoconstriction, and increased muscle blood flow.[59]

The specific mechanism whereby cigarette smoking either accelerates the development of CAD or precipitates its manifestations is yet to be defined. In patients with CAD, nicotine may contribute to the magnitude and frequency of reversible myocardial ischemia. There is increased oxygen consumption with the increased heart rate and blood pressure. The carbon monoxide inhaled also decreases the oxygen-carrying capacity of the blood. Carbon monoxide also may produce direct damage to the arterial endothelium. When a healthy person smokes a cigarette, blood flow increases to meet the increased demand.[59] In the presence of CAD, however, coronary blood flow cannot increase sufficiently to meet the increased demand because of a decreased coronary artery lumen size, which may cause angina pectoris or myocardial dysfunction.

Smoking may contribute to CAD through its effects on hemostasis and development of thrombosis, which is a factor in the atherogenic process and acute MI. Blood coagulates more easily in smokers than nonsmokers; fibrinogen levels are higher; platelets are reported in some studies to be more reactive,[60] and platelet survival is shortened in smokers as compared with nonsmokers.[59] Smokers also tend to have a relatively unfavorable lipoprotein pattern with a high total cholesterol to HDL ratio as compared with nonsmokers.[53]

The majority of smokers who quit do so without the help of structured groups or prescription medications.[61] Successful smoking cessation usually follows repeated attempts to quit.[62] There are several personal characteristics that are positively correlated with successful efforts to quit smoking: a high expectation of success, number and duration of past smoking cessation attempts, fewer cigarettes smoked per day, low stress, and traits such as a sense of personal control and security. Barriers to successful cessation include: lack of understanding about the health consequences of smoking, and fear of failure, nicotine withdrawal, and weight gain.[63]

Cigarette smoking meets the criteria for drug dependence described in the Surgeon General's report, "The Health Consequences of Smoking."[54] Several methods exist to assist with smoking cessation. A review of smoking cessation programs conducted by the U.S. Department of Health and Human Services identified certain factors that improved success: (1) use of multiple cessation methods, which can address the behavioral and pharmacologic components of addictions; (2) payment, as in commercial programs, which increases commitment; (3) the presence of illness or risk factors that improve motivation to quit; and

(4) good maintenance procedures, which provide ongoing support to the ex-smoker.[64]

Among medical patients, the rate of spontaneous quitting is 1% per year, but this rate can be increased severalfold with minimal health care provider intervention, such as simple instructions to stop smoking. Further treatment may require pharmacologic or behavior therapy, or both.[65]

Behavior therapy often is critical to successful smoking cessation. These methods are categorized into four types: (1) self-help methods, self-help aids, and mass media approaches; (2) health professional–directed minimal interventions, such as brief counseling, hypnosis, or single-session acupuncture; (3) comprehensive smoking cessation programs; and (4) either method 2 or 3 combined with a pharmacologic aid such as Nicorette gum or clonidine. Self-help methods including books, cassettes, or tapes are readily available to smokers. The use and efficacy of these approaches have not been thoroughly studied.[65]

Nasopuncture and auriculopuncture are the two primary methods of acupuncture used for smoking cessation. There are few published studies on the efficacy of acupuncture and most of these are methodologically flawed. Godenick,[66] in a review of these studies, concluded that there is no substantive evidence that acupuncture relieves withdrawal symptoms or promotes smoking cessation.

Studies on the effectiveness of hypnosis as a treatment for smoking also are difficult to evaluate because of poor study design and weak follow-up. Schwartz,[64] however, in a review of smoking cessation methods, concluded that the skill and experience of the therapist and multiple sessions appear to improve quit rates.

Behavioral methods for smoking cessation include aversive methods and self-management techniques. Aversive methods include rapid smoking and mild electric shock. Self-management methods include nicotine fading, gradually reducing the number of cigarettes smoked over time, and relaxation techniques. A recent review of these methods concluded that the best success rates have been achieved by a combination of aversive and self-management methods. Data indicate that aversion therapy is effective in initiating smoking cessation, whereas, abstinence is better helped by self-management strategies.[66]

Pharmacologic therapies to assist smoking cessation include receptor antagonists (such as mecamylamine), nonreceptor antagonists (such as clonidine), and nicotine substitution therapy. Mecamylamine decreases the satisfaction and other effects of smoking. Clonidine decreases the severity of the craving for nicotine and that of nicotine-withdrawal symptoms, probably by acting on alpha adrenergic receptors of the central nervous system.[50] In a recent clinical trial, clonidine therapy for 6 weeks was found to be more effective than a placebo in assisting smoking cessation, although the benefit was observed only in women.[67]

The most effective pharmacologic approach for smoking cessation has been nicotine-substitution therapy. In some studies, nicotine gum has been shown to be useful in helping subjects quit smoking.[68] The gum is most effective when used as a component of a comprehensive program including behavioral therapy.[69] Side effects from the gum such as hiccups and nausea may be controlled by lowering the dose of nicotine and by slow and paced chewing.[70]

A number of methods or a combination of them can help smokers to achieve abstinence. Programs with an effective maintenance component have the best long-term success. Social support, training in coping strategies, and using substitutes such as exercise may enhance long-term maintenance.[64]

## Glucose Intolerance

Coronary heart disease is more prevalent in patients with adult onset diabetes mellitus, although the precise mechanisms are unclear. Patients with diabetes have more connective tissue degeneration, which expedites atheroma formation. Men with glucose intolerance have a 50% greater risk of developing CAD than those without it whereas in women the risk is more than doubled, which equalizes the risk of CAD in men and women with diabetes.

## Physical Inactivity

A relationship exists between physical inactivity and increased risk of CAD. The strength of this relationship, however, is lower than those of hypertension, smoking, and hypercholesterolemia. Physical activity favorably influences certain risk factors, such as reducing blood pressure in some individuals, assisting in weight loss, and increasing HDLs. Physical activity, then, may have an indirect effect on CAD by reducing other risk factors.

Investigators have studied the effects of occupational and leisure time physical activity on CAD morbidity and mortality. More than 35 years ago Morris and colleagues[71] reported that physically active London transit workers and postal carriers had fewer CAD events than bus drivers and sedentary postal clerks. Follow-up work showed that the conductors had one-half the CAD mortality rate of the drivers.[72] These differences are significant when considering the mild form of exercise involved in collecting tickets or delivering mail. It was later determined, however, that the bus drivers weighed more than the conductors, which may have contributed to the difference in heart disease rates.[73]

Among the most well-controlled occupational studies was an investigation of Israeli workers living on farm settlements.[74] Many extraneous variables were eliminated because all subjects were of the same ethnic origin, lived in the same environment, ate the same diet in communal dining halls, and received similar medical care. There were no differences in body weight and cholesterol levels within the sample. In a 15-year retrospective survey of more than

10,000 men and women who were 40 to 64 years of age, there was a 2.5 and 3.1 greater incidence of CAD for men and women, respectively, who were engaged in sedentary work compared with those engaged in physical work.

A prospective study of 6351 longshoremen[75,76] demonstrated a strong inverse relationship between energy expenditure at work and CAD morbidity and mortality. The death rate for heart disease was about one half for the men who expended 8500 kcal per week or more (cargo handlers who loaded and unloaded ships) compared with those less physically active (foremen and clerks). This difference remained significant when cigarette smoking, systolic blood pressure, and body weight were excluded.

The Framingham study[77] used a subjective measure of physical activity based on recall of daily activities. The index used by this study was the product of hours spent at each physical activity level and a weight based on oxygen consumption of that activity. Men with the highest scores on this index had fewer deaths related to CAD than those who were less active, even when other risk factors were excluded. The significant relationship diminished for women when adjustment was made for age.

The largest body of evidence on the relationship between exercise and reduced CAD risk originates from studies of 17,000 Harvard alumni by Paffenbarger and colleagues.[78-80] The age-adjusted incidence of CAD was inversely related to energy expenditure as measured by responses to mail questionnaires. Men who expended less than 2000 kcal per week had a 64% greater risk than men who had a greater energy expenditure. In addition, alumni who had been college athletes and did not continue exercising had a higher risk for CAD, compared with alumni who were physically active, and had not been athletes in college. The implication of this study is that current physical activity is the relevant factor in determining the influence of exercise on the risk of CAD. Frequent follow-up of these alumni has demonstrated that exercise is inversely related to mortality, especially death from cardiovascular diseases.

One of the proposed mechanisms for the reduced incidence of CAD in those who regularly exercise is an increase in HDL. Wood and colleagues[81] followed for 1 year 81 healthy sedentary men aged 30 to 55 who were randomly assigned to a running program or to remain sedentary. The runners had a higher fitness level, as measured by maximum oxygen consumption, and less body fat than the sedentary controls. In addition, total cholesterol, LDL, and triglycerides were reduced, and HDL were increased in the runners. Opposite changes were observed in the sedentary subjects. These changes in lipid measurements, however, were not significant. Data from the group who averaged running at least 8 miles per week revealed an increase in HDL that was significant. Thus, beneficial lipoprotein changes may be related to quantity and quality of exercise. Significant increases in HDL also were found in 40 men, ages 29 to 56 years, who had CAD and engaged in a cardiac rehabilitation program.[82] The exercise consisted of aerobic activities during three 20-minute periods 5 days a week for 3 weeks. Nonsmoking participants had the greatest HDL increases, but no comparison group was included.

In addition to favorably altering lipid metabolism, exercise produces other effects that reduce CAD risk. Resting heart rate decreases as a result of exercise training, and blood pressure may be reduced in both normotensive and hypertensive individuals, producing an increase in myocardial oxygen supply and a reduction in myocardial oxygen consumption.[62,83-85] Additional cardiovascular benefits of exercise training include an increase in stroke volume, cardiac output, and arteriovenous oxygen difference. Individuals who exercise regularly also are more likely to engage in other healthy behaviors that contribute to a lower risk, such as eating moderately, coping more effectively with stress, and avoiding smoking.

Parents and educators should emphasize to children the importance of regular physical activity and exercise. Children must be encouraged to participate in school-related and community physical education programs that address the health benefits of exercise. This early exposure to exercise helps to form lifelong physical activity habits.

When adults decide to initiate an exercise program for the prevention of CAD, they should be encouraged first to obtain a physical examination. Ideally, this examination includes a graded maximum exercise test to determine aerobic capacity and evaluate cardiovascular status.

An exercise prescription may be provided based on an individual's functional capacity. An exercise prescription should address the type, intensity, duration, and frequency of physical activity. The type of exercise is any activity that uses large muscle groups and is aerobic in nature, such as running, jogging, walking, swimming, bicycling, rowing, cross-country skiing, skating, or jumping rope. These are considered to be endurance or dynamic forms of exercise. The intensity of training should be 65% to 90% of one's age-related maximum heart rate (220 minus the age). An individual should begin by exercising at 65% of his maximal heart rate and increase the intensity as conditioning effects, such as a lower resting heart rate, are observed. The duration of exercise is 15 to 60 minutes of continuous or intermittent aerobic activity. The duration depends on the intensity of the activity, thus lower intensity activity should be performed for a longer period of time. The frequency of activity is 3 to 5 days per week. Conditioning effects may be observed after the first 6 to 8 weeks of an exercise program.[86]

## Personality Factors

For many years CAD has been thought to be more prominent among individuals subject to chronic anxiety or stress. Subsequently personality type A was noted to be more prone to CAD. The characteristics of type A behavior include aggressiveness, ambition, competitive drive, and a chronic sense of urgency. Anger and hostility, key components of the type A behavior pattern, are associated with CAD.[87,88] It remains to be shown whether modification of behavior patterns is possible or whether it is effective in altering risk.

## Stress

Inability to cope with stress is related, either directly or indirectly, to cancer, lung ailments, accidental injuries, cirrhosis of the liver, and suicide—six of the leading causes of death in the United States.[89]

Stress may be experienced by the individual in a variety of ways, including muscle tightness, stomach discomfort, feelings of tension and anxiety, tachycardia, and diaphoresis. A number of personal factors affect an individual's ability to cope with stress, including the sense of being in control of one's life, having a network of friends or family or a social support system, and such personality factors as flexibility and optimism.

The relationship of stress to the development or progression of cardiovascular disease is not well established. It is known that blood pressure rises in response to acute psychologic and physiologic stress, but there has been no consistent research support for the hypothesis that persistent elevation of blood pressure may occur in chronically stressed individuals.[90]

Theorell[91] studied the demand/control model of Karasek, which postulates that excessive demands in a structure that prevents the individual from influencing the handling of the demands or from developing new skills are associated with elevated cardiovascular risk. In two studies, Theorell investigated changing psychosocial situations at work and the relationship to possible changes in blood pressure. In both studies, Theorell observed that as demands increased concomitant with a decrease in decision-making, systolic blood pressure increased. Theorell concluded that the sympathoadrenomedullary system has a role in physiologic reactions to adverse psychosocial situations. Additionally, the adrenocortical system plays an important role, although other studies have not correlated in any simple way cortisol with blood pressure or other cardiovascular risk factors.

Stress is often an aggravating factor that contributes to a number of coronary risks. For example, some people smoke in response to stress, others abuse alcohol or drugs, and others overeat. Management of stress can facilitate reduction of other risk factors, such as overweight, smoking, and high blood pressure.

The indirect approach to stress reduction includes such activities as exercise, listening to music, reading, and pet therapy. Almost every form of exercise performed regularly and rhythmically is useful in relieving the tension produced by stress.[92] This effect is achieved by relieving the muscle spasms caused by job stress, preventing the participants from thinking about their jobs, and increasing their feelings of well-being and self-esteem.

The direct approach for reducing stress includes physical massage, muscle tensing and relaxing exercises, biofeedback, self-hypnosis, rhythmic breathing, and time management. Therapeutic relaxation has a variety of forms, including transcendental meditation (TM) and yoga. The "relaxation response," coined by cardiologist H. Benson, can be achieved just by following four simple steps: assume a comfortable position, close your eyes, concentrate on a single word, sound, or phrase, and cast off all other thoughts. Biofeedback teaches one to use technology to measure and regulate physiologic variables and restores a sense of self-control to the individual. Time management is a direct method of stress reduction that is commonly introduced in the work setting. It focuses on setting priorities, improving functional time, and reducing perceptions of time urgency.

## Obesity

Although this is a controversial issue, most epidemiologic studies show a positive relationship between obesity (any weight greater than 20% over ideal weight) and morbidity and mortality from CAD among those under 50 years of age. It has primarily been considered as a risk in conjunction with its effects on other characteristics such as hypertension, but most data suggest that obesity makes an independent contribution to coronary heart disease risk, at least up to age 50.[1]

Studies of the relationship between obesity and CAD in women are more equivocal than data reported for men.[93] Obesity in women appears to be a less significant independent risk factor. In one study, the overall prevalence of obesity as one of several risk factors in young women with CAD was 21%, but only 5% of women had obesity as the sole risk factor. The comparison of obese women younger than 45-years old with nonobese women of the same age showed no statistically significant differences between the two groups when the data were adjusted for cigarette smoking, hypertension, oral contraceptive use, and prior preeclampsia. Recent data suggest that distribution of body fat rather than overall obesity may be a better indicator of CAD risk, with truncal rather than peripheral obesity being more detrimental.[93,94]

## Caffeine and Alcohol Intake

Although there is substantial literature describing the deleterious effects of caffeine, the association between caffeine use and cardiovascular risk has not been established, and the evidence is conflicting.

The influence of alcohol on cardiovascular risk continues to be debated. Several epidemiologic studies have shown that drinking alcohol in moderation reduces the risk of CAD.[95]

A recent study, however, which followed 7729 middle-aged men in Britain over 6½ years, showed no direct link between alcohol consumption and decreased incidence of CAD.[96]

This controversy has been fueled by recent evidence on the effect of alcohol on lipoprotein subfractions. Although it is known that regular use of alcohol can increase HDL levels, it is uncertain whether it raises HDL-2, the subfraction associated with protection from CAD.[97] Continued support, therefore, for the belief that moderate alcohol use has a "protective" effect should be based on stronger evidence than is currently available.

## Other Risk Factors

Additional signs associated with increased risk of coronary heart disease are electrocardiographic abnormalities at rest and in response to exercise, and hyperuricemia. Some major risk factors may be determined by familial or genetic factors. The tendency toward development of hypertension, diabetes, and hyperlipidemia may be inherited. Also, certain habits and lifestyles such as smoking, overeating, and lack of exercise may be passed down in a family. There may also be other inherited traits, currently unmeasurable, that affect one's risk. It is vitally important to recognize that risk is multifactorial, that the influence of two or more factors may be synergistic, and that risk is influenced by any given factor's degree of abnormality, not just its presence or absence. The emphasis for the future is on primary prevention, which includes risk factor education, basic research support, and acceptance by the public or responsibility for their own health maintenance. Secondary risk factors, including myocardial infarction and dysrhythmias, will be discussed in subsequent chapters.

## Summary

The most important primary prevention strategies for coronary artery disease are (1) better nutrition, (2) increase in physical activity, (3) cessation of smoking, (4) weight reduction, (5) effective stress management, (6) moderate alcohol consumption (a limit of 50 grams or 2 to 3 average drinks per day), and (7) control of hypertension. Nearly one in five Americans has a genetic susceptibility to hypertension.[98] The best strategy is one that includes each of these goals, a comprehensive "lifestyle change" strategy.

## PREVENTION IN THE COMMUNITY

Primary preventive strategies can be implemented singularly or in combination in a number of settings and through community and national health information programs. In general, health education programs aimed at providing information and altering the behavior of large groups of individuals are the most cost-effective.

## Home

The importance of beginning preventive strategies in childhood cannot be overemphasized. Although many heart, lung, and blood diseases are not manifest until middle-age or later, their development begins during childhood and adolescence.[99] The fatty streaks and fibrous plaques that apparently result in end-stage cardiovascular disease have frequently been observed in children and youth.[40] It is also true that individuals with higher than average blood pressure as teenagers are more likely to have elevated blood pressure as adults.

The majority of unhealthy behaviors seen in adults are learned during childhood and have their origins in the home. Eating habits, exercise patterns, smoking, use of alcohol, attitudes that relate to self-confidence and to society, management of stress, involvement with others, and decision-making abilities are all first learned in the home. Obesity, like other coronary risk factors, is more difficult to correct in adults than in children. It has been demonstrated that children of parents who set examples conducive to health are more likely to assume a healthy lifestyle than if the opposite were true. Primary prevention programs in the home must, therefore, involve both children and adults.

### School

Based on the results of pediatric epidemiologic studies, it is clear that the foundation for adult heart diseases is established in childhood.[100,101] Therefore screening for cardiovascular risks factors and specific health programs must be introduced into the educational system.

Numerous school-site programs recently have been implemented. A major focus is smoking prevention, since smoking is often initiated among adolescents. An assessment of school-based smoking prevention programs in the United States showed that these programs are consistently effective in delaying the onset of smoking, however, they have not often demonstrated the long-term effects of preventing smoking. A panel of the National Cancer Institute proposed minimum components for smoking prevention programs, which include instruction about social consequences, short-term physiologic effects of tobacco use, and social influences on tobacco use (peer, parent, and media influences), and training in refusal skills. The minimum length for these programs should be two, five-session blocks provided in separate school years between sixth and ninth grades. Programs should include peer and parental involvement, and teacher training.[102]

In 1983 the "Tobacco-Free Schools" project was initiated jointly by the American Lung Association of Minnesota and the Minnesota Department of Education. The project, which encourages local school districts to adopt tobacco-free policies, establishes nonsmoking as the norm in schools for both adults and students. It assumes that prevention education is more effective when programs, school policies, and adult models provide a consistent message that tobacco use is unhealthy and unacceptable.[103]

In addition, the American Cancer Society, the American Lung Association, and the American Heart Association began a 12-year collaborative program in 1988 aimed at including at least one third of the country's 3 million first-graders in the Smoke-Free Class of the year 2000. Specific lesson plans have been developed for participating schools.[104]

As a result of the data accumulated from the Bogulusa Heart Study on cardiovascular risk factors in children,[46] a program called "Heart Smart" was initiated to provide cardiovascular health education for elementary schoolchildren. The long-term goal of the program is to reduce cardiovascular risk factors in children through a health promotion program that facilitates adoption of healthy lifestyles. The program includes the modification of specific school activities, such as school lunch, physical education, school health services, and staff inservice education. A strong physical education program, "Super Kids–Super Fit," teaches aerobic activities and encourages children to adopt exercise as a lifelong habit. The school lunch program is an intervention to reduce sodium, fat, and sugar intake by modification of recipes and menus. Both formative and summative evaluation procedures are being used to assess the "Heart Smart" program.[105]

The American Heart Association provides resources to assist teachers at the kindergarten through high school levels with cardiovascular health education. The School-Site Program is a series of five self-contained packages designed to guide students in making heart-healthy diet decisions. Materials provided for each level represent a creative approach to education, which include audiovisuals, hands-on experiences, group activities, games, charts, songs, buttons, and pledge cards. A manual, which contains directions and additional background information is provided for teachers.

The inclusion of cardiovascular health concepts into school curricula at all levels is essential for positively influencing cardiovascular morbidity and mortality. Recognition by parents and educators that the onset of cardiovascular disease begins in childhood is needed, and health promotion programs that encourage adoption of healthy lifestyles should be integrated into the school system. Ideally, cardiovascular health should be taught in a variety of courses, such as science, biology, physical education, and social studies. Aerobic exercise should be a consistent focus in physical education, and school-lunch programs can model heart-healthy food choices.

### Work Site

Industry has taken increasing interest and played a growing role in health promotion and disease prevention among employees. The first National Survey of Worksite Health Promotion Activities conducted in 1988, surveyed a random sample of all private sector worksites with 50 or more employees.[106] Of the 1358 responding worksites, 65.5% had one or more areas of health promotion activity. Overall prevalence by type of activity included health risk assessment (29.5%), smoking cessation (35.6%), blood pressure control and treatment (16.5%), exercise/fitness (22.1%), back problem prevention and care (28.5%), and off-the-job accident prevention. Health promotion activities increased with worksite size and varied considerably by types of industries.[106]

With 100 million adult Americans at work every day, the worksite is an ideal setting for offering preventive health services and health education programs aimed at the prevention of CAD. Development of secondary prevention strategies also is important.

Prevention and promotion programs in the workplace are numerous and diverse. For example, Johnson & Johnson and IBM have comprehensive employee health promotion programs that include health checkups, exercise, and "lifestyle" classes for smoking cessation and stress management. Ford Motor Company runs a cardiovascular risk education and intervention program at its world headquarters in Dearborn, Michigan, with testing, risk assessment, and group sessions to motivate employees to decrease their risk factors. The Massachusetts Mutual Life Insurance Company provides a program in which education, detection, and follow-up of hypertensives is available at the worksite, and community physicians treat employees at the company's expense. General Foods has a fully-equipped gym with a staff of professional trainers at its headquarters in White Plains, New York.[107] The list of large corporations with fitness programs is extensive.

Worksite health promotion programs have had varying degrees of success. Massachusetts Mutual Life has recouped more than one half the cost of its program in reduced absenteeism alone. The Dallas school district reduced absenteeism by 1.25 days for teachers who participated in a comprehensive health promotion program.[108] Lockheed Missiles and Space Company reduced the rate of high blood pressure among one group of 7000 employees from 17% to 1.7% after it introduced an educational program aimed at improving diet and cutting stress and smoking. Tenneco Inc. employees who adhere to the company's exercise program have demonstrated higher job performance ratings than those who do not adhere to the program.[107] Tenneco Inc. also found that health care costs were lower among exercisers than nonexercisers.[109]

A primary motivation for the development of worksite health promotion programs is the potential financial benefit to employers. Employers now pay approximately one half of the nation's health care bill. There is strong evidence that poor employee health behaviors are associated with increased health care costs. Additional business costs that are adversely affected by preventable illness in workers include life insurance, absenteeism, disability insurance, workman's compensation, decreased productivity, and turnover. A recent review of the literature through 1986 examined the economic implications of workplace health promotion programs.[110] In general, the claims of programs

profitability are based on anecdotal evidence or analyses that included methodologic flaws. The authors recommend the development of a new research-based body of knowledge to clearly document the economic merits of health promotion programs.

## Community

During the past 20 years a number of community-wide health promotion demonstration programs have been undertaken, both in the United States and in other industrial nations. The Stanford Health Disease Prevention Program,[111,112] was originally a 2-year experimental program in three California communities whose major objective was to determine whether intensive educational efforts could reduce cigarette smoking, blood cholesterol levels, and high blood pressure. Two communities were exposed to a mass media campaign designed to influence adults to change their living habits in ways that could reduce the risk of heart attack and stroke. In one of these towns the media campaign was supplemented with intensive face-to-face instruction for people identified as being at high risk. A third community, which was relatively isolated from the media shared by the two communities, served as a control. After 2 years the overall risk of cardiovascular disease in the control community increased about 7%, while in the other two towns there was a substantial (15% to 20%) decrease in risk. In the community that had the media campaign plus personal instruction, the initial improvement was greater than in the other experimental town, and health education was more successful in reducing cigarette smoking. At the end of the second year the decrease in risk was roughly the same in both experimental communities. The program concluded that intensive face-to-face instruction and counseling seem important for changing such behaviors as smoking and inadequate diet; however, where resources are limited, mass media education campaigns are an effective influence in reducing the risk of cardiovascular disease.

The Five City Project is a major outgrowth of the original Stanford Heart Disease Project, designed to stimulate and maintain lifestyle changes that would result in reduction of cardiovascular disease risk in the community. The project recognized the need to reach persons who do not speak English, and it developed health promotion messages for Spanish radio stations. Field trials underway seek to determine the impact of educational programs in the community on changes in cardiovascular risk factors and morbidity and mortality.[113]

The North Karelia Project in Finland, begun in 1972, was the first major community-based cardiovascular disease prevention program. The program activities were primarily educational, aiming to teach the community how to adopt healthy lifestyles and reduce cardiovascular risk. Other strategies included development of a hypertension screening process and environmental changes such as smoking restrictions and introduction of low-fat food products. Follow-up surveys have indicated that health behaviors and risk factors changed over a 5-year period, with a decreased risk of 17% for cardiovascular disease in men and 12% in women. In addition, approximately 17,000 hypertensives were recruited to the hypertension register as a result.[114]

Other community-based intervention trials have included the Interuniversity study on Nutrition and Health in Belgium, the Pawtucket Heart Health Project (Rhode Island), and the Minnesota Heart Health Program.[115-117]

Recently, many communities have passed local initiatives requiring all public places to restrict smoking to designated areas. Future research will demonstrate the comparative effect of community-wide behavioral restrictions versus educational efforts alone.

Based on the results of these demonstration programs, community wide programs have been implemented. Program initiatives arise both from organizational and individual efforts. Many programs are jointly sponsored and publicized by voluntary organizations working in the community.

Prevention of cardiac disease through nutritional intervention is widely seen. Within many communities restaurants provide heart healthy meals that follow the American Heart Association dietary guidelines. Participating restaurants work with volunteer dieticians to modify both the food served and the manner of preparation to meet heart healthy guidelines. Guides to restaurants offering heart healthy menus are distributed by local organizations and are advertised as having heart healthy menu selections. Food Festivals,[118] such as the week-long event in September sponsored by the Chicago Heart Association, are held to focus public attention of AHA dietary guidelines and their impact on cardiovascular health. Stores allow volunteers to work at information displays promoting proper nutrition and to give cooking demonstrations and tours when appropriate. Corporate and nonprofit institutional cafeterias use heart healthy menus for the week, and provide nutritional information to their employees. An annual heart healthy recipe contest has encouraged development of recipes using the nutritional guidelines. These recipes are then distributed through the area. The American Heart Association has recently developed a program called Culinary Hearts Kitchen. The program is a demonstration course on cooking meals low in calories, cholesterol, fat and sodium.[119]

Video messages of 45 to 60 seconds on the selection and use of lean meats and poultry are being developed. These videos are being tested in grocery stores to target consumers who may not read nutritional information. They are intended to inform the consumer at the point of purchase with the goal of increasing purchases of lean protein sources.[118]

Cookbooks directed at adults and children are available with heart healthy recipes. Some cookbooks combine nutritional information from the cardiovascular, diabetic, and cancer literature.

The prevention and detection of hypertension also is a community based activity. Church-based hypertension screening and counseling programs have targeted medically underserved areas. Church members are trained to conduct blood pressure screening and present education concerning risk factors. Appropriate referrals are then made as necessary.[118] These are but a few examples of the programs designed to have community impact on cardiovascular health. Information concerning programs of this nature can be obtained from local voluntary associations.

## NATIONAL PRIORITIES

Although the government has important responsibilities in national health education, since there is no established health policy governing lifestyle and behavior, the implementation and impact of government-sponsored programs is often disappointing. For example, the Department of Health and Human Services' National Institutes of Health has increased awareness about hypertension among the population and may have influenced hypertensive people to seek medical care for their disease. Yet Medicare (also housed within the Department of Health and Human Services) does not provide reimbursement for the cost of the necessary drugs.[120] The National Clearinghouse on Smoking and Health has implemented a rigorous educational program for smoking cessation and the present Surgeon General has made reducing cigarette smoking a priority goal. However, the Department of Agriculture continues its unchallenged subsidization of tobacco crops.

One of the most important issues in the ambiguity of national policy concerning health promotion issues is that no single government agency has control. At the federal level, 12 departments, 17 independent agencies, and 3 quasi-official agencies have health-related responsibilities or functions. Food and nutrition programs are administered by the Department of Agriculture, occupational safety and health programs by the Department of Labor, environmental control programs by the Environmental Protection Agency, and so on.

This does not mean that effective health promotion programs have not emanated from the federal government. The National Conference on Health Promotion Programs in Occupational Settings (1979), the National Conference on Nutrition Education (1979), the National Conference on Physical Fitness and Sports for All (1980), Regional Forums on Community Health Promotion (1979), Promoting Health through the Schools (1980), and the National Children and Youth Fitness Study (1985) are all examples of federally sponsored health promotion efforts.[121,122] What is needed at this point is for public policy to be consistent, to be coordinated among the various bureaucracies and for some of the goals established in *Healthy People*[123] to be implemented at the policy level.

Policy as it relates to cigarette smoking can be used as an example. If the federal government is convinced that it is harmful to the health of Americans and truly wishes to change smoking behavior to improve disease risk, then a policy that restricts tobacco advertising (especially the kind that glamorizes smoking to young people), increases cigarette taxes, eliminates tobacco price supports, makes the purchase of cigarettes by children more difficult, and reduces taxes that feed into Medicare and Medicaid for nonsmokers and raises them for smokers would be in order.

## RESEARCH NEEDS IN HEALTH PROMOTION

A comprehensive approach to health promotion has been described as an essential part of a primary prevention program directed against the premature onset of coronary artery disease. Given the acceptance of disease prevention and health promotion by the American people, the scientific evidence on which these concepts are based must be strengthened; program evaluation techniques must be refined; ways must be found to allocate resources fairly; the needs of special populations must be accommodated; new organizational structures must be developed—all these and many more issues must be carefully and intelligently considered for all levels of society.

Preventive strategies must be tested through longitudinal, multidisciplinary, invasive studies of the intersection of high-risk groups and high-risk situations against control groups. Research is also needed to identify the developmental determinants of unhealthful behavior during childhood and adolescence. Genetic research is already making inroads in this regard, adding to the knowledge base information about the genes involved in heart disease, especially those responsible for the body's use and disposal of fats. More studies on the impact of risk factor reduction on women, the elderly, and ethnic groups are also necessary.

Many ramifications of health education are still unknown. For example, what kinds of national education models will work most effectively on the heterogeneous U.S. population? Will benefits accrue rapidly or slowly? Will they be temporary or permanent? Will they occur in the general population or only in high-risk groups? Unfortunately, there are major weaknesses in much of the evaluation of patient education: oversimplification of the behavior and causes of behavior that must be influenced by patient education; failure to make explicit the theoretic or assumed connection between educational interventions and behavioral or health results; and limited analyses of data, which leave many questions unanswered.[124] These issues are further complicated by the lack of reimbursement for patient education in the health care delivery system.

Clearly, successful health education programs offer great promise; consumers will assume more responsibility for adopting health practices that protect health and prevent illness or complications, and they will make more timely and appropriate use of health resources. Such changes should result in increased patient satisfaction, improved quality of life, better use of health care providers, fewer hospital admissions, and shorter hospital stays, thus helping to control rising health care costs.

## REFERENCES

1. American Heart Association: 1989 Heart Facts, Dallas, TX, 1989, The Association.
2. Wolintsky H: A new look at atherosclerosis, Cardiovasc Med 1:41, 1976.
3. Ross R: The pathogenesis of atherosclerosis—an update, N Engl J Med 314:488, 1986.
4. Roberts WC: Coronary thrombosis and fatal myocardial ischemia, Circulation 49:1, 1974.
5. Mcgill H: The pathogenesis of atherosclerosis, Clin Chem 34:833, 1988.
6. Ross R: The pathogenesis of atherosclerosis—an update, N Engl J Med 314:488, 1986.
7. Hillis LD and Braunwald E: Coronary-artery spasm, N Engl J Med 299:695, 1978.
8. Rosenblatt A and Selzer A: The nature and clinical features of myocardial infarction with normal coronary angiogram, Circulation 55:578, 1977.
9. Bigger JT and others: Prevalence and significance of arrhythmias in 24 hour ECG recordings made within one month of acute myocardial infarction. In Kulbertus HE and Wellers HJ, editors: The first year after a myocardial infarction, Mount Kisco, NY, 1983, Futura Publishing Co, Inc.
10. Kaplan NM and Stamler J: Prevention of coronary heart disease, Philadelphia, 1983, WB Saunders Co.
11. Gillum RF and Feinleib M: Coronary heart disease in the elderly, Compr Ther 14(8):66-73, 1988.
12. Joint National Committee: The 1988 report of the joint national committee on detection, evaluation, and treatment of high blood pressure, Arch Intern Med 148:1023, 1988.
13. Brest AN: Antihypertensive therapy in perspective, part 1, Mod Conc Cardiov Dis 57:65, 1988.
14. Kannel WB: Role of blood pressure in cardiovascular morbidity and mortality, Prog Cardiov Dis 17:5, 1974.
15. Castelli WP: Cardiovascular disease and multifactorial risk: challenge of the 1980s, Am Heart J 106:1191, 1983.
16. Schmieder RE, Messerli FH, and Ruddel H: Risks for arterial hypertension, Cardiol Clin 4:57, 1986.
17. Havlik RJ and others: Weight and hypertension, Ann Intern Med 98:855, 1983.
18. Raison J and others: Extracellular and interstitial fluid volume in obesity with and without associated systemic hypertension, Am J Cardiol 57:223, 1986.
19. Kaplan NM: Clinical hypertension, Baltimore, 1986, Williams & Wilkins.
20. Niarchos AP, Weinstein DL, and Laragh JH: Comparison of the effects of diurectic therapy and low sodium intake in isolated systolic hypertension, Am J Med 77:1061, 1984.
21. Potter JF and Beevers DG: Pressor effect of alcohol in hypertension, Lancet 1:119, 1984.
22. Mellerowicz H and Smodlaka VN: Ergometry, Baltimore, 1981, Urban and Schwarzenberg.
23. Conway J: Hemodynamics of essential hypertension, Physiol Rev 64:617, 1984.
24. Fitzgerald W: Labile hypertension and jogging: new diagnostic tool or spurious recovery? Br Med J 282:542, 1981.
25. Health and Public Policy Committee, American College of Physicians: Biofeedback for hypertension, Ann Intern Med 102:709, 1985.

26. Patel C and others: Trials of relaxation in reducing coronary risk: four-year follow-up, Br Med J Clin Res 290:1103, 1985.

27. Engel BT, Glasgow MS, and Gaarder KR: Behavioral treatment of high blood pressure. III. Follow-up results and treatment recommendations, Psychosom Med 45:23, 1983.

28. Lawrence L and McLemore T: NCHS Advance data, vital and health statistics of the national center for health statistics, Washington DC, 1983, US Department of Health and Human Services, No 88, March 16, 1983.

29. Cutler J and others: Beliefs and practices by primary care physicians and the public regarding hypertension, Circulation 70 (suppl II):II-281, 1984.

30. Veterans Administration Cooperative Study Group on Antihypertensive Agents: Effects of treatment on morbidity in hypertension. III. Influence of age, diastolic pressure, and prior cardiovascular disease: further analysis of side effects, Circulation 45:991, 1972.

31. Hypertension Detection and Follow-up Program Cooperative Group: Five-year findings of the Hypertension Detection and Follow-up Program. I. Reduction in mortality of persons with high blood pressure, including mild hypertension, JAMA 242:2562, 1979.

32. Medical Research Council Working Party: MRC trial of treatment of mild hypertension: principal results, Br Med J Clin Res 291:97, 1985.

33. Brewer H and others: Apolipoprotein and lipoproteins in human plasma: an overview, Clin Chem 34:84, 1988.

34. Schaefer E and others: Genetics and metabolism of lipoproteins, Clin Chem 34:89, 1988.

35. Mannihen V, Elo O, and Frick MH: Lipid alterations and decline in the incidence of coronary heart disease in the helsinki heart study. JAMA 260:641, 1988.

36. Martin MJ and others: Serum cholesterol, blood pressure, and mortality: implications from a cohort of 361,662 men, Lancet 2:933, 1986.

37. Stamler J, Wentworth D, and Neaten J: Is the relationship between serum cholesterol and risk of death from CHD continuous and graded? JAMA 256:2823, 1988.

38. Lipid Research Clinics Program: The Lipid Research Clinics coronary primary prevention trial results. I. Reduction in the incidence of coronary heart disease, JAMA 251:351, 1984.

39. Frick MH and others: Helsinski heart study: primary-prevention trial with gemfibrozil in middle-aged men with diplipidemia, N Engl J Med 317:1237, 1987.

40. Mannimen V and others: Lipid alterations and decline of coronary heart disease in the Helsinki heart study JAMA, 260:641, 1988.

41. Canover PL and others: Fifteen years mortality in coronary drug project patients: long term benefits with niacin, Am Cardiol 8:1245, 1986.

42. Goodman D and others: Expert panel on detection, evaluation, and treatment of high blood cholesterol in adults, NIH publication No 88-2925, 1988.

43. Bush T, Fried L, and Barret-Connor: Cholesterol, lipoproteins, coronary heart disease in women, Clin Chem 34:B60, 1988.

44. Castelli W: Cardiovascular disease in women, Am J Obstet Gynecol 1553, 1988.

45. Perlman J and others: Cardiovascular risk factors, premature heart disease, and all cause mortality in a cohort of northern California women, Am J Obstet Gynecol 1568, 1988.

46. Newman WP and others: Relation of serum lipoprotein levels and systolic blood pressure to early atherosclerosis: the Bogalusa heart study, N Engl J Med 314:138, 1986.

47. Weidman W and others: Diagnosis and treatment of primary hyperlipidemia in childhood, Circulation 74:1181A, 1986.

48. Davidson D and others: School-based blood cholesterol screening, J Ped Health Care 3:3, 1989.

49. Sempos C and others: The prevalence of high blood cholesterol levels among adults in the United States, JAMA, 262:45, 1989.

50. Glassman AH and others: Cigarette smoking, smoking withdrawal, and clonidine, Science 226:864, 1984.

51. Blum C and Levy R: Current therapy for hypercholesterolemia, JAMA, 261:3582, 1989.

52. Healthy people: The Surgeon General's report on health promotion and disease prevention, publication 79-55071A, US Department of Health, Education and Welfare, Public Health Service, 1979.

53. Stokes J and Rigotti N: The health consequences of cigarette smoking and the internist's role in smoking cessation, Adv Intern Med 33:431, 1988.

54. Reducing the health consequences of smoking: 25 years of progress. A report of the Surgeon General US Department of Health and Human Services Public Health Service, Centers for Disease Control, Center for Chronic Disease Prevention and Health Promotion, Office on Smoking and Health, DHHS Publication No (CDC) 89-8411, 1989.

55. State legislated actions on tobacco issues. A public policy project sponsored by AHA, ALA, ACS. Oct 1989.

56. Kannel WB, McGhee DL, and Castelli WP: Latest perspective on cigarette smoking and cardiovascular disease: the Framingham Study, J Cardiac Rehab 4:266, 1984.

57. Mulcahy R and others: Factors influencing long term prognosis in male patients surviving a first coronary attack, Br Heart J 37:158, 1975.

58. Jajich CL, Ostfeld AM, and Freeman DH: Smoking and coronary heart disease mortality in the elderly, JAMA 252:2831, 1984.

59. Benowitz N: Pharmacologic aspects of cigarette smoking and nicotine addiction, N Engl J Med 319:1318, 1988.

60. Siess W and others: Plasma catecholamines, platelet aggregation and associated thromboxane formation after physical exercise, smoking or norepinephrine infusion, Circulation 66:44, 1982.

61. Fielding JE: Smoking: II. Health effects and control, N Engl J Med 313:555, 1985.

62. Pickering TG: Exercise and hypertension, Cardiol Clin 5:311, 1987.

63. Joseph A and Byrd JR: Smoking cessation in practice, Prim Care 16:83, 1989.

64. Schwartz J: Review and evaluation of smoking cessation methods: the US and Canada, 1978-1985. US Department of Health and Human Services. Public Health Service, National Institute of Health, NIH Publication No. 87-2940, April 1987.

65. Godenick M: A review of available smoking cessation methods, 1989, Maryland Med J April, P 277, 1989.

66. Godenick M: A review of available smoking cessation methods, 1989. Part II, Maryland Med J April, P 377, 1989.

67. Glassman AH and others: Heavy smokers, smoking cessation, and clonidine: results of a double blind randomized trial, JAMA 259:2863, 1988.

68. Hughes JR and Miller SA: Nicotine gum to help stop smoking, JAMA 252:2855, 1984.

69. Buchkremer G and others: Combination of behavioral smoking cessation with transdermal nicotine substitution, Addict Behav 14:229, 1989.

70. Schneider NG and others: Nicotine gum in smoking cessation: a placebo-controlled, double-blind trail, Addict Behav 8:253, 1984.

71. Morris JN and others: Coronary heart disease and physical activity of work, Lancet 2:1053, 1953.

72. Morris JN and others: Incidence and prediction of ischaemic heart disease in London busmen, Lancet 2:552, 1966.

73. Morris JN: Uses of epidemiology, New York, 1975, Churchill Livingstone.

74. Brunner D and others: Physical activity at work and the incidence of myocardial infarction, angina pectoris and death due to ischemic heart disease: an epidemiological study in Israeli collective statements (kibbutzim), J Chronic Dis 27:217, 1974.

75. Paffenbarger RS and Hale WE: Work-activity and coronary heart disease mortality, N Engl J Med 292:545, 1975.

76. Paffenbarger RS and others: Work-energy level, personal characteristics, and fatal heart attack: a birth cohort effect, Am J Epidemiol 105:200, 1977.
77. Kannel WB and Sorlie P: Some health benefits of physical activity: the Framingham study, Arch Intern Med 139:857, 1979.
78. Paffenbarger R and others: Physical activity as an index of heart attack risk in college alumni, Am J Epidemiol 108:161, 1978.
79. Paffenbarger RS and others: A natural history of athleticism and cardiovascular health, JAMA 252:491, 1984.
80. Paffenbarger RS and others: Physical activity, all-cause mortality, and longevity of college alumni, N Engl J Med 314:605, 1986.
81. Wood PD and others: Increased exercise level and plasma lipoprotein concentrations: a one-year, randomized, controlled study in sedentary, middle-aged men, Metabolism 32:31, 1983.
82. Cowan GO: Influence of exercise on high-density lipoproteins, Am J Cardiol 52:13B, 1983.
83. Paffenbarger RS and others: Physical activity and incidence of hypertension in college alumni, Am J Epidemiol 117:245, 1983.
84. Blair SN and others: Physical fitness and incidence of hypertension in healthy normotensive men and women, JAMA 252:487, 1984.
85. Haskell WL: Overview: health benefits of exercise. In Matarazzo JD and others, editors: Behavioral health—a handbook of health enhancement and disease prevention, New York, 1984, John Wiley & Sons.
86. American College of Sports Medicine: Guidelines for exercise-testing and prescription, Philadelphia, 1986, Lea & Febiger.
87. Matthews KA and others: Competitive drive, pattern A, and coronary heart disease: a further analyses of some date from the Western Collaborative Group Study, J Chron Dis 30:489-498, 1977.
88. Dembroski TM and others: Components of type A, hostility and anger. In Relationship to angiographic findings, J Psychosom Med 47:219-233, 1984.
89. Wallis C: Stress: can we cope? As modern pressures take their toll, doctors preach relaxation, Time p 43, June 6, 1983.
90. Harlan WR: Rationale for intervention on blood pressure in childhood and adolescence. In Matarazzo JD and others, editors: Behavioral health—a handbook of health enhancement and disease prevention, New York, 1984, John Wiley & Sons, Inc.
91. Theorell T: On biochemical and physiological indicators of stress relevant to catdiovascular illness, Eur Heart J 9:705-708, 1988.
92. Maslow AH: Eupsychian management, Homewood, IL, 1965, Dorsey Press, p 129.
93. Burkman RT: Obesity, stress, and smoking: their role as cardiovascular risk factors in women, Am J Obstet Gynecol 158:1592-1597, 1988.
94. Pepine CJ: Acute myocardial infarction. In Brest AN, editor: Cardiovascular clinics, Philadelphia, 1989, FA Davis Co.
95. Dyer AR and others: Alcohol consumption and 17-year mortality in the Chicago Western Electric Company study, Prev Med 9:78, 1980.
96. Shaper AG and others: Alcohol and ischaemic heart disease in middle aged British men, Br Med J 294:733, 1987.
97. Eichner E: Alcohol, stroke and coronary artery disease, Am Fam Physician 37(3):217, 1988.
98. O'Donnel MP and Ainsworth TH, editors: Health promotion in the workplace, New York, 1984, John Wiley & Sons, Inc.
99. Little JA: Coronary prevention and regression, studies updated, Can J Cardiol 4(A):11A, 1988.
100. Kolbe LJ and Newman IM: The role of school health education in prevention heart, lung, and blood diseases, School Health Res. 54(6):15, 1984.
101. Berenson GS and others: Cardiovascular risk factors in children and early prevention of heart disease, Clin Chem 34:B115, 1988.
102. Glynn TJ: Essential elements of school-based smoking prevention programs, J Sch Health 59:181, 1989.
103. Griffin GA and others: Tobacco-free schools in Minnesota, J Sch Health 58:236, 1988.
104. Turn-of-century high school class may turn tide against tobacco use, JAMA 260:13, 1988.
105. Downey AM and others: Implementation of "Heart Smart", a cardiovascular school health promotion program, J Sch Health 57:98, 1987.
106. Fielding JE and Piserchia PV: Frequency of worksite health promotion activities, Am J Public Health 79(1):16, 1989.
107. Fitness, corporate style: companies are racing to invest in employee wellness, Newsweek p 96, Nov 5, 1984.
108. Baun S and others: Health promotion for educators: impact on absenteeism, Prev Med 15:166, 1986.
109. Baun W, Bernacki E, and Tsni, S: A preliminary investigation: effect of a corporate fitness program on absenteeism and health care cost, J Occup Med 28:18, 1986.
110. Warner K and others: Economic implications of workplace health promotion programs: review of the literature, J Occup Med 30:106, 1988.
111. Farquhar JW and others: Community education for cardiovascular health, Lancet 1:1192, 1977.
112. Maccoby J and others: Reducing the risk of cardiovascular disease: effects of a community-based compaign on knowledge and behavior, J Community Health 3:100, 1977.
113. Farquhar JW and others: The Standord Five City Project: an overview. In Matarazzo JD and others, editors: Behavioral health—a handbook of health enhancement and disease prevention, New York, 1984, John Wiley & Sons, Inc.
114. Puska P: Community-based prevention of cardiovascular disease: the North Karelia Project. In Matarazzo JD and others, editors: Behavioral health—a handbook of health enhancement and disease prevention, New York, 1984, John Wiley & Sons, Inc.
115. Kittel F: The interuniversity study on nutrition and health. In Matarazzo JD and others, editors: Behavioral health—a handbook of health enhancement and disease prevention, New York, 1984, John Wiley & Sons, Inc.
116. Lasater T and others: Lay volunteer delivery of a community-based cardiovascular risk factor change program: the Pawtucker Experiment. In Matarazzo JD and others, editors: Behavioral health—a handbook of health enhancement and disease prevention, New York, 1984, John Wiley & Sons, Inc.
117. Blackburn H and others: The Minnesota Heart Health Program: a research and demonstration project in cardiovascular disease prevention. In Matarazzo JD and others, editors: Behavioral health—a handbook of health enhancement and disease prevention, New York, 1984, John Wiley & Sons, Inc.
118. American Heart Association of Metropolitan Chicago: Chicago, IL, 1989.
119. American Heart Association National Center: Dallas, TX, 1989.
120. Bauer KG: Federal government policies and activities in health promotion. In Faber MM and Reinhardt AM, editors: Promoting health through risk reduction, New York, 1982, Macmillan Publishing Co.
121. Faber MM and Reinhardt AM: Promoting health through risk reduction, New York, 1982, Macmillan Publishing Co.
122. Gilbert GG, Davis RL, and Damberg CL: Current federal activities in school health education, Pub Health Rep 100:499, 1985.
123. US Department of Health, Education, and Welfare: Healthy people: the Surgeon General's report on health promotion and disease prevention, US Public Health Service Pub No 79-55071, Washington DC, 1979, US Government Printing Office.
124. Bishop JE: Probing the cell: scientists are learning how genes predispose some to heart disease, Wall Street Journal, February 6, 1986.

# CHAPTER 7

# Care of the Cardiac Patient

Joann M. Pillion

The coronary care unit (CCU) has been credited with a major contribution to reduced mortality associated with myocardial infarction (MI) and its complications; however, in recent years the validity of this claim has been questioned. Some studies have suggested that admission to a CCU favorably influenced the mortality rate; others have failed to show benefits.[1-8] At a time when modern technology and scientific research are expanding the ability of health professionals to diagnose and treat patients with acute myocardial infarction, some investigators are questioning the necessity of admitting all patients with chest pain and possible diagnosis of MI to the CCU. As health care costs rise and private and governmental agencies investigate the validity of these rising costs, it is small wonder that research teams have questioned the value of managing all patients with suspected acute MI in hospital CCUs. The basic premise for CCUs seems sound: the CCU has generally been considered an indispensable component of any acute care hospital. The introduction of the CCU coincided with a remarkable reduction in mortality from MI in North America and there are data to suggest that mortality caused by MI can be reduced if patients enter an emergency medical system with a CCU as soon as possible after the onset of illness.[1] The two activities most likely to positively influence mortality are the prevention of ventricular fibrillation and its successful management when it does occur. The three categories of patients who benefit most from treatment in a CCU are those who have (1) angina at rest, (2) an MI in progress, or (3) an extension of the infarction.

Scientific and technologic advances have created an increasingly complex environment for the care of the cardiac patient. In an effort to improve patient care services, new or more specialized health practitioners have been introduced into the milieu of coronary care. Many units now employ monitor and cardiovascular technicians whose primary responsibility is maintenance of the equipment used in patient care. Many of these technicians are also responsible for monitoring cardiac rhythms and initiating appropriate therapy. A variety of respiratory, physical, and occupational therapists are also involved. Dieticians and pharmacists are often employed solely for the hospital's cardiac patient population. Cardiovascular nurse clinicians and cardiovascular clinical nurse specialists are commonplace in many CCUs and have varying responsibilities related to patient care and staff development. Physicians seek consultation from specialists who have advanced knowledge and skill in cardiovascular nuclear radiology, electrocardiography, echocardiography, electrophysiology, and arteriography. Associated with these specialists are a variety of additional technicians who interact with the patient.

The proliferation of health practitioners in coronary care introduces the potential for fragmentation of patient care and loss of focus on the patient as a whole being. This concern led the NIH Consensus Conference on Critical Care to conclude that "nurses are the key element in critical care."[9] To prevent fragmentation and to promote effective, efficient, and holistic care for the cardiac patient, collaboration and cooperation are essential among all care providers. The primary physician and nurse have the responsibility to seek advice and assistance as appropriate from other health practitioners, the patient, and the family, and to use their contributions as they make decisions concerning patient care. The physician and nurse together need to develop a comprehensive plan that encompasses the goals and activities of all who interact with the patient.

MI is one manifestation of coronary artery disease; other manifestations of this disease include heart failure, pulmonary edema, cardiogenic shock, dysrhythmias, and sudden cardiac death. The purpose of this chapter is to present a comprehensive approach to planning and implementing the care of the patient exhibiting one or more of these complications of coronary artery disease, based on the patient's individual needs from admission to discharge. Such an approach is important because patients are likely to be moved from one hospital area to another as their condition improves. Needs change as the patient and family adjust to the suddenness of admission to a CCU and as they plan for discharge and resumption of their normal activities. Of course, recovery is not always uneventful and the patient and family must address crises as they occur.

## PRIORITIES IN ADMISSION TO THE CCU

Patients are admitted to a CCU for rapid management of existing problems, surveillance for and early management of dysrhythmias, and initial rehabilitation. At the time of admission it is important to collect baseline data for initiating therapy and for comparison at later stages in the patient's course (Fig. 7-1).

```
                                                    Stamp here with
                                                     patient's plate
                                                    _____

                              ADMISSION NOTE
Admission status: Clinic _____ ER _____ Date _____ Time _____
Married _____ Single _____ Widowed _____ Divorced _____
Race and nationality _____ Religion _____ Age _____

Patient history

Chest pain _____ Onset _____ Duration _____ Location _____
   Radiation _____ Subjective description _____
Associated acute events:
   Loss of consciousness _____ Duration _____ Cardiac arrest _____
   Palpitations _____ GI _____ Perspiration _____ Anxiety _____

   Dyspnea _____
Medications taken or administered and time _____
Medical history and risk factors (check those appropriate):
   Myocardial infarction _____ Angina _____ Obesity _____
   Weight loss _____ Cerebrovascular accident _____ Alcohol _____
   Respiratory _____ Hypertension _____ Glaucoma _____ Diabetes _____
   Smoking _____ Prostatic hypertrophy _____ Blood transfusion _____
   Gout _____ Surgery _____ Reaction to anesthesia _____
Postcardiopulmonary resuscitation _____ Contraindications to anticoagulation _____
   Other _____

Personal information

   Height _____ Weight _____ Dentures _____ Glasses _____ Contacts _____
   Sleeping habits _____ Usual diet _____
   Food, medication, environmental allergies (especially to streptokinase) _____
   Prostheses _____ Family history _____

Physical examination

   General appearance _____ Mental status _____
   Vital signs: Temperature _____ Pulse _____ Respiration _____
   Blood pressure: Right _____ Left _____
   Lungs: Aeration _____ Wheezes _____ Crackles _____
   Cardiovascular: Heart sounds _____ Quality _____ Rhythm _____
      Lifts _____ Heaves _____ Thrills _____ Murmur _____ Rub _____
      Gallop _____
   Pulses (all extremities) _____ Neck Veins _____ Abdomen _____
   Skin: Color _____ Temperature _____ Cyanosis _____ Edema _____
   Clubbing _____ Other _____

                              Signature _____

Insert ECG strip here.
```

**Fig. 7-1**  Sample form for admission note to the CCU.

## Immediate Monitoring of Cardiac Rate and Rhythm

It is essential that electrodes be applied to the patient immediately on admission in order to detect abnormal cardiac rhythms, which may be life-threatening. A brief explanation of the purpose of the electrodes should be given to the patient at this time. As the patient becomes stabilized, the monitoring equipment can be discussed with the patient more thoroughly. *Rate meter alarms should always be set* to alert the staff to any tachydysrhythmia or bradydysrhythmia.

## Establishing Intravenous Access

An indwelling catheter is inserted and secured in place as a means of administering fluids, pain medication, and emergency drugs should they be required. A heparin lock is particularly advantageous because it minimizes the amount of fluid necessary for maintaining intravenous IV access; in patients with heart failure it is important to limit fluid intake.

## Relief of Pain and Anxiety

The effects of pain and anxiety may be synergistic and result in an increased myocardial oxygen demand by an already compromised heart. Therefore it is vital that both pain and anxiety be promptly alleviated. The physician will usually prescribe analgesics and nitrates for relief of pain, and these should be administered as needed.

Morphine sulfate is often used to alleviate pain and anxiety but may be contraindicated if second-degree AV block or sinus bradycardia is present. If morphine sulfate is given and the degree of AV block or sinus bradycardia worsens, atropine may be administered to counteract its effects. After morphine is given, it is important that blood pressure, heart rate, and respiratory rate be carefully monitored for any adverse effects. Brief explanations to the patient about activities and equipment may assist in re-

---

### CORONARY CARE UNIT INFORMATION

While you, a family member, or friend are in the CCU, you may hear terms such as *coronary, electrocardiogram* (ECG), or *congestive heart failure* and be uncertain as to what they mean about the patient's condition. This may be a time when you have a lot of questions and anxieties.

The CCU staff understands this and has prepared this information sheet to help you understand what goes on in a CCU. If you want to know more about heart disease, there is literature available in our unit on request. Also we will be glad to try to answer any questions you may have.

#### Patient care

A CCU is for the "intensive" care of cardiac patients. This CCU has 16 beds and is attended 24 hours a day by registered nurses who are specially trained to read ECGs and recognize any early signs of complications. From the time a patient arrives in the unit until he is transferred to a room, there is a nurse near the bedside to render the care needed.

Because of the serious nature of heart disease, a patient is placed in the CCU during the critical phase of the heart's condition and remains there until this critical phase is over, usually 3 to 5 days. Progress is followed continuously with special monitoring equipment at each bedside and at the nurses' station to record the patient's ECGs, which indicate the heart rhythms.

While in the CCU, patients need only their necessary personal belongings. Shaving equipment (razor with nurse's approval), cosmetics, toilet articles, eyeglasses, and small change may be kept in the bedside drawer. Male patients may wear pajama bottoms. Female patients do not need their night gowns, since it is preferred that a hospital gown be worn. A small radio and reading materials are allowed if approved by the physician. Television, flowers, and suitcases are not allowed.

When the physician approves transfer out of the CCU, the patient is usually taken to a room on another floor. Transferring patients is usually done during the day, but if an emergency situation arises and a bed is needed in the unit during the night, a patient may have to be moved then.

Visiting is permitted from 10 AM to 8 PM for members of the patient's immediate family or significant others. Because of the nature of the patient's illness, no more than two visitors should be in the patient's room at one time. *If emergency situations exist, visitation may be refused.*

#### Phone

There is a pay phone available. Direct calls to the unit are not permitted. Families may leave their phone numbers at the desk in the CCU.

#### Chaplain

This service is available on request at any time by contacting a CCU nurse or the chaplain's office.

#### Waiting rooms

The waiting room is open only until 8:30 PM. Those who wish to stay during the night must use the waiting room in the emergency department.

If you have questions, please contact a CCU nurse.

*The CCU Staff*

---

**Fig. 7-2** Sample fact sheet given to families of patients in the CCU.

lieving anxiety. A mild sedative such as diazepam may be prescribed to reduce anxiety and stress. Opiates and sedatives, however, should be given cautiously, if at all, to confused and restless patients suffering from shock or heart failure. Family visits may contribute to or mitigate against stress and anxiety and should be carefully monitored for these effects. A booklet about the CCU that is tailored to the individual is helpful to families in understanding what is being done and why (Fig. 7-2).

## Supplemental Oxygen

Even in patients with uncomplicated infarctions, hypoxemia may be present and necessitate the use of oxygen. Most often a binasal cannula administering 1 to 2 L/min is sufficient. Application of a lubricant or emollient to the nares helps to prevent irritation and maintain skin integrity. Measurement of arterial blood gas levels[10] 30 minutes after initiating oxygen therapy provides a baseline for arterial oxygenation. Arterial blood gas levels are measured as necessary to guide oxygen administration and maintain acid-base balance.

## Decrease in Myocardial Oxygen Consumption

Recovery of the myocardium after an ischemic episode requires that the workload and subsequent oxygen demand of the heart be reduced. This is accomplished generally through bed rest and assistance with activities of daily living. While complete bed rest for several weeks was once thought to be necessary for the healing of the infarction, current regimens are less restrictive. The concept of METs is frequently used to determine appropriate activity following myocardial infarction. An MET is a unit of measurement for oxygen uptake, with 1 MET representing an oxygen uptake of 3.5 ml/kg of body weight per minute. Sitting quietly in a chair requires 1 MET, while slow walking requires 3 METs. In the CCU, activities that require 1.5 to 2 METs are generally permitted. Other protocols for increasing activity may include gradually increasing exercise to a level that raises the heart rate 20 beats per minute or less above resting heart rate. The systolic blood pressure (SBP) also increases with exercise, and activity should be adjusted so that SBP does not increase by more than 30 mm Hg above resting pressure.

## Completion of Database

As soon as possible after admission, information necessary to complete the database should be obtained. The patient history and physical examination should be completed (see Chapter 2), paying particular attention to the following:

A. Patient history
B. Physical examination
1. Inspection of skin for color, diaphoresis, and other abnormalities.
2. Palpation of chest area for unusual movements, excursion, cardiac enlargement, apical impulse, and other signs.
3. Percussion of chest for areas of dullness and of liver for edge and size. Cardiac borders are seldom defined by percussion.
4. Auscultation of blood pressure, carotid arteries (bruit), apical heart rate, heart sounds, pericardial friction rub, gallops, and murmurs. The murmur of papillary muscle dysfunction may occur in the acute phase of MI as a result of ischemia and/or infarction of the papillary muscle. The murmur of mitral regurgitation results when the injured papillary muscle fails to contract properly, allowing blood to regurgitate into the left atrium during systole. The murmur is often transient, but it may be permanent if the papillary muscle does not heal completely. A ventricular septal defect murmur may also occur during the first 10 days after infarction and is a very loud grade 4 or 5 systolic murmur. There is usually an accompanying systolic thrill, and the murmur is best heard along the lower left sternal border. The appearance of this murmur is an ominous event prognostically, sudden in onset, and frequently accompanied by profound cardiogenic shock. It is also important to auscultate the lungs for crackles, rhonchi, wheezes, and increased or decreased breath sounds. Note the rate, character, and depth of respirations. These data are necessary to evaluate the presence or absence of congestive heart failure and are useful for comparison should this be a consideration at a later date.

C. Supportive data
1. Serum cardiac isoenzyme levels should be measured initially and then daily for 3 days to document any abnormal increase in serum levels. Should the patient have a sudden exacerbation of pain with associated ECG changes, cardiac enzyme level measurements may be indicated to assist in determining whether the previous infarction has continued.
2. Arterial blood gas levels may be measured initially and then as needed (depending on the patient's condition) to determine the adequacy of oxygenation and acid-base balance.
3. Fluid and electrolyte balance should be monitored. It is imperative that fluid intake and output be accurately measured. Equally important is that an accurate daily weight of the patient be taken at the same time each day on the same scale. This can help to determine the minimum weight gain that occurs in the early stages of heart failure or when other indicators, such as the chest x-ray film, are still normal. Personnel must be reminded to actually measure rather than to estimate intake, just as all output is measured. It should also be remembered that fluids, such as tube feedings, those used to flush the Swan-Ganz catheter and arterial lines, and those from any other sources, must be included in the

patient's total fluid intake measurement. Output should include bleeding and drainage from any site, as well as urine and stool. The patient's state of hydration may also be evaluated by the skin tone.

4. Edema may be a late sign of congestive failure and should be added to the database already gathered on the fluid balance of the patient. The extent of peripheral edema should be measured by palpation once it appears, and comparative evaluations should be performed frequently to determine changes in edema noted in the periphery. Edema in a bedridden cardiac patient is frequently noted in dependent areas such as the sacrum or genitalia.

5. The dietary regimen, if different from the patient's usual diet, should be explained to the patient and family. Cardiac patients are usually placed on a low-sodium, low-fat, low-cholesterol diet. In some cardiac patients sodium restriction may be unnecessary or impractical; these patients are given food with the usual sodium content. A soft diet may be prescribed with frequent small feedings, although some physicians prefer clear liquids on the first day, followed by full liquids on the second day. Because metabolic demands increase following ingestion of food, the quantity of food at each serving should be kept small. Studies show that hot and cold liquids are not detrimental, so their exclusion from diets is unnecessary. Decaffeinated coffee and tea are permitted. The relationship between caffeine intake and heart problems has not been clearly established. Mathewson,[10] for example, has concluded that there is no relationship between caffeine intake and MI but there is a relationship between caffeine intake and dysrhythmias in the ischemic heart.

6. A 12-lead ECG (see Chapter 4) should be performed initially in the emergency room or in the CCU. A copy should be maintained on the patient's chart for comparison with later tracings, which are performed daily for 3 days and with every exacerbation of chest pain, and/or developing dysrhythmia. Personnel in the CCU should be adept at obtaining and interpreting the 12-lead ECG in a patient with MI.

Medical and nursing diagnoses are derived from the compiled data and serve as the basis for planning medical and nursing therapies.

## EQUIPMENT
### Monitoring System

In the CCU the first equipment with which the patient is likely to come in contact is the monitoring system. For a patient who has suffered an MI or who has had a pacemaker implanted, careful monitoring of cardiac performance is essential. The cardiac monitor simplifies such care by continuously displaying the cardiac rhythm, blood pressure, and other parameters not readily followed by other means. Because most dysrhythmias occur during the first 48 to 72 hours after infarction and 80% to 90% of patients who have myocardial infarctions experience dysrhythmias, constant surveillance is vital.

**Components.** The cardiac monitor is an instrument that displays electrical activity during the cardiac cycle as a wave pattern across a screen. An example of the basic components of cardiac monitors is shown in Fig. 7-3.

**Oscilloscope.** The screen on which the patient's electrocardiographic pattern appears is an oscilloscope

**Digital display.** An electronic mechanism averages the number of ventricular complexes per minute, and this rate is shown on the rate scale indicator. Also, each QRS complex is indicated by an audible beep and flashing light. If the pulse rate can be relayed to a console at the nursing station, the bedside monitor beep should be silenced so that the patient does not hear it.

**Rate meter.** Integrated with the alarm system is the rate meter, which signals if the heart rate goes above or below predetermined limits. The limits vary according to the routine of a particular unit, based on the sensitivity of the electrodes and monitoring system. For example, the alarm may be triggered to sound at either 25 beats above or below an individual patient's average heart rate, or it may be set to sound automatically at the high-low values of 150 beats/min and 50 beats/min.

**Alarm control system.** When the heart rate falls below or rises above the preset levels, audio and visual alarms alert the staff. Each time an alarm is triggered, the staff must observe the patient and make a prompt decision regarding the cardiac rhythm.

When the CCU personnel depend on an alarm system for warning, the rate limit indicators and alarm system must be checked regularly—not only for accuracy but also to be sure that the system is operative. There are situations when the limit settings are temporarily turned off in the patient's room. At these times personnel must depend on visual observation of the oscilloscope and the related clinical picture. For instance, the limit settings are turned off to prevent false alarms from electric interference resulting from the use of a high-power machine (e.g., a direct write-out ECG machine, or a portable x-ray machine). False alarms may also be triggered by manipulation of the chest electrodes when repositioning them to other sites on the chest or when bathing the patient. The patient's welfare is endangered if the alarm limit settings remain off; therefore it is essential to check these settings periodically.

When such an alarm system is not available, personnel must develop some other means of being alerted to changes in rhythm on the monitor oscilloscope. Only through an adequate method of observation can significant changes be identified and further rhythm disturbances prevented.

**Sweep speed.** The rate at which the electronic beam

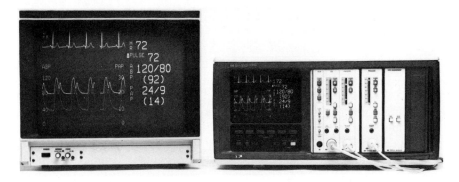

**Fig. 7-3** Monitoring system shows oscilloscope, digital and numerical display, and wave forms. (Reprinted with permission of Hewlett-Packard Co., Palo Alto, CA.)

sweeps across the screen can be controlled, and the sweep can be set at trace speeds of 25 mm/second (beam sweeps across standard screen in 6 seconds) or 50 mm/second (the 3-second sweep position). The 6-second position is generally used for routine monitoring. The 3-second position often provides for better interpretation of the rhythm or the pressure waveform by spreading the complexes.

Filter. The filter reduces extraneous muscular artifacts. However, when a 12-lead ECG is recorded from the monitor, the filter must be switched off, since it may distort the ST segment.

Central console. Individual bedside monitors in a CCU are connected to a central console at the nursing station to permit continuous observation of the ECG patterns from all the monitors.

Additional components. Complementary parts can be added to the basic monitoring system as necessary. For example, a direct write-out ECG machine can be located in the central station; this is triggered to record the cardiac rhythm automatically during alarm situations or on demand. Such recordings may be used to demonstrate the patient's response to antidysrhythmic therapy.

Some monitor systems have memory tapes that store a predetermined duration of the patient's ECG, which can then be recalled at will. This allows a printout of the cardiac rhythm recorded over the previous 60 seconds. At the time of alarm some monitors printout memory storage and then the current rhythm from the time of trigger. Memory mechanisms, however, erase after a period of time; therefore at the moment of an alarm, personnel must decide whether to record the stored memory information or the current rhythm. Use of 24-hour tape monitoring simplifies this problem. The monitoring system may also include multichannel recorders to monitor central venous, pulmonary artery, pulmonary capillary wedge, and arterial pressures, and other physiologic parameters. In some centers this information can be stored and retrieved from a computer. Also many new monitoring systems use computer analysis for dysrhythmia interpretation.

## Electrodes

Topical electrode patches are commonly used for patient monitoring. The following steps are involved in preparing the skin and in applying the electrodes:

1. At the sites chosen for electrode placement, clean the skin thoroughly with alcohol to remove all residues. If necessary, shave the hair at these sites.
2. The skin of some patients may require abrasion at the electrode sites to obtain an adequate ECG signal. If this is the situation, abrade each site by rubbing the area with a gauze pad.
3. Apply adhesive electrode pads and press them against the skin at the prepared sites. For extra adhesion a strip of nonallergenic tape may be applied over electrodes.

Placement of electrodes. The most commonly used leads for cardiac monitoring are II, $V_1$, or $MCL_1$ (modified chest lead). The lead that best displays the QRS complexes and P waves (and pacing stimuli if pacing is used) is used for monitoring.

A positive electrode, a negative electrode, and a ground electrode are required to record one bipolar lead. The location for these electrodes determines the lead recorded by the monitor. For example, a modification of lead $V_1$ ($MCL_1$) is recorded by placing the negative electrode just under the outer quarter of the left shoulder and the ground electrode beneath the right clavicle, with the positive electrode being placed at the fourth right intercostal space at the right sternal border (the usual $V_1$ position).

Many of the computerized monitoring systems use lead II for interpretation. The negative electrode is placed just under the outer quarter of the right shoulder and the ground electrode is positioned in the left lower abdominal area (left leg position).

To prevent their interfering with the physical examination, the chest electrodes should be placed away from the area near the apex of the heart. Placement of the electrodes on the chest reduces motion and muscle artifacts and allows the patient more freedom of movement than does limb-lead monitoring. Electrodes should be repositioned daily to prevent local skin irritation caused by prolonged contact of the hypertonic electrode paste with one point of the skin surface.

The modified $V_1$ chest lead has the added advantage over the other chest leads (often haphazardly positioned on the chest) of giving a maximum amount of information about rhythm disturbances and conduction. The $MCL_1$ provides an easily recognized recording of the sequence of ventricular activation and therefore furnishes maximum information to discriminate between right and left bundle branch block and between PVCs and aberrant supraventricular complexes (see Chapter 4).

The electrode wires from the patient are attached to a connector unit pinned to the patient's gown. From this unit a cable leads to the monitor where the electrode wires are connected to their respective terminals: positive wire to positive terminal, negative wire to negative terminal, and ground wire to ground terminal. In certain machines the electrode terminals are specifically labeled. In other machines it is necessary to be familiar with the terminal connections. Incorrect matching of electrodes and terminals will change the lead that is to be monitored.

### Interference with Monitoring

External voltage and patient movements generally are responsible for interference that occurs in a properly operating monitoring system. External voltage interference (alternating 60-cycle current) appears on the screen as a smooth thickening of the baseline resulting from the 60 tiny peaks/second (Fig. 7-4, A). Inadequate grounding of the monitor and other equipment or improper electrode placement and connection may produce this type of interference.

Because the cardiac monitor registers muscle potential, any sudden voluntary or involuntary movement by the patient can cause interference. For example, coughing or turning over in bed may precipitate a wandering baseline and erratic or irregular fluctuations on the oscilloscope (Fig. 7-4, B). Placing the electrodes in areas of limited muscular activity will reduce this problem.

In the tense, nervous, or cold patient, the monitor may display a harsh, jagged, uneven oscillation about the baseline. Another patient activity that can simulate ventricular fibrillation is tooth-brushing. Personnel must be careful not to interpret these baseline undulations as signifying fibrillatory waves.

### Electric Hazards

The electric equipment employed in a CCU increases the potential of electric shock hazard for both the patient and the equipment operator. Therefore it is important that CCU personnel have a basic understanding of the principles of current flow, current source, and grounding.

When ground connections of equipment are not at the same potential (zero volts or a few millivolts above zero), leakage current may flow between the source and its ground. Current will flow through the patient if he serves as a link in this circuit. Skin offers resistance to current flow and therefore protects the heart from electric shock. If the voltage is high enough or skin resistance has been lowered or eliminated, ventricular fibrillation may result. On some equipment, built-in isolation circuits isolate patients from the ground and the power line, thus preventing any conductive pathways. However, an intracardiac catheter or fluid column bypasses the skin and the protection from current flow that it affords, making the patient highly vulnerable to electric shock. Alternating current (AC)

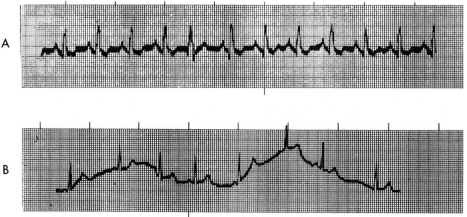

**Fig. 7-4** **A,** ECG tracing that shows external voltage interference (alternating 60-cycle current) appearing as a smooth thickening of the baseline as a result of the 60 tiny peaks per second. **B,** ECG tracing in which patient interference (e.g., coughing and turning) is shown by a wandering baseline.

**TABLE 7-1** Effects of electric current

| 60-Cycle Current (1-Second Duration) Delivered Through Skin | | 60-Cycle Current (1-Second Duration) Leading to Heart | |
|---|---|---|---|
| Millamperes | Effects | Microamperes | Effects |
| 1 | Threshold of perception; tingling | 20 to 50 | Ventricular fibrillation |
| 16 | "Let go" current; muscle contraction | | |
| 50 | Pain; possible fainting; mechanical injury | | |
| 100-3000 | Ventricular fibrillation | | |
| 6000 or greater | Sustained myocardial depolarization followed by normal rhythm; temporary respiratory paralysis; burns | | |

power-line current levels of only millionths of amperes, undetectable when applied to the skin, can induce ventricular fibrillation if contact with the myocardium is made.

Any AC power-line—operated device from which some of the current flows through the metal frame, case, or other exposed parts may serve as a current source. It may be an electric bed with a broken or missing ground connection or any device with two-wire power cords (two-pronged plugs) such as TV sets, bed lamps, or electric fans. The patient may lie in the path of the current source and ground directly by touching the electric device, or the patient may ground indirectly by making physical contact with another person who touches the defectively grounded instrument. Either situation causes the patient to become a conductive pathway and allows current to flow through him to ground.

Equipment operators should be cautious when using electronic equipment near water, steam pipes, radiators, or plumbing fixtures. Such pipes and fittings are excellent electric grounds. Consequently any electric device near them, including the power cords, plugs, and wall receptacles, that exposes the user to live current can be extremely hazardous if the operator simultaneously contacts both the device and a grounded pipe or faucet. The operator then becomes the link between the current source and the ground that the current seeks. The resultant shock may not be fatal, but serious injury can result from the violent muscular reaction in "letting go" (Table 7-1).

Personnel may detect tingling sensations when touching or brushing against a piece of electronic equipment. The voltage necessary to produce this sensation is only one thousandth of an ampere. Under ordinary circumstances this is harmless; however, this voltage is nearly 50 times the amount necessary to produce ventricular fibrillation if current flows directly to the patient's heart.

Clearly, many considerations are necessary to ensure electric safety. Awareness of potential hazards, prompt correction of faulty equipment, and regular safety inspection checks are all needed. Personnel should be thoroughly briefed in the following rules for electric safety in the CCU:

A. All equipment should be grounded. This means that a pathway of least resistance is available for the currents within the machine to flow to ground.
 1. All equipment must have three-pronged plugs that connect the hospital ground to the equipment chassis.
 2. Adaptors fitting a three-prong plug into a two-slot electric outlet should not be used.
 3. Extension cords should not be used to connect electronic equipment. If extensions are necessary, use only three-pronged grounding-type cords.
B. Wet surfaces conduct current. Therefore hazards such as wet sheets and wet floors should be eliminated.
C. Safety inspection checks should be routine. A qualified electric technician should check all equipment for faulty or missing ground connections and hazardous voltages. (Remember that equipment can still operate with defective ground connections.)
D. When two instruments are in use near a patient, connect them to the same power receptacle.
E. Never plug or unplug equipment or turn on a light while any part of your body or the patient's is in contact with water, steam pipes, radiators, or plumbing fixtures.
F. Prevent equipment cords from kinking, draping on pipes and plumbing, or lying on wet surfaces.
G. Report tingling sensations emitted from objects such as a bed frame or an instrument case. Unplug the equipment that is not necessary to support the life of the patient; correct this condition immediately in equipment necessary for life support.
H. When using an intracavitary lead, connect the electrode catheter to the V lead of the ECG machine, since this circuit has a high electric resistance in relation to ground. Anyone or anything electrically grounded must not touch the V-lead electrode terminals.
I. Additional precautions should be taken for patients with temporary cardiac pacemakers.

1. The electrodes at the end of the pacemaker should be well insulated. On older models a rubber glove is used to cover the exposed terminals at the junction with the external power source. Most newer models are adequately insultated.

2. When possible, use external battery pacemakers that are isolated from the power-line sources.

3. Personnel should wear rubber gloves when connecting or disconnecting the battery pacemaker and when adjusting electrodes at the end of the catheter.

4. Patients should use battery-operated razors rather than razors that require electricity.

## COMPLICATIONS OF CORONARY ARTERY DISEASE

The most common complications of coronary artery disease are angina and myocardial infarction. The clinical syndromes of heart failure, pulmonary edema, cardiogenic shock, dysrhythmias, and sudden cardiac death usually occur as a complication of myocardial ischemia or infarction. In addition, psychologic alterations may be noted at any point during the illness.

### Angina Pectoris

Angina pectoris is a syndrome characterized by chest discomfort that occurs as a result of transient myocardial ischemia. This myocardial ischemia is a result of an imbalance of myocardial oxygen supply and demand, either a decreased supply or an increased demand, or both. An inadequate supply of oxygen can be caused by coronary artery obstruction, usually because of artherosclerosis. However, coronary artery spasm or coronary artery thrombosis also may cause or contribute to the obstruction. Severe anemia and hypoxia also can cause a decrease in myocardial oxygen supply. There are many clinical conditions that can cause an increased demand for myocardial oxygen including tachycardias, hypertension, valvular stenosis, left ventricular hypertrophy and hyperthyroidism.[11]

Various types of anginal pain occur. Exertional, or stable, angina is initiated by exertion, is predictable at a certain level of activity, and is associated with a fixed coronary obstruction. Variant angina produces symptoms similar to stable angina, but it is caused by coronary artery spasm.[11] Some patients with coronary artery spasm are found to have normal coronary arteries,[12] however may patients with spasm also have some degree of stenosis. Variant angina usually occurs at rest, often during the night or early morning, frequently happening at the same time each day. On ECG, ST segments are elevated during the attack and return to normal with pain relief.[13] Variant angina may be stable, as in Prinzmetal's angina,[14] but more often it is unstable.

Unstable angina, also called *crescendo angina, preinfarction angina,* or *progressive* angina, can be defined as any new onset of angina, acceleration of previously stable angina, or severe, prolonged ischemic pain at rest.[14] Unstable angina is thought to be caused by acute changes, such as fissuring of the intracoronary plaque, thrombus formation,[15-17] or spasm.[18] These events cause transient myocardial ischemia. Unstable angina also is called *unstable myocardial ischemia,* and acute myocardial infarction is an extreme form of unstable ischemia.[19]

Although the term *angina pectoris* literally means chest pain, perhaps it should be referred to as discomfort because many patients may deny experiencing chest pain. Rather, they often refer to vague sensations, feelings, or aches. These unpleasant feelings have been described in a variety of ways, including a sense of pressure or burning, squeezing, heaviness, smothering, and very frequently as "indigestion." Since the discomfort of angina is usually located in the retrosternal region, patients will often illustrate the nature and location of their symptoms by placing a clenched fist against their sternum. Often angina pectoris is not confined to the chest but may radiate to the neck, jaw, epigastrium, shoulders, or arms. Most often it radiates to the left shoulder and left arm. Occasionally, angina may produce discomfort in an area of radiation without affecting the retrosternal region.

Attacks of exertional angina are typically preceded by an elevation of blood pressure or heart rate or both. During the attack, pulse rate and blood pressure usually increase further, presumably as a consequence of anxiety and as a physiologic response to pain. In some instances, however, blood pressure and pulse may fall dramatically as a result of vagally mediated reflexes. More important than the location is the duration of the pain and the circumstances under which it occurs. Angina pectoris lasts usually only a few minutes if the precipitating factor is relieved. Attacks are often induced by effort and *during* rather than after exertion. Exertion during cold weather or following meals is particularly likely to produce pain. Anxiety, smoking, stressful situations, worry, anger, hurry, and excitement are common precipitating factors. Patients have described the following situations as producing chest pain: running to catch a bus, driving in heavy traffic, nightmares, painful stimuli, sexual intercourse, and straining at stool.

Angina typically lasts from 1 to several minutes and usually no more than 3 to 5 minutes. It is relieved by rest, by nitroglycerin, or by any influence that will drop arterial pressure or heart rate and equalize the supply of blood and nutrients with the demand.

Diagnosis. The diagnosis of angina pectoris is usually made from a characteristic history because frequently there are few abnormalities found through physical examination and the ECG may be normal at rest. It is best to allow patients to describe symptoms without using suggestive terms. Time and patience are necessary to explore the patient's lifestyle, habits, and emotions to obtain a clear picture of the pain and the extent of incapacitation.

On physical examination, the patient's blood pressure and pulse should be measured, because hypertension and/or tachycardia can be precipitating factors.[20] Also, signs of congestive heart failure such as rales, an $S_3$ gallop, peripheral edema, and neck vein distention may be present.[20] During episodes of angina, the patient may be diaphoretic and restless. Heart rate, blood pressure, and respiratory rate may be elevated but may return to normal with pain relief.[20]

A 12-lead ECG may show ST segment or T wave changes in the affected leads. These changes may be caused by transmural ischemia, such as in an acute MI or coronary artery spasm. Return of the ST segment and T wave to baseline after relief of the angina indicates that coronary artery spasm was the precipitating factor.[19]

Also useful in the diagnosis of angina are stress testing,[21] radionuclide studies, and Holter monitoring. In addition, cardiac catheterization is indicated to accurately determine the extent of coronary artery disease in patients with severe unstable angina. In order to document the presence of coronary artery spasm, ergonovine maleate[22] can be injected into the coronary artery during cardiac catheterization to induce spasm.

**Treatment.** The first principle in treatment of angina pectoris is to minimize the discrepancy between the demand of the heart muscle for oxygen and the ability of the coronary circulation to meet this demand. Accordingly, patients must learn to pace themselves so that physical activity is kept below the threshold of discomfort. Moderate exercise performed below the angina threshold should be encouraged. Additional measures include adopting a diet designed to achieve the individual's ideal weight and the cessation of smoking. Hypertension, if present, should be treated.

Pharmacologic treatment is directed at two objectives; first, relief from symptoms when they occur and, second, prevention of angina. For the first objective, nitroglycerin taken sublingually is the treatment of choice. For prevention, beta-adrenergic blocking agents are prescribed to slow the heart rate and attentuate the contractile response to physical or emotional activity. Longer-acting nitrates such as isosorbide dinitrate (Isordil) or nitrol paste exert an action for 2 to 4 hours and are very effective. Reichek and others[23] have found that transdermal nitroglycerin patches did not offer 24 hours of stable antianginal protection. During sustained transdermal treatment, patients develop tolerance to nitroglycerin, and antianginal efficacy was diminished. An intermittent dosage schedule is recommended to avoid nitrate tolerance.

Recent reports indicate that vasodilators acting principally on the arterial system (e.g., hydralazine or prazosin) may attenuate the hypertensive response to exertion and aid in preventing angina. Calcium-blocking agents (e.g., nifedipine, verapamil, and diltiazem) are another group of potent vasodilators for coronary and peripheral arteries that also have the ability to decrease afterload and myocardial contractility. The combination of nitrate therapy and calcium blockers has been extremely effective.[24] Other investigators have demonstrated improved LV function, improved exercise tolerance, and delayed onset of chest pain with combination therapy consisting of nitrates, beta-adrenoreceptor-blocker therapy and calcium antagonists.[25]

Other general measures for the management of angina include sedation, relief of anxiety, and supervised exercise programs designed to enhance physical condition and thereby reduce the blood pressure and heart rate response to exercise.[26,27]

In addition to nitrates, beta blockers and calcium channel blockers, heparin and thrombolytic therapy may be considered for patients with unstable angina.[18,19] Angioplasty[19] and coronary artery bypass surgery[28] provide good relief of symptoms and prolong life in selected subgroups of patients.

### Acute Myocardial Infarction

An MI is an ischemic event that occurs over several hours and can induce ischemic injury and necrosis (cell death) in myocardial tissue (Fig. 7-5). Tissue damage occurs in a wavelike fashion; the center of the infarct is the area of necrosis, and this is surrounded by an area of injured myocardium, which in turn is surrounded by an area of ischemic tissue. The most common cause of MI is coronary arterial thrombosis,[29] which is often superimposed on an already atherosclerotic vessel; another cause of MI is coronary artery spasm. The initial goals of treatment are to confirm the diagnosis and to preserve ischemic myocardium.

Chest pain is the presenting symptom in most patients

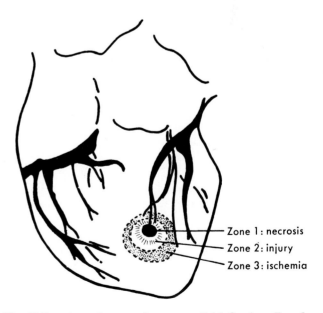

**Fig. 7-5**   Tissue damage after myocardial infarction. *Zone 1,* Necrotic tissue; *zone 2,* injured tissue; *zone 3,* ischemic tissue.

with acute MI. The pain is frequently severe, but there may be minimal discomfort and, on occasion, none. It is usually substernal and may radiate to the epigastric region, the jaw, shoulders, elbows, or forearms. The pain is usually described as a heaviness, tightness, or constriction but occasionally as indigestion or a burning sensation. It usually persists for 30 minutes or longer, often until potent analgesics have been administered. In its classic presentation the symptoms of MI are more severe than typical angina. On the other hand, the symptoms of infarction may be subtle, and very often severity and duration of pain do not distinguish between prolonged angina, coronary insufficiency (prolonged ischemia), and MI.

In addition to chest pain, patients with MI may experience shortness of breath, sweating, weakness or extreme fatigue, nausea, vomiting, and severe anxiety. On physical examination they may show evidence of overactivity of the sympathetic nervous system, including tachycardia, sweating, and hypertension. Alternatively, evidence of vagal hyperactivity may predominate with bradycardia and hypotension. Many patients look surprisingly normal. Hypotension with tachycardia and peripheral cyanosis suggests a markedly reduced cardiac output and shock. In some patients normal blood pressure is maintained, but an $S_3$ gallop and pulmonary rales indicate acute left ventricular failure. Murmurs related to mitral insufficiency or a ruptured interventricular septum may develop and a pericardial friction rub may be heard. Heart sounds are usually diminished in intensity, and particularly with anterior infarction a paradoxical parasternal systolic lift can be felt inside the apex region.

The diagnosis of MI is initially made on the basis of the patient's history and ECG tracings and finally confirmed with cardiac enzymes. Ancillary but nonspecific findings of infarction include low grade fever, elevation of the white blood cell count, and elevation of the erythrocyte sedimentation rate. The ECG may show typical findings of infarction or nonspecific changes of the ST segment or T wave. Rarely, if ever, are serial ECGs normal in a patient with documented infarction.

With necrosis of heart muscle, enzymes that are normally confined within the myocardial cell leak out and appear in peripheral blood; serum glutamic-oxaloacetic transaminase (SGOT), lactate dehydrogenase (LDH), and creatine phosphokinase (CPK) are the enzymes measured most frequently. LDH and CPK appear in more than one form and are referred to as isoenzymes. The isoenzymes of LDH and CPK are distributed differently in different tissues so that elevations of the "heart" isoenzymes are more specific evidence of heart muscle necrosis than elevation of either the total CPK or LDH. Elevations of CPK-MB and of LDH-1 (the predominant heart isoenzymes) are typically observed in MI.

Radionuclide imaging techniques used to confirm the diagnosis of MI have received considerable attention.

These imaging methods include thallium 201 scintigraphy and technetium-99m pyrophosphate imaging.[30-33] Myocardial uptake of thallium 201 depends on blood flow; with decreased blood flow an area of diminished activity is visualized. Because a single study cannot differentiate between ischemic and necrotic myocardium, serial studies are necessary and the first thallium 201 study should be done within 6 hours after the onset of symptoms. In conjunction with other findings noted above, serial thallium 201 images can be used to diagnose an MI as well as to estimate the location and extent of decreased coronary perfusion and resulting necrosis.

Dipyridamole-thallium 201 scintigraphy has been useful in identifying subsets of patients at high risk for future cardiac events after an MI. Dipyridamole is a potent coronary vasodilator. When used in conjunction with thallium 201, it simulates an exercise thallium 201 test.[34,35] In studies with 51 patients, Leppo and others,[36,37] found that dipyridamole-thallium scintigraphy had 93% sensitivity and 80% specificity for coronary artery disease and was a useful predictor of postmyocardial infarction events.

The radionuclide imaging test using technetium 99m pyrophosphate is regarded as a fairly sensitive technique for confirming myocardial damage. The isotope is taken up by necrotic cells within 12 to 18 hours after the onset of infarction; uptake persists for 4 to 5 days and then typically decays. Even small areas of infarction can be identified by appropriate scanning equipment from the "hot spot" produced on the scintigram. For optimum results the test should be done between 48 and 72 hours after the onset of infarction.

Because wall motion abnormalities and wall thinning correlate with ischemia and infarction, two-dimensional echocardiography may be used to assess the ischemic heart. Systolic wall thickening is normally seen. Systolic wall thinning is seen when the infarct involves more than 20% of the transmural thickness. Although echocardiographic wall motion abnormalities seem to consistently overestimate infarct size, echocardiography can give a reasonable estimate of overall left ventricular function. Echocardiography is also useful in determining acute and chronic mechanical complications of infarction. The acute complications easily defined include a ruptured mitral valve, papillary muscle dysfunction, papillary muscle rupture, ventricular septal rupture, cardiac rupture, and pericardial effusion. The chronic complications consist of aneurysm formation and intracavitary clot formation.[38-40]

It is useful to distinguish between patients with complicated and uncomplicated acute MI, since nearly all deaths occur in the former group, whereas those patients in the latter group have an excellent prognosis and are candidates for early mobilization and discharge. The conditions that identify the complicated group include the following:

1. *Persistent Pain.* Pain that persists or recurs is fre-

quently associated with unusually high enzyme elevations or secondary rises and suggests that ischemia persists and infarction is in a process of evolution.

2. *Serious Dysrhythmia.* Nearly all patients with acute infarction experience some transient alterations of rhythm. The alterations considered serious include ventricular fibrillation or ventricular tachycardia, second or third degree heart block, and new atrial flutter or fibrillation.[41] In addition, sinus tachycardia ($\geq 100$ beats/min) that persists for more than 24 to 48 hours in the absence of fever should alert those caring for the patient to the possibility of heart failure.[42]

3. *Pulmonary Edema.* Pulmonary edema produces a sense of breathlessness, wet rales on examination, and typical changes on the chest x-ray film. It is accompanied by a significant rise in pulmonary artery and wedge pressure and indicates acute left ventricular failure.

4. *Persistent Hypotension.* The arterial systolic blood pressure may drop below 90 mm Hg without accompanying signs of shock. Often this is an early and transient finding associated with bradycardia and other signs of vagal overactivity. Alternatively, it may reflect an inadequate blood volume. When hypotension persists despite an adequate heart rate and central venous pressure, it usually signifies a markedly reduced cardiac output.

In a study of 500 patients with acute MI, the sample was classified on the basis of the presence or absence of complications during the first 4 days of hospitalization.[43] Among the group who were *not* free of complications through the fourth day, most either died subsequently in the hospital or suffered a serious late complication. Patients who were free of complications for the first 4 days appeared to be candidates for early mobilization and early discharge. Among patients without complications discharged on the seventh hospital day, there were no serious complications or deaths at home during early follow-up. DeBusk and associates demonstrated a similar low complication rate among patients discharged early after uncomplicated MIs.[44]

MI patients can be further classified according to whether they had nontransmural or transmural infarcts. In the past, patients with nontransmural infarcts were thought to follow an uncomplicated course. Evidence suggests that patients with nontransmural infarctions are actually at higher risk for complications and sudden death after discharge from the hospital.[45] In view of these findings, survivors of nontransmural infarction are especially appropriate candidates for early functional assessment and arteriography.

Low level exercise testing before discharge has proven to be of value in predicting patients at high risk for subsequent complications. Evidence indicates that patients who develop either ST segment abnormalities, angina pectoris, or abnormal blood pressure responses during low level exercise testing are at higher risk of developing cardiac complications.[46,47] Nishimura and associates[48] found that wall motion studies using two-dimensional echocardiography may be helpful in identifying subsets of patients at high risk for complications.

**Treatment.** In the early stages of acute MI, pain, anxiety, and alterations of rhythm dominate the clinical picture. After establishing a route for intravenous therapy and ECG monitoring, morphine should be given in doses that eliminate or greatly reduce chest pain and relieve anxiety. Excessive bradycardia with a pulse rate below 50 to 55 beats/min, particularly if accompanied by hypotension and ectopic beats, should be treated with atropine.[49]

The greatest threat to life in the early hours after MI is ventricular fibrillation. In approximately 50% of patients, episodes of ventricular fibrillation are preceded by ventricular premature beats. The high prevalence of premature beats and the fact that fibrillation is sometimes not heralded by these changes has led in recent years to the use of prophylactic antidysrhythmic therapy in some centers. Lidocaine is given as an initial bolus (75 to 100 mg), followed by a continuous intravenous infusion.

Because a decrease in arterial $PO_2$ caused by ventilation perfusion inequalities is common, oxygen is administered to all patients. Most physicians also advocate giving routine low-dose subcutaneous heparin to reduce the possibility of thromboembolic complications.[50]

In patients who have persistent or recurrent pain despite therapy, efforts are made to balance the oxygen supply and demand and hence to diminish ischemia. For example, if sinus tachycardia persists and signs of left ventricular failure are absent, propranolol in doses of 0.05 to 0.10 mg/kg can be given to reduce heart rate. Although this treatment has been shown to eliminate pain and reduce ST segment elevation, the hemodynamic response needs to be monitored closely.[51] Other patients with persistent or recurrent pain have elevated arterial blood pressure. Reducing blood pressure with propranolol or nitroprusside has a favorable effect in these patients. Finally, in patients with left ventricular failure and elevated pulmonary artery and wedge pressures, vasodilators such as nitroprusside or IV nitroglycerin will "unload" the ventricle and often reduce pain and ST segment elevation.

IV nitroglycerin has been demonstrated to be efficacious in limiting complications (pump failure, chest pain) of an acute MI. Nitroglycerin is an excellent coronary vasodilator, whereas sodium nitroprusside may have deleterious effects on the ischemic heart. Nitroprusside dilates the intramyocardial resistance arteries supplying the normal myocardium. Since resistance vessels supplying the ischemic areas are already presumably maximally dilated, dilating other resistance vessels further would shunt blood from the ischemic areas to normal areas, resulting in a "coronary steal" phenomenon. Consequently, IV nitro-glycerin is the preferred drug.[52,53]

MI is a dynamic process in which the ultimate fate of ischemic but still viable heart muscle is not determined until several hours after the onset of symptoms. Survival after MI depends on the size of the infarction and residual left ventricular function.[54] The primary objective of therapy following an MI is to reestablish myocardial perfusion and thereby minimize necrosis and ischemic damage. Current revascularization techniques include thrombolytic therapy, percutaneous transluminal coronary angioplasty, and coronary artery bypass surgery (CABG)[55] (see Chapter 12 for more information on CABG).

**Thrombolytic therapy.** Because most MIs are caused by coronary arterial thrombosis, the goal of thrombolytic therapy is to lyse the intracoronary clot, restore blood flow, and thereby salvage ischemic myocardium, limit the size of the infarction and preserve left ventricular function.[56,57] Currently, there are four thrombolytic agents approved for use by the Food and Drug Administration: streptokinase, urokinase, recombinant tissue plasminogen activator (rt-PA), and anistreplase.

Thrombolysis can be initiated by the activation of plasminogen, a serum protein that is a precursor of the enzyme plasmin. Plasminogen activators are chemicals that convert plasminogen into plasmin. Plasmin breaks down fibrin, causing the clot to dissolve. This also produces fibrin degradation products, which are potent anticoagulants (Fig. 7-6).[58]

Streptokinase is a proteolytic enzyme synthesized by streptococcal bacteria. When this enzyme is injected into humans, it combines with circulating plasminogen to form streptokinase-plasminogen complex, which activates plasminogen to form plasmin. The net effect of the therapy is to produce a hypocoagulable state. Streptokinase can be given via the IV or intracoronary routes. The IV route allows for much quicker administration of the drug. Potential adverse effects include allergic reactions such as fever, rash, and, rarely, anaphylactic shock. Hypotension, sometimes requiring vasopressors, can occur.[58,59] There have been many studies in which streptokinase was used as a thrombolytic agent. Data from two large clinical trials, the GISSI study and ISIS-2, revealed a 50% increase in survival with the use of streptokinase as opposed to traditional medical therapy.[60,61] The GISSI study also showed a higher survival rate in patients who received streptokinase therapy early during the infarct episode. In addition, the ISIS-2 trial demonstrated a higher survival rate with the combination of streptokinase and oral aspirin than with either drug alone.[62]

Urokinase is another proteolytic enzyme; it is made from cultured kidney cells. It also works by converting plasminogen to plasmin, causing a systemic lytic state. Urokinase can be given as an intracoronary infusion or an IV bolus.[58] It is nonantigenic and no adverse effects have been

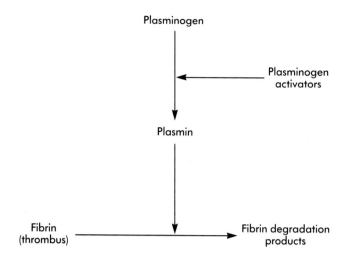

**Fig. 7-6** The role of plasminogen activators in the process of thrombolysis.

reported. Like streptokinase, it has a more pronounced effect on the hemostatic system and a longer half-life than rt-PA.[59]

Tissue plasminogen activator is a naturally occuring protein with a very high affinity for fibrin. In the presence of fibrin, t-PA converts fibrin-bound plasminogen to plasmin at the surface of a clot. The plasmin then breaks down the fibrin and the clot dissolves. Therefore, t-PA is clot-specific,[63] whereas streptokinase and urokinase have a hypocoagulable effect on the entire circulatory system. This enzyme can now be mass-produced with recombinant DNA techniques, and it is called recombinant tissue type plasminogen activator (rt-PA). Advantages of rt-PA include the fact that it has a short half-life, it is clot-specific in its action, and it causes no allergic reactions.[59] A disadvantage is the relatively high cost for the drug, more than 10 times the cost of streptokinase.[64] The incidence of bleeding complications is about the same for rt-PA as for streptokinase. Several studies have shown a 70% to 75% efficacy for rt-PA to successfully lyse a coronary thrombus, and two studies have demonstrated that rt-PA has a higher efficacy than does streptokinase.[65-67] Large multicenter trials, such as the TIMI trial and the European Cooperative Group, are evaluating the relative value of the various thrombolytic agents, as well as percutaneous transluminal coronary angioplasty.

Investigations of new thrombolytic agents are underway. Anisoylated plasminogen streptokinase activator complex, anistreplase, has recently been approved by the FDA for clinical trials as a thrombolytic agent. It is a combination of streptokinase and plasminogen and will be marketed under the name *eminase*. One clinical advantage of eminase is that it can be given intravenously in less than 5 minutes, whereas, rt-PA must be given intravenously over several hours.[68,69] Initial studies with recombinant single-chain urokinase type plasminogen activator (SCU-PA) and the combination of urokinase-type plasminogen activator and urokinase indicate that these reagents are effective at restoring patency in 70% to 80% of the patients evaluated.[70,71]

Not all MI patients are candidates for thrombolytic therapy. In order for thrombolytic therapy to be beneficial, the drug should be administered within 4 to 6 hours from the onset of symptoms: the earlier the treatment is initiated, the greater the benefit derived. Patients must meet the ECG criteria of ST elevation of at least 0.1 mV in 2 leads. Most centers exclude patients older than 65 or 70 years because of a higher incidence of intracranial hemorrhage in this population.[72] although some investigators have recently recommended including high-risk patients such as the elderly and patients with pulmonary edema.[73] Contraindications are related to an increased risk of bleeding such as recent active internal bleeding, history of CVA, recent history of major surgery or trauma, prolonged CPR, hypertension, history of a bleeding disorder, or puncture of a noncompressible vessel.[72,74,75] In addition, clinical factors such as older age, female sex, low body weight, and low fibrinogen and fibrin degradation product levels are believed to increase the risk of bleeding.[76] In the major clinical trials, the number of bleeding complications reported has been very low. The major bleeding complication is hemorrhagic stroke, which occurs in approximately one out of every 200 to 250 patients regardless of the thrombolytic agent used.[73]

Thrombolytic therapy is initiated in conjunction with other pharmacologic agents for acute MI. A heparin bolus and drip are usually given to prevent any further clot formation, with the infusion titrated to keep the partial thromboplastin time (PTT) 1½ to 2 times normal. Lidocaine is used prophylactically to prevent dysrhythmias caused by the infarction or reperfusion. Antiplatelet drugs such as aspirin, sulfinpyrazone, and dipyridamole have been tried to help prevent reocclusion and reinfarction. In view of current research, and if there are no contraindications, it is recommended that one aspirin a day be given to MI patients.

The most definitive method for determining if reperfusion has been successfully achieved by thrombolytic therapy is by cardiac catheterization. However, certain clinical signs have been associated with reperfusion. These clinical markers include an abrupt cessation or reduction of chest pain, resolution of ST segment elevation, reperfusion dysrhythmias, and a rapid peaking of CPK enzymes. The most common dysrhythmias associated with reperfusion are ventricular tachycardia, sinus bradycardia, accelerated idioventricular rhythm (AIVR), and premature ventricular contractions.[74,79]

The most frequent complications of thrombolytic therapy are related to bleeding. The additional use of heparin to prevent further clot formation may also contribute to these complications. Periaccess site bleeding from cardiac catheterization can be a problem.[59] Intracranial hemorrhage occurs in 0.5% of patients receiving thrombolytic therapy. There may also be gingival bleeding, epistaxis, hemoptysis, and bleeding from recent cuts and abrasions.[74] Internal bleeding, such as gastrointestinal or retroperitoneal bleeding, occurs less frequently. Any serious bleeding episode may necessitate the immediate discontinuation of the thrombolytic agent and heparin infusion. Blood transfusions may be required.

Coronary artery reocclusion may be caused by rethrombosis, coronary artery spasms or incomplete lysis of the thrombus. With coronary artery occlusion, the myocardium is again at risk. Signs and symptoms of ischemia, such as chest pain, nausea, diaphoresis, and ECG changes may occur.[80] Cardiac catheterization, PTCA, or a repeat dose of rt-PA may be required.

Frequent and careful monitoring of the patient receiving thrombolytic therapy is required. Many of the observations are necessary because of the increased risk of bleeding caused by the thrombolytic agents and concomitant heparin infusion. The PTT should be monitored frequently. The patient's neurologic status should be evaluated frequently and checked for any changes in level of consciousness or complaints of headache that may indicate an intracranial bleed. All puncture and access sites should be checked for bleeding or hematoma formation. The patient's gums and nose should be checked for bleeding and the skin should be inspected for bleeding, bruises, or ecchymotic areas. In addition, the urine, stool, sputum, and emesis should be checked for blood. Unnecessary arterial and venous punctures should be avoided and heparin locks used for blood sampling. Intramuscular (IM) injections should not be given while the patient is in a hypocoagulable state. It is important to assess for signs of internal bleeding such as a drop in hemoglobin or hematocrit levels, a sudden change in vital signs, restlessness, a rapidly distending abdomen, low back pain, or diminished peripheral pulses. Direct pressure should be applied for at least 30 minutes (or until bleeding stops) to all puncture sites and then a sterile pressure dressing should be applied. The patient should be handled gently to prevent bruising.[80]

During thrombolytic therapy, observe the patient for any signs of reperfusion such as a cessation of chest pain, resolution of ST segment elevation, early peaking of CPK enzymes, or dysrhythmias. Monitor the patient closely for signs of myocardial ischemia including chest pain, nausea, diaphoresis, shortness of breath, or ECG changes.

In addition to the intense monitoring of the patient receiving thrombolytic therapy, psychologic support of the patient and his or her family is important. Anxiety and fear are common reactions during an MI. The potential risks of thrombolytic therapy may increase those reactions. It is important to provide a calm, reassuring atmosphere and give clear, simple explanations of treatments and activities.

Percutaneous transluminal coronary angioplasty. Percutaneous transluminal coronary angioplasty (PTCA) is a nonoperative procedure that uses a balloon catheter to increase the luminal diameter of stenotic coronary arteries and thereby increase blood flow distal to the stenosis. Improvement in coronary blood flow following PTCA is associated with decreased symptoms and increased exercise tolerance in patients with angina pectoris.[81] PTCA may also prevent reocclusion following thrombolytic therapy for acute MI. Consequently, PTCA has gained wide acceptance as an effective therapy for selected patients with symptomatic coronary artery disease.

Dotter and Judkins first used a percutaneously introduced catheter in 1964 to dilate peripheral atherosclerotic lesions.[82] In 1977 Gruetzig applied percutaneous transluminal angioplasty to a highly selected subgroup of patients with stable angina and a discrete proximal, noncalcific stenosis of a single coronary artery.[83] Technical advancements in percutaneous catheters, guidewires, and balloons have expanded the range of indications for PTCA. Patients with unstable angina, multivessel disease, multiple stenoses in single vessels, and stenoses in coronary artery bypass grafts have been successfully treated.

The use of PTCA has increased for several reasons. When compared with coronary artery bypass grafting (CABG), PTCA is psychologically and physically much less traumatic. The recovery period for PTCA is short: less than 24 hours of bed rest is required after the procedure. The patient is usually discharged from the hospital within 3 days after angioplasty. Although the number of patients who return to work after successful angioplasty is not significantly different from patients who have undergone CABG, the length of time until return to work is shorter in PTCA patients.[84]

**Equipment.** Basic equipment used during angioplasty includes a balloon, pacing and guiding catheters, and a transducer system for monitoring ventricular and coronary artery pressures. The balloon catheter has two lumens; the central lumen is used for injection of contrast media and for pressure monitoring, and the outer lumen is used for balloon inflation and deflation. Gold markers, visible under fluoroscopy, are positioned at both ends of the balloon to define its alignment within the lesion.

As a precautionary measure, a pacing catheter is placed prior to angioplasty. If the right coronary artery is to be dilated, third-degree AV block may result while the artery is occluded. If the left anterior descending artery is occluded during angioplasty, an idioventricular rhythm may occur.

The guiding catheter is a large, single-lumen one used to position the balloon catheter. A modern angioplasty catheter system is shown if Fig. 7-7.

**Mechanism.** Initially, the main mechanism of PTCA was thought to be the compression and relocation of atherosclerotic plaque. Several human cadaver and animal studies now suggest that balloon inflation during angioplasty causes the plaque to split at its thinnest and weakest point.[85-88] This split may extend into internal elastic membrane, and further balloon dilatation may stretch the media and adventitia of the vessel,[89] causing an arterial wall tear

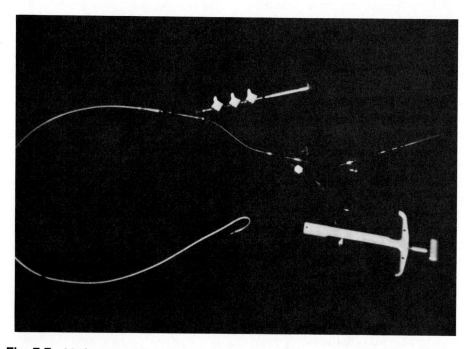

**Fig. 7-7** Modern steerable guidewire equipment used for coronary angioplasty. (Courtesy of Dr. Richard Stack, Duck University Medical Center.)

to occur in the direction of blood flow. The subsequent healing process is not well understood; presently it is thought that some of the plaque may dissolve in the bloodstream. Arterial wall fibers may cause retraction of the split, and endothelial cells may promote healing of the exposed inner surface of the vessel.[90]

**Selection of patients for PTCA.** The results of the history, treadmill test, and coronary angiogram are used to determine a patient's suitability for PTCA. Ideally, the stenosis should be less than 10 mm in length, not involve a major vessel bifurcation, and be free of angiographic filling defects.[91] The ideal candidate for PTCA has a single, proximal, concentric, noncalcific coronary artery lesion in the setting of persistent angina despite medical therapy. Patients whose symptoms are controlled by medical therapy may do just as well on medical therapy as they would with PTCA.

PTCA may be performed in patients over 65 years of age, although the success rate is lower in this age group than in younger patients. The complication rate of PTCA in the elderly is higher than in younger patients, with death occurring in 2.2% of all patients over the age of 65 according to the National Heart, Lung, and Blood Institute Registry as compared with 0.7% of patients under 65. Excluding death, the complication rate for both age groups is the same.[92]

Not all lesions are considered for angioplasty. An increased frequency of coronary occlusion and an inability to localize and effectively use the dilating balloon make lesions that are excessive in number and length and distal in location high risk. If tortuosity of the vessel precludes easy placement of the steerable guidewire, the patient should not be considered a candidate for angioplasty. In most centers patients with left main disease are not candidates. Individual patients' coronary arteriograms must be evaluated to make these decisions. The box above lists indications and precautions for PTCA.

**Procedure.** In most cases a diagnostic cardiac catheterization precedes PTCA by one or more days. Although the angioplasty procedure is very similar to cardiac catheterization, the patient may express new fears concerning balloon dilatation and possible emergent coronary artery bypass grafting. Therefore it is important to thoroughly explain the procedure to the patient. The family or support system of the patient should be included in the teaching so they have an understanding of the procedure and can provide the support the patient needs.

The patient is allowed nothing by mouth from midnight until after angioplasty to minimize the risk of emesis and aspiration during the procedure. Both groins are cleansed and shaved. Routine laboratory tests obtained prior to angioplasty include hemoglobin, hematocrit, coagulation studies, electrolytes, BUN, and creatinine. Blood is typed and screened in case emergency surgery is required.

The operating suite should be notified in advance of all

---

## INDICATIONS AND PRECAUTIONS FOR PTCA

**INDICATIONS**

1. Stenosis that is:
   a. Less than 10 minutes in length
   b. Proximal
   c. Single
   d. Concentric
   e. Noncalcific

**PRECAUTIONS**

1. Stenosis that:
   a. Involves a major vessel bifurcation
   b. Has angiographic filling defects
   c. Is tortuous
2. Multivessel disease
3. Coronary artery bypass grafts
4. Excessive number of stenoses
5. Chronic total coronary artery lesions
6. Left main disease (contraindicated in most medical centers)

---

angioplasty cases. A room should be prepared and a cardiothoracic team must be mobilized in the event of any complications of angioplasty that require immediate surgery.

Because platelet adhesion is thought to be the cause of early restenosis after angioplasty, low molecular weight dextran or a combination of aspirin and dipyridamole may be given before the procedure. However, the effectiveness of these drugs has not been proved. Diphenhydramine is commonly administered before angiography to reduce the risk of allergic reaction to contrast media. Long-acting nitrates and calcium channel blockers may be given before angioplasty.

Once in the angiography laboratory, the patient is prepped and draped, using sterile technique. After the femoral vein is located with a large-bore needle, an introducer sheath is inserted and the pacing catheter is advanced to the level of the inferior vena cava. A second needle is used to locate the femoral artery. An introducer sheath is placed in the artery, and the guiding catheter is advanced to the level of the coronary ostium. To prevent spasm, 200 mcg to 300 mcg of intracoronary nitroglycerin and/or sublingual nifedipine may be given. A steering device on the distal end of the guidewire system directs the guidewire into the coronary circulation and across the atherosclerotic lesion. Once in place and verified by fluoroscopy, the balloon is advanced along the guidewire and across the lesion. Gold markers at each end of the balloon assist in determining proper placement within the vessel, and pressure gradients across the lesion may then be measured. The guiding catheter measures proximal pressure while the dilating catheter measures distal pressures; the difference in pressures is termed the *pressure gradient*. A large lesion that significantly obstructs blood flow causes a greater decrease

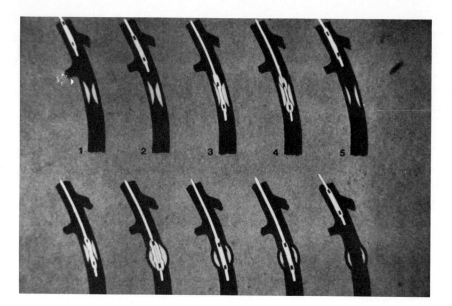

**Fig. 7-8** Balloon compression of atherosclerotic lesion. (Courtesy of Dr. Richard Stack, Duke University Medical Center.)

in pressure distal to the lesion and, consequently, a greater pressure gradient.

The balloon is then inflated at pressures from 2 to 10 atmospheres for 10 to 60 seconds (Fig. 7-8). One or more inflations at varying pressures may be performed. With the guidewire across the lesion in case of sudden reocclusion, the results are assessed by arteriography. The pressure gradient measured after successful angioplasty should be significantly lower. Pressure gradients may be distorted by the presence of the balloon catheter or guidewire across the lesion, contrast media, or collateral blood flow.[89] With these limitations in mind, some investigators do not rely on pressure gradients to determine success after PTCA. Fig. 7-9 shows coronary arteriograms before and after PTCA.

If angioplasty is successful, the catheters are removed. Because heparin is given during angioplasty, clotting times will be elevated after the procedure. The sheaths are left in place to prevent bleeding, and the patient is returned to his or her room. To decrease the risk of sudden arterial reocclusion after PTCA, intravenous heparin may also be given after the procedure. The heparin may be discontinued several hours to 24 hours after PTCA. When coagulation times return to normal, the sheaths may be removed, after which the patient should lie flat for approximately 6 hours to promote healing of the femoral artery puncture site. The patient should be watched closely for signs of bleeding in the groin area. Pedal pulses should be checked frequently in case thrombosis of the femoral artery occurs. Blood pressure is taken frequently to monitor for hypotension.

Most important, the patient should be monitored for chest pain, which is common after PTCA and may be caused by abrupt occlusion or restenosis of the dilated coronary artery, coronary artery spasm, or pulmonary embolism. When chest pain occurs, an ECG should be obtained and nitrates and calcium-channel blockers should be administered. If the ECG reveals ST segment elevations and chest pain is not relieved by medication, occlusion should be suspected and emergent repeat PTCA or CABG should be performed. After medication, if ST elevations return to baseline and pain subsides, spasm should be considered and medication continued. Since ST depressions on ECG indicate possible restenosis, urgent repeat PTCA should be performed. Pulmonary embolism should be considered if no cardiac source of chest pain is found. The usual source of pulmonary emboli after PTCA is the femoral vein puncture site. When pulmonary embolism is documented, systemic anticoagulation should be initiated. If no organic source of chest pain is found, anxiety is probably the cause and the patient should be reassured.

**Complications.** Complications associated with PTCA are similar to those of cardiac catheterization. Dye reaction, hypotension, bradycardia, blood loss, and hematoma may occur. Each of these can usually be treated effectively and results in minor morbidity. Other complications—such as coronary artery dissection, occlusion, spasm, embolism, perforation, or rupture—result from the angioplasty procedure. An ischemic event, such as MI or prolonged angina, also may occur during PTCA.

Major complications such as MI, emergency surgery, and in-hospital death occurs in 5% to 10% of patients. Minor complications include prolonged angina, bradycardia, transient ventricular dysrhythmias, or excessive blood loss.[93,94]

Restenosis is a significant long-term complication as-

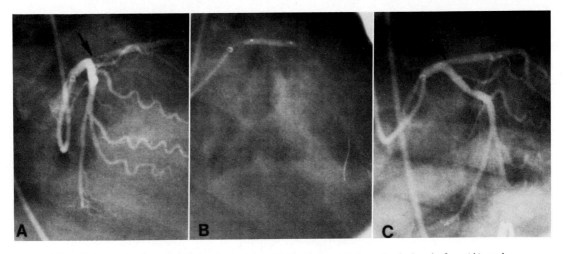

**Fig. 7-9** Coronary arteriograms during PTCA. Arrows denote the lesion before (**A**) and after (**C**) dilatation. **B,** The balloon inflated within the lesion. (Courtesy of Dr. Richard Stack, Duke University Medical Center.)

sociated with PTCA. It is defined as greater than 30% in the narrowing of the stenotic site at follow-up angiography or a 50% reduction in luminal diameter when compared with the initial improvement obtained at angioplasty.[95] Restenosis occurs in approximately 25% to 30% of patients, but a wide range (13% to 47%) has been reported.[95-97] Restenosis can only be documented by coronary arteriography, but recurrence of symptoms after PTCA may suggest restenosis.[95] Most coronary restenosis after successful PTCA occurs in the first 6 to 8 months after the procedure.[91] A repeat PTCA usually results in the same or improved success rate as the first procedure.[98]

Several antiplatelet agents are used routinely to help prevent restenosis, although their effectiveness has not yet been documented. Aspirin alone or in combination with dipyridamole is frequently used to reduce platelet adhesion to the endothelium of the dilated coronary vessel.

Because acute closure and restenosis affect approximately 30% of the patients who have undergone PTCA, current research is focused on alleviating these problems. Techniques under investigation include intracoronary stents, atherectomy devices, and laser angioplasty.

Intracoronary stents are metal coil or tubular mesh devices that are placed in the area of the coronary lesion to keep the vessel open. The stents are either self-expanding or balloon expandable. Anticoagulation is required to prevent thrombus formation. Currently, four types of stents are undergoing clinical investigations.[99,100]

Atherectomy and rotational devices have been developed to leave a smoother intraarterial surface. The directional atherectomy device and the transluminal extraction device physically remove plaque from the inside of the vessel, thereby improving blood flow.[101]

Laser angioplasty works by vaporizing solid matter, such as an atheromatous plaque, to gas. The continuous wave or pulsed wave laser energy is transmitted through a flexible, fiberoptic catheter. Lasers currently under investigation include the argon, Nd:YAG (neodymium:yttrium-aluminum-garnet), excimer, and pulsed dye systems.[101-103]

**Complications.** A pericardial rub is heard in about 25% of patients with transmural infarction, usually on the third to fifth day. Within 1 to 4 weeks after infarction, pericarditis with effusion and fever develop in about 2% to 5% of patients. This is known as *Dressler's syndrome* and is thought to result from an autoimmune response. Pericarditis, early or late, is generally treated symptomatically. Use of aspirin, indomethacin, or even steroids may be required; anticoagulation should be discontinued unless there is an overriding reason to continue its use, such as an overt pulmonary embolus. Pulsus paradoxus is evaluated to detect early signs of potential cardiac tamponade.

Prolongation of the PR interval and Wenckebach cycles are common after posterior and inferior infarctions. They usually regress or can be treated with atropine. Third degree AV block and conditions associated with a high incidence of progression to complete block, for example, Mobitz type II second-degree block or new bifascicular bundle branch block, especially associated with PR prolongation, are regarded as indications for insertion of a temporary transvenous pacemaker. Use of the pacemaker is then determined primarily by the ventricular rate and the patient's hemodynamic response. (See Chapter 11.)

### Heart Failure

Heart failure may be defined as a state in which the cardiac output is insufficient to meet the metabolic needs of the body. It can occur when the cardiac output is normal, increased, or decreased. In most cases, patients with heart failure have a decreased cardiac output. Congestive failure is manifested by retention of fluid and the formation of edema. Low output failure occurs when the heart is unable to meet the metabolic demands of tissues, even if they are normal. A number of cardiac disorders can result in low output failure. For example, MI affecting a large area of the left ventricle or stenosis or insufficiency of the cardiac valves can impair the heart's ability to pump. Constrictive pericarditis or pericardial effusion can restrict the ability of the heart to fill and empty.

Less commonly, heart failure occurs when peripheral demands exceed even the capacity of a normal heart to adequately perfuse the tissues. This is called *high output failure* and can occur in severe anemia, sepsis, thyrotoxicosis, and in patients who have arteriovenous fistulas.

The usual defect in heart failure is a decrease in the pumping ability of the heart. Patients with early or mild heart disease may show no significant abnormalities at rest because of reserve in cardiac function. Despite a normal cardiac output at rest, cardiac output with exercise is subnormal, and the patient shows a decreased exercise tolerance.

The factors that affect cardiac output are preload, afterload, heart rate, and contractility. Preload is defined as the amount of blood delivered to the ventricles during diastole (venous return). Afterload is the force the heart pumps against (systemic vascular resistance). Contractility is the force of contraction of the heart (see Chapter 1). As the heart begins to fail, a large number of compensatory mechanisms are set in motion in an effort to maintain cardiac output at a level that is adequate to meet the metabolic needs of the body. Most of these mechanisms are the same as those used by normal persons during exercise or during periods of increased stress. The principal initial adjustments are a reflex increase in sympathetic nerve discharge and a decrease in parasympathetic activity. These autonomic alterations, affecting the heart, arteries and veins, result in the increase of systemic vascular resistance and arterial pressure (afterload). Venous tone increases, which in turn increases venous pressure and helps maintain venous return (preload).

An increase in heart rate (tachycardia) by itself may increase cardiac output. Above a certain rate, however, cardiac output may begin to decrease. This rate is about 170 to 180 beats/min for most normal young individuals. In trained athletes the rate may be 200 to 220, whereas in patients with myocardial disease the rate limit may be 120 to 140. A decrease in cardiac output above a certain heart rate is caused by a shortening of diastole, which limits the time for adequate filling of the ventricles and for coronary blood flow. Slow heart rates allow more complete diastolic filling.

When cardiac output falls for whatever reason, the kidney retains salt and water as an early compensatory mechanism. This is caused in part by sympathetic stimulation, which produces renal vasoconstriction and a reduction in renal blood flow. Sympathetically mediated activation of the renin-angiotensin system triggers aldosterone release and causes more sodium retention. Expansion of the intravascular blood volume results in increases in the end-diastolic volume and pressure and ultimately in leaking of fluid from the vascular bed and edema formation (Table 7-2).

A major long-term hemodynamic adjustment to heart failure is ventricular hypertrophy. This is thought to be caused by a chronic increase in the systolic force or tension developed by the myocardial fibers. Although the contractility of hypertrophied myocardium is lower than normal for each unit of muscle and is associated with an imbalance between energy production and energy usage, the hypertrophied myocardium may maintain compensation because the total mass of myocardium is increased. If the pumping capacity (contractility) of the ventricle is restored by hypertrophy, tachycardia and edema may no longer be present.

## TABLE 7-2  Edema formation

| Organ | Edema | Description |
| --- | --- | --- |
| Skin | Dependent edema, pitting type | Increased venous pressure forces fluid through capillary walls into subcutaneous tissues; in ambulatory patients edema localized in dependent parts of body (hands and feet); patients in bed may lose edema of legs and feet, have it only in presacral region |
| Liver | Hepatomegaly | Increased pressure in hepatic veins causes accumulation of fluid in liver, which becomes enlarged and tender |
| Pleural cavity | Pleural effusion; hydrothorax | Venous congestion forces fluid into pleural cavity |
| Pericardial cavity | Pericardial effusion | Fluid accumulation in pericardial cavity |

## Left Ventricular Failure

The heart is really comprised of two pumps in series, the right ventricle and the left ventricle. Certain events may alter the function of one of these pumps without affecting the other. In acute myocardial infarction, for example, the primary insult is usually to the left ventricle. When the ability of the left ventricle to pump blood is compromised without compromise to the right ventricle, a temporary imbalance in the output of the two sides of the heart results. The right side of the heart continues to pump blood into the lungs. At the same time, the left side of the heart is unable to move the blood adequately into the systemic circulation.

The blood backs up into the left atrium and the pulmonary vessels and increases the pressure in the left side of the heart and the pulmonary vessels. Consequently, one of the first symptoms associated with acute left ventricular failure is dyspnea. If dyspnea occurs when the patient is recumbent, it is called orthopnea and is usually relieved by sitting up. Dyspnea is the symptomatic manifestation of increased work of breathing related to pulmonary venous engorgement and increased pulmonary blood volume.

Paroxysmal nocturnal dyspnea, which is a form of acute pulmonary edema, is almost a specific sign of left ventricular failure. The patient awakens suddenly at night, extremely breathless, and seeks relief by sitting up or running to an open window for fresh air. When the patient goes to sleep, the metabolic needs of the body may decrease. As a result, the cardiac output that had previously been inadequate may now be adequate to supply the body's needs. Fluid that had been pocketed away is mobilized into the vascular system, thus increasing the blood volume. The blood volume and a redistribution of this volume to the lungs resulting from the recumbent position are major factors in causing nocturnal dyspnea.

As the heart's compensatory mechanisms fail, the already-elevated diastolic filling pressure and left atrial pressure continue to increase. To maintain flow, the pressure in the pulmonary veins and capillaries exceeds the intravascular osmotic pressure (approximately 30 mm Hg), and fluid rapidly leaks into the interstitial regions of the lung tissue. Pulmonary edema greatly reduces the amount of lung tissue available for the exchange of gases and consequently results in a dramatic clinical presentation characterized by extreme dyspnea, cyanosis, and severe anxiety. This is called *acute pulmonary edema* and is considered a medical emergency.

In the early stages of pulmonary edema, the patient appears anxious, restless, or vaguely uneasy. Wheezing, orthopnea, diaphoresis, and pallor appear as left ventricular failure progresses. A third heart sound may be heard as the distensibility of the ventricle decreases. Sinus tachycardia and increased systemic arterial pressure are common as neural reflexes attempt to correct the imbalance. If these physiologic compensations fail, hypotension may occur,

rales develop from alveolar edema, and copious blood-tinged, frothy sputum is expectorated. As the accumulation of pulmonary interstitial and intraalveolar fluid progresses, arterial hypoxemia and cyanosis occur in varying degrees. Arterial blood gases may show the presence of hypoxia with a drop in the $_pO_2$. The chest x-ray typically shows mottling from the hilar regions, which may cover both lung fields. With the elevation of the pulmonary venous pressure, diffuse interstitial edema results and is seen as cloudy lung fields. In severe pulmonary edema, Kerley-B lines appear and possibly a total "white out" of the lung fields. This deterioration in pulmonary function is reflected in the patient's mental status. Anxiety progresses to mental confusion and eventually to stupor and coma. The patient is literally drowning in his own secretions. See Table 7-3 for treatment of acute pulmonary edema.

## Right Ventricular Failure

Usually right ventricular failure follows left ventricular failure. Right heart failure without left heart failure may be caused by pulmonary hypertension secondary to lung disease or recurrent pulmonary emboli and is referred to as *cor pulmonale*. In either case, pulmonary hypertension presents an increased resistance to right ventricular ejection and a resulting increase of right ventricular end-diastolic and right atrial pressures. This impedes venous return. Clinical manifestations include: (1) distention of the neck veins, which appear full even when the head is raised (normally these empty when the head is elevated to a 45-degree angle), (2) a distended and often tender liver, and (3) peripheral edema (Table 7-2). When the accumulation of fluid becomes extensive and generalized, the patient is said to have anasarca. Other consequences of congestive heart failure include pleural effusions, ascites jaundice caused by hepatic engorgement, and ultimately cardiac cachexia.

**Treatment of heart failure.** Treatment of patients with heart failure requires an understanding of the condition(s) that lead to this clinical state and of the mechanisms that produce congestion.

When heart failure results from certain specific mechanical problems such as aortic or mitral valve stenosis or insufficiency, persistent uncontrolled dysrhythmias, severe anemia, hypertension, or a congenital cardiac lesion, therapy is directed at correcting the cause. It is important to recognize that regardless of the cause of heart disease, infections, dysrhythmias, anemia, thyrotoxicosis, and pregnancy may each place a sufficient added burden on the heart to precipitate heart failure. Thus appropriate treatment of these conditions may convert a patient with heart disease from a decompensated to a compensated state.

Heart failure has previously been defined as a condition in which the cardiac output is not sufficient to meet the metabolic demands of the body. Essentially all of the situations that aggravate heart failure do so by increasing the metabolic demands on a heart that is not capable of re-

TABLE 7-3   Treatment of acute pulmonary edema

| Therapy | Principle | Precaution |
|---|---|---|
| Supplemental oxygen by face mask, nasal cannula, or, rarely, intermittent positive pressure breathing (IPPB) or continuous positive airway pressure (CPAP) | Supplemental oxygen raises $p_{O_2}$ levels | Patient may not be able to tolerate a face mask; always administer oxygen with humidification to avoid airway drying; IPPB and CPAP may increase the patient's work of breathing and anxiety level |
| Place patient in high Fowler's position | Sitting up increases lung volume and vital capacity, and decreases venous return and work of breathing | In presence of hypotension, Fowler's position is avoided or used cautiously |
| Morphine sulfate intravenously | Morphine decreases anxiety, respiratory rate, and venous return (preload) | May cause respiratory depression; contraindicated in the presence of severe pulmonary disease |
| Preload reduction: vasodilators may be used to reduce preload; nitroglycerin is usually the drug of choice; sodium nitroprusside may be used if the patient is extremely hypertensive | Nitroglycerin and sodium nitroprusside cause venous vasodilatation and reduce preload and afterload; nitroglycerin has a more pronounced effect on the venous system | Monitor blood pressure closely; hypotension and reflex tachydysrhythmias may occur |
| Tourniquets (tight enough to occlude venous return but not impair arterial pressure) may be applied to three extremities and rotated every 15 minutes | Tourniquets cause pooling of blood in the extremities, decreasing venous return | Prolonged constriction of extremities causes pain and loss of function; release tourniquets, one at a time, at 15 minute intervals |
| Decrease intravascular volume: diuretics such as furosemide, ethacrynic acid, or bumetanide are used; phlebotomy of 300 to 500 ml | A decrease in intravascular volume improves ability of lungs to exchange gases and decreases cardiac work | Monitor blood pressure and intake and output; diuretics can cause volume and electrolyte depletion |
| Aminophylline, intravenously, for bronchospasm caused by bronchiolar congestion | Aminophylline dilates bronchioles and is a venous vasodilator | May cause tachydysrhythmias, nausea, vomiting, headache, and hypotension |

sponding with an adequate ouput. A favorable response in patients with heart failure often can be obtained by rest. Defining the level of physical activity that a patient can tolerate without precipitating failure is a major objective of subsequent follow-up and treatment.

In addition to prescribing rest and defining the level of physical activity a patient can tolerate, a second focus of therapy is improving cardiac performance and cardiac output. Obviously if tight aortic stenosis or another structural defect is present, surgery is indicated. On the other hand, digitalis, which increases the contractility of heart muscle, has a favorable effect on cardiac performance and output. In most instances of heart failure it is used routinely with beneficial results. In acute MI with heart failure, the evidence of benefit from digitalis is minimal. Furthermore, because of a potentially increased sensitivity to toxic manifestations of digitalis excess, its use in this situation is still controversial.

In patients with a severely decompensated congestive heart, the renin-angiotensin system is activated, resulting in the maintenance of elevated systemic vascular resistance (afterload). Captopril inhibits this renin-angiotensin mechanism, reducing afterload and resulting in clinical improvement of congestive heart failure.[104] Vasodilator agents are an important addition to the treatment of heart failure. This class of agents includes nitrates, nitroprusside, hydralazine, minoxidil, and prazosin.[105,106] Some are designed for intravenous use and some for oral use. Some act predominantly on the arterial system, and others exert significant actions on veins as well. The principle for using these agents is to reduce arterial resistance (afterload) which is accompanied by an increase in cardiac output, a decrease in left atrial and pulmonary venous pressure, and a decrease in left ventricular end-diastolic volume (preload) and pressure. These agents have proven very useful in the treatment of acute heart failure in MI, in heart failure associated with severe mitral insufficiency, and in chronic heart failure caused by myocardial disease. The benefits of vasodilator therapy are greatest when left atrial and pulmonary pressures are elevated. Vasodilators are not useful and may even be detrimental in patients with a normal or reduced left ventricular filling pressure.

Two additional agents used in the treatment of congestive heart failure are melrinone and amrinone. These are nonadrenergic, nonglycoside agents with combined positive inotropic and vasodilating properties. Intravenous amrinone causes an increase in cardiac output and a decrease in the pulmonary capillary wedge pressure, right atrial pressure, and systemic vascular resistance. Subsequently, the myocardial oxygen consumption rate is also decreased. No major change in the blood pressure or heart rate is observed. Amrinone has been comparable to dobutamine and dopamine as inotropic therapy in heart failure.[107-109] Melrinone has shown similar results in the treatment of congestive heart failure.[110]

The third focus in the treatment of patients with heart failure is achieving and maintaining an appropriate blood volume. As noted before, several compensatory mechanisms invoked when cardiac output is insufficient affect sodium and water balance by the kidney. The net effect of these influences is sodium (and water) retention and a diminished ability to excrete a sodium load. A normal sodium intake of 5 g to 8 g/day cannot be tolerated by most patients with heart failure and should be reduced to 2 g/day or even less. Diuretics promote the excretion of sodium and hence water by the kidneys through one or more of several specific actions. Thiazide diuretics inhibit sodium transport primarily in the distal or cortical segment of the nephron. Loop diuretics such as ethacrynic acid and furosemide are very potent and act on both the cortical and medullary segments of the nephron. Spironolactone is a diuretic that specifically antagonizes the effect of aldosterone on the collecting duct. Triamterene has an action on sodium transport identical to spironolactone, but its action is not dependent on blocking aldosterone. In general thiazides and loop diuretics also cause potassium loss, whereas spironolactone and triamterene do not. These agents vary in potency but with appropriate selection and dosage can promote a diuresis in patients with edema caused by heart failure and with chronic use can diminish the tendency of patients with heart failure to retain salt and water.

Mild to moderate heart failure in patients with acute infarction is usually managed successfully with limitation of physical activity, oxygen, morphine, careful attention to fluid balance with optimization of pulmonary artery wedge pressure, and the use of vasodilators and diuretics when indicated.

## Cardiogenic Shock

When oxygen and other nutrients become unavailable to the cells of the body, shock may occur. Shock is a descriptive term denoting a clinical picture that develops in the presence of inadequate tissue perfusion. Cardiogenic shock is defined as shock caused by decreased cardiac output. Acute MI is the most common cause of cardiogenic shock. Other causes of cardiogenic shock include acute valvular insufficiency, dysrhythmias and cardiac tamponade. It can also occur with tension pneumothorax, pulmonary embolism, and open heart surgery. It occurs in about 15% of patients hospitalized with acute MI. The clinical picture is characterized by (1) a systolic blood pressure of less than 90 mm Hg or at least 30 mm Hg lower than the prior basal level and (2) signs of impaired tissue perfusion such as pallor, cyanosis of varying degrees, cool clammy skin, mental confusion or obtundation, and a urine output of less than 20 ml/hr. Cardiogenic shock caused by acute MI is thought to evolve over a period of hours or days as more and more myocardium becomes necrosed.[113] With conservative management, the mortality rate is 80% to 90%.[114] Reperfusion therapy and aggressive treatment of heart failure are recommended.[113,114]

Cardiogenic shock occurs in three stages. In the first stage, compensated hypotension, the body tries to compensate for the fall in cardiac output by increasing the rate and force of contraction of the heart. Constriction of peripheral blood vessels occurs, resulting in shunting of blood to the brain, heart, and kidneys. The second stage of cardiogenic shock, uncompensated hypotension, occurs when these compensatory mechanisms fail. The body cannot maintain an adequate arterial blood pressure or perfusion of vital organs, and cardiac, cerebral, and renal ischemia occur. Further vasoconstriction and hypoperfusion occur, leading to tissue hypoxia and metabolic acidosis. Unless the shock can be reversed, the third and irreversible stage of cardiogenic shock occurs: microcirculatory failure and cellular membrane injury. This results in irreversible organ damage and death.[112]

It is important to quickly and accurately diagnose cardiogenic shock and institute appropriate therapy to reverse this process. Hemodynamic monitoring is useful, not only in the diagnosis of cardiogenic shock but also as a means of assessing the effectiveness of treatment.

**Hemodynamic assessment.** Most coronary care units have developed means of measuring hemodynamic status by the bedside without increasing risk or discomfort for the patient. With the aid of fluoroscopy or a pressure recorder or both, a balloon-tipped, flow-directed catheter is inserted into the subclavian or brachial vein and directed into the right ventricle and pulmonary artery (Fig. 7-10, A and B). A multipurpose flow-directed pulmonary arterial catheter permits monitoring of the pulmonary arterial pressure, pulmonary capillary wedge pressure, central venous pressure, and cardiac output. In addition, the standard thermistor catheter can be modified to include electrodes for atrial, ventricular, and atrioventricular sequential pacing and for recording intraatrial and intraventricular ECGs.

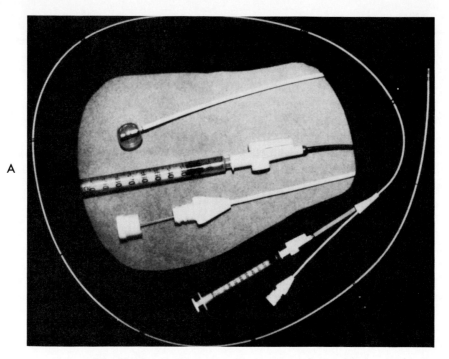

**Fig. 7-10** A, The Swan-Ganz flow-directed catheter.

**Pulmonary artery (PA) pressure.** The pulmonary artery waveform evidences a sharp rise during ejection of blood from the right ventricle after the pulmonary valve opens. This pressure rise is followed by a slow decrease in pressure during the ejection of blood from the right ventricle until the pulmonic valve closes, indicated by the dicrotic notch. The pressure continues to decrease until systole occurs again.

Normal PA systolic pressure is 20 to 30 mm Hg, and normal PA diastolic pressure ranges from 5 to 16 mm Hg. The normal mean PA pressure ranges from 10 to 20 mm Hg. The PA systolic pressure normally equals the right ventricular systolic pressure (Fig. 7-11). The pulmonary artery end-diastolic pressure (PAEDP) should be almost equal to the mean pulmonary capillary wedge pressure (PCWP) in the absence of pulmonary vascular disease.

Elevation of PA pressure may occur during (1) increased pulmonary blood flow, as in a left-to-right shunt resulting from atrial or ventricular septal defect, (2) increased pulmonary arteriolar resistance resulting from primary pulmonary hypertension or mitral stenosis, and (3) left ventricular failure resulting from any cause.

**Pulmonary capillary wedge pressure (PCWP).** Since there is normally a direct relationship among PAEDP, PCWP, and LVEDP, an elevated PAEDP or PCWP reflects the elevated LVEDP that occurs when the left ventricle can no longer adequately pump blood.

The PCWP reflects the elevated LVEDP that occurs when the left ventricle can no longer adequately pump blood.

The PCWP is normally 4 to 12 mm Hg. PCWP exceeding 12 mm Hg may occur as a result of left ventricular failure, mitral stenosis, or mitral insufficiency, in addition to other possible causes.

**Pulmonary artery end-diastolic pressure (PAEDP).** Since the PAEDP is approximately equal to the PCWP and because the PAEDP is an accurate reflection of LVEDP (Fig. 7-12), the PAEDP can be used as an alternative measurement of LVEDP in most patients, even in the presence of pulmonary venous hypertension. At the time of catheter insertion, the PAEDP can be compared with the PCWP. If the difference is less than 5 mm Hg, the PAEDP can be used as an accurate estimation of the LVEDP,[115] eliminating the need for wedging the catheter. A PAEDP or PCWP measurement of greater than 12 mm Hg is considered abnormal. The balloon-tipped catheter may also aid in establishing the cause of heart failure or shock, as well as in evaluating the effectiveness of the therapy. For example, in a state of hypotension caused by hypovolemia, infusing normal saline, whole blood, or low weight molecular dextran elevates the systemic pressure. In this case the PAEDP and PCWP, initially low, will return to normal when the blood volume has been restored. If the PAEDP is elevated because of heart failure, effective therapy should lower the pressure readings that were initially elevated.[116]

The use of the central venous pressure (CVP) to measure right atrial pressure (RAP) is no longer considered sufficiently accurate because the relationship between the RAP and LVEDP is inconsistent. Therefore PAEDP and

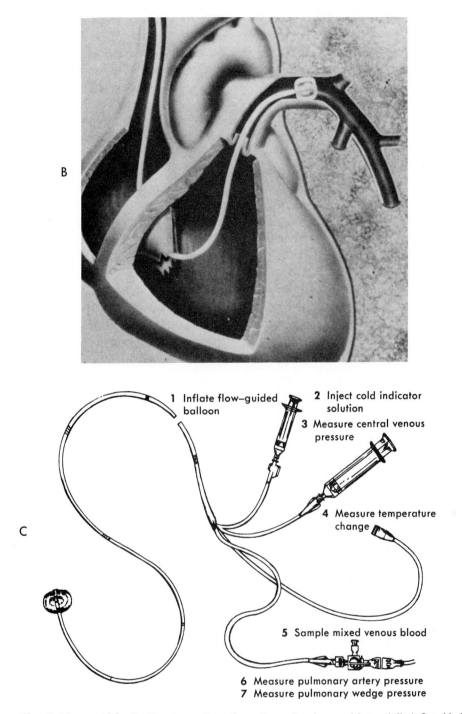

1 Inflate flow-guided balloon
2 Inject cold indicator solution
3 Measure central venous pressure
4 Measure temperature change
5 Sample mixed venous blood
6 Measure pulmonary artery pressure
7 Measure pulmonary wedge pressure

**Fig. 7-10, cont'd    B,** The Swan-Ganz flow-directed catheter with *partially inflated* balloon is passed through the superior vena cava and into the right atrium, where the balloon is then inflated to its maximum recommended capacity. Continued catheter advancement propels the balloon-tipped catheter into the right ventricle, pulmonary artery, and finally into the wedged position that is evidenced by a characteristic change in pressure waveform. **C,** The Swan-Ganz flow-directed thermodilution catheter. (**A** and **C** reproduced with permission of Edwards Laboratories, Division of American Hospital Supply Corp., Santa Ana, Calif.)

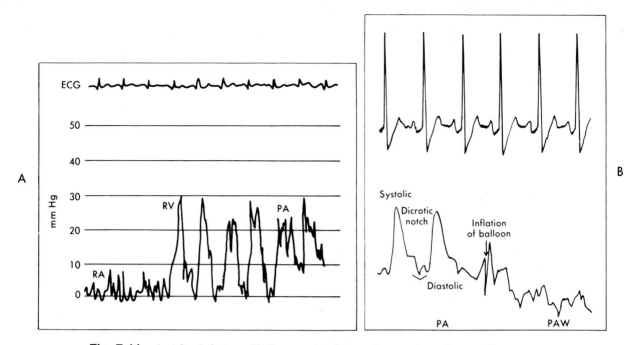

A

B

**Fig. 7-11** **A,** After inflation of balloon at tip of Swan-Ganz catheter, intracardiac pressure identifies right atrium *(RA)*, *right ventricle (RV)*, and pulmonary artery *(PA)* as catheter is advanced. Right ventricle is characterized by higher systolic but similar diastolic pressure value when compared with right atrial pressure. Pulmonary artery pressure shows same systolic value as that in right ventricle but diastolic pressure is higher than that in either right ventricle or atrium. Catheter whip or artifact is produced by exaggerated motion of catheter with inflated balloon and usually disappears with deflation of balloon. **B,** PA pressure waveform via balloon-tip catheter. Note balloon inflation and subsequent change to pulmonary artery wedge (PAW) waveform. (**A,** modified from Rackley CW and Russell R: Invasive techniques for hemodynamic monitoring, Dallas, 1973, by permission of the American Heart Association. **B,** modified from Daily EK and Schroeder JS: Techniques in bedside hemodynamic monitoring, St Louis, 1976, Mosby–Year Book, Inc.)

PCWP, rather than CVP, should be used as major guides in the treatment of heart failure and shock.

As the clinical features of heart failure worsen, they are usually accompanied by an elevation of the PAEDP and PCWP, a drop in cardiac output, a drop in arterial and right atrial oxygen saturations, and a widening of the oxygen difference between arterial and venous blood samples, commonly referred to as the A-V oxygen difference. The drop in arterial oxygen tension is a sign of abnormal lung function and is thought to result, at least in part, from elevation of left atrial pressure. Changes in pulmonary function include (1) abnormalities of diffusion, particularly of oxygen, (2) a redistribution of pulmonary blood flow into the less well-ventilated upper lobes, and (3) intrapulmonary shunting. Not only is the arterial oxygen tension reduced in patients with acute infarction and shock, but it also fails to increase to expected values with the administration of oxygen, until pulmonary congestion has cleared.[117]

When right atrial oxygen saturation is reduced, a widened A-V oxygen difference and a low cardiac output can

be suspected. If arterial oxygen saturation remains at normal levels, reduced right atrial oxygen saturation reflects increased extraction of oxygen during the passage of blood from the arterial to the venous circulation. A widened A-V oxygen difference reflects this increased extraction and indicates a reduced cardiac output. Right atrial or pulmonary artery oxygen saturation can be useful indices of circulatory failure in patients with acute infarction. In addition to the bedside techniques for measuring pulmonary artery and pulmonary capillary wedge pressure, the simple test of determining whether the right atrial or pulmonary artery oxygen saturation is above or below 65% is a useful guide to therapy. The use of this variable is based on the Fick equation for measuring cardiac output (CO).

$$\text{Cardiac output} = \frac{\text{Oxygen consumption}}{\text{A-V oxygen difference}}$$

Most pulmonary artery catheters are equipped with a thermistor (temperature) electrode to measure cardiac output using the principle of thermodilution. The procedure involves the injection of cold or room temperature solution

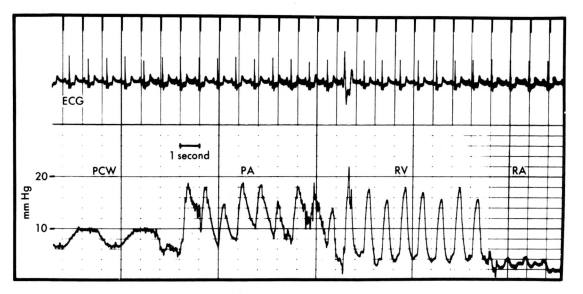

**Fig. 7-12**  Simultaneous recording of ECG and pulmonary capillary wedge *(PCW)*, pulmonary arterial *(PA)*, right ventricular *(RV)*, and right atrial *(RA)* pressures. The pulmonary arterial catheter was initially in a wedged position, with the balloon inflated. The balloon was then deflated, and the catheter was slowly withdrawn through the right heart chambers. Note the cyclic respiratory effects in the pressure signals. The PCW and PA end-diastolic pressures are equal. (From Mantle JA and others: Advances in the treatment of heart failure. In Rackley, CF, editor: Critical care cardiology: cardiovascular clinics, vol 11, No 3, Philadelphia, 1981, FA Davis Co.)

into the right atrium or superior vena cava.[118,119] The temperature change is perceived by the thermistor electrode in the pulmonary artery. Cardiac output is inversely proportional to the temperature change, that is, the greater the cardiac output the less the temperature change. The use of such a catheter facilitates measurement of the cardiac output and eliminates the need for a systemic arterial blood sample to determine cardiac output (Fig. 7-11, **C**). Normal cardiac chamber oxygen values are found in Fig. 7-13. Normal cardiac output is 4 to 8 L/min. However, in the assessment of cardiac performance, the cardiac index (CI)—which is the CO adjusted for body size and is calculated by dividing the cardiac output by the patient's body surface area (BSA)—is a more useful indicator. The BSA is calculated by obtaining the patient's height and weight and plotting them on a Dubois BSA chart. Normal cardiac index is 2.5 to 4.2 L/min/m². In cardiogenic shock, the cardiac index is below 2.2 L/min/m².[114]

**Measurement of PA pressure and PCWP.** The method used to record PA pressure and/or PCWP from the standard strain gauge pressure transducer differs among institutions. Special points to consider in maintaining the catheter and measuring pressures include the following:

A. Obtaining measurements
   1. Record pressures at regular intervals as specified by the physician and as necessary. Evaluate changes and report to the physician as appropriate.
   2. Calibrate equipment before each measurement.

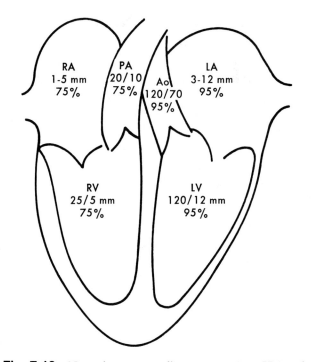

**Fig. 7-13**  Normal average cardiac pressures (mm Hg) and normal oxygen content (%) in each chamber.

3. Irrigate line before each measurement by pulling red rubber Intraflo plunger for 5 seconds (or manually if an Intraflo catheter is not used).

4. Measurements should be taken using the phlebostatic axis, which is located at the midaxillary line at the sixth intercostal space.

B. Maintaining the catheter
   1. Maintain patency of the catheter.
     a. Irrigate automatically with 3 ml of D5W or normosol and heparin solution per hour, using an Intraflo catheter and maintaining pressure bag at 300 mm Hg.
     b. Irrigate manually every hour by pulling the red rubber Intraflo plunger for 5 seconds.
     c. Measure irrigating solution used at the end of each shift as part of IV intake.
     d. Change the dressing as described in section on arterial catheters.
     e. Observe for signs of infection and/or phlebitis at the insertion site.
   2. Observe the complexes for changes in fluctuations.
     a. Flattened complex: a possible wedging of the catheter in a pulmonary arteriole, which could result in pulmonary infarction. Turn the patient and ask the patient to cough and take some deep breaths; this may dislodge a catheter stuck in a wedge position. The physician should be notified so that the catheter can be repositioned.
     b. Irregular complex: an irregular fluctuation with no clear pressure wave form, indicating the need for irrigation with a 10 ml syringe. If this complex continues, the catheter is probably of no value and should be removed.
     c. Unobtainable wedge pattern: when the balloon is inflated and no wedge pattern is noted. Either the balloon is ruptured or the catheter is out of position. The physician should be notified to reposition or remove the catheter.
     d. No complex: check all stopcocks for proper position and follow with recalibration if needed.

### Care of the Patient and Pulmonary Artery Equipment

1. Following insertion of the pulmonary artery catheter, apply a sterile dressing to the site and change it at least every 48 hours. Note the condition of the site, including presence of active bleeding and signs of infection.

2. Immobilize the extremity to prevent accidental dislodgement of the catheter. Tape the catheter to the extremity to stabilize the catheter. A padded armboard or wooden device promotes comfort and immobilizes the extremity.

3. Check the extremity for circulatory insufficiency and bleeding at least every hour.

4. Observe the catheter frequently for leakage and proper stopcock position. Care should be taken to return the stopcock to the off position when drawing blood from the catheter.

5. The balloon should always remain deflated with a syringe attached, except when the PCWP is being read.

6. After the catheter is removed, observe the site closely for bleeding and infection until healing is complete. Apply a sterile dressing to the site.

**Potential problems in use of pulmonary artery catheters.** There are several complications that may occur from the use of a pulmonary artery catheter. The major complication, pulmonary hemorrhage, may result if the balloon is inflated when the catheter tip is in a small arterial branch; however, careful adherence to proper procedures for balloon inflation will minimize this risk. The catheter tip may become wedged in a distal branch after repeated inflations, which may lead to a pulmonary infarction. When the catheter tip is withdrawn from the wedged position, it often recoils into the right ventricle or right atrium and must be repositioned.[115] There are particular changes in the PA waveform configuration that indicate that the catheter has slipped into the right ventricle (see Fig. 7-11, *A*). Other complications that are associated with pulmonary artery catheters include dysrhythmias, thrombosis, intracardiac knotting, ruptured balloon, valve damage, and infection.[120]

**Measuring arterial pressure.** In addition to hemodynamic monitoring, arterial pressure monitoring is useful for the continuous assessment of blood pressure, as well as rapid access for frequent blood specimens.

When monitoring arterial pressure directly, personnel must carefully observe the following precautions to obtain meaningful values:

1. Standardize, balance, and calibrate the monitoring equipment at least once every 8 hours and after position changes or movements that might alter the calibration. Instructions for this procedure accompany the individual manufacturer's equipment.

2. An Intraflo device provides continuous flushing with a prescribed flow rate of a solution of D5W or normosol with heparin. The catheter should be flushed manually to clear the line after blood is drawn or if blood is in the line for any reason. The pulse waveform will become dampened or flattened somewhat if impairment of flow occurs.

3. Prevent catheter displacement by fastening the arterial catheter securely to the skin. The catheter may be sutured to the skin after insertion.

4. Prevent blood from entering the transducer. Blood in the transducer will dampen the pressure reading and may damage the transducer.

5. Observe the extremity in which the catheter is inserted every 1 to 2 hours for bleeding and check for circulatory insufficiency by capillary refill, skin

temperature, and distal pulses. Check the arterial catheter frequently for leakage and proper stopcock position.

6. Apply a sterile dressing to the site, and change it at least once every 48 hours. Avoid the use of antimicrobial ointments at the insertion site. Povidone-iodine ointment at the insertion site is recommended to prevent infection. When a translucent dressing is applied, the dressing change can be done every 3 to 5 days unless conditions warrant more frequent changes.

7. Observe the site for infection when changing dressings. Should the catheter remain in the artery longer than 48 to 72 hours, observation of the site at least every 8 hours is imperative.

8. Immobilize the extremity to prevent accidental dislodgement of the catheter. If an armboard or wooden device is used, proper padding will prevent stasis changes of skin and increase comfort.

9. Exercise care when drawing blood from the catheter. The stopcock must be returned to the original position to ensure proper operation and prevent leakage.

10. After removing the catheter, apply direct pressure to the artery for 10 to 15 minutes or longer until bleeding ceases. The site should be covered with a sterile pressure dressing for 24 hours.

11. After the catheter is removed, observe the site for signs of bleeding, infection, and circulatory insufficiency until healing is complete. If any of these are noted, immediate attention should be given to correction of the condition.

**Treatment of shock.** The current term to describe the problem of patients in cardiogenic shock with or without congestive heart failure is *pump failure*. Most studies indicate a mortality rate of at least 80% in cardiogenic shock during the course of acute MI; unfortunately, current therapeutic measures have not affected these figures.

Although the primary therapeutic goals are to increase cardiac contractility and to maintain renal blood flow, there is no clear-cut regimen for the treatment of cardiogenic shock that can be applied to all patients since therapy depends on the specific findings in the individual patient. Therefore for the physician to direct treatment intelligently, as much clinical and hemodynamic information as possible should be available.

Therapy, as well as the natural evolution of the shock state, may change these values; therefore measurements should be repeated as often as necessary. Clinical management of the patient in cardiogenic shock is divided into general and specific measures as follows:

A. General therapeutic measures
  1. Have patient assume a supine position with a pillow. Trendelenburg position is not recommended for treating cardiogenic shock.

  2. Relieve pain with intravenous morphine doses (5 to 10 mg initially) just sufficient to be effective. Large doses of morphine sulfate should be avoided if possible. Observe for lowering of arterial pressure.

  3. Insert a Foley catheter to measure hourly urine output as an index of kidney function. Maintain urine output at a minimum of 20 ml/hour to prevent renal failure.

  4. Insert an intraarterial needle or catheter to monitor arterial blood pressure, blood gases, pH, cardiac output, A-V oxygen difference, and peripheral resistance.

  5. Insert a balloon-tipped flow-directed catheter to monitor PAEDP and PCWP as a reflection of left ventricular performance.

B. Specific therapeutic goals
  1. Correct dysrhythmias and establish appropriate heart rate. If the heart rate is above normal but not in the abnormal tachycardia range, no special therapy is necessary. If the rate is abnormally slow, the use of atropine in patients with MI may be considered. For the symptomatic (ventricular ectopic systoles, hypotension) patient with sinus bradycardia, atropine is clearly indicated. Also Isuprel in a continuous infusion may be indicated to increase heart rate. However, Isuprel may increase myocardial oxygen consumption. For the asymptomatic patient with sinus bradycardia, it would appear best not to administer atropine, but to monitor closely. When atropine is indicated, initial doses should be in the range of 0.4 to 0.6 mg IV, repeating with 0.2 to 0.4 mg if the initial dose does not produce the desired effect. If atropine does not raise the heart rate sufficiently to eliminate the symptoms accompanying the slower rate or if the cause of the low heart rate is complete heart block, then AV sequential pacing should be considered.

  2. Correct hypovolemia. Elderly patients with MI are prime candidates for relative hypovolemia, especially if they have been receiving diuretics or are on a low sodium diet. The acute stages of acute MI are associated with a reduced fluid intake because of pain, resulting from analgesic therapy, nausea, and vomiting. Further routes of fluid loss are profuse sweating, diarrhea secondary to medication, vigorous treatment with diuretics, and phlebotomy. Consequently, patients showing evidence of low cardiac output with hypotension and oliguria may be given a trial of fluid loading particularly if PAEDP and PCWP are low. Patients with evidence of severe pulmonary congestion are not suitable for this therapy. With low PAEDP and PCWP values, normal saline, blood products, or low molecular dextran may be infused until the PCWP reaches 15

to 18 mm Hg. Current experience indicates that PCWP should be kept slightly elevated in patients with cardiogenic shock.

3. Correct hypoxemia. Hypoxia with $PO_2$ values below the level of 70 to 75 mm Hg while the patient is receiving nasal oxygen indicates that the patient should probably be intubated and given positive pressure or volume assistance and 100% oxygen.

4. Correct acidosis. When circulatory impairment exists, the metabolic activity of the perfused cells of the body changes, and lactic acid and other metabolic products are released into the vascular system and ineffectively metabolized as a result of which systemic acidosis develops. This state contributes to poor tissue perfusion and is indicated by the blood pH. The complication is treated with intravenous sodium bicarbonate, taking precautions not to produce sodium overload.

5. Improve cardiac contractility. Use of digitalis in the management of cardiogenic shock is not well supported by existing data. Experimental studies show that the positive inotropic effect of digitalis preparations improves contractility but significantly increases myocardial oxygen demand.[121,122] Other agents that enhance the state of cardiac contractility have been employed in cardiogenic shock. In patients with adequate filling pressures and normal or increased peripheral resistance, dopamine hydrochloride, dobutamine, or amrinone can cause a significant increase in cardiac output. Dopamine has a strong inotropic effect and causes renal vasodilatation at low doses. Dobutamine increases contractility, stroke volume, and cardiac output, and decreases systemic vascular resistance.[123-125] Amrinone has no effect on blood pressure or heart rate but decreases PCWP, systemic resistance, and myocardial oxygen consumption ($MVO_2$).

6. Improve circulation. Clinical estimates of the degree of increased peripheral resistance usually present in the shock syndrome can be made from the degree of increased venous pressure, the amount of decrease in pulse pressure, the decrease in cutaneous blood flow with cold and cyanotic extremities, the poorly palpable peripheral pulses in spite of bounding pulsations, urine flow, and the clinical appearance of the patient. If these findings persist, a dangerously inappropriate prolonged period of peripheral vasoconstriction may exist. If the patient exhibits signs of the shock syndrome with a low or normal calculated peripheral resistance, an infusion of a drug with combined alpha and beta adrenergic properties may be considered. Norepinephrine (Levarterenol, Levophed) is used to increase arterial blood pressures and improve perfusion of ischemic areas of myocardium that are functionally depressed. The elevated pressure may open existing or latent coronary collateral channels, which require a relatively high pressure to maintain blood flow through them, bypassing concomitant areas of arterial atherosclerosis. Consequently this drug improves myocardial function and increases cardiac output. However, at the same time, it increases cardiac afterload (resistance against which the ventricle pumps) and thus myocardial oxygen consumption. Therefore the use of this agent should be aimed at producing the desired balance between coronary perfusion and afterload.

Vasodilators are used to decrease preload and afterload in patients with cardiogenic shock. A decrease in preload, caused by venous dilatation, causes a decrease in pulmonary congestive pressure and a decrease in myocardial oxygen consumption. A reduction in afterload improves left ventricular ejection and stroke volume. Commonly used vasodilators include nitroprusside and intravenous nitroglycerin. Current studies of these drugs show promise in patients with an increased pulmonary capillary wedge pressure and signs of left ventricular failure. They should not be used if arterial pressure is below 90 mm Hg unless they are used in conjunction with dopamine to maintain an adequate blood pressure.

**Intraaortic balloon pumping.** In addition to pharmacologic therapy, intraaortic balloon pumping (IABP), also referred to as *counterpulsation,* may be required to treat cardiogenic shock. IABP can improve cardiac output, reduce evidence of myocardial ischemia, relieve pain, and reduce ST segment elevation. Other indications for intraaortic balloon counterpulsation include severe congestive heart failure, medically refractory ischemia, ventricular septal defects, and left main coronary stenosis. In most instances, the intraaortic balloon pump provides additional protection for the myocardium until surgery can be done.

In this procedure the balloon is inserted percutaneously into the femoral artery and positioned in the descending aorta just below the origin of the left subclavian artery. The catheter is connected to a console that controls the inflation and deflation of the balloon with helium. The balloon is inflated and deflated in a cyclic fashion, according to the cardiac rhythm of the patient. An ECG and arterial waveform are used to time the inflations and deflations of the balloon. The balloon is inflated during diastole, increasing aortic diastolic pressure and coronary perfusion, and thus improving myocardial oxygen supply. Balloon inflation during diastole (and the resulting increased pressure) does not affect the left ventricle because the aortic valve is closed.[114] The intraaortic balloon is deflated during ventricular systole and thus partially empties the aorta. The effect is to decrease the resistance to ventricular ejection (afterload), allowing the left ventricle to eject blood with less effort. This decreases myocardial work and myocardial oxygen consumption.

Timing of the inflation and deflation of the balloon are correlated with the ECG and/or the arterial waveform. On the ECG, the R wave triggers balloon deflation. Inflation is triggered on the downslope of the T wave or a set time interval after the R wave. The arterial waveform may be used for manual adjustment or "fine tuning" of the balloon pump. Inflation should be adjusted first and should occur at the beginning of diastole, represented by the dicrotic notch on the arterial waveform. Deflation should occur at the very end of diastole or just prior to ventricular systole.[126] Pumping options on the balloon console range from 1:1 (every heartbeat is assisted) to 1:8 (every eighth beat is assisted). The usual therapeutic option is 1:1. Adjustment of timing should be done in the 1:2 mode (or greater) to allow comparison of an assisted beat to an unassisted beat. Timing should be assessed every hour and with any change in the patient's condition.

Complications of IABP therapy include arterial wall injury, compromise of peripheral circulation, bleeding, and infection.[127] Arterial wall injury may occur during insertion of the balloon or as a result of catheter dislodgement and migration. Compromise of the peripheral circulation may be caused by plaque dislodgement, thrombus formation, gas emboli, improper placement or migration of the balloon, or incorrectly timed counterpulsation.[127] It is important to assess pulses and temperature and sensation of extremities before and at least every hour after insertion of the balloon. The head of the bed should be elevated no more than 30 degrees. The affected leg should not be flexed. The patient should be turned every 2 hours by log-rolling technique. Anticoagulant therapy (usually heparin) is required to prevent thrombus formation. Close monitoring of PT, PTT, hemoglobin, hematocrit, and platelet levels is required, and the insertion site should be observed frequently for bleeding. The patient should be monitored for signs of internal bleeding such as tachycardia, hypotension, a drop in hemoglobin or hematocrit, and low back pain, which may be a sign of retroperitoneal bleeding. IABP therapy may cause stress ulcers to occur. For this reason, all stools and nasogastric drainage should be checked for occult blood. Antacids and/or histamine 2 antagonists may be used to neutralize or block the secretion of excess stomach acids. Strict attention to sterile technique is necessary to prevent infection in an already compromised patient. Dressings should be changed daily and as needed and the insertion site should be checked for redness, swelling, or drainage. The Foley catheter should be taped to the opposite leg to avoid contamination of the IABP insertion site.[127] The patient's temperature should be monitored every 4 hours. It is also important to provide emotional support to the patient and family. Clear, simple explanations of the equipment and procedures used in IABP therapy should be given and the patient and family should be provided with frequent updates on the patient's progress.

## Dysrhythmias

Dysrhythmias can compromise cardiac function by reducing cardiac output and coronary blood flow, increasing the myocardial need for oxygen, predisposing the patient to the development of more serious dysrhythmias, and complicating therapy. Therefore prompt prevention and control of dysrhythmias and the states predisposing to them (acidosis, electrolyte imbalance, early cardiac failure, pain, and anxiety) decrease the incidence of more serious dysrhythmias and should improve the chances for survival after MI. Awareness of these facts underscores the importance of detecting dysrhythmias through cardiac monitoring.

Dysrhythmias can be divided into two categories: acutely life-threatening and potentially life-threatening. Acutely life-threatening dysrhythmias include ventricular fibrillation, ventricular tachcardia without a pulse, and asystole. Potentially life-threatening dysrhythmias include ventricular tachycardia with a pulse and its precursors, supraventricular tachydysrhythmias and bradydysrhythmias. Because of the life-threatening nature of some dysrhythmias, it is necessary that the staff be certified in basic cardiac life support (BCLS) as defined by the American Heart Association or the American Red Cross. Personnel must also be trained to perform other procedures, including preparation of medication, recording times of events and medication given, and assisting as necessary with activities during the resuscitation effort.

Certification in the skills of advanced cardiac life support (ACLS) is also important for coronary care personnel. ACLS includes all the skills of basic cardiac life support in addition to the techniques of endotracheal intubation, venipuncture, dysrhythmia interpretation, and drug administration.

## Defibrillation and Cardioversion

Transthoracic defibrillation delivers electric energy to the heart by means of metal paddles placed on the intact chest or placed directly on the heart when the chest is opened, as during cardiac surgery. This procedure depolarizes the excitable myocardium, thereby interrupting reentrant circuits and discharging automatic pacemaker foci to establish electric homogeneity. Defibrillation successfully restores sinus rhythm if the sinus node becomes the first automatic focus to fire after the electric shock and thus controls the packing function of the heart.

By synchronizing the capacitor to discharge during the downslope of the R wave or with the S wave, the vulnerable period of the ventricle (an interval of 20 to 40 msecs near the apex of the T wave) may be avoided. This minimizes but does not completely eliminate the danger of precipitating ventricular fibrillation with the DC shock. Defibrillation with synchronization of the R wave is called *cardioversion*. However, if synchronization cannot be established rapidly and immediate defibrillation is indicated, the shock is delivered asynchronously. Immediate defibrillation using 200 joules is the mandatory treatment for ventricular fibrillation and ventricular tachycardia without a pulse. If defibrillation is unsuccessful, IV drug therapy should begin with epinephrine, followed by lidocaine, procainamide, or bretylium tosylate.[128]

However, if the tachydysrhythmia does not terminate promptly, imediate defibrillation should be performed us-

ing 200 to 300 joules. If this is unsuccessful, a third shock is delivered using 360 joules. Short, limited bursts of ventricular tachycardia are treated medically. As a general rule any supraventricular tachydysrhythmia that produces signs or symptoms, such as hypotension, angina, or congestive heart failure, and does not respond promptly to medical therapy should be terminated electrically. Cardiopulmo-

**VENTRICULAR FIBRILLATION and
PULSELESS VENTRICULAR TACHYCARDIA**

Witnessed Arrest
↓
Check Pulse—If No Pulse
↓
Precordial Thump
↓
Check Pulse—If No Pulse

Unwitnessed Arrest
↓
Check Pulse—If No Pulse

CPR Until a Defibrillator Is Available
↓
Check Monitor for Rhythm—if VF or VT
↓
Defibrillate, 200 Joules*
↓
Defibrillate, 200-300 Joules*
↓
Defibrillate With up to 360 Joules*
↓
CPR If No Pulse
↓
Establish IV Access
↓
Epinephrine, 1:10,000, 0.5-1.0 mg IV Push†
↓
Intubate If Possible‡
↓
Defibrillate With up to 360 Joules*
↓
Lidocaine, 1 mg/kg IV Push
↓
Defibrillate With up to 360 Joules*
↓
Bretylium, 5 mg/kg IV Push§
↓
(Consider Bicarbonate)‖
↓
Defibrillate With up to 360 Joules*
↓
Bretylium, 10 mg/kg IV Push§
↓
Defibrillate With up to 360 Joules*
↓
Repeat Lidocaine or Bretylium
↓
Defibrillate With up to 360 Joules*

This sequence was developed to assist in teaching how to treat a broad range of patients with VF or pulseless VT. Some patients may require care not specified herein. This algorithm should not be construed as prohibiting such flexibility. The flow of the algorithm presumes that VF is continuing.
*Check pulse and rhythm after each shock. If VF recurs after transiently converting (rather than persists without ever converting), use whatever energy level has previously been successful for defibrillation.
†Epinephrine should be repeated every 5 minutes.
‡Intubation is preferable. If it can be accomplished simultaneously with other techniques, then the earlier the better. However, defibrillation and epinephrine are more important initially if the patient can be ventilated without intubation.
§Some may prefer repeated doses of lidocaine, which may be given in 0.5 mg/kg boluses every 8 minutes to a total dosage of 3 mg/kg.
‖The value of sodium bicarbonate is questionable during cardiac arrest, and it is not recommended for the routine cardiac arrest sequence. Consideration of its use in a dose of 1 mEq/kg is appropriate at this point. One half of the original dose may be repeated every 10 minutes if it is used.

**Fig. 7-14**  ACLS algorithms. (Reprinted with permission of American Heart Association, Dallas, TX.)

nary resuscitation (CPR) is performed during this period as indicated by patient condition. See ACLS algorithms for ventricular tachycardia and fibrillation (Fig. 7-14).

An elective cardioversion may be done wherever resuscitative aids, such as suction, intubation equipment, medications, and experienced personnel trained in airway management, are available. The cardioversion procedure is listed below.

1. Explain the procedure to the patient and obtain written *informed* consent.
2. Withhold diuretecs and short-acting digitalis preparations for 24 to 36 hours. However, it has been suggested that discontinuing digitalis in nontoxic, normokalemic patients may not be necessary. If indicated, obtain a serum potassium or serum digitalis level. Hypokalemia enhances electric instability and may in-

## ASYSTOLE (Cardiac Standstill)

If Rhythm Is Unclear and Possibly Low Amplitude Ventricular Fibrillation, Defibrillate as for VF. If Asystole is Present
↓
Continue CPR
↓
Establish IV Access
↓
Epinephrine, 1:10,000, 0.5-1.0 mg IV Push*
↓
Intubate When Possible†
↓
Atropine, 1.0 mg IV Push (Repeated in 5 min)
↓
(Consider Bicarbonate)‡
↓
Consider Pacing

This sequence was developed to assist in teaching how to treat a broad range of patients with asystole. Some patients may require care not specified herein. This algorithm should not be construed to prohibit such flexibility. The flow of the algorithm presumes asystole is continuing.
*Epinephrine should be repeated every 5 minutes.
†Intubation is preferable; if it can be accomplished simultaneously with other techniques, then the earlier the better. However, CPR and the use of epinephrine are more important initially if the patient can be ventilated without intubation. (Endotracheal epinephrine may be used.)
‡The value of sodium bicarbonate is questionable during cardiac arrest, and it is not recommended for the routine cardiac arrest sequence. Consideration of its use in a dose of 1 mEq/kg is appropriate at this point. One half of the original dose may be repeated every 10 minutes if it is used.

## ELECTROMECHANICAL DISSOCIATION

Continue CPR
↓
Establish IV Access
↓
Epinephrine, 1:10,000, 0.5-1.0 mg IV Push*
↓
Intubate When Possible†
↓
(Consider Bicarbonate)‡
↓
Consider Hypovolemia,
Cardiac Tamponade,
Tension Pneumothorax,
Hypoxemia,
Acidosis,
Pulmonary Embolism

This sequence was developed to assist in teaching how to treat a broad range of patients with EMD. Some patients may require care not specified herein. This algorithm should not be construed to prohibit such flexibility. The flow of the algorithm presumes that EMD is continuing.
*Epinephrine should be repeated every 5 minutes.
†Intubation is preferable; if it can be accomplished simultaneously with other techniques, then the earlier the better. However, epinephrine is more important initially if the patient can be ventilated without intubation.
‡The value of sodium bicarbonate is questionable during cardiac arrest, and it is not recommended for the routine cardiac arrest sequence. Consideration of its use in a dose of 1 mEq/kg is appropriate at this point. One half of the original dose may be repeated every 10 minutes if it is used.

**Fig. 7-14, cont'd** ACLS algorithms.

*Continued.*

crease the likelihood of dysrhythmias after cardioversion.[129]

3. Withhold food and drink for 6 to 8 hours before cardioversion.

4. Perform a thorough physical examination, including vital signs, mentation, and palpation of pulse

5. Obtain a 12-lead ECG before and after cardioversion, as well as a rhythm strip or oscilloscopic monitoring (or both) during procedure.

6. Maintain a patent IV access.

7. If the patient has dentures, remove them.

8. Allow the patient to breathe oxygen for 5 to 15 minutes before and then immediately after DC shock if not contraindicated; this promotes myocardial oxygenation. During cardioversion the presence of oxygen with electric arcing may encourage combustion.

9. Employ the synchronous discharge mode on the difibrillator/cardioverter. The QRS complex recorded on the oscilloscope must be tall to ensure that it alone triggers the capacitor discharge. Determine the accuracy of synchronization by discharging several test shocks before applying the paddles to the patient.

10. Administer diazepam or other medication (such as methohexital [Brevital] or misonidazole [Versed]) prescribed to produce transient amnesia or light sleep.

11. Apply electrode paste liberally but not excessively to the polished surface of the paddles (or use gel defibrillation pads), and then place them in firm contact with the chest wall at points distant from the monitoring electrodes. The paddles may be positioned (1) anterioposteriorly in the left infrascapular region and over the upper sternum at the third interspace, or (2) anteriorly to the right of the sternum at the second intercostal space and in the left midclavicular line at the fifth intercostal space.

12. Employing the minimum effective electric energy level

## SUSTAINED VENTRICULAR TACHYCARDIA

| No Pulse | Pulse Present |
|---|---|
| ↓ | |
| Treat as VF | |

Pulse Present branches into Stable* and Unstable†*

**Stable***
↓
O₂
↓
IV Access
↓
Lidocaine, 1 mg/kg
↓
Lidocaine, 0.5 mg/kg Every 8 min
Until VT Resolves, or
up to 3 mg/kg
↓
Procainamide, 20 mg/min
Until VT Resolves,
or up to 1000 mg
↓
Cardiovert as in
Unstable Patients‡

**Unstable†***
↓
O₂
↓
IV Access
↓
(Consider Sedation)†
↓
Cardiovert 50 Joules§‖
↓
Cardiovert 100 Joules§
↓
Cardiovert 200 Joules§
↓
Cardiovert With up to
360 Joules§
↓
If Recurrent, Add Lidocaine
and Cardiovert Again Starting
at Energy Level
Previously Successful; Then
Procainamide or Bretylium¶

This sequence was developed to assist in teaching how to treat a broad range of patients with sustained VT. Some patients may require care not specified herein. This algorithm should not be construed as prohibiting such flexibility. The flow of the algorithm presumes that VT is continuing.
*If the patient becomes unstable (see Footnote † for definition) at any time, move to the "Unstable" arm of the algorithm.
†Unstable = symptoms (e.g., chest pain, dyspnea), hypotension (systolic <90 mm Hg), congestive heart failure, ischemia, or infarction.
‡Sedation should be considered for all patients, including those defined in Footnote † as unstable, except those who are hemodynamically unstable (e.g., hypotensive, in pulmonary edema, or unconscious).
§If hypotension, pulmonary edema, or unconsciousness is present, unsynchronized cardioversion should be done to avoid delay associated with synchronization.
‖In the absence of hypotension, pulmonary edema, or unconsciousness, a precordial thump may be employed prior to cardioversion.
¶Once VT has resolved, begin an IV infusion of the antidysrhythmic agent that has aided resolution of the VT. If hypotensive, in pulmonary edema, or unconscious, use lidocaine if cardioversion alone is unsuccessful, followed by bretylium. In all other patients, the recommended order of therapy is lidocaine, procainamide, and then bretylium.

**Fig. 7-14, cont'd**   ACLS algorithms.

**BRADYCARDIA**

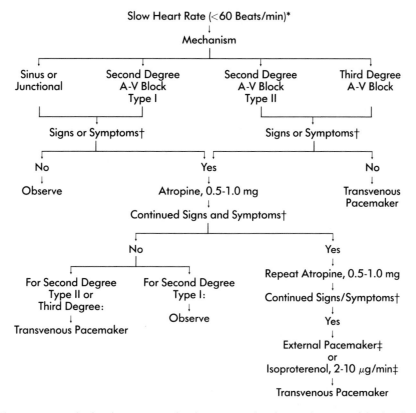

This sequence was developed to assist in teaching how to treat a broad range of patients with bradycardia. Some patients may require care not specified herein. This algorithm should not be construed to prohibit such flexibility.

*A chest thump or a cough may stimulate cardiac electric activity and result in improved cardiac output and may be used at this point.

†Hypotension (BP <90 mm Hg), PVCs, altered mental status or symptoms (e.g., chest pain, dyspnea), ischemia, or infarction.

‡Temporizing therapy.

**PAROXYSMAL SUPRAVENTRICULAR TACHYCARDIA**

| **Unstable** | **Stable** |
|---|---|
| ↓ | ↓ |
| Synchronous Cardioversion 75-100 Joules | Vagal Maneuvers |
| ↓ | ↓ |
| Synchronous Cardioversion 200 Joules | Verapamil, 5 mg IV |
| ↓ | ↓ |
| Synchronous Cardioversion 360 Joules | Verapamil, 10 mg IV (in 15-20 min) |
| ↓ | ↓ |
| Correct Underlying Abnormalities | Cardioversion, Digoxin, β-Blockers, Pacing as Indicated (See Text) |
| ↓ | |
| Pharmacologic Therapy + Cardioversion | |

If conversion occurs but PSVT recurs, repeated electric cardioversion is *not* indicated. Sedation should be used as time permits.

This sequence was developed to assist in teaching how to treat a broad range of patients with sustained PSVT. Some patients may require care not specified herein. This algorithm should not be construed as prohibiting such flexibility. The flow of the algorithm presumes PSVT is continuing.

**Fig. 7-14, cont'd**    ACLS algorithms.

*Continued.*

**ACUTE SUPPRESSIVE THERAPY
for VENTRICULAR ECTOPY**

Assess for Need for
Acute Suppressive Therapy
↓

→ Rule Out Treatable Cause
→ Consider Serum Potassium
→ Consider Digitalis Level
→ Consider Bradycardia
→ Consider Drugs

Lidocaine, 1 mg/kg
↓
If Not Suppressed,
Repeat Lidocaine, 0.5 mg/kg Every 2-5 min,
Until No Ectopy, or up to 3 mg/kg Given
↓
If Not Suppressed,
Procainamide 20 mg/min
Until No Ectopy, or up to 1000 mg Given
↓
If Not Suppressed,
and Not Contraindicated,
Bretylium, 5-10 mg/kg Over 8-10 min
↓
If Not Suppressed,
Consider Overdrive Pacing

Once Ectopy Resolved, Maintain as Follows:
    After Lidocaine, 1 mg/kg . . . Lidocaine Drip, 2 mg/min
    After Lidocaine, 1-2 mg/kg . . . Lidocaine Drip, 3 mg/min
    After Lidocaine, 2-3 mg/kg . . . Lidocaine Drip, 4 mg/min
    After Procainamide . . . Procainamide drip, 1-4 mg/min (Check Blood Level)
    After Bretylium . . . Bretylium Drip, 2 mg/min

This sequence was developed to assist in teaching how to treat a broad range of patients with ventricular ectopy. Some patients may require therapy not specified herein. This algorithm should not be construed as prohibiting such flexibility.

**Fig. 7-14, cont'd** ACLS algorithms.

reduces complications; therefore the starting level for most dysrhythmias is around 50 joules or less (Fig. 7-15). The energy necessary to terminate some dysrhythmias, such as atrial flutter or ventricular tachycardia, may be considerably less. If unsuccessful, this initial level may be increased to 100 joules and then by 100-joule increments until a level of 360 joules is reached. Make sure that all personnel have moved away from the patient and the bed before discharging the defibrillator, and call out "all clear."

13. Record the postshock rhythm to determine whether the procedure was successful. $V_1$ or $MCL_1$ lead recording is preferable. An oscilloscope interpretation is frequently unreliable.

14. Continue rhythm monitoring and close observations of cardiovascular and pulmonary status for 2 to 3 hours until the patient's condition is stable after cardioversion.

15. Precautions
    a. When digitalis excess is suspected, electric cardioversion should be deferred and the dysrhythmia treated with medication intially to prevent production of serious ventricular tachydysrhythmias and failure to terminate the digitalis-related dysrhythmia.
    b. Emergency drugs and equipment needed for pacing, intubation, or suction must be available.
    c. If using electrode paste, avoid coating the paddles excessively or placing them too near monitoring electrodes, which may allow a spark to jump and burn the skin. Local skin inflammation caused by the paddles is best treated with a topical steroid preparation.

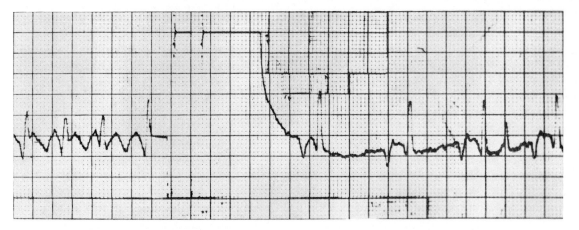

**Fig. 7-15** Termination of atrial flutter. Direct current countershock was administered at 50 watt-seconds. The synchronized discharge occurred on R wave and terminated the flutter rhythm.

d. Certain dysrhythmias may occur after cardioversion; therefore monitoring the rhythm must continue for 2 to 3 hours. Other complications may include embolic episodes, which occur in 1% to 3% of patients after the dysrhythmia is converted to sinus rhythm.

Electrophysiologic monitoring. When the modified pulmonary artery catheter is in the right atrium at the junction of the superior vena cava, stable ECGs of high quality can be obtained. These high-fidelity ECGs allow rapid and accurate diagnosis of various complex dysrhythmias. Because of the limited noise in the ECG signal, continuous quantitative interval measurements by a computerized system are possible. Moreover, the stable intracavitary electrode position provides a reliable atrial pacing site for converting supraventricular tachycardias, for maintaining an adequate rate during sinus bradycardia, and for suppressing ventricular premature beats by rapid atrial pacing rates.[115] This multipurpose catheter provides safe and convenient monitoring for long periods of time in patients with unstable cardiopulmonary problems.

### Circulatory Arrest

Resuscitation begun during the first 3 to 4 minutes following circulatory arrest usually prevents irreversible cerebral damage. Ventricular fibrillation, rather than ventricular asystole, commonly precipitates the arrest. However, a recent study reported sudden death in ambulatory monitored patients secondary to bradydysrhythmias.[139] Defibrillation procedures should be initiated in a CCU within 30 seconds of onset of the arrest. Prompt reversion to sinus rhythm often prevents the biochemical derangements that accompany ventricular fibrillation, eliminates the need for endotracheal intubation, and significantly increases the success rate of resuscitation attempts. After a successful resuscitation, it is important that measures be taken to prevent recurrence of the cardiac arrest. Prophylactic lidocaine and cardiac pacing can be used to prevent extrasystoles and/or bradycardia, since these dysrhythmias may presage the occurrence of ventricular tachycardia/fibrillation.

When the monitor alarm is activated or the dysrhythmia is observed on the oscilloscope, personnel must correlate the observed rhythm with the patient's clinical status by rapidly evaluating the patient's orientation, respirations, pupils, and carotid or femoral pulses. Loose leads can produce a rhythmic pattern simulating ventricular fibrillation. Moreover, a lidocaine reaction can mimic the disoriented state seen in tachydysrhythmias associated with inadequate cardiac output. The importance of careful diagnosis cannot be overemphasized.

### Resuscitation*

1. Establish unresponsiveness by shaking the patient and calling his name. If there is no response, call for help.
2. Place patient in a supine position with a board or firm mattress under the chest.
3. Open the patient's airway using the head-tilt and chin-lift method or head-tilt and neck-lift method. The chin-lift method is preferred.
4. Look, listen, and feel for breathing. If the patient is breathing, keep the airway open, but do not begin other CPR techniques.
5. If the patient is not breathing, administer two breaths of about 1.5 seconds each into victim's mouth after pinching the nostrils and sealing the mouth.[131]
6. Check the patient's carotid pulse. If present, con-

---

*For further information refer to the American Heart Association or the American Red Cross guidelines for cardiopulmonary resuscitation

tinue to administer only breathing a rate of one breath every 5 seconds.

7. If the patient has no palpable pulse, begin cycles of 5 external cardiac compressions (at rate of 80 to 100/min) and 1 breath if two people are resuscitating, or cycles of 15 compressions (at a rate of 80 to 100/min) and 2 breaths if only one person is resuscitating the patient. Check for correct hand positioning.

8. After 4 cycles of ventilation and compression, check for return of patient's pulse and spontaneous breathing. If there is no pulse or spontaneous breathing, repeat the process.

9. Do not stop CPR for more than 7 seconds once it has begun. Pause every 4 cycles (after the initial pause noted in No. 8) to check for carotid pulse, spontaneous breathing, and pupillary reaction to light.

10. At the same time one or more people provide cardiorespiratory support, someone else sets up the defibrillator if the patient's rhythm is unknown or is known to be ventricular tachycardia or fibrillation. If only one person is present, he or she must decide between instituting CPR and attempting to defibrillate the patient. If the defibrillator is close at hand and the patient can be treated with it in 15 to 30 seconds, it is probably best for the single resuscitator to choose defibrillation rather than beginning CPR alone. *(It is extremely critical that DC shock not be delayed when CPR has begun, an intubation attempted, an ECG recorded, or a physical examination [other than, for example, a brief palpation of pulses] performed. Rapid application of DC shock is usually the most important therapeutic maneuver in this situation.)*

11. As soon as the defibrillator is made ready (this should take no more than 30 seconds), apply the paddles for a quick-look. Most defibrillators have monitoring capability; their paddles act as electrodes that display and record the rhythm disturbance. The defibrillator is then charged to the appropriate energy level (Fig. 7-16) and the electric countershock is delivered.

12. Patients with ventricular fibrillation and pulseless ventricular tachycardia are defibrillated or cardioverted immediately at 200 joules. If this shock is unsuccessful, a second shock is delivered at 200 to 300 joules. If the second shock is unsuccessful, a third shock is delivered at 360 joules (see ACLS algorithms). These shocks should be delivered as quickly as possible. Remember to check for a pulse after each countershock. Failure to restore an effective rhythm after delivery of a properly administered countershock at high intensity suggests that complicating problems such as hypoxia, acidosis, or drug toxicity may be present. If possible, these conditions should be corrected before the next countershock is delivered. Sodium bicarbonate may be given to treat acidosis.

13. IV fluid is started if it is not already running.

14. It is helpful to have a drug list such as the one shown in Table 7-4 taped to the emergency cart. Medications most likely to be needed are prepared at the first opportunity.

15. Repetitive shocks may not be effective in the presence of fine fibrillatory waves on the ECG. Giving

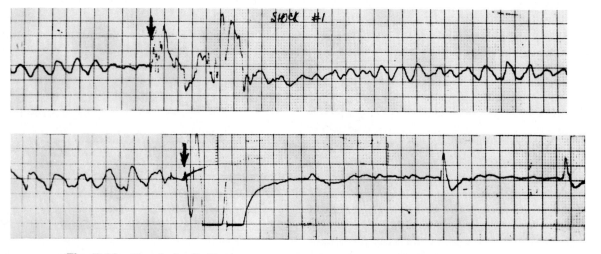

**Fig. 7-16** Ventricular fibrillation was treated with application of unsynchronized countershock at 200 joules in top strip (noted by arrow). Because countershock was unsuccessful, as noted in continuous strip, countershock was again applied at 300 joules (arrow in second strip). Rhythm then converted to idioventricular mechanism.

**TABLE 7-4** Drugs commonly used in cardiac arrest: how supplied, usual dose (average adult)

| Drug | Concentration and Volume of Prefilled Syringe | Dose | Infusion Rate | Remarks |
|---|---|---|---|---|
| Atropine sulfate | 0.1 mg ml in 10 ml syringe | 0.5-1.0 mg = 5-10 ml | | Repeat at 5-minute intervals to achieve desired rate; generally, do *not* exceed 2 mg |
| Bretylium tosylate | 50 mg/ml in 10 ml ampule | 5 mg/kg 350-500 mg as initial dose | 500 mg in 5% dextrose in water (in 250 ml = 2 mg/ml; in 500 ml = 1 mg/ml) Infusion: 1-2 mg/min | Infusion started after loading dose to control recurrent ventricular tachycardia or ventricular fibrillation |
| Calcium chloride 10% | 100 mg/ml in 10 ml syringe | 50 mg = 5 ml | | May repeat dose every 10 minutes as needed |
| Dopamine | 200 mg in 5 ml ampule | | 200 mg in 250 ml dextrose in water = 800 µg/ml Infusion: 2-10 µg/kg/min | |
| Epinephrine 1:10,000 | 0.1 mg/ml in 10 ml syringe | 0.5 mg-1.0 mg = 5-10 ml IV or intratracheal | 1 mg in 5% dextrose in water (in 250 ml = 4 µg/ml; in 500 ml = 2 µg/ml) Infusion: 1 µg/min for maintenance of BP | Avoid intracardiac injection; repeat dose every 5 minutes as needed in cardiac arrest |
| Isoproterenol | 0.2 mg/ml in 5 ml ampule | | 1 mg in 5% dextrose in water (in 250 ml = 4 µg/ml; in 500 ml = 2 µg/ml) Infusion: 2-20 µg/min Titrate | Beware of PVCs |
| Lidocaine | For IV bolus: 1% (10 mg/ml) in 10 ml = 100 mg 2% (20 mg/ml) in 5 ml = 100 mg For infusion after bolus: 4% (40 mg/ml) in 25 ml = 1 g | 1%: 75 mg = 7.50 ml 2%: 75 mg = 3.75 ml | 2 g in 500 ml 5% dextrose in water (or 1 g in 250 ml) = 4 mg/ml Infusion: 1-4 mg/min | For breakthrough ventricular ectopy: additional 50 mg bolus every 5 minutes to suppress, or total of 225 mg; increase drip to 4 mg/min |
| Procainamide | For IV bolus: 100 mg/ml in 10 ml ampule For infusion after bolus: 500 mg/ml in 2 ml ampules | 20 mg/min until: a) Dysrhythmia suppressed b) Hypotension c) QRS widens by 50% d) Total 1 g administered | 1 g in 250 ml 5% dextrose = 4 mg/ml Infusion: 1-4 mg/min | Monitor ECG and blood pressure; administer cautiously in patients with acute MI |
| Sodium bicarbonate | 1 mEq/ml in 50 ml = 50 mEq | 1 mEq/kg or 75 ml initial dose (average-size adult) according to pH | | Repeat according to pH |

From Textbook of advanced cardiac life support, American Heart Association, 1983. Reprinted with permission of the American Heart Association, Dallas, TX.

the patient 5 ml of epinephrine 1:10,000 solution intravenously may convert these fine waves to large coarse, fibrillatory waves. In some cases lidocaine alone or in combination with epinephrine may assist in defibrillation. Procainamide IV and/or bretylium tosylate IV may also be tried.[132]

16. After successful conversion to sinus rhythm, continuous infusion with the antidysrhythmic drug, such as lidocaine, procainamide, or bretylium, should be instituted for maintenance therapy.[132]

17. If the rhythm is known to be ventricular asystole, CPR should be initiated immediately (see Nos. 1 to 9 and administer epinephrine. See below.)

18. After establishing IV access, epinephrine, 0.5 to 1.0 mg of a 1:10,000 solution, is administered intravenously. If this is unsuccessful, atropine 1.0 mg may be administered intravenously. Atropine may be repeated in 5 minutes.

19. The patient should be intubated. If the patient is intubated prior to establishing IV access, epinephrine and atropine may be given by the endotracheal route.

20. External and/or transvenous pacing may be attempted.

21. Electromechanical dissociation (EMD) is also a form of cardiac arrest (see Nos. 1 to 9). The highest priority is to maintain the patient while searching for a correctable cause, such as hypovolemia, cardiac tamponade, tension pneumothorax, hypoxemia, acidosis, or pulmonary embolism. See ACLS algorithm for EMD (Fig. 7-14).

22. At the first opportunity an episode sheet is completed, and clinical events and a drug tally are recorded.

**Control of environment.** Regulation of the environment facilitates the rapidity and efficiency of the resuscitation procedure. The corridor to the patient's room must be free from obstacles. The patient's room should have adequate lighting with electric outlets visible from the door. Furniture should not block traffic from the room door to the patient's bed. Flowers, if allowed in the CCU, should be set on a shelf away from the bed so that they will not be knocked off the table during an emergency.

Note: A fully stocked, adequately maintained emergency cart is imperative in every unit. It should include all drugs and equipment needed in an arrest and should not be cluttered with unnecessary items. The emergency cart and equipment should be checked each shift.

**Postresuscitative care.** In the aftermath of a successful resuscitation it seems natural for CCU personnel to relax; however, meticulous attention to the patient's hemodynamic status, blood gas levels, and electrolyte balance continues to be important in maintaining clinical stability and in preventing recurrence. This is a time too during which the patient's family should be encouraged to visit when

appropriate. The family should be prepared for changes in the patient or new equipment in use, such as a ventilator.

## Sudden Cardiac Death

Sudden cardiac death is the loss of life occurring within 1 hour of the onset of cardiovascular symptoms in a patient previously free of symptoms who has not suffered circulatory collapse during the preceding 24 hours, and in whom no other cause of death is identified either by history or by autopsy.[133] Sudden cardiac death accounts for approximately 1000 deaths in the United States every day.[134]

Ventricular fibrillation is the most common dysrhythmia recorded at the onset of cardiopulmonary resuscitation in patients who have out-of-hospital cardiac arrest or in patients who die suddenly.[135-138] In one study[137] bradydysrhythmias were present in nearly one third of the patients, a frequency that is much higher than that found in other studies.[135,136,138] Since bradydysrhythmias commonly occur when there has been delay in initiating emergency care,[135] it is unclear how often they actually cause sudden death. For example, combined data from eight monitored patients who did not have evidence of acute MI showed that ventricular fibrillation caused sudden death in seven patients and severe bradydysrhythmias in only one patient.[139-141] An ECG depicting a cardiac arrest caused by the spontaneous onset of rapid ventricular tachycardia that degenerated into ventricular fibrillation is shown in Fig. 7-17. Ventricular dysrhythmias are the most likely cause of sudden death in patients who have an acute MI but die before being hospitalized.

Most patients who have coronary artery disease and develop sudden cardiac death demonstrate no recent thrombi in the coronary arteries at postmortem examination.[142,143] Moreover, the majority of patients successsfully resuscitated from sudden death do not have an acute MI.[144] In patients who are resuscitated from out-of-hospital sudden death, the presence of an acute MI has important prognostic significance: of 424 survivors of ventricular fibrillation, the 1-year mortality in patients who had an acute MI was 2%, and in patients who did not have an infarction the mortality was 22%.[145] These data confirm the observation that the occurrence of ventricular fibrillation in the coronary care unit in patients who have an acute MI does not increase the risk of sudden death in these patients after hospital discharge.[146]

The difference in long-term survival after resuscitation for a patient who had and one who did not have an acute MI may be partially explained by the fact that the transient electrophysiologic and biochemical alterations that occur in the ventricle during an acute MI may result in ventricular fibrillation. When the acute phase of the infarction resolves, such patients have a low recurrence rate of ventricular fibrillation most likely because their hearts no longer have the electrophysiologic/anatomic capability to develop and/or sustain ventricular dysrhythmias. In contrast, patients

Sustained ➡

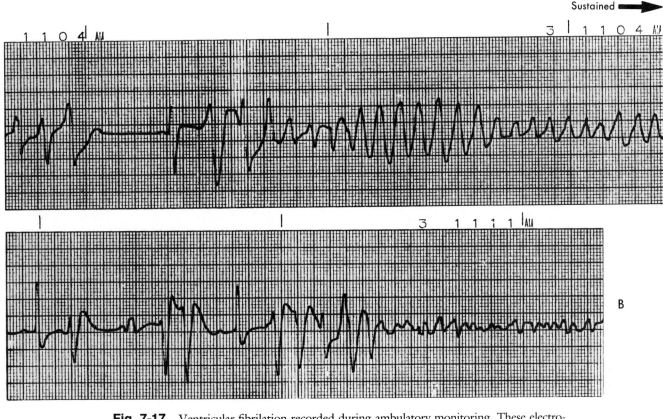

A

B

**Fig. 7-17**  Ventricular fibrillation recorded during ambulatory monitoring. These electrocardiographic tracings occurred during an in-hospital, 24-hour, ambulatory recording on a patient who had a previous out-of-hospital cardiac arrest. **A,** The onset of rapid (approximately 300 beats/min) ventricular tachycardia that degenerated into ventricular fibrillation; the patient was successfully defibrillated to sinus rhythm. **B,** Seven minutes later a second episode of ventricular fibrillation occurred after a short run of ventricular tachycardia; defibrillation again restored sinus rhythm.

who have ventricular fibrillation without infarction have a relatively high risk of recurrent ventricular fibrillation. The high recurrence rate in these patients may be related to the fact that the "arrhythmogenic" area of the ventricle does not become infarcted and remains capable of initiating or sustaining ventricular dysrhythmias.

Although sudden cardiac death occurs most often in patients who have coronary artery disease, it also occurs in patients with a variety of other cardiac conditions[132,133,149-150] such as hypertrophic cardiomyopathy, dilated cardiomyopathy, mitral valve disease, and primary electric disease (which is the presence of cardiac dysrhythmias with no other cardiac abnormalities found during physical examination, echocardiograhy, or cardiac catheterization).

Patients who have a prolonged QT interval are at increased risk for sudden cardiac death.[150] The upper limit for QT duration corrected for heart rate (QTc) is usually given as 0.44 seconds. Although a QTc interval ≥0.44 seconds can occur in patients without dysrhythmias, there

is a congenital disorder called *prolonged QT syndrome* that occurs in patients with[151] or without deafness[152,153]; this disorder is associated with a predisposition to develop ventricular tachycardia or ventricular fibrillation. Sudden cardiac death in patients with an acquired prolonged QT interval may be caused by hypokalemia and quinidine-like antidysrhythmic drugs. A connection between prolonged QT interval and sudden death has been dramatically demonstrated in patients receiving a liquid protein diet.[154,155]

**Risk factors for sudden cardiac death.** Risk factors for sudden cardiac death include the presence of complex PVCs, ventricular tachycardia, or left ventricular dysfunction. Simple (uniform, infrequent) and complex (multiform, frequent) PVCs commonly occur in patients who have coronary artery disease. The prevalence of complex PVCs increases directly with the number of diseased coronary arteries and with the severity of left ventricular dysfunction.[156-158] Although the presence of complex PVCs increases the risk of subsequent sudden death, most patients who have complex PVCs do not die suddenly. Ven-

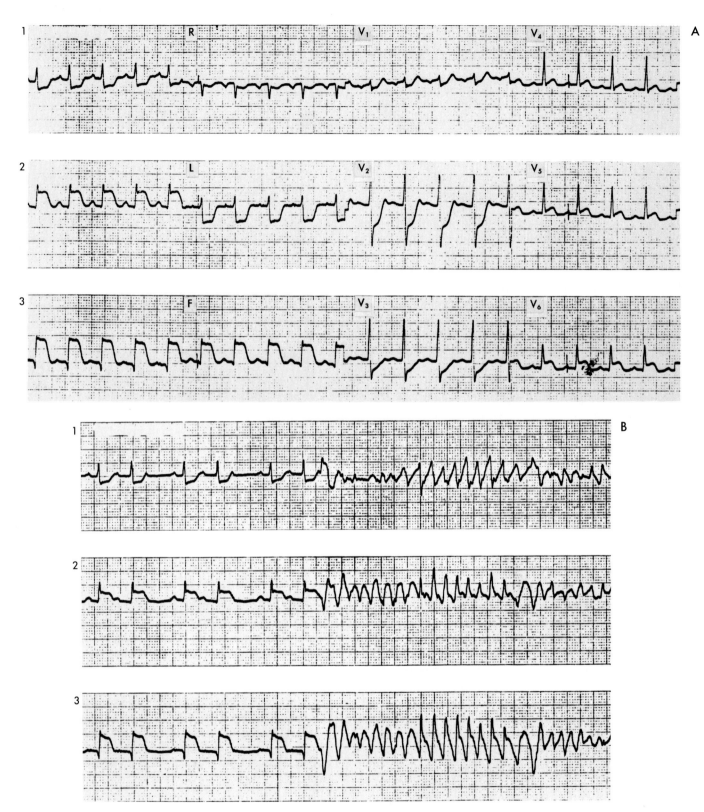

**Fig. 7-18** Ventricular fibrillation in the presence of an acute myocardial infarction. **A,** A 12-lead ECG demonstrating a current of injury pattern (that is, ST elevations) in leads II, III, aVF, and V₄ to V₆. This patient later developed Q waves in these leads. In both **A** and **B** the three leads arranged vertically were recorded simultaneously (e.g., I, II, and III). **B,** A rhythm strip taken simultaneously for leads I, II, and III. Wenckebach AV block occurs on the left, and rapid ventricular tachycardia that degenerates into ventricular fibrillation is seen on the right.

tricular fibrillation is often preceded by ventricular tachycardia,[138,139,159,160] (Fig. 7-18) but it is not known how frequently ventricular tachycardia degenerates into ventricular fibrillation.

Sudden death also occurs in patients who have nonsustained ventricular tachycardia that is associated with few or no symptoms.[161,162] In some cases nonsustained ventricular tachycardia may progress to sustained ventricular tachycardia, and this may lead to the development of ventricular fibrillation. The occurrrence of a sustained ventricular tachycardia may depend on multiple factors such as myocardial ischemia, increased left ventricular dimension, electrolyte disorders, or autonomic disturbances.

Patients who have an acute MI are at increased risk of developing subsequent sudden death if they have congestive heart failure while still in the coronary care unit[146,163] or have a low cardiac ejection fraction (determined by radionuclide angiography) prior to hospital discharge.[156] As noted in the previous section, complex PVCs commonly occur in patients who have myocardial dysfunction, and the two abnormalities compound the risk for sudden death.[164,165] This risk is greatest in patients who have congestive heart failure and complex PVCs but is lower for patients who have only congestive heart failure or complex PVCs.[165] Other clinical factors related to an increased risk of sudden death include psychologic stress,[166] increasing age, hypertension, and diabetes.[167]

Diagnosis. Several diagnostic tests are used to determine the cause of the dysrhythmia in survivors of sudden cardiac death. Holter monitoring is commonly used to document the presence of dysrhythmias and to evaluate the effectiveness of antidysrhythmic drugs. The ECG monitor is worn by the patient for 24 hours and the patient is encouraged to pursue his or her normal activities. Exercise stress testing may also be used to detect dysrhythmias. A third test used to determine the cause of dysrhythmias is the signal-averaged ECG. The signal-averaged ECG is a noninvasive procedure, similar to a standard 12-lead ECG, that can be used to detect late potentials (low-amplitude, high-frequency signals that may occur at the end of the QRS). The presence of late potentials seems to indicate an increased risk of reentrant tachycardias and sudden death.[168]

Treatment of ventricular dysrhythmias. Ventricular tachydysrhythmias may be controlled by a variety of therapies that include drugs, pacemakers, cardioverter/defibrillators, and surgery. Probably the most difficult task in caring for patients who have ventricular dysrhythmias is deciding *whether* to treat them rather than which treatment modality to use. Since the risk of sudden death is not the same for all ventricular dysrhythmias, treatment to suppress ventricular dysrhythmias should be guided by the relative risks of sudden death in a particular dysrhythmia. The assumption, although often difficult to prove, is that abolition of the dysrhythmia will prevent death; obviously,

the decision to treat a patient must be made from the data obtained on the patient and sound clinical judgment. Of the ventricular dysrhythmias, the lowest risk of sudden death occurs in patients who have PVCs but no structural heart disease, and the highest risk occurs in patients who have sustained ventricular tachycardia and severe congestive heart failure; as a rule, the former group should not receive antidysrhythmic therapy (assuming that the patient is asymptomatic,), whereas the latter group requires therapy. In general, drug therapy is not recommended for any patient with asymptomatic PVCs, but patients who have sustained ventricular tachycardia should be treated. If nonsustained ventricular tachycardia causes substantial symptoms in patients with or without structural heart disease, it may be desirable to suppress the dysrhythmia; if the dysrhythmia is asymptomatic and occurs in otherwise healthy individuals, treatment may not be necessary, but careful follow-up of these patients is suggested.

In studies testing the effectiveness of therapy with beta-blocking drugs,[169-172] a significant decrease in sudden death occurred in patients treated with alprenolol, practolol, timolol, and metoprolol compared with control patients. The apparent benefits of beta blockers may be caused by their antisympathetic effects, membrane-active properties, their antiischemic effects, or a combination of multiple actions. Antidysrhythmic drug therapy is not without risks. Antidysrhythmic drugs commonly cause side effects[173] and in some patients can cause ventricular tachycardia and sudden death.[174,175] In some patients administration of type I antidysrhythmic drugs (for example, quinidine, procainamide, or disopyramide) may cause marked prolongation of the QT interval and result in a specific form of ventricular tachycardia, known as *torsade de pointes* (Fig. 7-19).

Electrophysiologic testing. One method employed to assess the efficacy of drug therapy in the suppression of spontaneous ventricular tachycardia/fibrillation is to monitor for variable time periods the patient's heart rhythm during therapy under normal activity and during stress testing.[176] If ventricular dysrhythmias are markedly suppressed during the monitoring period, the patient is discharged and further follow-up is done out-of-hospital. In many patients ventricular tachydysrhythmias are episodic, which precludes accurate assessment of drug efficacy by noninvasive monitoring techniques only; unfortuantely, out-of-hospital sudden death is not an uncommon sequela in these patients.

Electrophysiologic studies with programmed electric stimulation to induce ventricular tachycardia has been used to judge the ability of drugs to prevent ventricular dysrhythmias.[133,177-179] Thus patients who have ventricular tachycardia induced before but not after drug therapy usually have no recurrence of ventricular tachydcardia if they continue to take the dosage of the antidysrhythmic drug that prevented induction of ventricular tachycardia at electrophysiologic study.

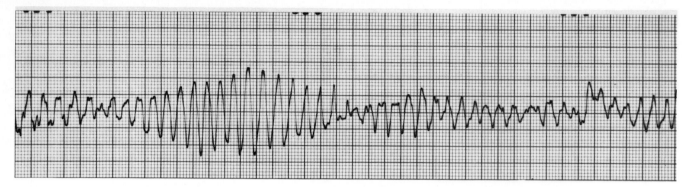

**Fig. 7-19** Torsades de pointes. This specific type of ventricular tachycardia usually occurs in the presence of a prolonged QT interval and is characterized by a QRS morphology that appears repeatedly to change its axis by 180 degrees.

An electrophysiologic study procedure is similar to a cardiac catheterization. Multielectrode catheters are inserted into a vein, usually the femoral, brachial, basilic, subclavian, or jugular, and the electrodes are positioned in various locations within the heart. Arterial cannulation is done only if left ventricular stimulation is required. The catheters are used to make simultaneous recordings of the electric activity of the heart (similar to ECGs). Pacing electrodes on the catheters are used to stimulate the heart (a process called *programmed electric stimulation,* or PES), and induce dysrhythmias, which also are recorded. The pacing electrodes can also be used to terminate a dysrhythmia by overdrive pacing. Cardioversion or defibrillation may be required if the dysrhythmia causes loss of consciousness or hemodynamic compromise.

The initial study is performed after withholding all antidysrhythmic medications. After obtaining baseline data, an antidysrhythmic drug may be infused, and the programed electric stimulation is repeated. Plasma drug levels of the antidysrhythmic agent used may be drawn during or after the study.

Many electrophysiologic studies may be required to ascertain which drug or combination of drugs effectively prevent dysrhythmia induction. It also is necessary to ensure that plasma drug levels are in a therapeutic range before initiation of the study. It may be necessary to return the patient to a drug-free state before evaluating the efficacy of the next drug. All of these factors influence the scheduling of repeat studies, which may range from 1 to 14 days.[180]

The care of the patient preparing for electrophysiologic study includes providing psychologic support. The sudden appearance of a cardiac dysrhythmia, especially one that is life-threatening, is often devastating to patients and frequently produces feeling of anger, anxiety, and depression. The thought of undergoing an invasive procedure magnifies these emotions.

It is very important for nurses and physicians to realize the emotional upheaval that occurs in patients with dysrhythmias and make attempts to help them cope with their feelings. Although patients may use a variety of coping mechanisms on their own, attempts should be made to make their environment calm, in or out of the electrophysiology laboratory. It is useful to bring patients to the laboratory on the day prior to the study to familiarize them with the surroundings. Patients often cannot remember what was explained to them in the laboratory at the end of the procedure, possibly because of their heightened emotional state, and therefore it is helpful to go over the study results with them shortly after they have been returned to their room.

Immediate post–electrophysiologic study care is similar to post–cardiac catheterization care: frequent vital signs, observation of insertion site, assessment of peripheral pulses, bedrest, and immobilization of the affected extremity. On initiation of antidysrhythmic drug therapy, the patient should be observed for signs and symptoms of drug toxicity or allergy. ECG monitoring is necessary to document any rhythm changes.

In summary, electrophysiologic testing in selected patients who have ventricular tachycardia/fibrillation is an important adjunct to testing drug efficacy. Ideally, the patient should be discharged while receiving the antidysrhythmic drug (or drugs) that totally suppresses ventricular tachycardia/fibrillation during electrophysiologic testing. Practically, however, the total suppression of ventricular tachycardia during electrophysiologic testing is not accomplished in many cases, and nonsustained or sustained ventricular tachycardia can still be induced. If patients continue to have hemodynamically unstable ventricular dysrhythmias with all drug combinations, they should be considered for alternative therapy such as surgery or the implantation of pacemakers or other electric devices,[181-187] such as the automatic implantable cardioverter defibrillator (AICD).

**Automatic implantable cardioverter defibrillator.** The automatic implantable cardioverter defibrillator (AICD) is

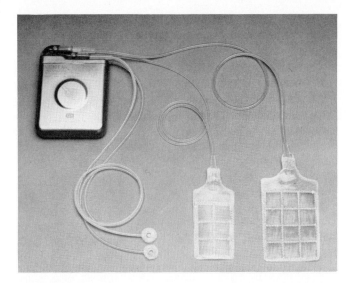

**Fig. 7-20**    Automatic implantable cardioverter defibrillator (AICD), pulse generator, and electrodes. (Reprinted with permission of CPI, St. Paul, MN.)

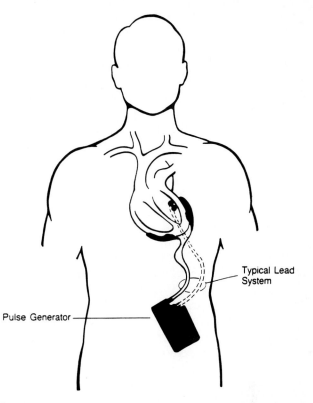

**Fig. 7-21**    Implanted AICD. (Reprinted with permission of CPI, St. Paul, MN.)

a miniaturized cardioverter defibrillator that is used to treat ventricular tachycardia and ventricular fibrillation. This device has dramatically improved the survival rate in sudden death patients. Currently, the AICD is used for patients who have survived at least one sudden death episode not associated with an MI and in whom conventional anti-dysrhythmic drug therapy has failed. Candidates for AICD implantation should have a life expectancy of at least 6 months. Patients who have frequent episodes of ventricular tachycardia or ventricular fibrillation are not candidates for AICD implantation because of early battery depletion.

The initial evaluation for AICD implantation includes the documentation of the dysrhythmia and an assessment of the cardiac anatomy by echo, multiple-gated blood pool scan (MUGA), and cardiac catheterization. A baseline electrophysiologic study, serial drug tests, and an exercise test may be done. Psychologic evaluation is also important. Optimum candidates demonstrate emotional maturity, stability, and a willingness to cooperate during the extensive follow-up that is required after implantation.[188]

The AICD device consists of a pulse generator and four electrodes (Fig. 7-20). The titanium pulse generator is approximately 11 × 7 × 2 cm, and it weighs 0.25 kg (about ½ lb). It contains the circuitry, capacitors, and a lithium battery. One set of electrodes is used for sensing the QRS waveform and delivering the shock when required. This set of electrodes can consist of (1) a left ventricular patch electrode sewn onto the epicardium and a spring electrode inserted transvenously into the superior vena cava near the right atrium or (2) a right atrial and a left ventricular patch sewn onto the epicardium. The sec-

ond set of electrodes is for rate sensing. These electrodes may be inside a single bipolar transvenous lead that is placed in the right ventricle, or they may be inside two epicardial screw-in electrodes (Fig. 7-21).

The AICD has two sensing systems, one for sensing heart rate and one for sensing QRS morphology. The rate-sensing system determines the patient's heart rate. In order for the cardioverter defibrillator to deliver a charge, the heart rate must exceed a set cutoff rate. The cutoff rate is set by the manufacturer and is usually in the range of 120 to 200 beats/min. Ideally, the patient's cutoff rate should be below the rate of his or her ventricular tachycardia but greater than his or her maximum sinus rate. The morphology sensing system allows the AICD to differentiate ventricular tachycardia and ventricular fibrillation from sinus rhythms. However, some sinus rhythms with wide QRSs may be mistaken for ventricular tachycardia by the AICD but these rhythms should not meet the rate criteria.[126] Some AICD models may be programed only to meet the rate criteria; whereas, other models are required to meet the rate cutoff, as well as QRS morphology.

Once the rate cutoff (and the morphology criteria, if required) has been met, the AICD takes 10 to 35 seconds to charge and deliver the first shock of approximately 25 joules. If the dysrhythmia continues, the device charges and delivers a second, third, and fourth shock of 30 joules. After the fourth shock, the AICD must sense at least 35 seconds of a nonventricular rhythm to reset for the next four-shock cycle. In most instances, the AICD is successful with the first shock.[188] If the AICD is unsuccessful after the cycle of four shocks for a life-threatening dysrhythmia, external countershock must be applied immediately. Newer models of the AICD deliver a five-shock cycle.

There are four surgical options for the placement of the epicardial and patch leads. A median sternotomy approach is used when patients are undergoing additional cardiac surgery such as coronary artery bypass grafting. The left lateral thoracotomy, left subcostal, and subxyphoid approaches also can be used. Once the epicardial leads and patches are in place, the wires are tunneled under the skin and connected to the pulse generator, which is pocketed in the paraumbilical area. Once the system is in place, intraoperative testing is performed to ensure that the AICD can terminate the induced dysrhythmia. The cardioverter/defibrillator electrodes may be repositioned to determine optimum placement.[189]

The AICD can be activated and deactivated with a magnet. The device is implanted in the deactivated mode, then activated for intraoperative testing. The AICD is then deactivated for completion of surgery. To activate the AICD, a doughnut-shaped magnet is placed over the right corner of the pulse generator for 30 seconds. An audible beeping tone, synchronized to the QRS, should be heard. To deactivate the AICD, the magnet is placed over the pulse-generator. After 30 seconds the beeping should change to a continuous tone. In caring for a patient with an AICD, it is important to note whether the AICD is in the active or inactive mode. A device called an *Aidcheck* is used to determine battery life and the total number of shocks delivered through the lead system.[188]

Potential complications of AICD implantation include infection, subclavian vein thrombosis, lead dislodgement, pericarditis, and pacemaker interactions.[190] Unipolar pacemakers emit large signals that may cause double sensing by the AICD.

Before the patient is discharged, another electrophysiologic study is performed. The dysrhythmia is induced to determine that the AICD is functioning properly. This also allows the patient to experience a shock in a controlled environment. Some patients describe the shock as feeling like a blow or kick to the chest. If someone is touching the patient during a shock, that person may feel a tingling or buzzing sensation. In addition to an electrophysiologic study, exercise testing may be performed to determine that the exercise-induced sinus tachycardia is less than the AICD cutoff rate.

### Predischarge instructions following AICD implantation

1. Activity limitations: avoid contact sports, which could cause lead fracture; some states have laws prohibiting persons with dysrhythmias from driving.

2. Avoid strong magnetic fields (arc welding, electrocautery, airport metal detectors, radio frequency transmitters), which may interfere with the functioning of the AICD. If the beeping tone is heard, walk away in the opposite direction. The magnetic field may inactivate the AICD.
3. Observe incision and report any signs of infection.
4. Avoid restrictive clothing around the waist, which may cause lead fracture.
5. Report first shock to physician.

The patient's family should be encouraged to learn CPR; and the patient and his or her family should be instructed about when to notify the physician or call EMS.

## PSYCHOLOGIC ADJUSTMENT TO CORONARY HEART DISEASE

The emotional, behavioral, and social impact of a heart attack is often profound and, for many patients, may be even more debilitating than the limitations imposed solely by the physical effects of the disease. Psychologic adaptation begins when symptoms are first noticed and continues throughout hospitalization and the subsequent return home. Three phases of the illness will be discussed: prehospital, hospital, and posthospital.

### Prehospital Phase

Probably the most common reaction of the patients to the first signs of illness is simply to do nothing and hope that the symptoms go away. The average time between symptom onset and admission to a medical facility is about 3 hours, although patients may delay seeking help for more than 24 hours.[191]

Approximately 55% to 65% of the time between symptom onset and hospital arrival involves what has been termed *decision time*. During this period patients become aware of their symptoms and may engage in various behaviors designed to provide themselves with relief: they may rest, take medication, or discuss the problem with spouse or friends. An additional 25% of the time between symptom onset and entry into the medical facility involves the period of *medical preparation*. It is during this time sequence that the physician is contacted and arrangements are made for subsequent hospital care. The remaining 10% is time required for transportation to the hospital and is typically referred to as *transportation time*.

Since more than half of all deaths following MI occur within the first 4 hours, it is important that the interval between symptom onset and medical care be reduced. Longer time to respond to symptoms appears to be unrelated to demographic factors such as age, sex, or socioeconomic status. Psychologic factors appear to play a predominant role, especially in the decision time. Denial, that is, the tendency to ignore or minimize the true significance of the symptoms, seems to be the most common reaction and often leads to incorrectly attributing the symptoms to such noncardiac factors as indigestion or dysfunction in other organ systems.[197]

## Hospital Phase

Admission to the hospital is an unmistakable sign to the patient that something is wrong and that medical intervention is required. The single most important emotional feature of patients in the initial acute phase of their illness is extreme fear and anxiety. The content of anxious thought usually focuses on the realization of the possibility of sudden death, concerns about being abandoned and out of control, and the conscious preoccupation with symptoms such as shortnesss of breath, chest pain, fatigue, or irregular heart rhythm. Depression, hostility, and agitation also are observed in many patients. Cassem and Hackett[192] have developed a model for the temporal sequence of emotional reactions in patients with coronary heart disease (CHD), based on reasons for psychiatric referral in the Coronary Care Unit (CCU). The sequence is graphically displayed in Fig. 7-22. The patient feels heightened anxiety during the first 2 days of hospitalization and subsequently becomes depressed for a few days. Anxiety and depression both decline after 5 or 6 days as a result of the mobilization of two main defense mechanisms: denial and repression. Isolation of affect is a third common defense mechanism that helps the patient cope with the illness. This process involves the acknowledgement of the reality of the situation, but the affective or emotional component of this awareness is unconscious. Although the majority of patients do not require formal psychiatric intervention, a substantial number do experience significant emotional distress. Many patients have confronted death for the first time, they are frightened and depressed over the perceived loss of physical health, they are prone to worry about future employment, family relations are disrupted, and their financial security may be threatened.

While patients with CHD often tend to avoid admitting fears and worries during brief interviews, more intensive contact in which the patient is given an opportunity and permission to discuss feelings and problems in a supportive, nonthreatening environment can be extremely therapeutic. Most patients will welcome a chance to "get things off their chest," and the process often promotes feelings of reassurance and relief.

Patient teaching is another important aspect of the hospital phase. Frequently patients have trouble assimilating and retaining all the information presented to them. However most want to know about their condition (in varying degrees of detail); so it is often useful to sit down with the patient and spouse to review the important aspects of cardiac care. It is imperative to *listen* as well as to talk with the patient. Patients will communiate what they know and what they want to know if given an opportunity. Disguised fears and anxieties and misconceptions about their illness also can become apparent. For example, the statement "I guess this means I'll never go back to work" may reflect apprehension about remaining autonomous, anxiety about beng dependent on others, and uncertainty about the realistic limitations of the illness. Such statements should be explored and discussed with the patient.

Patient instruction is an extremely important activity and has been shown to increase the patient's knowledge and to improve subsequent psychosocial and medical adjustment. It should be noted, however, that patients differ in their receptivity to health information, and that the amount of responsibility and information given to a patient

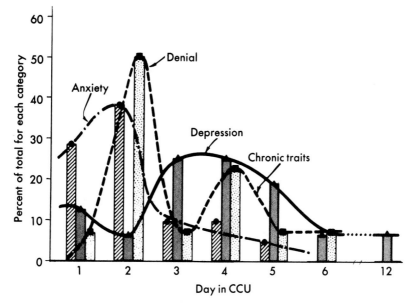

**Fig. 7-22** Hypothesized course of emotional behavioral reactions in the CCU. (From Cassem NH and Hackett T: Ann Intern Med 75:9, 1971.)

must be carefully determined by taking into account the patient's ability to comprehend and use the information.

A number of research investigations have attempted to relate stressful experiences in the CCU to subsequent recovery. In general, data suggest that the CCU equipment, activities, and procedures do not result in any long-term maladjustment in coronary patients.[193] However at least one study[194] has shown that witnessing a coronary crisis in the CCU can result in physiologic arousal (that is, heightened systolic blood pressure) and increased subjective anxiety.

## Posthospital Phase

After about a week on the CCU the patient is transferred to a ward with less supervision but remains under intensive medical care for the next 1 to 2 weeks. The posthospital phase begins with the patient's discharge from the hospital and for all practical purposes continues indefinitely thereafter. During this phase the responsibility for the patient's care shifts from the hospital team of physicians, nurses, physical therapists, and others to the patient and family.

It has been widely documented that psychologic and behavioral factors affect the course of recovery and that psychologic problems are seldom resolved during the acute period of hospitalization. For example, research has documented that at 6 months to 1 year after discharge from the hospital, as many as 88% of the patients sampled were anxious or depressed, 50% reported disturbed sleep, 20% did not return to work, and 83% complained of excessive weakness.[195] Heart disease also affects the family, and marital conflicts, often centering around medical instructions (concerning such areas as diet, medication, and sexual activity), are not uncommon.[196]

Unlike the structured hospital setting, the return home often means that the patient is unsupervised and that no concrete, specific guidelines are made available. The patient may be uncertain about the extent to which physical activity is permissible, and the advice "take it easy" is too often misunderstood or is so general as to be of no real value. Concern about sexual functioning, apprehensiveness about returning to work, and awareness of diminished energy and strength are not uncommon.

In general, emotional distress reaches its peak during the patient's convalescence. There appear to be at least five main problem areas that affect a substantial number of coronary patients: (1) excessive concerns about health and the fear of dying, (2) organic problems, (3) emotional problems, (4) continuation of personality problems from the time before the illness, and (5) developmental issues and existential concerns.

## Excessive Concerns about Health

Once a person has experienced a myocardial infarction (MI), good health can no longer be taken for granted. Many patients become sensitized to their bodily function-

ing. In extreme cases patients may become preoccupied with their health and overrreact to even minor discomfort.

Fear and anxiety about death are common reactions to a heart attack. Most people do not think about their own deaths very much. However, the occurrence of a heart attack serves as a reminder of our mortality and raises a cultural expectation of death. This expectation is founded in clinical fact, since patients with CHD have higher mortality rates than their healthy age-matched counterparts. Thus a diagnosis of coronary disease may be viewed as a "hex word," suggesting that death is imminent.[197]

Losses are considered to be less disruptive when they are "scheduled" or when the events are perceived as being subject to schedule.[198] Anxiety about death as a major loss is also related to attitudes about aging. Expectations for decline, loss, or death are far more inconsistent for the later years of life than for the early years. Thus for the young, society expects continued growth and the pattern of change is predictable. As people grow older, however, the pattern of development becomes ambiguous and expectations become unclear. The lack of clear positive expectations for development during the adult years also contributes to the attribution of normative loss. However, an MI may be more traumatic for a young person than for an older individual whose MI, which heralds aging, is more often expected. Disability and death are seen as more appropriate to the elderly than to the young and public policy decisions predictably follow this attitude.[199]

For many patients, a heart attack represents significant *loss:* loss of income, loss of family and friends, loss of job, loss of status, and loss of independence, as well as loss of health. As a result of these actual and/or threatened losses, grief reactions are not unusual. The patient's reactions may parallel the stages observed among patients with cancer: denial, anger, depression and, ultimately, acceptance.[200] These "states of dying" have not been fully confirmed, however, and some of the conceptual and methodologic deficiencies have been described elsewhere.[201]

In the past, it was felt that health professionals should not talk with cardiac patients about anything that might disturb or excite them. As a consequence, the post-MI patient's fears and anxieties were often denied or ignored. More recently, however, the importance of effective communication with the coronary patient has been recognized. Specifically, affective empathy is considered extremely important along with acceptance of the patient's feelings.

*Cardiac neurosis* is a term often used to describe a situation in which the patient has become completely debilitated by the illness. Fear of leaving home or anxiety over physical exertion may be present, and even minor symptoms are thought to be emergencies or precursors of a fatal cardiac event. Encouragement and support, firm and concrete guidelines for progressive physical exercise, and regularly scheduled medical checkups appear to be very therapeutic for these patients.

## Organic Problems

Impaired cognitive functioning is present in a small proportion of patients with coronary disease. Patients who undergo bypass surgery have a higher incidence of cognitive changes. In addition to the effects that the disease process may have on cognitive functions, advancing age contributes to a general decline in mental abilities. Aging is associated with a decline in cognitive functioning, and cardiac disease is most common in the latter half of the life cycle. Research has suggested that "crystallized" abilities, such as a person's vocabulary or fund of information, may remain intact, whereas "fluid" abilities, such as problem-solving or verbal reasoning skills may deteriorate more quickly as a result of the combined effects of aging and organic damage.

## Emotional Problems

Depression is a common complaint that is often characterized by sadness, crying spells, sleep disturbance (such as early morning awakening), excessive fatigue and weakness, and low energy. Anxiety is also fairly common, although the defense mechanisms of repression, denial, and isolation of affect often protect the patient from consciously experiencing the subjective discomfort associated with anxiety. Most patients do not suffer from significant and debilitating anxiety a year after MI. For patients whose symptoms persist, however, anxiolytic or antidepressant medication (such as doxepin hydrochloride [Sinequan] or Xanax) is often helpful in reducing symptoms.

CAD may evoke feelings of vulnerability and worthlessness. The patient may become dependent or unconsciously allow himself or herself to become passive as a result of the socially acceptable role as patient. Encouraging the patient to talk about feelings and to become more physically active are important aids to treatment. The importance of exercise therapy is now widely recognized.

## Problems Continuing from Earlier Years

Most patients who develop CAD are not psychiatric patients. However patients with significant emotional problems also develop heart disease. Problems that have developed over the course of a lifetime rarely improve after a heart attack. People who are prone to depression can be extremely affected by a sudden decline in their health. Similarly, people who tend to act impulsively or who show an inability to tolerate life's frustrations may exhibit a continuation of past behaviors: they may continue to overeat, overdrink, or overindulge themselves in ways that have a negative effect on their health and on those around them.

In brief, individuals who have problems before their illness are likely to have problems after their illness. Marriages are seldom improved when one member becomes sick, and often CAD may cause additional problems for couples and families.

## Developmental Issues and Existential Concerns

Familial, cultural, and spiritual values become more important as one grows older, and illness often brings about a reevaluation of what is meaningful, not only in terms of what happens after death but also in terms of what happens before death. An MI may make a patient seek to avoid feelings of helplessness and hopelessness and may stimulate a renewed interest in people. It is not uncommon for patients to review their lives and to reflect on opportunities chosen and neglected. Some patients adopt a new philosophy about life and shift from material to more spiritual interests.

Patients with CHD are often in their middle years and must face developmental issues common to middle age. The most important issues facing middle-aged and older adults is how to cope with loss; for the MI patient, the most obvious loss is that of physical prowess and functional abilities. This may threaten the individual's self-concept and may lead to forced dependence on others.

As one gets older, the experience of illness becomes more frequent, and it is more difficult to compensate for lost friends. Patients may feel lonely, isolated, deserted, and experience the loss of shared memories. Retirement also can be traumatic. It means an end of a phase of life, and with loss of work is often a loss of a sense of autonomy and power. Loss of relationships with coworkers, of social status, and of income are also experienced.

Talking about life requires someone who is willing to listen. Although professional help is often useful, a patient should also be encouraged to talk with spouse, relatives, and friends.

## Treatment Considerations

Most published research on the psychologic treatment of MI patients has been about treatment in the form of group psychotherapy. To date, results have been mixed. Several studies have demonstrated improved psychologic well-being in the treatment group compared with a no-treatment control group, and at least one study[202] has reported a significantly lower mortality in the treated group. However, it has been noted that group treatment of cardiac patients does not follow a process similar to group treatment of psychiatric patients (see recent reviews by Blanchard and Miller[203] and Gil and Blumenthal[204]). Educational and supportive groups appear to be preferable to self-exploratory or psychoanalytically oriented groups.

Several recent studies have employed behavioral techniques, including progressive muscle relaxation training and stress management techniques. The main behavioral treatments for patients with coronary disease appear to be those that attempt to remove the source of stress or modify the patients' perceptions and reactions to stress. *Progressive muscle relaxation,* in which the patient is taught to tense and relax muscles, is an example of a technique that counteracts the effects of a stressful environment. Other behavioral techniques for treating stress reactions include *cognitive restructuring,* in which the patient is taught to reinterpret events to make them less stressful, and *systematic desensitization,* in which the patient learns to relax to counteract the emotional or physical symptoms during exposure to situations that evoke symptoms. *Biofeedback,* a treatment designed to teach patients control of autonomic nervous system functions, has been used successfully to treat a variety of cardiovascular disorders including cardiac dysrhythmias, hypertension, and peripheral vascular disease. However the effectiveness of behavioral techniques in actually prolonging the life of patients with coronary disease has not been established. *Type A modification* has also gained widespread recognition, and recent data have suggested that reductions in type A behavior may be associated with decreased risk of recurrent CAD events.[205]

Recovery from a heart attack is a complex process. Social, psychologic, and medical factors are all important and interrelated. Successful treatment is most likely to be achieved by the collaborative efforts of nurses, physicians, psychologists, physical therapists, and vocational counselors. The key ingredient is an interest in and commitment to victims of a disease with important psychosocial as well as physical consequences.

## CARE ISSUES
### Sociocultural Considerations

Because the United States is a pluralistic society, health professionals must be prepared to work with patients from various cultures and to present health care in ways that are appropriate for individual patients. In addition, when professionals understand specific factors that influence individual health behaviors, they are in a better position to meet patients' needs. Knowledge of cultural backgrounds can help personnel anticipate differences in values, religion, dietary practices, lines of authority, family life patterns, and beliefs and practices related to health and illness. Total care can only become a reality when patients are seen in the framework of their individual cultural patterns.[206,207]

A minority culture frequently speaks English only as a second language. Persons who are bilingual may manifest a communication pattern that uses a combination of their native language and English, resulting in idiomatic speech. Because they have difficulty understanding and following medical jargon and staff directions, patients often feel devalued by staff members. Many patients express feelings of inferiority because of the inability to speak English or because they speak English incorrectly. Because of language difficulty, many patients are unable to read and comprehend consent forms or explanations of therapies.

Role expectations for the health professional vary. In general, they are based on sex, age, educational preparation, and the ethnic identity of the staff. Greater courtesy and deference have been accorded to female nurses than to their male counterparts, and disapproval has been expressed by patients when health professionals did not fulfill sex role expectations. Age is an important consideration in providing care. Many subcultures maintain a reverence for the elderly that has become minimized in our youth-dominated society. The elderly patient expects to be treated respectfully and in a formal manner, and the behavior of some younger staff has been viewed as callous and disrespectful.

In many subcultures health is not viewed as a high priority. The illness episode is viewed as a small part of a person's life. It is often difficult to gain cooperation for preventive health behaviors such as diet as part of blood pressure control and cessation of smoking to prevent heart and lung disease.

### Daily Care

Once potential problems have been assessed, daily care of the patient can be based on the data obtained. Important components in daily care of the patient include relief of anxiety and pain, monitoring of blood gas levels and fluids, decreasing the myocardial work load, continuation of dietary recommendations, and prevention and/or early detection of complications.

If the patient experiences pain, it is important to note the frequency, duration, quality, quantity, location, associated factors such as diaphoresis and dyspnea, and alleviating factors. This information should be recorded on the patient's chart, accompanied by an ECG rhythm strip. Furthermore, a 12-lead ECG should be obtained and evaluated for changes from the initial ECG, and the patient's physician should be notified. If the physician has prescribed nitrates and analgesics, they should be given to the patient, and the nurse should monitor the patient's vital signs and respiratory characteristics. If the pain is not relieved, the physician should be notified so that the duration of pain and the increased oxygen demand on the heart can be decreased as soon as possible.

Once established, the need for supplemental oxygen should be evaluated often during the acute phase of the illness. Arterial blood gas samples should be drawn at intervals to evaluate acid-base balance.

Flow sheets that record many values are useful in maintaining a graphic representation of the patient's progress (Fig. 7-23). Some CCUs prefer a separate flow sheet for arterial blood gas levels, especially for people who require frequent arterial blood gas analysis.

Limiting myocardial work continues to be an important component of daily patient care. Activities should be gradually increased according to the plan of rehabilitation and the patient's stage of recovery. Patients are now being mobilized earlier than in previous years, since prolonged bed rest may not prevent but may actually promote development of complications following MI. The patient must, however, be assisted in all activities, especially during the acute phase of the illness.

| | Date:<br>Time: | 7-3 | 3-11 | 11-7 | 7-3 | 3-11 | 11-7 |
|---|---|---|---|---|---|---|---|
| **Chest** | | | | | | | |
| Chest pain | | No | | | | | |
| $R_x$ and response | | - | | | | | |
| Gallops/murmurs | | S3 | | | | | |
| 1 + edema | | 1+pedal | | | | | |
| Jugular venous<br>   distention | | No | | | | | |
| Breath sounds | | Bilateral | | | | | |
| Crackles | | Inspiratory | | | | | |
| Rhonchi | | No | | | | | |
| Wheezes | | RUL | | | | | |
| Cough | | Yes | | | | | |
| Dyspnea | | No | | | | | |
| Cyanosis | | No | | | | | |
| Other | | | | | | | |
| **Abdomen** | | | | | | | |
| Nausea/vomiting | | No | | | | | |
| Appetite/diet | | Not hungry | | | | | |
| Bowels/guaiac | | No | | | | | |
| Abdominal distention | | No | | | | | |
| Hepatomegaly | | No | | | | | |
| Other | | | | | | | |
| **Rhythm** | | | | | | | |
| Basic rhythm | | NSR | | | | | |
| Arrhythmias | | Occ. PVCs | | | | | |
| Conduction defect | | No | | | | | |
| Emotional status | | Quiet<br>Appears<br>depressed | | | | | |
| Other | | | | | | | |
| **Vital signs** | | Bed bath/bed rest | | | | | |
| Bath/activity level | | up to B.S.C. | | | | | |
| Temperature/weight | | 99.4°/206 lbs. | | | | | |
| Apical/radial pulse | | 82/82 | | | | | |
| Respirations | | 20 at rest | | | | | |
| Blood pressure | | 138/84 R. arm | | | | | |
| Pedal pulses | | 3+bilateral | | | | | |
| Cardiac output | | N.A. | | | | | |
| Right atrial pressure | | N.A. | | | | | |
| Pulmonary artery pressure | | N.A. | | | | | |
| Pulmonary capillary wedge<br>   pressure | | N.A. | | | | | |
| Time | | 7 A.M. | | | | | |
| **Laboratory data** | | | | | | | |
| Enzymes | | CK-MB-7%, $LDH_1 > LDH_2$ | | | | | |
| Blood gases | | N.A. | | | | | |
| Other | | | | | | | |
| **I and O** | | | | | | | |
| Intake | | | | | | | |
|    Oral | | 740 cc | | | | | |
|    IV | | 280 cc | | | | | |
|    Total | | 1020 | | | | | |
|    Total 24 hours | | | | | | | |
| Output | | | | | | | |
|    Urine | | 530 cc | | | | | |
|    Emesis/Gomco | | N.A. | | | | | |
|    Total | | | | | | | |
|    Total 24 hours | | 530 | | | | | |
| Signature | | | | | | | |

**Fig. 7-23**   CCU summary flow sheet.

Initial dietary recommendations are usually maintained throughout the acute phase of illness and often throughout hospitalization and convalescence.

As previously discussed, fluid and electrolyte balance is vital during the acute phase of the MI. Accurate measurement of intake and output levels, daily weight readings, evaluation of hydration, presence of pulmonary findings such as crackles, and edema are all important components in the evaluation of fluid and electrolyte balance.

Techniques such as recording daily weight and accurate intake and output measurements are aimed at preventing congestive heart failure or detecting it early. Except in an emergency, all fluids should be administered via microdrip, and drugs such as lidocaine should be placed in a reliable automatic drip-control device and checked frequently to determine whether the proper amount of fluid is being delivered. A heparin lock may be substituted when it is necessary to continue IV medications.

Each of these components should be evaluated and care planned accordingly. Goals should be set with the patient for his care. Reevaluation and further planning are performed in relation to changes in the patient's status.

Antiembolic hose on the legs also may be used to prevent venous stasis. They must be applied with equal pressure from the foot to above the knee, checked frequently, and removed 2 or 3 times a day. Lotion or powder may be applied to the skin. The patient should be instructed not to cross his legs or ankles in order to prevent venous stasis. Sometimes the elastic stockings roll down over the knee and create a tourniquet effect on the leg; if this occurs, it should be corrected promptly. The legs should be observed for redness, swelling, heat, red streaks, and a positive Homans' sign. This sign occurs as a slight pain at the back of the knee or calf where the ankle is forcibly dorsiflexed and is indicative of incipient or established thrombosis in the veins of the leg. Should any evidence of embolization be observed, the patient's physician should be notified.

The exercise program is a necessary component of the total rehabilitation effort. An exercise program can help prevent the complication engendered by inactivity, such as respiratory complications, venous stasis, joint stiffness from immobility, and the weakness resulting from loss of muscle tone. Furthermore, exercise therapy promotes relaxation by decreasing tension and aids the patient psychologically.

An exercise program with appropriate program goals and priorities for implementation should be planned with the patient for use throughout hospitalization and after discharge. Structured in progressive stages, the exercise program should be individualized according to the patient's tolerance. Initially the patient may be assisted in performing passive exercises. A footboard is useful for the patient to exercise his leg muscles. Tolerance to exercise at each stage should be observed, evaluated, and recorded. When the patient is out of bed for the first time, medical personnel should record the patient's supine and standing blood pressures.

## Transfer from CCU

Patients experiencing minimum or no complications are generally transferred to an intermediate care unit by the third day after MI. Adequate preparations are important to minimize any emotional or physiologic reactions that may accompany transfer. Because the CCU is viewed by some patients as a safe atmosphere, they may be reluctant to leave. Others may anticipate moving to an environment they view as less restrictive. Whatever the reaction may be, it is important that the personnel in the CCU provide explanations of the regimens to be followed that can be reinforced by the staff in the intermediate care unit.

Because the actual transfer may be planned or sudden, the patient should be informed about the elements of transfer before the anticipated time of transfer. The patient should be aware that the staff in the intermediate care unit will be given a verbal report concerning his illness, progress, and potential problems for which they should be alert.

The following suggestions will ease the patient's transition from the CCU to the intermediate care area:

1. Have the intermediate care area prepared with all the equipment needed by the patient.
2. Monitor cardiac activity by telemetry to provide rapid detection of potential dysrhythmic problems.
3. Provide a proposed guideline of educational activities for the patient to participate in during the remainder of hospitalization.
4. Provide the patient and family with information on routines appropriate to efficient operation of the unit, such as visiting policies, educational opportunities, activity routines, and the purpose of specialized equipment.

Several terms have evolved to describe an area designed to allow closely supervised convalescence for patients who have been transferred from the CCU. This area provides more intense observation and care than a routine medical unit but less than that provided in a CCU. Synonyms for this area include *step-down unit, liberalized cardiac unit,* and *intermediate care unit.* Regardless of the name selected, this unit has these multiple purposes:

1. Continued patient monitoring to allow for immediate recognition of cardiac dysrhythmias and conduction disturbances
2. Immediate cardiopulmonary resuscitation
3. Safe, supervised, early mobilization
4. Reduction in costs
5. Environment conducive to psychologic and physical recovery
6. Education and reeducation concerning abilities and disabilities related to heart disease
7. Continuation of the planned rehabilitation program

Studies have shown that some patients who suffer acute

MI continue to be at risk even after surviving the first few hazardous days after onset.[34] In fact mortality during the later in-hospital phase of the illness, when the patient is usually no longer being cared for in the CCU, may be as high as that in the CCU for some groups of patients. This situation is the basis for the concept of intermediate coronary care, whereby patients can be located in an area that is usually close to the CCU. This unit has monitoring and resuscitative equipment and is staffed with personnel sufficiently prepared to provide routine as well as emergency cardiopulmonary care.

The following groups of patients have been shown to be at increased risk of catastrophic cardiac events during hospitalization and after discharge from the CCU[208]:

1. Patients with anterior infarctions involving large portions of the left ventricle and interventricular septum
2. Patients who while in the CCU exhibit circulatory failure in the form of cardiogenic shock, pulmonary edema, and congestive heart failure
3. Patients with preexisting cardiovascular disease, prior infarction, and fascicular block
4. Patients who exhibit dysrhythmias that are primarily ventricular in origin, such as premature ventricular systoles, or are indicative of heart failure, such as atrial fibrillation or flutter and/or persistent sinus tachycardia
5. Patients with severe left ventricular dysfunction
6. Patients with functional abnormalities, such as exercise-induced ischemia noted as at least 2 mm of ST segment depression or angina at heart rates less that 135 and exercise intolerance noted as exercise capacity of less than 4 metabolic equivalents (METs)

Although current data indicate that people who fall within the categories listed above have a 2 to 6 times greater chance of late in-hospital sudden death, this cannot be predicted with complete accuracy. However, these patients have had a slightly longer stay in the CCU (1 to 2 days longer) and tend to be 3 to 4 years older than their counterparts who survive hospitalization. These facts alone support the need for accurate assessment and interpretation of data to prevent and treat the complications that contribute to this high late in-hospital mortality.[209]

### Priorities during Intermediate Care

During the period of intermediate care, attention is focused on activity tolerance, educational strengths and deficits, and the patient's physical and psychologic status.

One goal of intermediate care is supervised early mobilization. Consistent with this expectation is a gradual increase in physical activity during the remainder of hospitalization, enabling the patient to reach the activity levels required for self-care when he returns home. The activities allowed include progressively increased self-care, increas-

ing time spent sitting up in a chair, and body motion and strength-building exercises. The patient should increase his ambulation daily until he can walk about the hosptial unit without tiring.

These physical activities are alternated with rest periods. Exercise should always be avoided after meals, when a large percentage of cardiac output is diverted to digest food. Criteria for decreasing the level of activity include the following:

1. Chest pain or dyspnea
2. Heart rate exceeding 120 beats/min
3. Occurrence of a significant dysrhythmia
4. Decrease in systolic blood pressure of 20 mm Hg
5. Increased ST segment displacement on the ECG or monitor[14]

Assessment of the patient's educational strengths and deficits should be determined soon after admission to the intermediate care unit so that planned teaching can be completed before discharge. In many instances personnel with special knowlege and skill in psychologic evaluation can be of tremendous assistance in determining how best to motivate patients and facilitate their learning. For some patients denial, depression, and despair are patterns of behavior that prevent optimum benefit from educational efforts. Individuals who have psychologic expertise can be of help in dealing with these exceptional patients and their families. This period immediately following the CCU experience has been recognized as the time when patients are most receptive to changes in lifestyle. Lifelong habits can be changed at this point more easily than later when the emotional impact of the acute event has subsided. Personnel must take full advantage of this receptive period.

### Preparation for Discharge

Bauknecht[210] reported in a study that investigated changes in patterns of referrals from hospitals to home health care that patients are being released from the hospital earlier in their convalescent period. Some patients are being discharged directly from intensive care units while still requiring respirators, suction machines, nasogastric tubes, urinary catheters, intravenous therapy, and continuous oxygen.[210-211]

The average length of stay for the uncomplicated MI patient has decreased. This shortened hospital stay has impinged on the time available for patient education and patient comprehension. Written materials are especially useful to patients and families both in helping them to understand information that is given to them by personnel and in reminding them of the information once they are at home. Written materials should cover information needed by the patient to comply with prescriptions related to medications, diet, physical activity, and health behaviors. Although providing such information does not ensure compliance, it is necessary that the patient know how he can best contribute to his recovery.

**Medications.** Prescriptions and details of the drug regimen should be explained to both the patient and a responsible family member. Prescriptions should be labeled, and actions and side effects of each drug noted. The patient should be assisted to adjust the medication schedule to the usual lifestyle at home to ensure maximum adherence to the regimen.

**Nutrition.** The desired dietary modifications of calories, cholesterol, fats, and sodium should be explained. Demonstration of food preparation consistent with the dietary regimen and the patient's eating preferences and habits is desirable.

**Physical activity.** An activity prescription should be individualized for each patient based on his prior level of activity and job requirements. It is the responsibility of the health team to prescribe and initially supervise the type of exercise, determine its duration and schedule, and warn against overexercising and describe its signs.

**Smoking.** Patients who smoke should be discouraged from continuing this practice. Many self-help programs are available to assist in smoking cessation. Moreover, health care personnel should set an example by not smoking.

**Sexual activity.** It is important that the patient and partner receive information about resuming sexual relations. Often patients and their partners do not ask questions because of embarrassemnt or fear and make false assumptions about returning to previous sexual behavior. It is the responsibility of the health care team to ensure that this information is provided and that the patient and partner be allowed to express concerns and ask any questions they may have. Patients and their partners should learn when it will be safe to engage in sexual intercourse and that sexual activity should commence when the patient is rested and not after a heavy meal or alcohol consumption.

**Follow-up care.** Patients should receive information about a follow-up visit to the physician. In addition, the patient should know that chest pain, palpitations, shortness of breath, syncope or presyncope should be reported at once. It is important that family members learn about available community emergency services and how to obtain help if needed. Moreover, family members should be encouraged to acquire CPR skills.

**Community resources.** The local heart association, vocational rehabilitation center, Veterans Administration, and other organizations may be of help to the patient. Other people, such as the social worker, public health nurse, dietitian, physical therapist, chaplain, occupational therapist, and psychologist may be asked for assistance and advice. Many communities have developed "coronary clubs," in which interested postmyocardial infarction patients, their families, and health care workers meet at regular times for guidance in care and education. This offers an opportunity to teach basic cardiac life support to the former patient and his family. Guest speakers may discuss topics such as nutrition, exercise, sexuality, basic cardiac life support, and antismoking techniques.

## REFERENCES

1. McGregor M: Myocardial ischemia: towards better use of the coronary care unit, Am J Med 76:887, 1984.
2. Wheeler DJ: Unresolved questions concerning coronary care units, Clin Invest Med 4(1):13, 1981.
3. Hofvendahl S: Influence of treatment in a coronary care unit on prognosis in acute myocardial infarction, Acta Med Scand 519(suppl):1, 1971.
4. Astvad K and others: Mortality from acute myocardial infarction before and after establishment of a coronary care unit, Br Med J 1:567 ,1974.
5. Hill JD, Holdstock G, and Hampton JR: Comparison of mortality of patients with heart attacks admitted to a coronary care unit and ordinary medical ward, Br Med J 2:811, 1977.
6. Armstrong A and others: Natural history of acute coronary heart attacks: a community study, Br Heart J 34:67, 1972.
7. Goldman L and others: Evidence that hospital care for acute myocardial infarction has not contributed to the decline in coronary mortality between 1973-1974 and 1977-1978, Circulation 65:936, 1982.
8. Gordis L, Naggan L, and Tonascia J: Pitfalls in evaluating the impact of coronary care units on mortality from myocardial infarctions, Johns Hopkins Med J 141:287, 1977.
9. National Institutes of Health (NIH) Consensus Development Conference on Critical Care, vol 4, No 6, 1983.
10. Mathewson M: Rule: give only decaffeinated coffee to cardiac patients, Crit Care Nurs 4:12, 1984.
11. Cooke DH: When angina destabilizes, Emerg Med 20:9, 1988.
12. Cheng TO and others: Variant angina of Prinzmetal with normal coronary arteriograms: a variant of the variant, Circulation 47:476, 1973.
13. Hillis LD and Braunwald DE: Coronary artery spasm, N Engl J Med 299:695, 1978.
14. Amsterdam EA: Unstable angina, medical management, Pract Cardiol 14:10, 1988.
15. Sherman CT and others: Coronary angioscopy in patients with unstable angina pectoris, N Engl J Med 315:913, 1986.
16. Falk E: Unstable angina with fatal outcome: dynamic coronary thrombosis leading to infarction and/or sudden death, Circulation 71:699, 1985.
17. Holmes DR and others: Coronary artery thrombosis in patients with unstable angina, Br Heart J 45:411, 1981.
18. Maseri A and others: Coronary vasospasm as a possible cause of myocardial infarction: a conclusion derived from the study of "preinfarction angina," N Engl J Med 299:1271, 1978.
19. Bashour TT and others: Unstable myocardial ischemia, Pract Cardiol 15:10, 1989.
20. Wilson DB and Vacek JL: Angina and coronary artery disease, Postgrad Med 84:7, 1988.
21. Webster MWI and Sparpe N: Exercise testing in angina pectoris: the importance of protocol design in clinical trials, Am Heart J 117:2, 1989.
22. Schroeder JS and others: Provocation of coronary spasm with ergonovine maleate: new test results with 57 patients undergoing coronary arteriography, Am J Cardiol 40:487, 1977.
23. Reichek N and others: Antianginal effects of nitroglycerin patches, Am J Cardiol 54:1, 1984.
24. Mukharji J and others: Early positive exercise test and extensive coronary disease: effect of antianginal therapy, Am J Cardiol 55:267, 1985.
25. Ho SWC and others: Effect of beta adrenergic blockade in results of exercise testing related to extent of coronary artery disease, Am J Cardiol 55:258, 1985.
26. Hoekenga D and Abrams J: Rational medical therapy for stable angina pectoris, Am J Med 76:309, 1984.
27. Flaherty J: Unstable angina: rational approach to management, Am J Med 76:52, 1984.

28. Rahimtoola RH: Coronary bypass surgery for unstable angina, Circulation 69:842, 1984.

29. Alpert JS: The pathophysiology of acute myocardial infarction, Cardiovasc Clin 19:2, 1988.

30. Pitt B: Clinical application of myocardial imaging with radioisotopes in the evaluation and management of patients with coronary artery disease, Adv Cardiol 26:30, 1980.

31. Wackers FJT: Current status of radionuclide imaging in the management and evaluation of patients with cardiovascular disease, Adv Cardiol 27:40 ,1980.

32. Wackers FJT: Radionuclide evaluation of patients in the CCU, Adv Cardiol 27:105, 1980.

33. Willerson JT and others: Radionuclide imaging in acute myocardial infarction, Cardiovasc Med 3:69, 1978.

34. Held AC: Dipyridamole-thallium imaging, Arch Intern Med 145:1927, 1985.

35. Riesman S: Dipyridamole thallium testing: an alternative form of stress testing in patients unable to exercise, Chest 88:321, 1985.

36. Leppo JA and others: Dipyridamole-thallium-201 scintigraphy in the prediction of future cardiac events after acute myocardial infarction, N Engl J Med 310:1014, 1984.

37. Leppo JA and others: Serial thallium 201 myocardial imaging after dipyridamole infusion: diagnostic utility in detecting coronary stenoses and relationship to regional wall motion, Circulation 66:649, 1982.

38. Lieberman AN and others: Two dimensional echocardiography and infarct size: relationship of regional wall motion and thickening to the extent of myocardial infarction in the dog, Circulation 63:739, 1981.

39. Kisslo J and others: Serial wall changes after acute myocardial infraction by two dimensional echo, Circulation 60(suppl 11):151, 1979.

40. Pandian N and Kerber R: Two dimensional echocardiographic assessment of wall thinning and its relation to perfusion during graded coronary stenosis, Am J Cardiol 47:1384, 1981.

41. Waugh RA: Immediate and remote prognostic implications of fascicular block during acute myocardial infarction, Circulation 47:765, 1973.

42. Crimm A and others: prognostic significance of ioslated sinus tachycardia during first 3 days of acute myocardial infarction, Am J Med 76:983, 1984.

43. McNeer JF and others: Hospital discharge the week after acute myocardial infarction, N Engl J Med 298:229, 1978.

44. DeBusk RF and others: Medically directed at-home rehabilitation soon after clinically uncomplicated acute myocardial infarction: a new model for patient care, Am J Cardiol 55:251, 1985.

45. Cannon DS and others: The short and long term prognosis of patients with transmural and nontransmural infarction, Am J Med 61:452, 1976.

46. Haskell N and DeBusk R: Cardiovascular response to repeated treadmill exercise testing soon after myocardial infarction, Circulation 60:1247, 1978.

47. Starling MR and others: Exercise testing early after myocardial infarction: predictive value for subsequent unstable angina and death, Am J Cardiol 46:909, 1980.

48. Nishimura RA and others: Prognostic value of predischarged 2-dimensional echocardiogram after acute myocardial infarction, Am J Cardiol 53:429, 1984.

49. Rackley E and others: Modern approach to myocardial infarction: determination of prognosis and therapy, Am Heart J 101:75 ,1981.

50. Ewy GA: Anticoagulation in patients with acute myocardial infarction, Pract Cardiol 4:25, 1978.

51. Mueller H and Ayers S: Propanolol in the treatment of acute myocardial infarction, Circulation 49:1078, 1974.

52. Cohn JN and others: Effect of short term infusion of sodium nitroprusside on mortality rate in acute myocardial infarction complicated by left ventricular failure, N Engl J Med 306:1129, 1982.

53. Chiarello M and others: Comparison between the effects of nitroprusside and nitroglycerin on ischemic injury during acute myocardial infarction, Circulation 54:766, 1976.

54. Muller JE and others: National Heart, Lung and Blood Institute multicenter investigation of the limitation of infarct size (MILIS) design and methods of the clinical data: an investigation of beta-blockade and hyaluronidase for the treatment of acute myocardial infarction. Monograph 100. Dallas, 1984, The American Heart Association.

55. Kovach R and Goldverg S: Interventional treatment in evolving myocardial infarction, Cardiology 76:158, 1989.

56. Hugenholtz PG and Suryapranata H: Thrombolytic agents in early myocardial infarction, Am J Cardiol 63:94E, 1989.

57. Misinski M: Pathophysiology of acute myocardial infarction: a rationale for thrombolytic therapy. Part 2, Heart Lung 17:6, 1988.

58. Kleven MR: Comparison of thrombolytic agents: mechanism of action, efficacy and safety. Part 2, Heart Lung 17:6, 1988.

59. Topol EJ: Thrombolytic therapy for myocardial infarction, Pract Cardiol 14:3, 1988.

60. Gruppo Italiano per lo Studio Streptochinase nell'Infarto Miocardico (GISSI): Effectiveness of intravenous thrombolytic treatment in acute myocardial infarction, Lancet 1:397, 1986.

61. ISIS Collaborative Group: Intravenous streptokinase given within 0-4 hours of onset of myocardial infarction reduced mortality in ISIS-2, Lancet 1:502, 1987.

62. ISIS-2 (Second International Study of Infarct Survival): Randomized trial of intravenous streptokinase, oral aspirin, both or neither among 17,187 case of suspected acute myocardial infartion, JACC 12:6, 1988.

63. Verstraete M and others: Pharmacokinetic and systemic fibrinogenolytic effects of recombinant human tissue-type plasminogen activator (rt-PA) in humans, J Pharmacol Exp Ther 235:506, 1985.

64. Sun M: The coming competition among clot-busting drugs, Science 240:1267, 1988.

65. Verstraete M and others: Randomized trial of intravenous recombinant tissue-type plasminogen activator versus intravenous streptokinase in acute myocardial infarction, Lancet 1:842, 1985.

66. Topol EJ: Advances in thrombolytic therapy for acute myocardial infarction, J Clin Pharmacol 27:735, 1987.

67. Collen D and others: Coronary thrombolysis with recombinant human tissue-type plasminogen activator: a prospective, randomized, placebo-controlled trial, Circulation 70:1012, 1984.

68. Anderson JL: Use of APSAC in the management of acute myocardial infarction: current status, Pract Cardiol 14:12, 1988.

69. Bassand J and others: Multicenter trial of intravenous anisoylated plasminogen streptokinase activator complex (APSAC) in acute myocardial infarction: effects on infarct size and left ventricular function, J Am Coll Cardiol 13:988, 1989.

70. Collen D and others: Biological and thrombolytic properties of proenzyme and active forms of human urokinase-III: thrombolytic properties of natural and recombinant urokinase in rabbits with experimental jugular vein thrombosis, Thromb Haemost 52:27, 1984.

71. Werf Van den F and others: Coronary thrombolysis with recombinant single-chain urokinase-type plasminogen activator in patients with acute myocardial infarction, Circulation 74:1066, 1986.

72. Wasserman AG and Ross AM: Patient selection for thrombolytic therapy, Am J Cardiol 64:17B, 1989.

73. Bates ER: Expanding indications for thrombolytic therapy in AMI, Pract Cardiol 15:4, 1989.

74. Giebel RA and others: t-PA therapy in acute myocardial infarction, JEN 14:4, 1988.

75. Sanders M and Kostis JB: Emergency reperfusion during acute myocardial infarction, Pract Cardiol 14:3, 1988.

76. Faxon DP: The risk of reperfusion strategies in the treatment of patients with acute myocardial infarction, J Am Coll Cardiol 12:52A, 1988.

77. Cairns JA: Antiplatelet drugs and the secondary prevention of myocardial infarction, Pract Cardiol 14:3, 1988.

78. Fuster V and others: Antithrombotic therapy after myocardial reperfusion in acute myocardial infarction, J Am Coll Cardiol 12:78A, 1988.

79. Henderson E: Assessment of successful reperfusion after thrombolysis. Part 2, Heart Lung 17:6, 1988.

80. Magee M: Nursing care of the patient receiving thrombolytic therapy. Part 2, JEN 15:2, 1989.

81. Kent K and others: Improved myocardial function during exercise after successful percutaneous transluminal coronary angioplasty, N Engl J Med 306:441, 1982.

82. Dotter CT and Judkins MP: Transmittal treatment of arteriosclerotic obstruction: description of a new technique and a preliminary report of its application, Circulation 30:654, 1964.

83. Gruentzig AR, Senning A, and Siegenthaler WE: Nonoperative dilatation of coronary artery stenosis: percutaneous transluminal coronary angioplasty, N Engl J Med 301:61, 1979.

84. Holmes DR and others: Return to work after coronary angioplasty: a report from the National Heart, Lung, and Blood Institute Percutaneous Transluminal Coronary Angioplasty Registry, Am J Cardiol 53:48C, 1984.

85. Pasternak RC and others: Scanning electron microscopy after coronary transluminal angioplasty of normal canine coronary arteries, Am J Cardiol 45:591, 1980.

86. Simpson JB and others: Coronary transluminal angioplasty in human cadaver hearts (abstract), Circulation 58(suppl II):11, 1978.

87. Block PC and others: Morphology after transluminal angioplasty in human beings, N Engl J Med 305:382, 1981.

88. Block PC and others: Transluminal angioplasty: correlation of morphologic and angiographic findings in an experimental model, Circulation 61:778, 1980.

89. Stack RS and others: Interventional cardiac catheterization, Invest Radiol 20:333, 1985.

90. Zarins CK and others: Arterial disruption and remodeling following balloon dilatation, Surgery 92:1086, 1982.

91. Block P: Percutaneous transluminal coronary angioplasty: role in the treatment of coronary artery disease, Circulation 72(6):161, 1985.

92. Mock MB and others: Percutaneous transluminal coronary angioplasty (PTCA) in the elderly patient: experience in the National Heart, Lung, and Blood Institute PTCA Registry, Am J Cardiol 53:890, 1984.

93. Cowley MG and others: Acute coronary events associated with percutaneous transluminal coronary angioplasty, Am J Cardiol 53:12C, 1984.

94. Corros G and others: Percutaneous transluminal coronary angioplasty: report of complications from the National Heart, Lung, and Blood Institute PTCA Registry, Circulation 67:723, 1983.

95. Holmes DR and others: Restenosis after percutaneous transluminal coronary angioplasty (PTCA): a report from the PTCA Registry of the National Heart, Lung, and Blood Institute, Am J Cardiol 53:77C, 1984.

96. Scholl JM and others: Recurrence of stenosis following percutaneous transluminal coronary angioplasty, Circulation 64(suppl IV):193, 1981.

97. Jutzy KR and others: Coronary restenosis rates in a consecutive patient series one year post successful angioplasty, Circulation 66(suppl II):331, 1982.

98. Maler B and others: Repeat coronary angioplasty, JACC 4:463, 1984.

99. Lembo NJ and Roubin GS: Intravascular stents, Cardiol Clin 7:4, 1989.

100. Ellis SG and Topol EJ: Intracoronary stents: will they fulfill their promise as an adjunct to angioplasty? JACC 13:6, 1989.

101. Sanborn TA: New interventional techniques for atherosclerotic disease, Prim Cardiol 15:8, 1989.

102. Litvak F and others: Role of laser and thermal ablation devices in the treatment of vascular diseases, Am J Cardiol 61:81G, 1988.

103. Sanborn TA: Laser angioplasty: Peripheral and coronary applications—coronary angioplasty, Cardiovasc Clin 19:2, 1988.

104. Dzau VJ and others: Sustained effectiveness of converting enzyme inhibition in patients with severe congestive heart failure, N Engl J Med 302(25):1371, 1980.

105. Cohn JN: Choice and rationale for vasodilators treatment of hypertension or relief of heart failure, Cardiovasc Rev Rep 1:686, 1980.

106. Mason DT and others: Treatment of acute and chronic congestive heart failure by vasodilator-afterload reduction, Arch Intern Med 140:1577, 1980.

107. Mancini D, LeJentel T, and Sonnenblack E: Intravenous use of amrinone for the treatment of the failing heart, Am J Cardiol 56:8P, 1985.

108. Benotti J and others: Comparative inotropic therapy in heart failure, Circulation 68(suppl 3):128,1983.

109. Taylor SH and others: Intravenous amrinone in left ventricular failure complicated by acute myocardial infarction, Am J Cardiol 56:29B, 1985.

110. Simonton CA and others: Melrinone in congestive heart failure: acute and chronic hemodynamic and clinical evaluation, J Am Coll Cardiol 6:453, 1985.

111. Blake P: Precision moves that counter cardiogenic shock, RN 52:5, 1989.

112. Hurst J and others: The heart, arteries and veins, ed 6, New York, 1986, McGraw-Hill Book Co.

113. Ayres SM: The prevention and treatment of shock in acute myocardial infarction, Chest 93(suppl):1, 1988.

114. Gunnar RM and others: Managing cardiogenic shock, Patient Care 23:2, 1989.

115. Mantle J: Cardiovascular evaluation and therapy in unstable patients. In Kinney M and others, editors: AACN's clinical reference for critical care nursing, New York, 1981, McGraw-Hill Book Co.

116. Ratshin RA and others: Hemodynamic elevation of left ventricular function in shock complicating myocardial infarction, Circulation 45:127, 1972.

117. Rotman M and others: Pulmonary artery diastolic pressure in acute myocardial infarction, Am J Cardiol 33:357, 1974.

118. Larson CA and Woods SL: Effect of injectate volume and temperature on thermodilution cardiac output measurements in acutely ill adults (abstract), Circulation 66(suppl 2):98, 1982.

119. Vennex CV, Nelson DH and Pierpont DL: Thermodilution cardiac output in critically ill patients: comparison room-temperature and iced injectate, Heart Lung 13:574, 1984.

120. Masters S: Complications of pulmonary artery catheters, Crit Care Nurse 9:9, 1989.

121. Shubin H and Weil MH: Practical considerations in the management of shock complicating acute myocardial infarction: a summary of current practice, Am J Cardiol 26:603, 1970.

122. Loeb HS and Gunnau RM: Treatment of pump failure in acute myocardial infarction, JAMA 245:2093, 1981.

123. Holzer J and others: Effectiveness of dopamine in patients with cardiogenic shock, Am J Cardiol 32:79, 1973.

124. Loeb HS and others: Acute hemodynamic effects of dopamine in patients with shock, Circulation 44:163, 1971.

125. Keung ECH and others: Dubotamine therapy in myocardial infarction, JAMA 245:13, 1971.

126. Vinsant MO and Spence MI: Commonsense approach to coronary care, ed 5, St Louis, 1989, Mosby—Year Book, Inc.

127. Fenton M: Intra-aortic balloon pump therapy, Crit Care Nurse 5:4, 1985.

128. Textbook of advanced cardiac life support, Dallas, 1987, American Heart Association.

129. Spence M: Cardioversion. In Miller S and others, editors: Methods in critical care, Philadelphia, 1980, WB Saunders Co.

130. Clark MB, Dwyer EM, and Greenberg H: Sudden death during ambulatory monitoring, analysis of six cases, Am J Med 75:801, 1983.

131. Standards & guidelines for cardiopulmonary resuscitation (CPR) and emergency cardiac care (ECC), JAMA 255:2905, 1986.

132. Pedersen DH and others: Ventricular tachycardia and ventricular fibrillation in a young population, Circulation, 60:988, 1979.

133. Skale BT and others: Survivors of cardiac arrest: prevention of recurrence by drug therapy as predicted by electrophysiologic testing versus ECG monitoring, AM J Cardiol 57:113, 1986.

134. Lown B: Sudden cardiac death: the major challenge confronting contemporary cardiology, Am J Cardiol 43:313, 1979.

135. Cobb LA, Werner JA, and Trobaugh GB: Sudden cardiac death. I. A decade's experience with out-of-hospital resuscitation, Mod Concepts Cardiovasc Dis 49:31, 1980.

136. Liberthson RR and others: Prehospital ventricular defibrillation: prognosis and follow-up course, N Engl J Med 291:317, 1974.

137. Myerburg RJ and others: Clinical, electrophysiologic, and hemodynamic profile of patients resuscitated from prehospital cardiac arrest, Am J Med 68:568 ,1980.

138. Pratt CM and others: Analysis of ambulatory electrocardiograms in 15 patients during spontaneous ventricular fibrillation with special reference to preceding arrhythmia events, J Am Coll Cardiol 2:789, 1983.

139. Lahiri A, Balasubramanian V, and Raftery EB: Sudden death during ambulatory monitoring, Br Med J 1:1676, 1979.

140. Gradman AH, Bell PA, and DeBusk RF: Sudden death during ambulatory monitoring: clinical and electrocardiographic correlations: report of a case, Circulation 55:210, 1977.

141. Denes P, and others: Sudden death in patients with chronic bifascicular block, Arch Intern Med 137:1005, 1977.

142. Spain DM and Bradess VA: The relationship of coronary thrombosis to coronary atherosclerosis and ischemic heart disease (a necropsy study covering a period of 25 years), Am J Med Sci 240:701, 1960.

143. Myers A and Dewar HA: Circumstances attending 100 sudden deaths from coronary artery disease with coroner's necropsies, Br Heart J 37:1133, 1975.

144. Braum RS, Alvarez H III, and Cobb LA: Survival after resuscitation from out-of-hospital ventricular fibrillation, Circulation 50:1231, 1974.

145. Cobb LA, Werner JA, and Trobaugh GB: Sudden cardiac death. II. Outcome of resuscitation; management, and future directions, Mod Concepts Cardiovasc Dis 49:37, 1980.

146. Bigger JT and others: Risk stratification after acute myocardial infarction, Am J Cardiol 42:202 ,1978.

147. Elharrar V and Zipes DP: Cardiac electrophysiologic alterations during myocardial ischemia, Am J Physiol 233:H329, 1977.

148. Opie LH, Nathan D, and Lubbe WF: Biochemical aspects of arrhythmogeneisis and ventricular fibrillation, Am J Cardiol 43:131, 1979.

149. Maron BJ and others: Sudden death in young athletes, Circulation 62:218, 1980.

150. Moss AJ and Schwartz PJ: Sudden death and the idiopathic long QT syndrome, Am J Med 66:6, 1979.

151. Jervell A and Lange-Nielsen F: Congenital deaf-mutism, functional heart disease with prolongation of the QT interval, and sudden death, Am Heart J 54:59, 1957.

152. Romano C, Gemme G, and Pongiglione R: Aritimie cardiache rare dell'eta pediatrica, Clin Pediatr (Bologna) 45:656, 1963.

153. Ward O: A new familial cardiac syndrome in children, J Irish Med Assoc 54:103, 1964.

154. Singh BN and others: Liquid protein diets and torsade de pointes, JAMA 240:115, 1978.

155. Isner JM and others: Sudden, unexpected death in avid dieters using the liquid-protein modified-fast diet: observations in 17 patients

156. Schulze RA, Strauss HW, and Pitt B: Sudden death in the year following myocardial infarction: relation to ventricular premature contractions in the late hospital phase and left ventricular ejection fraction, Am J Med 62:192,1977.

157. Calvert A, Lown B, and Gorlin R: Ventricular premature beats and anatomically defined coronary heart disease, Am J Cardiol 39:627, 1977.

158. Schulze RA Jr and others: Left ventricular and coronary angiographic anatomy: relationship to ventricular irritability in the late hospital phase of acute myocardial infarction, Circulation 55:839, 1977.

159. Lie KI and others: Observations on patients with primary ventricular fibrillation complicating acute myocardial infarction, Circulation 52:755, 1975.

160. Lie KI and others: Early identification of patients developing late in-hospital ventricular fibrillation after discharge from the coronary care unit: a 5½ year retrospective and prospective study of 1,897 patients, Am J Cardiol 41:674, 1978.

161. Meinertz T and others: Significance of ventricular arrhythmias in idiopathic dilated cardiomyopathy, Am J Cardiol 53:902, 1984.

162. Miles WM and others: Management of patients with asymptomatic nonsustained ventricular tachycardia directed by electrophysiologic study, Clin Res 34(2):326A, 1986.

163. Christensen D and others: Sudden death in the late hospital phase of acute myocardial infarction, Arch Intern Med 137:1675, 1977.

164. Bigger JT and others, and Multicenter Post-Infarction Research Group: The relationships among ventricular arrhythmias, left ventricular dysfunction, and mortality in the 2 years after myocardial infarction, Circulation 69:250, 1984.

165. Ruberman W and others: Ventricular premature beats and mortality after myocardial infarction, N Engl J Med 297:750, 1977.

166. Brodsky MA and Allen BJ: Stress cardiac arrhythmias and sudden cardiac death, Pract Cardiol 15:7, 1989.

167. Lown B and others: Sudden cardiac death: management of the patient at risk, Curr Prob Cardiol 4:1, 1980.

168. Stevens LL and Buckingham TA: Late potentials: a method for screening patients at risk for sudden cardiac death, Crit Care Nurse 9:5, 1989.

169. Green KG and others: Improvement in the prognosis of myocardial infarction by long-term beta-adrenoreceptor blockade using practolol, Br Med J 3:735, 1975.

170. Wilhelmsson C and others: reduction of sudden deaths after myocardial infarction by treatment with alprenolol: preliminary results, Lancet 2:1157, 1974.

171. The Norwegian Multicenter Study Group: Timolol-induced reduction in mortality and reinfarction in patients surviving acute myocardial infarction, N Engl J Med 304(14):801, 1981.

172. Olsson G and others: Long-term treatment with metoprolol after myocardial infarction: effect on 3-year mortality and morbidity, J Am Coll Cardiol 5:1428, 1985.

173. Kosowsky BD and others: Long-term use of procainamide following acute myocardial infarction, Circulation 47:1204, 1973.

174. Selzer A and Wray HW: Quinidine syncope: paroxysmal ventricular fibrillation occurring during treatment of chronic atrial arrhythmias, Circulation 30:17, 1964.

175. Minardo JD and others: Drug associated ventricular fibrillation: analysis of clinical features and QTc prolongation, J Am Coll Cardiol 7:158A, 1986.

176. Graboys TB and others: Long-term survival of patients with malignant ventricular arrhythmia treated with antiarrhythmic drugs, Am J Cardiol 50:437, 1982.

177. Naccarelli GV and others: Role of electrophysiologic testing in managing patients who have ventricular tachycardia unrelated to coronary artery disease, Am J Cardiol 50:165, 1982.

178. Fisher JD and others: Serial electrophysiologic-pharmacologic testing for control of recurrent tachyarrhythmias, Am Heart J 93:658, 1977.

179. Prystowsky EN: Electrophysiologic testing in patients with ventricular tachycardia: past performance and future expectations, J Am Coll Cardiol 1(2):558, 1983.

180. Mercer ME: The electrophysiology study: a nursing concern, Crit Care Nurs 7:2, 1987.

181. Gallagher JJ: Surgical treatment of arrhythmias: current status and future directions, Am J Cardiol 41:1035, 1979.

182. Guiraudon G and others: Encircling endocardial ventriculotomy: a new surgical treatment for life-threatening ventricular tachycardias resistant to medical treatment following myocardial infarction, Ann Thorac Surg 26:438, 1978.

183. Josephson ME, Harken AH, and Horowitz LN: Endocardial excision: a new surgical technique for the treatment of recurrent ventricular tachycardia, Circulation 60:1430, 1979.

184. Mirowski M and others: Clinical treatment of life-threatening ventricular tachyarrhythmias with the automatic implantable defibrillator, Am Heart J 102:265, 1981.

185. Fisher JD, Mehra R, and Furman S: Termination of ventricular tachycardia with bursts of rapid ventricular pacing, Am J Cardiol 41:94, 1978.

186. Zipes DP and others: Clinical transvenous cardioversion of recurrent life-threatening ventricular tachyarrhythmias: low energy synchronized cardioversion of ventricular tachycardia and termination of ventricular fibrillation in patients using a catheter electrode, Am Heart J 103:789, 1982.

187. Zipes DP and others: Early experience with the implantable cardioverter, N Engl J Med 311:485, 1984.

188. Moser SA and others: Caring for patients with implantable cardioverter defibrillators, Crit Care Nurse 8:2, 1988.

189. McCrum AE and Tyndall A: Nursing care for patients with implantable defibrillators, Crit Care Nurse 9:9, 1989.

190. Baba LN: Automatic implantable cardioverter defibrillators (AICD). Proceedings National Teaching Institute, Newport Beach, CA, 1989, AACN.

191. Gentry WD and Haney T: Emotional and behavioral reaction to acute myocardial infarction, Heart Lung 4:738, 1975.

192. Hackett TP and Cassem NH: Factors contributing to delay in responding to the signs and symptoms of acute myocardial infarction, Am J Cardiol 24:651, 1969.

193. Doehrman SR: Psychosocial aspects of recovery from coronary heart disease: a review, Soc Sci Med 11:199, 1970.

194. Bruhn JG and others: Patients' reaction to death in a coronary care unit, J Psychosom Res 14:65, 1970.

195. Wishnie HA, Hackett TP, and Cassem NH: Psychological hazards of convalescence following myocardial infarction, JAMA 215:1292, 1971.

196. Cassem NH and Hackett TP: Psychological rehabilitation of myocardial infarction patients in the acute phase, Heart Lung 2:382, 1973.

197. Weisman AD and Hackett TP: Predilection to death: death and dying as a psychiatric pattern, Psychosom Med 23:232, 1961.

198. Glasser BG and Strauss AL: Time for dying, Chicago, 1967, Aldine Publishing Co.

199. Kastenbaum R: Dying and death: a life span approach. In Birren JE and Shaie KW, editors: The handbook of the psychology of aging, New York, 1986, Van Nostrand Reinhold Co, Inc.

200. Kübler-Ross E: On death and dying, New York, 1969, Macmillan Publishing Co, Inc.

201. Kastenbaum R and Costa PT: Psychological perspectives on death. In Rosenwage MR and Porter LW, editors: annual review of psychology, Palo Alto, CA, 1977, Stanford University Press.

202. Ibrahim MA and others: Management after myocardial infarction: a controlled trial of the effects of group psychotherapy, Int J Psychiatry Med 5:253, 1974.

203. Blanchard EB and Miller ST: Psychological treatment of cardiovascular disease, Arch Gen Psychiatry 34:1402, 1977.

204. Gil K and Blumenthal JA: Behavior modification in the primary and secondary prevention of coronary heart disease, Cardiol Pract 1:274, 1985.

205. Friedman M and others: Alteration of type A behavior and reduction in cardiac recurrences in postmyocardial infarction patients, Am Heart J 108:237, 1984.

206. Tripp-Reimer T, Brink PJ, and Saunders JM: Cultural assessment: content and process, Nurs Outlook 32:78, 1984.

207. Graison B, O'Leary L, and Wagner J: Cultural assessment . . . how well do we know our patients, J Nephrol Nurs 1:132, 1984.

208. Dennis C: Which MI patient has second-event risk? Hosp Pract 19(9):50, 1984.

209. Vedin A and others: Prediction of cardiovascular deaths and nonfatal reinfarctions after myocardial infarction, Scand J Rehabil Med 201:309, 1977.

210. Bauknecht VL: Testimony cites impact of DRG system, Am Nurse 17(10):3, 1985.

211. Andreoli KG and Musser LA: Trends that may affect nursing's future, Nurs Health Care 6:47, 1985.

# CHAPTER 8

# Valvular Heart Disease

Erin L. Abramczyk
Mary-Michael Brown

The heart has four valves: aortic, mitral, pulmonic, and tricuspid. These valves are responsible for ensuring the one-way, forward flow of blood through each heart chamber and for preventing backflow of blood within the heart.

Diseases of these valves result in two major problems: valvular stenosis and valvular regurgitation (or insufficiency). Valvular stenosis is the narrowing of the valve orifice, which hinders the unobstructed, forward movement of blood from a heart chamber. Some causes of valvular stenosis include rheumatic fever, congenital malformations of the valve, idiopathic calcification, myxomas, bacterial vegetations, and thrombus. Valvular insufficiency or regurgitation is the leaking of blood in a backward direction because of abnormally formed, floppy, stretched, inflamed, infected, or lesion-lined valve leaflets that prevent tight valve closure. Because of the high pressures in the left side of the heart, the aortic and mitral valves are the ones most commonly affected by disease. The pulmonic and tricuspid valves are affected less often; however, these valves can be diseased significantly and may even result in death. Pulmonic valve dysfunction, when present, is often associated with congenital malformations.

Nurses who care for patients afflicted with valvular heart disease are challenged to understand the complex nature of these illnesses. It is important for nurses to appreciate that valvular heart disease may be a chronic or an acute problem and may be manifested at any time in the life cycle. Nurses must be aware of the different types of valvular heart disease and which valves are typically affected. Nurses must be knowledgeable about the various treatment options available to patients, and they must be able to identify the disastrous complications that may accompany valvular heart disease. Finally, nurses must accurately estimate patients' understanding of their illness and the degree of family support available. It becomes essential, therefore, that nursing care be based on an understanding of the structure and function of the heart valves and the causes and treatments for the malfunction.

This chapter will describe the location and function of each of the heart valves; discuss manifestations of valvular disease; review the physical findings and diagnostic evaluation of valvular disease; and consider the medical, surgical, and nursing treatment of the patient with valvular heart disease.

## STRUCTURE AND FUNCTION OF VALVES

Although there are four valves in the heart, structurally and functionally there are actually two types: semilunar and atrioventricular. The semilunar type are the aortic and pulmonic valves; they are named for their half-moon shape. Each of the semilunar valves consists of three pocketlike cusps of equal size. These cusps are smooth and thin and arise from the arterial wall (see Fig. 1-3).

The mitral and tricuspid valves are called atrioventricular (AV) valves because of their placement between the atria and ventricles. The AV valves are composed of four major structures: annulus, cusps, chordae tendineae, and papillary muscles. These valves originate from the annulus, a somewhat ill-defined ring of fibrous tissue around the AV orifice. The AV valves have three or four cusps, which are thin, membranous, trapezoid structures. The tricuspid valve usually has three or four cusps: one anterior, one medial, and one or two posterior. The mitral (or bicuspid) valve has four cusps. Two are large cusps called the *anterior* (or *aortic*) and *posterior* (or *mural*) cusps, and two are small *commissural* cusps.

Chordae tendineae are strong, tendonlike cords that attach the ventricular surface of the cusps to the papillary muscles and allow the valve leaflets to balloon upward and against each other.[1] The papillary muscles are located at the base of the ventricles and pull the chordae and the AV valves together and downward at the beginning of the ventricular systole. This downward pull on the chordae prevents the eversion of valve leaflets during ventricular systole.

It is important to keep these basic valve structures in mind because valvular disease affects one or more of these structures. Treatment is aimed at modifying or replacing one or more of the dysfunctional structures to alleviate the manifestations of valvular heart disease.

TABLE 8-1  Physiologic dynamics of acquired valvular heart disease

| Valve Disease | Causes | Signs | Symptoms |
|---|---|---|---|
| Aortic stenosis | Rheumatic heart disease<br>Atherosclerosis<br>Calcification | Harsh, systolic, crescendo-decrescendo murmur at the second intercostal space, right sternal border<br>Increased point of maximum impulse<br>Paradoxically split $S_2$ | Angina pectoris<br>Dysrhythmias<br>Myocardial infarction<br>Syncope<br>Fatigue<br>Cough<br>Dyspnea on exertion<br>Orthopnea<br>Paroxysmal nocturnal dyspnea<br>Pulmonary edema |
| Aortic regurgitation | Rheumatic heart disease<br>Deceleration blunt chest trauma<br>Syphilis<br>Arthritic disease<br>Infective endocarditis<br>Aortic valve sclerosis<br>Hypertension<br>Aortic aneurysm<br>Calcification<br>Dysfunction of an aortic valve prosthesis<br>Senile dilatation of the annulus | Chronic:<br>High-pitched, blowing diastolic decrescendo murmur at the third or fourth intercostal space, right sternal border<br>Systolic hypertension<br>Diastolic hypotension<br>Capillary beds flush and pale with each pulse<br>Water hammer pulse<br>Head bob with pulse<br>PMI downward and to the left<br>Diastolic thrill at the suprasternal notch<br>Acute:<br>Soft murmur<br>Tachycardia<br>$S_3$ | Chronic:<br>Palpitations<br>Fatigue<br>Cough<br>Dyspnea on exertion<br>Orthopnea<br>Paroxysmal nocturnal dyspnea<br>Pulmonary edema<br>Angina pectoris<br>Night sweats<br>Headaches<br><br>Acute:<br>Fatigue<br>Cough<br>Dyspnea on exertion<br>Orthopnea<br>Paroxysmal nocturnal dyspnea<br>Pulmonary edema |
| Mitral stenosis | Rheumatic heart disease<br>Tumor<br>Left atrial thrombus<br>Bacterial vegetations<br>Calcification | Low-pitched, rumbling diastolic murmur at the apex<br>Opening snap<br>Atrial fibrillation<br>Hepatomegaly<br>Ascites<br>Jugular venous distention<br>Peripheral edema | Dyspnea<br>Interstitial and alveolar pulmonary edema<br>Orthopnea<br>Paroxysmal nocturnal dyspnea<br>Hemoptysis<br>Hoarseness |
| Mitral regurgitation | Rheumatic heart disease<br>Endocarditis<br>Prolapse<br>Dilated left ventricle<br>Calcification<br>Trauma<br>Dysfunction of a mitral valve prosthesis<br>Rupture/dysfunction of a papillary muscle | Chronic:<br>High-pitched, blowing systolic murmur at the apex<br>PMI downward and to the left<br>Atrial pulsation at the third left intercostal space<br>Atrial fibrillation<br>Jugular venous distention<br>Hepatomegaly | Chronic:<br>Fatigue<br>Exhaustion<br>Palpitations<br>Atypical chest pain<br>Dysphagia<br>Symptoms of mitral stenosis |

From Schakenbach LH: Physiologic dynamics of acquired valvular heart disease, J Cardiovasc Nurs 1(3):14, 1987.

**TABLE 8-1**  Physiologic dynamics of acquired valvular heart disease—cont'd

| Valve Disease | Causes | Signs | Symptoms |
|---|---|---|---|
| Mitral regurgitation—cont'd. | | Acute:<br>  High-pitched, blowing systolic murmur at the apex<br>  Sinus tachycardia<br>  $S_4$<br>  Widely split $S_2$ | Acute:<br>  Pulmonary edema<br>  Symptoms of mitral stenosis |
| Pulmonic stenosis | Rheumatic heart disease<br>Cancer | Harsh, systolic crescendo-decrescendo murmur at the second intercostal space, left sternal border<br>Widely split or absent $S_2$<br>Jugular venous distention<br>Peripheral edema<br>Hepatomegaly<br>Ascites | Dyspnea on exertion<br>Fatigue |
| Pulmonic regurgitation | Infective endocarditis<br>Tumors<br>Syphilitic aneurysm of the pulmonary artery | With elevated pulmonary pressures:<br>  High-pitched blowing, diastolic murmur at the mid left sternal border<br>Jugular venous distention<br>Peripheral edema<br>Hepatomegaly<br>Ascites<br>Without elevated pulmonary pressures:<br>  Medium-pitched, diastolic decrescendo murmur with inspiration<br>Jugular venous distention | With elevated pulmonary pressures:<br>  Dyspnea on exertion<br>  Fatigue |
| Tricuspid stenosis | Rheumatic heart disease<br>Atrial myxomas<br>Cancer | Low-pitched, rumbling diastolic, decrescendo murmur at the fourth intercostal space (increasing in intensity with inspiration), left sternal border<br>Jugular venous distention<br>Peripheral edema<br>Hepatomegaly<br>Ascites | Fatigue<br>Neck pulsations |
| Tricuspid regurgitation | Rheumatic heart disease<br>Infective endocarditis<br>Right ventricular dilatation<br>Trauma<br>MI<br>Triscuspid valve prolapse<br>Left heart failure<br>Pulmonary hypertension<br>Cancer<br>Right atrial myxoma | High-pitched, blowing systolic murmur at the fourth intercostal space, left sternal border or at the xyphoid region (increases with inspiration)<br>Left parasternal lift<br>Hepatomegaly<br>Splenomegaly<br>Right bundle branch block<br>Ascites<br>Peripheral cyanosis | Fatigue<br>Jaundice<br>Anorexia |

## MURMURS OF VALVULAR HEART DISEASE

When the cardiac cycle proceeds normally, the valves open to let blood flow from one chamber to the next and close to keep blood from leaking backward[2] (see Chapter 1). The sound produced as blood flows through a stenotic or regurgitant valve is called a murmur. The murmur is a result of the turbulent blood flow through a diseased valve, and these abnormal sounds are characteristic of valvular heart disease.

There are two major types of murmurs: systolic (or ejection) and diastolic murmurs. Chapter 2 details the cardiac cycle and the various features of cardiac murmurs. Table 8-1 describes the murmurs associated with each valvular disease.

## AORTIC VALVE DISEASE

The aortic valve is located between the left ventricle and the aorta. The aortic valve opens to facilitate forward flow of blood during ventricular systole and closes to prevent the backflow of blood from the aorta into the left ventricle during ventricular diastole.

### Aortic Stenosis

**Definition.** Aortic stenosis is a narrowing of the aortic valve orifice, which obstructs the ejection of blood from the left ventricle. This obstruction leads to a high-pressure gradient between the left ventricle and aorta during systolic ejection.[3] Isolated aortic stenosis affects men 3 times more often than women.[4]

**Etiology.** The three major causes of aortic stenosis are (1) congenital abnormalities, (2) rheumatic fever, and (3) idiopathic calcification. Aortic stenosis of congenital origin, such as unicuspid, bicuspid, multicuspid, or unequal aortic valve leaflets, is generally seen in patients younger than 30 years of age.[3] These congenital aberrations of the aortic valve make the valve leaflets more susceptible to the normal stress of cardiac hemodynamics. This increased stress and turbulent blood flow cause injury, predisposing the valvular leaflets to the development of fibrosis and calcification. The aortic valvular orifice then becomes rigid and narrowed. See Table 8-1 for more information on the causes of aortic stenosis.

Rheumatic disease affects patients from childhood through the seventh decade and causes the commissures of the valve to fuse, retract, and shorten the leaflet edges.[3] Although the aortic valve may be affected by rheumatic disease, the mitral valve is more frequently affected. However, improved treatment of streptococcal sore throat has markedly decreased the incidence of rheumatic valvular disease in the United States. Rheumatic fever is seen more commonly in developing countries. Idiopathic calcification most often affects patients in their seventh decade. Calcified deposits cause the valve leaflets to fuse and become fibrotic.[3]

**Pathophysiology.** Normally, the aortic valve orifice is 2.6 to 3.5 cm².[5] A valve orifice narrowed to 0.5 cm² may still prove functional if the stenosis develops over several years and the left ventricle is able to compensate.[6]

As the orifice of the aortic valve gradually becomes narrowed, the left ventricle compensates by exerting more pressure against the valve. Hypertrophy of the left ventricle develops concentrically without ventricular wall dilatation, which normalizes the systolic force of the ventricular wall. This concentric hypertrophy results in a near normal ejection fraction and cardiac output.[3] As the aortic valve orifice continues to narrow and the left ventricle attempts to compensate, a pressure gradient occurs between the aorta and the left ventricle. When the aortic valve orifice narrows to 0.4 cm² with a peak systolic pressure gradient above 50 mm Hg, a critical obstruction is reached.[5] The left ventricle dilates and the left atrium enlarges with an increase in pressure to overcome the ventricular dilatation. The higher pressure in the left atrium is reflected backward through the pulmonary vasculature to the right side of the heart. Right ventricular pressure, right atrial pressure, and central venous pressure increase. Eventually, the left side and the right side of the heart fail (see Fig. 8-1).

**Signs and symptoms.** Fatigue, chest pain, syncope, and dyspnea on exertion are the classic manifestations of aortic stenosis. Approximately 50% of patients experience chest pain (exertional angina) caused by underlying coronary artery disease or a disproportion of myocardial oxygen demand and supply during strenuous activities.[3,5] The already thickened and stretched left ventricle cannot meet the challenge of the increasing cardiac demand during exercise.

Syncope affects between 15% and 30% of patients with aortic stenosis as a consequence of a dysrhythmia, or from an abrupt fall in the patient's systemic vascular resistance

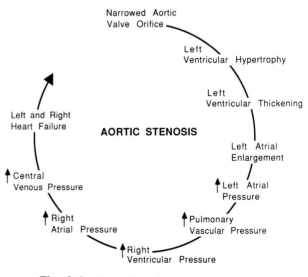

**Fig. 8-1** Pathophysiology of aortic stenosis.

with a fixed cardiac output.[5] Dyspnea on exertion occurs as a sequela of left ventricular dysfunction. Increases in left ventricular end-diastolic pressure cause an increased left atrial pressure, which is reflected back into the pulmonary vascular system. As the left ventricular failure worsens, the patient will experience cough, orthopnea, paroxysmal nocturnal dyspnea, and fatigue.

On examination, the patient appears pale, fatigued, and has a narrow pulse pressure. The murmur of aortic stenosis is a loud, harsh, crescendo-decrescendo systolic ejection murmur heard best at the second intercostal space, at the right sternal border[3,5,7] (see Table 8-1).

**Diagnostic evaluation.** The ECG reveals left ventricular hypertrophy, first degree atrioventricular block, and a left bundle branch block pattern.[3,5,6] The chest roentgenogram evidences left ventricular enlargement, a poststenotic dilatation of the aorta, calcification of valve cusps, and pulmonary congestion. The echocardiogram reveals left ventricular thickening and reduced mobility, and if present, calcification of the cusps. Nuclear scans can assess ventricular function and myocardial performance and determine the ejection fraction at rest and following exercise. The cardiac catheterization estimates the severity of obstruction by determining the gradient and evaluates left ventricular function. This study can determine the presence of valvular lesions as well as the presence or absence of coronary artery disease.

**Treatment.** Medical treatment of aortic stenosis consists of providing antibiotic prophylaxis against infective endocarditis. When patients require dental or other procedures requiring instrumentation (urinary catheterizations, prostatic manipulation, abortions)[3] or surgery, they should receive antibiotic coverage before and after the procedure.

Nitrates, used to relieve chest pain, should be administered cautiously because of the potential development of syncope and orthostatic hypotension. Digoxin and diuretics may be prescribed for controlling left ventricular dysfunction and dyspnea; however, the best treatment for aortic stenosis is to relieve the mechanical obstruction.

Balloon valvuloplasty is a nonsurgical procedure available to the elderly or to patients who present as high surgical risks. These patients may have severe left ventricular dysfunction, severe coronary artery disease, or chronic pulmonary disease.[5,8] Under fluoroscopy, a balloon-tipped catheter is directed to the aortic valve and inflated and deflated repeatedly. This dilatation may separate fused commissures or fracture calcified valve cusps, thus reducing the stenotic obstruction. Leaflet tearing, valve ring disruption, and restenosis of the valve may result from a valvuloplasty and emergent valve replacement becomes necessary.[9] While valvuloplasty may be a viable alternative to surgical valve replacement, the long-term results are still unknown.

Surgical treatment of aortic stenosis is indicated for asymptomatic patients who develop a gradient greater than 50 mm Hg and for patients who develop congestive heart failure, angina, or exertional syncope.[10]

An aortic commissurotomy may be performed for aortic stenosis, particularly in young patients. However, most of these patients eventually require replacement of the valve.[10]

Aortic valve replacement requires the use of extracorporeal circulation and selection of a valvular prosthesis. There are two kinds of prosthetic valves: mechanical and biologic.

Mechanical valves include the ball-and-cage (Starr-Edwards), the tilting disc (Bjork-Shiley, Lillehei-Caster, Medtronic Hall), and the central flow disc (St. Jude) (see Fig. 8-2). Mechanical valves are high-profile valves, which means they are more suitable for the larger orifices of the aortic and mitral valves. Mechanical valves are durable but also thrombogenic, requiring long-term anticoagulation.

Bioprostheses are made from pig or calf tissue. Porcine valves are excised aortic pig valves, which are preserved in glutaraldehyde. Bovine valves are made from calf pericar-

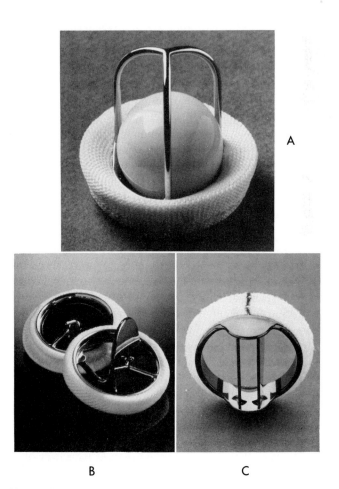

**Fig. 8-2** **A,** Starr-Edwards prosthetic valve; **B,** Medtronic Hall prosthetic valve. **C,** St. Jude Medical Heart Valve. (**B,** Courtesy of Medtronic, Minneapolis, MN; **C,** Courtesy of St. Jude Medical, Inc., St. Paul, MN.)

dium, which is cut into three pieces and mounted on a stent to form three valve leaflets.[11] The Carpentier-Edwards and Hancock valves are examples of porcine valves. The Ionescu-Shiley is a bovine pericardial graft.

The advantage of a bioprosthesis is the low risk of thromboembolic complications without anticoagulation. The disadvantage is the tendency of the bioprosthesis to degenerate.[10] Approximately 20% of patients with a bioprosthetic aortic valve require a second valve replacement within 8 years.[10]

Human allografts, or homografts (valves removed and prepared from cadavers), show less degenerative changes than other tissue valves, but more data are needed on the long-term results.[10]

Selection of the type of prosthetic valve is determined by the surgeon who measures the size of the valve orifice during surgery. Patients with a life expectancy of greater than 10 years generally receive mechanical valves. Patients with a questionable ability for compliance with anticoagulation, liver dysfunction, or a stated desire to bear children receive a bioprosthesis.

Nursing treatment is based on a holistic assessment of the patient and determining the individual's response to aortic stenosis. Decreased activity tolerance, alterations in comfort (chest pain, syncope), potential for infection, and anxiety related to knowledge deficit are problems commonly seen in patients with aortic stenosis.

For patients who have had an aortic valve replacement, potential for injury (thromboembolism, anticoagulation), potential for noncompliance, and potential for infection are the major nursing problems. Patients with bioprostheses can expect to be anticoagulated with warfarin (Coumadin) for approximately 6 weeks following valve replacement. Patients with mechanical valves are anticoagulated for the rest of their lives with warfarin, often in conjunction with dipyridamole (Persantine). Nurses must scrutinize the patient's understanding of the necessity for and the hazards of anticoagulation. Nurses must also assess the patient's ability and desire to comply with the therapeutic prescriptions.

Antibiotic prophylaxis against infective endocarditis is always indicated for surgical or dental procedures. See Table 8-2 for a list of possible nursing problems and treatment strategies.

## Aortic Regurgitation

**Definition.** Aortic regurgitation is the backward flow of blood from the aorta into the left ventricle during ventricular diastole.

**Etiology.** Rheumatic fever and syphilis have previously been identified as the major causes of aortic regurgitation; however, in recent years, antibiotics have exerted control over this problem.[10] Connective tissue disorders such as Marfan's syndrome, rheumatoid arthritis, and ankylosing spondylitis are responsible for changes in the annulus or leaflets causing leaflet malalignment and regurgitation. Aortic stenosis is also capable of causing aortic regurgitation because fixed and stenotic leaflets may allow the backflow of blood.[10]

Aortic dissection, infective endocarditis, trauma, and unsuccessful valvular surgery are causes of acute aortic regurgitation. Chronically elevated blood pressure and arteriosclerosis may cause mild aortic regurgitation.[7,10]

**Pathophysiology.** Aortic regurgitation, whether developing acutely or as a chronic problem, produces a volume overload for the left ventricle. During ventricular diastole, the backward flow of blood from the aorta is added to the blood that is emptied from the left atrium. When aortic regurgitation develops over several years, the increase in left ventricular end-diastolic volume results in a more forceful left ventricular contraction. The force of contraction is maintained by left ventricular hypertrophy and dilatation. Eventually, the hypertrophied ventricle can no longer support the force of contraction needed to eject blood. Under these circumstances, left ventricular end-diastolic pressure increases and is reflected backward to the left atrium, pulmonary vasculature, and right heart. Pulmonary congestion and right heart failure ensue.

If aortic regurgitation develops acutely, the left ventricle does not have the opportunity to hypertrophy and to increase the force of contraction to eject blood from the left ventricle. An increase in left ventricular end-diastolic volume causes an elevated left ventricular end-diastolic pressure. This pressure may actually exceed left atrial pressure and cause the mitral valve to close prematurely.[7] These hemodynamic changes produce pulmonary venous hypertension and pulmonary edema[10] (see Fig. 8-3).

**Signs and symptoms.** The person with mild aortic regurgitation may be asymptomatic. Signs and symptoms vary greatly, depending on the severity of the disease. The

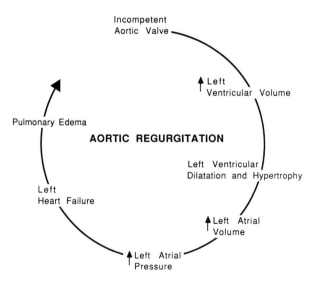

**Fig. 8-3** Pathophysiology of aortic regurgitation.

**TABLE 8-2** Nursing treatment of valvular heart disease

| Problem | Treatment |
| --- | --- |
| 1. Anxiety, related to dyspnea | Apply oxygen as needed. Administer diuretics and vasodilators as prescribed. Place patient in a comfortable position such as semi-Fowler's. Use relaxation techniques as needed. |
| Anxiety, related to knowledge deficit | Explain the function of the diseased valve and the cause of the dysfunction. Carefully review the medical and/or surgical plan. Clarify the patient's misconceptions, and answer the patient's questions. |
| Anxiety, related to alterations in comfort (chest pain, syncope) | Discuss reasons for chest pain and syncope. Discuss avoidance measures (minimize strenuous activities, exertion). Assist patient to rise slowly from a supine position to an upright position to avoid syncope and orthostatic hypotension. Carefully administer diuretics and vasodilators. Administer antidysrhythmic medication to maintain sinus rhythm. |
| 2. Decreased activity tolerance, related to decreased cardiac output | Assist patient in activities of daily living. Instruct patient to alternate periods of activity and rest. Consult caridac rehabilitation specialist for reconditioning exercises. Administer antidysrhythmic medications, diuretics, and vasodilators as prescribed. |
| 3. Fluid volume excess, related to dysfunctional valve | Provide bedrest. Administer prescribed diuretics. Monitor intake and output, daily weight, and laboratory values for electrolyte imbalances. |
| 4. Impaired gas exchange, related to fluid volume excess | Auscultate breath sounds frequently. Monitor chest roentgenogram for fluid volume excess. Notify physician for absent, unequal, diminished breath sounds, crackles, or wheezing. Notify physician for changes in the patient's baseline arterial blood gases. Provide supplemental oxygen or mechanical ventilation as needed. Administer diuretics as prescribed. Position patient comfortably (semi-Fowler's or high Fowler's). |
| 5. Potential for infection, risk factors: congenitally misshaped valve, intravenous drug abuse | Administer antibiotics as prescribed. Instruct patient about necessity of antibiotic prophylaxis with invasive procedures and about signs and symptoms of infection. Instruct intravenous drug abusers about fatality of infections in valve replacement recipients; instruct about cleaning used needles with bleach. |
| 6. Potential for injury, risk factors: anticoagulation, thrombus formation | Explain the use of warfarin and dypyridamole to patient. Administer warfarin as prescribed. Determine that the prothrombin time is 1.5 times greater than the control. Alert the physician of subtherapeutic prothrombin times. Instruct the patient to refrain from activities that may precipitate bleeding (use soft-bristled toothbrush, electric shaver; refrain from intense contact sports such as football, soccer, skiing). Instruct women of child-bearing age to contact their physician prior to attempting to become pregnant. Instruct patients to have their laboratory studies (blood work) drawn according to their scheduled appointments. |
| Potential for injury, risk factor: improperly seated prosthetic valve | Auscultate heart sounds postoperatively. Notify physician for changes in heart sounds or the presence of a new murmur. Monitor vital signs per the critical care unit's routine. Notify the physician for abrupt changes (increase heart rate, decreased blood pressure, decreased cardiac output). |
| 7. Potential noncompliance, risk factors: knowledge deficit; lack of economic resources | Review therapeutic regimen with the patient. Answer all questions; clarify misconceptions. Carefully explain the consequences of not adhering to the prescribed medical regimen. Ascertain the patient's ability to comply with the therapeutic plan. Note any discrepancies in subtherapeutic prothrombin times and verify that the patient is taking medication as prescribed. |

patient with chronic aortic regurgitation presents with the signs and symptoms of left ventricular failure: fatigue, dyspnea, and pulmonary edema. Patients may develop palpitations with exercise, neck pulsation, exertional chest pain, skin that appears warm and flushed, diaphoresis, dizziness, and increased systolic blood pressure with an ab-normally low diastolic blood pressure. Depending on cerebral blood flow, patients' neurologic status may vary markedly from an alert state to one of altered mentation and consciousness. Patients may complain of an awareness of their heart beat, particularly when lying on their left side. The patient with acute aortic regurgitation develops left ventricular failure and pulmonary edema. Physical abnormalities that may be found are the arachnodactyly of Marfan's syndrome and head bobbing with carotid pulsations.[10] A classic finding of aortic regurgitation is the "water-hammer" pulse, which manifests as a rapid disappearance of the pulse as arterial pressure suddenly falls in late systole and early diastole.

The diastolic murmur auscultated in chronic aortic regurgitation is high-pitched, blowing, and decrescendo heard best in the third or fourth intercostal space at the left or right sternal border.[10] If the patient sits forward and exhales, the murmur intensifies. A third or fourth heart sound may be heard depending on the degree of aortic regurgitation. Other murmurs, such as an Austin-Flint murmur, may also be auscultated. (See Chapter 2 for a discussion of murmurs.)

In acute aortic regurgitation, the murmur is soft and a third heart sound is audible (see Table 8-1).

**Diagnostic evaluation.** The electrocardiogram shows left ventricular hypertrophy (increased amplitude of the QRS and ST-T wave strain pattern).[10] Atrioventricular conduction is prolonged. Hypertrophic changes are not evident on the ECG with acute aortic regurgitation, but ST-T wave changes are consistent with myocardial ischemia.[10]

The chest roentgenogram shows dilatation of the left ventricle with elongation of the apex inferiorly and posteriorly (as seen in fluid volume overload). A prominent ascending aorta may be seen with Marfan's syndrome.

The echocardiogram visualizes vegetation formation on the valve leaflets that resulted from endocarditis. The amount of valvular regurgitation may also be quantified with this diagnostic study.

The cardiac catheterization estimates the severity of the regurgitation and evaluates the extent of left ventricular failure.[10] Radionucleide studies can demonstrate diminished performance of the left ventricle during exercise.

**Treatment.** Medical treatment of aortic regurgitation includes antibiotic prophylaxis against infective endocarditis. As with aortic stenosis, patients should receive antibiotics prior to and following dental or surgical procedures. Congestive heart failure is treated with diuretics, digoxin, vasodilators, and preload and afterload reducers.[10] Hydralazine has been successfully prescribed to control the regurgitant volume and improve the mechanical function of the left ventricle.[10]

Surgical treatment is indicated for patients with chronic aortic regurgitation who have developed symptoms. Asymptomatic patients who evidence left ventricular failure and patients with left ventricular end-diastolic pressure greater than 55 mm Hg also require surgery.[10] Surgical treatment is indicated for patients who develop aortic regurgitation acutely such as in aortic dissection or infective endocarditis.

The type of surgical prosthesis used depends on the patient's age, need for anticoagulation, and the durability of the valvular prosthesis. Mechanical valves carry a 2% to 3% incidence of thromboembolic and bleeding complications.[10] Porcine valves carry a 15% to 20% failure rate in 10 years.[10] There is a 1% to 2% incidence of prosthetic infective endocarditis regardless of the valvular prosthesis selected. Homografts may be especially useful in an infected valve.[10]

Nursing treatment of patients with aortic regurgitation is similar to care rendered to patients with aortic stenosis. One major point to remember is that aortic stenosis is a pressure overload disturbance, whereas aortic regurgitation is a fluid volume overload problem. Therefore nurses treat impaired gas exchange caused by fluid volume overload by administering diuretics, vasodilators, and preload and afterload reducing agents. Nurses assist patients to manage their anxiety by treating the patient's dyspnea and by addressing any knowledge deficit about the disease process and treatment. Nurses need to anticipate infection, hemorrhage, and thrombus formation in patients who are treated surgically to correct their aortic regurgitation (see Table 8-2).

## MITRAL VALVE DISEASE

The mitral valve is located between the left atrium and the left ventricle. During diastole, the mitral valve opens and permits blood to flow from the left atrium into the left ventricle. Immediately before ventricular systole, the mitral valve closes, preventing the leakage of blood from the left ventricle into the left atrium during the high-pressure phase of systolic ejection.

There are three types of mitral valve disease: mitral stenosis, mitral regurgitation, and mitral valve prolapse.

### Mitral Stenosis

**Definition.** Mitral stenosis refers to the narrowing of the mitral valvular orifice, producing an obstruction of blood flow from the left atrium, across the mitral valve, and into the left ventricle.

**Etiology.** Mitral stenosis is primarily a result of rheumatic fever. Myxomas, bacterial vegetations, thrombus, and calcification are less frequent causes.[12] The inflammatory processes of rheumatic fever cause the cusps of the valve to fibrose and thicken, thus decreasing the surface area of the opening (see Table 8-1).

**Pathophysiology.** The disease process of mitral stenosis begins with the formation of fibrous plaques on the mitral valve leaflets. These plaque aggregations lead to thickening, scarring, fusion, and contractures of the leaflets, and eventually the valve becomes calcified and stenotic. This calcification and fusion process decreases the valvular orifice and impedes blood flow through the mitral valve.

The chordae tendineae, which provide secondary channels for blood flow from the left atrium to the left ventricle,

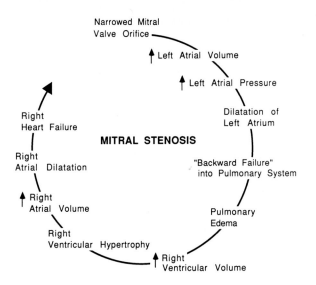

Narrowed Mitral
Valve Orifice

↑ Left Atrial Volume

↑ Left Atrial Pressure

Dilatation of
Left Atrium

**MITRAL STENOSIS**

Right
Heart Failure

Right
Atrial Dilatation

"Backward Failure"
into Pulmonary System

↑ Right
Atrial Volume

Pulmonary
Edema

Right
Ventricular Hypertrophy

↑ Right
Ventricular Volume

**Fig. 8-4** Pathophysiology of mitral stenosis.

also become inflamed and diseased in mitral stenosis. The chordae tendineae fuse, and further obstruction to blood flow across the mitral valve occurs.[3]

The normal mitral valve orifice is 5 cm². In mitral stenosis, the valvular opening may decrease to 1.5 cm². This narrowed opening causes an increased pressure in the left atrium, resulting in dilatation of the chamber.

A "backward" heart failure increases pressure in the pulmonary veins, capillaries, and arteries. Pulmonary arterial hypertension, which serves as a compensatory mechanism, may develop. As the pressure in the pulmonary capillaries exceeds the oncotic pressure, pulmonary edema develops. Eventually, the right ventricle hypertrophies, fails, and produces jugular venous distention, liver enlargement, ascites, and peripheral edema. Fig. 8-4 provides a summary of the sequelae of mitral stenosis.

**Signs and symptoms.** In acquired mitral stenosis, the symptoms appear gradually over a period of approximately 20 years.[3] Mitral stenosis primarily affects women in their third decade. In fact, two thirds of all patients with mitral stenosis are female. The most frequently occurring symptoms of mitral stenosis are dyspnea, fatigue, palpitations, cough, and hemoptysis. These are all signs of the "backward" failure into the pulmonary system and the right side of the heart. Less common symptoms include dysphagia, hoarseness, chest pain, embolic events, seizure, and cerebrovascular accident.

The decrease in cardiac output and cardiac reserve that results from mitral stenosis is directly proportional to the severity of the stenosis.[13] Generally, symptoms of mitral stenosis are not experienced at rest. However, the symptoms are worsened by exercise and are evidenced as pulmonary edema.

The murmur associated with mitral stenosis is a result of turbulent blood flow through and around the stenotic mitral valve. It is appreciated best at the apex. An opening snap may be auscultated, followed by a low-pitched diastolic rumble that may be intensified when the patient is placed in the left lateral recumbent position.

**Diagnostic evaluation.** The ECG evidences characteristically wide, notched P waves.[12] Atrial fibrillation occurs in 40% to 50% of patients with mitral stenosis. In atrial fibrillation, the atrium does not contract as completely or forcefully as it does in normal sinus rhythm. The loss of proper atrial contraction in atrial fibrillation increases the risk of thrombus formation and subsequent embolic events.

Chest roentgenograms of patients with mitral stenosis may reveal left atrial, right ventricular, and pulmonary artery enlargement.[12] Pulmonary capillary and alveolar wall thickening and fibrosis may be detected. Oxygen use is inhibited, and eventually lung capacity decreases.

The most useful noninvasive method for detection of mitral stenosis is the echocardiogram. The stenotic mitral valve appears thick and shows diminished motion and posterior leaflet movement. Valvular gradient data may be obtained by cardiac catheterization.[12]

**Treatment.** Medical treatment focuses on prophylactic antibiotic therapy to reduce the risk of recurrent rheumatic fever and endocarditis. Patients with mitral stenosis must receive antibiotics with any invasive procedure or dental surgery. Medical therapy includes diuretics for symptoms of congestive heart failure, a low-sodium diet, avoiding exertion (which may invoke symptoms), anticoagulation, and digoxin, quinidine, or synchronized cardioversion for atrial fibrillation. Caution should be taken when cardioverting any patient who has been in atrial fibrillation for a prolonged period of time, for fear of mobilizing thrombi. Balloon valvuloplasty has recently been employed in patients with mitral stenosis who are considered at high operative risk. Complications of valvuloplasty such as bleeding, inadvertent creation of atrial septal defects with the balloon catheter, and restenosis require more extensive evaluation.[12]

Surgical intervention is the only permanent method for reducing obstruction of a stenotic mitral valve. Valve replacement or valve repair are two surgical alternatives. In patients with pure mitral stenosis (those who develop mitral stenosis in their third decade), a mitral valve commissurotomy is the treatment of choice. If reconstruction of the valve is not appropriate, replacement of the stenotic mitral valve is indicated. (Refer to the section on surgical treatment of aortic stenosis for a discussion of valve prostheses.)

Generally, younger patients receive mechanical valve replacements. Long-term anticoagulation is indicated with these prostheses and is generally acceptable in young, otherwise healthy adults. Mechanical valves function for a longer period of time than bioprostheses before requiring replacement. Elderly patients receive bioprosthetic valves such as Carpentier-Edwards porcine (pig) valves, or Ionescu-Shiley bovine (cow) valves. Human allograft valves are not currently used for mitral valve replacement.

Nursing treatment primarily includes reduction of anxiety related to occurrence of symptoms of right heart failure, impaired gas exchange, and lack of knowledge of diagnosis. Counseling for activity intolerance and coping with the diagnosis are also important features of nursing intervention (see Table 8-2).

### Mitral Regurgitation

**Definition.** Mitral valve regurgitation is the backward leakage of blood from the left ventricle into the left atrium during the high-pressure ventricular systole. The incompetent or regurgitant mitral valve fails to provide a secure seal between the left atrium and the left ventricle.

**Etiology.** Historically, an overwhelming proportion of the cases of mitral regurgitation were attributed to rheumatic fever; however, current research indicates that mitral valve prolapse and coronary artery disease are the principal causes of mitral valve regurgitation.[12] Less common causes of acquired mitral regurgitation include Marfan's syndrome, calcification of the mitral valve annulus, Ehlers-Danlos syndrome, ischemic heart disease, MI, ventricular aneurysm, papillary muscle damage, and endocarditis.[12] Mitral regurgitation may also be congenital in origin.

Cardiomyopathy, or any other disease process that causes the left ventricle to hypertrophy, may increase the valvular orifice, thus disrupting the anchoring function of the papillary muscles. Mitral regurgitation may also be caused by calcification of the mitral ring. This calcification is common in elderly women.[13] The majority of patients with acquired mitral regurgitation are females.[3]

**Pathophysiology.** Mitral regurgitation results in an increased blood volume in the left ventricle and left atrium. Because the mitral valve does not close tightly during systole, blood flows into the left atrium and a smaller volume of blood is ejected into the aorta during left ventricular systole.[13] The inflammation and scarring from rheumatic fever produce rigidity and contraction of the valvular leaflets, fusion of the valve commissures, and shortening of the chordae tendineae. All of these changes culminate in a leaky, incompetent mitral valve.

As mitral regurgitation progresses, the increased volume in the left atrium creates left atrial enlargement. The posterior leaflet of the mitral valve is shifted posteriorly and loses its full range of motion, thus invoking an incompetent closure of valvular leaflets.[12]

Increased volume from the left atrium to the left ventricle results in left ventricular dilatation and hypertrophy. Despite attempts to adjust, the left ventricle fails, and this failure is reflected into the left atrium and the pulmonary system. The pulmonary system attempts to compensate for the greater volume by increasing lymphatic flow, thus in-

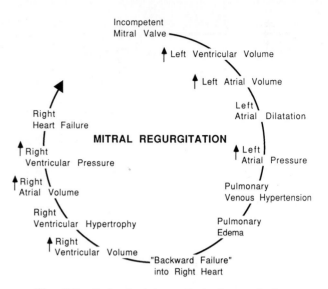

**Fig. 8-5** Pathophysiology of mitral regurgitation.

creasing pulmonary pressures. If the left atrial pressure reaches 30 to 40 mm Hg, pulmonary edema usually ensues.[13]

Over time, pulmonary edema may lead to pulmonary hypertension and failure of the right side of the heart. Pulmonary edema may also create a "backward" failure on the right side of the heart. The right ventricle enlarges to compensate for higher blood volumes and fails. Right ventricular failure causes right atrial failure, which culminates in ascites and peripheral edema. See Fig. 8-5 for a synopsis of mitral regurgitation.

**Signs and symptoms.** Fatigue, weakness, exhaustion, and cachexia occur when the cardiac output is significantly decreased from mitral regurgitation. Atrial fibrillation is a common symptom of mitral regurgitation. As the atrium dilates, a greater surface area is created, thus increasing the distance the cardiac conduction impulse must travel. The increased distance enhances the potential for the impulse to become abnormal, and for atrial fibrillation to develop. In the presence of atrial fibrillation, the heart's ability to function as a strong pump decreases, which further reduces cardiac output.[13] Other signs of mitral regurgitation include tachypnea, hypotension, and pulmonary edema.

The murmur associated with mitral regurgitation is a blowing, systolic sound appreciated best at the apex and radiating to the left axilla. In mitral regurgitation, the first heart sound is difficult to auscultate and may be absent. The second heart sound is split, and, occasionally, a third or fourth heart sound may be noted.[3]

**Diagnostic evaluation.** The ECG of the patient with mitral regurgitation evidences altered P wave and QRS complex amplitude. Atrial fibrillation is usually seen. Q waves from previous MIs may also be noted if the mitral regurgitation is the result of coronary ischemia. Several nonspecific ST changes may also be exhibited on the ECG. The chest roentgenogram will demonstrate left ventricular and left atrial enlargement. The echocardiogram evidences decreased ventricular wall motion, and the echo Doppler provides data for estimating the severity of the regurgitation.[13] Cardiac catheterization is useful in measuring the left ventricular end-diastolic pressure and demonstrating wall motion.

**Treatment.** Medical treatment of mitral regurgitation is aimed at alleviating the symptoms. Presence of symptoms is directly related to the severity of the disease. Medications prescribed include diuretics, digoxin, quinidine, and vasodilators to alleviate the symptoms associated with right-sided heart failure. Anticoagulation therapy may also be prescribed to decrease the risk of thrombus and subsequent embolus caused by atrial fibrillation. Restriction of symptom-producing activity is recommended and a low-sodium diet is also prescribed. Surgical treatment of mitral regurgitation is the same as surgical intervention for mitral stenosis.

Nursing treatment focuses on relieving anxiety related to the diagnosis of mitral regurgitation. Because the symptoms of mitral regurgitation may not be evidenced for many years, the patient needs to be knowledgeable about the signs and symptoms of mitral regurgitation. Nursing intervention for treatment of the symptoms of decreased cardiac output is also necessary for the nursing care of the patient with mitral regurgitation. Utilizing the interdisciplinary health care team is essential in providing holistic care for these patients (see Table 8-2).

## Mitral Valve Prolapse

**Definition.** Mitral valve prolapse, also known as Barlow's syndrome or floppy valve syndrome, occurs when one or more valvular leaflets protrude into the left atrium during ventricular systole. The posterior leaflet is most commonly involved. Mitral valve prolapse is the most widespread valvular disease in adults, occurring in 4% of the population.[3] The syndrome occurs in all age groups; however, it is most frequently found in women between 20 and 50 years of age.[14] This abnormality tends to occur in families and is probably carried in an autosomal dominant genetic pattern.[3]

**Etiology.** Mitral valve prolapse is hereditary, and it may also be a result of atrial and ventricular septal defects, patent ductus arteriosus, skeletal abnormalities, or Marfan's syndrome. Acquired mitral valve prolapse may be the result of endocarditis, myocarditis, coronary artery disease, cancer with myocardial metastases, muscular dystrophy and acromegaly, or collagen vascular diseases such as systemic lupus erythematosus.[12]

**Pathophysiology.** Regardless of the etiology of mitral valve prolapse, the posterior leaflet of the mitral valve protrudes into the left atrium during ventricular systole. This prolapse of the leaflet becomes significant because the posterior leaflet encompasses approximately two thirds of the entire orifice of the mitral valve.

**Signs and symptoms.** The most common symptom of mitral valve prolapse is chest pain. This pain may be related to the myocardial ischemia that may result from the tremendous pull that must be exerted by the papillary muscles on the damaged leaflet. Coronary artery spasm may also occur as a result of this force.[12] Other symptoms include dizziness, palpitations, dyspnea, and syncope. Skeletal abnormalities such as a pigeon breast, funnel chest, scoliosis, kyphosis, or straight back syndrome may be exhibited.

The murmur associated with mitral valve prolapse is a systolic click that is best appreciated at the apex along the left sternal border. Recent literature suggests that dysautonomia (dysfunction of the nervous system) may be linked to mitral valve prolapse.[14] Patients with mitral valve prolapse have significantly elevated levels of epinephrine and norepinephrine. These high levels of catecholamines may suggest why mitral valve prolapse patients have panic attacks, are susceptible to stress-induced dysrhythmias, and demonstrate altered blood pressure and pulse responses to position changes.[14] Mitral valve prolapse may rarely involve lethal dysrythmias, resulting in sudden death. In some patients, mitral valve prolapse may progress to mitral valve regurgitation and require surgical replacement of the regurgitant valve.

**Diagnostic evaluation.** Dysrhythmias are evident in the ECGs of 60% of patients with mitral valve prolapse. The most frequently occurring rhythm disturbances include bradycardia and atrioventricular blocks. Supraventricular tachycardias and premature ventricular contractions are also noted. There may be ST segment and T wave alterations and QT prolongation. The chest roentgenogram shows a normal cardiac silhouette. Echocardiogram evidences a floppy posterior mitral valve leaflet.

**Treatment.** Medical treatment includes propranolol for chest pain and dysrhythmias. Prophylactic antibiotic therapy may be used, although there is a low incidence of endocarditis related to mitral valve prolapse. All patients with mitral valve prolapse and any degree of mitral regurgitation should receive prophylactic antibiotics. Medical therapies for dyspnea and palpitations may be prescribed. Propranolol may be prescribed for mitral valve prolapse patients with hyperadrenergic symptoms, and low doses of barbiturates may be indicated for hypervagal patients. Psychotherapy may also be prescribed for patients with panic attacks. Asymptomatic patients with mitral valve prolapse may not require any treatment. No surgical treatment for mitral valve prolapse is indicated. The goal of nursing treatment is alleviating anxiety related to the diagnosis of mitral valve prolapse and the symptoms of dysautonomia. Nursing treatment must also include educating persons with mitral valve prolapse about the etiology and treatment of mitral valve prolapse (see Table 8-2).

## TRICUSPID VALVE DISEASE

The tricuspid valve is located between the right atrium and right ventricle and is closed during right atrial diastole to allow blood to collect in the right atrium. The tricuspid valve opens as pressure in the right atrium exceeds that in the right ventricle. As right ventricular diastole is completed, the tricuspid valve again closes in preparation for right ventricular systole. The closure of the tricuspid valve prevents backflow of blood from the higher pressured right ventricle into the lower pressured right atrium during ventricular systole.

### Tricuspid Stenosis

**Definition.** Tricuspid stenosis is the narrowing of the tricuspid valve orifice; this narrowing obstructs blood flow across the valve during the diastolic filling of the right ventricle.[15]

**Etiology.** The causes of tricuspid stenosis include rheumatic heart disease, carcinoid syndrome, atrial myxoma, and other diseases. Rheumatic heart disease, which causes a fibrous thickening and contracture of the valve leaflets, is usually associated with a concomitant mitral stenosis[7,15] (see Table 8-1).

Carcinoid syndrome results from a malignant tumor (usually gastrointestinal in origin) that causes fibrous tissue deposits to form on the tricuspid valve leaflets. The leaflets then become rigid and contracted, leading to tricuspid valvular stenosis.

Atrial myxomas mechanically obstruct the tricuspid valve as can right atrial thrombi and metastatic tumors.[15]

**Pathophysiology.** Tricuspid stenosis reduces diastolic blood flow across the valve. Right atrial pressure rises in an attempt to overcome this obstruction. The cardiac output is reduced because less blood fills the right ventricle, and hence, less blood reaches the left side of the heart.

The normal tricuspid valve area is 7 cm². A reduction in right ventricular filling occurs when the valve orifice is reduced to 1.5 cm² or less.[15] When right atrial pressure rises to 10 mm Hg or more, peripheral edema may be noted. Atrial fibrillation, which often accompanies tricuspid stenosis, further increases the right atrial pressure.

The hemodynamic effects of tricuspid stenosis, including increased right atrial pressure and reduced cardiac output, are actually worsened by the usually coexistent mitral stenosis (see Fig. 8-6).

**Signs and symptoms.** The major signs and symptoms of tricuspid stenosis are dyspnea and fatigue. Patients may evidence peripheral edema and neck pulsations as the internal jugular veins become distended.[15]

The murmur of tricuspid stenosis is a low-pitched diastolic rumble best heard at the fourth intercostal space, left sternal border. The murmur increases in intensity with

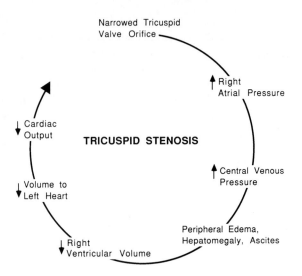

**Fig. 8-6** Pathophysiology of tricuspid stenosis.

inspiration as intrathoracic pressure is reduced and right ventricular filling increases.[7] The murmur is caused by turbulent blood flow across the narrowed valvular orifice (see Table 8-1).

**Diagnostic evaluation.** The ECG reveals large P waves in the absence of right ventricular enlargement.[15] The chest roentgenogram shows a prominent right atrium. The echocardiogram can identify fibrosis, calcifications, and obstruction of the valve. The echo Doppler technique can estimate the diastolic gradient across the valve. A cardiac catheterization confirms a gradient of greater than 1 mm Hg between the right atrium and right ventricle.

**Treatment.** Medical treatment of tricuspid stenosis consists of antibiotic prophylaxis to prevent infective endocarditis. Peripheral edema may not respond to diuretics, digitalis, and/or preload or afterload reduction since the edema is not the result of fluid volume overload, but a pressure overload.[15] Surgical treatment is indicated if tricuspid stenosis is severe. Because of the high thrombogenic rate associated with tricuspid valve replacement, anticoagulation with warfarin is warranted, often in conjunction with dipyridamole. Long-term anticoagulation, therefore, negates the benefit of a bioprosthesis, and hence mechanical valves are often used to replace a diseased tricuspid valve.[15] Preferred valves include the St. Jude valve, a tilting disc, or a ball-and-cage device.[15]

Nursing treatment of tricuspid stenosis is directed toward alleviation of the patient's anxiety. Such anxieties result from a lack of knowledge about valvular disease and treatment. Similarly, anxiety may be precipitated by dyspnea. Patients may suffer from a decreased activity tolerance, which is a consequence of low cardiac output. The potential for valve infection is a persistent problem; infective endocarditis may strike both a dysfunctional valve or a prosthetic replacement. Patients who are anticoagulated are at risk for injury (hemorrhage) and must be instructed about safety precautions; they must also be responsible for self-administration of warfarin or antiplatelet medications (see Table 8-2).

## Tricuspid Regurgitation

**Definition.** Tricuspid regurgitation is the backward flow of blood from the right ventricle into the right atrium through an incompetent valve during right ventricular contraction.

**Etiology.** The most common reason for tricuspid regurgitation is right ventricular dilatation and failure, which develops as a sequela to left ventricular failure and/or pulmonary hypertension. Concomitant aortic and mitral valvular disease are frequently responsible for this left ventricular failure and pulmonary hypertension. Right ventricular dilatation causes the valve orifice and annulus to stretch and enlarge, thus preventing the valve leaflets from closing completely (see Fig. 8-7).

Infective endocarditis causes the tricuspid valve leaflets to malalign because of vegetations along the cusps. Intravenous drug abuse is a major cause of infective endocarditis.[15] Other causes of tricuspid regurgitation include MI, blunt trauma to the chest (steering wheel injuries in automobile accidents or external compressions from cardiopulmonary resuscitation), carcinoid syndrome, and congenital anomalies (see Table 8-1).

**Pathophysiology.** The backward flow of blood into the right atrium increases right atrial pressure, which, in turn, increases systemic venous pressure. Because some blood escapes backward to the right atrium during right ventricular systole, not all blood reaches the left side of the heart. Cardiac output, therefore, is reduced. The right ventricle dilates and hypertrophies in an effort to eject more blood, but this dilatation and hypertrophy actually can worsen the tricuspid regurgitation. The right atrium then enlarges and frequently atrial fibrillation ensues, further reducing the cardiac output. This course is often complicated by pulmonary hypertension and left heart failure, which initially may have caused the tricuspid regurgitation.

**Signs and symptoms.** Patients with tricuspid regurgitation experience dyspnea, orthopnea, peripheral edema, and fatigue. Atrial fibrillation is common. Patients with infective endocarditis causing tricuspid regurgitation may be febrile. Other signs and symptoms include hepatomegaly, anorexia (from liver and intestinal venous congestion), and peripheral cyanosis (from a low cardiac output).[7]

The murmur of tricuspid regurgitation is high-pitched, blowing, and holosystolic; it is heard best at the fourth intercostal space at the left sternal border or xiphoid area. The murmur intensifies with inspiration.

**Diagnostic evaluation.** The ECG frequently shows atrial fibrillation or a right bundle branch block caused by right ventricular hypertrophy. The chest roentgenogram evidences both right atrial and right ventricular enlargement. The echocardiogram facilitates recognition of vegetative lesions, ruptured chordae and papillary muscles, and the back-and-forth movement of the valve.[15] The echo Doppler technique estimates the severity of the regurgitation. The cardiac catheterization reveals a prominent cv wave in the right atrium suggestive of tricuspid regurgitation.

**Treatment.** Medical treatment of tricuspid regurgitation is directed toward alleviation of right ventricular failure. A low-sodium diet, digitalis, diuretics, and vasodilators are used to treat right and left heart failure. If pulmonary hypertension and left heart failure are pesent, adding prostaglandin-E, dobutamine, and dopamine may help to dilate the pulmonary vasculature and increase the cardiac output.[15]

Surgical treatment of tricuspid regurgitation is based on the extent of concurrent mitral valvular disease. If mitral stenosis is critical, a mitral valve replacement is performed.[15] Intraoperatively, following the mitral valve surgery, the surgeon will determine if the tricuspid regurgitation has significantly improved. The surgeon also inspects the right atrium and vena cavae for moderate enlargement, an indication of the severity of tricuspid regurgitation. A tricuspid valve repair or replacement may ensue.

A repair or reconstruction of the valve leaflets (valvuloplasty) and the valve annulus (annuloplasty) is preferred since long-term results of these procedures are more favorable than complete valve replacement.[15] However, if the leaflets are hopelessly deformed, which may be seen with infective endocarditis, a tricuspid valve replacement is indicated.

As discussed in the surgical management of tricuspid stenosis, thrombogenesis remains a problem. Hence, the more durable mechanical valves may be favored since anticoagulation will still be necessary. The St. Jude, tilting

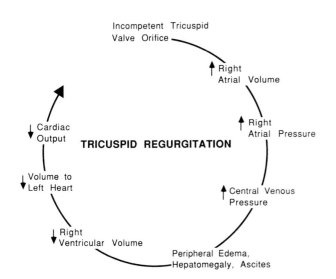

**Fig. 8-7** Pathophysiology of tricuspid regurgitation.

disc, and ball-and-cage prostheses are frequently used. A total tricuspid valvotomy may be performed in the case of infective endocarditis from intravenous drug abuse. While this procedure carries the risk of congestive heart failure, if the cessation of intravenous drug abuse is remote, implanting a mechanical valve will likely result in a fatal infection.

Nursing treatment is aimed at improving gas exchange related to the fluid volume overload seen in heart failure. Patients may also suffer from decreased activity tolerance related to a decrease in cardiac output; potential for infection, anxiety from dyspnea, and knowledge deficit about the disease process and treatment; and potential for injury from anticoagulation (see Table 8-2).

## PULMONARY VALVE DISEASE

The pulmonic valve is located between the right ventricle and the pulmonary artery; it prevents blood flow from the pulmonary artery into the right ventricle during diastole.[13] It is a semilunar valve with three similarly shaped cusps. Although the pulmonic valve may become diseased, the symptoms are generally not life-threatening because of the low pressures in the area where the pulmonic valve is located.

### Pulmonic Stenosis

**Definition.** Pulmonic valve stenosis refers to the obstruction of blood flow across a narrowed pulmonic valve during systole.

**Etiology.** Stenosis of the pulmonic valve is usually congenital. Acquired pulmonic stenosis rarely occurs, though it may be caused by rheumatic fever, cancerous valvular lesions, syphilis, endocarditis, and tuberculosis. The valvular changes that result from the inflammatory disease processes of rheumatic fever and endocarditis affect the mitral and aortic valves more often than the pulmonic valve, and usually cause pulmonic regurgitation. Pulmonic stenosis evolves slowly if it is a result of a metastatic carcinoid tumor.[7]

**Pathophysiology.** The inflammatory changes that occur from rheumatic fever and endocarditis cause a fibrous thickening of the cusps of the pulmonic valve, resulting in a decreased valvular orifice. The reduced opening of the stenotic valve causes a backward flow of blood into the right ventricle. Right heart failure follows from the increase in right heart volume and pressure. As the right side of the heart fails, a diminished cardiac output results. The pressure and volume in the right atrium also increase, resulting in venous engorgement, most notably hepatomegaly, jugular venous distention, and peripheral edema.[3] See Fig. 8-8 for the sequelae of events of pulmonic stenosis.

**Signs and symptoms.** Patients with pulmonic stenosis may remain asymptomatic for many years. The appearance of symptoms is directly proportional to the severity of the disease. The most frequently occurring symptoms are dys-

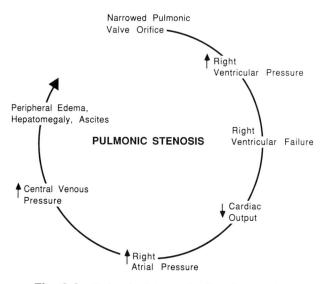

**Fig. 8-8** Pathophysiology of pulmonic stenosis.

pnea, fatigue, and syncope. If pulmonic stenosis is a consequence of rheumatic fever or other inflammatory diseases, patients may exhibit fever and pulmonary infections. Patients with pulmonic stenosis resulting from carcinoid tumors may evidence facial flushing, diarrhea, and bronchospasms, because of the release of serotonin by the tumor.[16]

The murmur auscultated in pulmonic stenosis is a sharp, systolic crescendo-decrescendo sound; it is best appreciated at the left sternal border at the second or third intercostal space. The second heart sound ($S_2$) is widely split or may be absent (see Table 8-1).

**Diagnostic evaluation.** Obtaining a thorough medical history of the patient is important in determining the cause of pulmonic stenosis (see Chapter 2). There are no definitive ECG abnormalities associated with pulmonic stenosis. However, if pulmonary hypertension is present, the ECG will evidence right axis deviation because of right ventricular hypertrophy and P wave morphologic changes related to right atrial enlargement.[16]

The chest roentgenogram reveals poststenotic dilatation, prominence of the pulmonary artery, and right ventricular hypertrophy. Echocardiography is the most valuable noninvasive tool for diagnosing pulmonic stenosis. The ECG detects lesions of and around the valve. The echo Doppler can ascertain the severity of the stenosis. Cardiac catheterization is not specifically useful in the diagnosis of pulmonic stenosis; however, a right-sided heart injection will demonstrate the outline of the pulmonic valve.[16]

**Treatment.** Medical treatment of pulmonic stenosis generally includes prophylactic antibiotics against recurrent endocarditis. If pulmonary emboli are suspected, anticoagulation is indicated. Vasodilator therapies including nitroglycerin and prostaglandin-E are employed to decrease the severity of pulmonary hypertension. Treatment of the symptoms of congestive heart failure may also be undertaken; such treatments include digoxin, diuretics, and a low-sodium diet.

Surgical replacement of a stenotic pulmonary valve is rare. However, a commissurotomy, or repair of the valve may be performed to alleviate the stenosis. Because of the high incidence of emboli associated with the mechanical valve prosthesis in the pulmonic valve position, bioprostheses are used when valves require replacement. Currently, a valvotomy, or removal of the valve and antibiotic prophylaxis seem to be the preferred treatments.[16]

Nursing treatment primarily focuses on patient education related to the diagnosis of acquired pulmonic stenosis. The symptoms of pulmonic stenosis usually remain dormant for many years; therefore a patient requires knowledge of the cause of the stenosis and preparation for the appearance of the symptoms. Nursing intervention to decrease the patient's anxiety related to the diagnosis of pulmonic stenosis is also indicated (see Table 8-2).

## Pulmonic Regurgitation

**Definition.** Pulmonic regurgitation denotes the backward leakage of blood from the pulmonary artery into the right ventricle during diastole. The regurgitant or incompetent pulmonic valve leaflets become scarred and do not close tightly, allowing blood to leak back into the right ventricle.

**Etiology.** Pulmonic regurgitation mainly occurs as a congenital defect. Acquired pulmonic regurgitation occurs more frequently than pulmonic stenosis, and it may result from any condition causing pulmonary hypertension; such conditions include mitral stenosis, chronic obstructive pulmonary disease, pulmonary embolism, endocarditis, valvotomy as treatment for pulmonic stenosis, sarcoma or myxoma tumors, and rarely, rheumatic fever or tuberculosis.[16]

**Pathophysiology.** In pulmonic regurgitation, the leaflets of the valve do not close firmly as a result of various disease processes. With endocarditis and cancerous tumor involvement, the cusps of the valve thicken, scar, and contract, thus permitting blood to flow through the gaps between the diseased cusps. If the valve has been removed, regurgitation obviously occurs. Elevated right ventricular pressure and hypertrophy ensue.[7] Eventually, the right ventricle fails, and a diminished quantity of blood is actually pumped into the pulmonary system. Increased volume and pressure back up into the right atrium, which causes right atrial hypertrophy and failure manifested by an elevated central venous pressure, jugular venous distention, and peripheral congestion and edema. Fig. 8-9 summarizes the sequelae of pulmonic regurgitation.

**Signs and symptoms.** The symptoms of pulmonic regurgitation will not be evidenced unless pulmonary hypertension exists concurrently. The patient with pulmonic regurgitation may remain asymptomatic for many years,

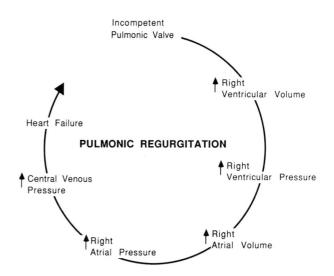

**Fig. 8-9** Pathophysiology of pulmonic regurgitation.

depending on the extent of the underlying disease. Isolated pulmonic regurgitation is usually tolerated without evidence of symptoms. Dyspnea, fatigue, and syncope, which result from pulmonary hypertension, are the most common symptoms.

The cardiac murmur associated with pulmonic regurgitation is high-pitched when pulmonary hypertension is present, or moderately-pitched without pulmonary hypertension. The murmur is a blowing sound most optimally auscultated at the fourth or fifth intercostal space at the left sternal border. If is often difficult to distinguish the murmur of pulmonic regurgitation from the murmur of aortic regurgitation (see Table 8-1).

**Diagnostic evaluation and treatment.** The diagnostic tools for pulmonic regurgitation are similar to those of pulmonic stenosis. A complete medical history to delineate the cause of the regurgitation is paramount (see Chapter 2). Treatment of pulmonic regurgitation is based on alleviating symptoms, usually with a medical regimen of diuretics, digoxin, and a low-sodium diet.

## SUMMARY

Valvular heart disease can affect one or more of the cardiac valves, producing either stenosis or regurgitation or both. The most frequent causes of dysfunction of the heart valves are rheumatic heart disease and infective endocarditis. Valvular heart disease occurs in all age groups and symptoms may develop suddenly or over a period of many years.

## REFERENCES

1. Schlant RC, Silverman ME, and Roberts WE: Anatomy of the heart. In Hurst JW and others, editors: The heart, ed 7, New York, 1990, McGraw-Hill.
2. Miracle VA: Anatomy of a murmur, Nursing 16:26, 1986.

3. Cavallo GAO: The person with valvular heart disease. In Guzzetta CE and Dossey BM, editors: *Cardiovascular nursing: bodymind tapestry,* St Louis, 1984, Mosby–Year Book, Inc.

4. Thibault GE, DeSanctis RW, and Buckley MJ: Aortic stenosis. In Eagle KA and others, editors: The practice of cardiology, ed 2, Boston, 1989, Little, Brown, & Co.

5. Vitello-Cicciu J and Lapsley DP: Valvular heart disease. In Kinney MR, Packa DR, and Dunbar SB, editors: AACN's clinical reference for critical-care nursing, ed 2, New York, 1988, McGraw-Hill.

6. Netter FH: The CIBA collection of medical illustrations: the heart, vol 5, Summit, NJ, 1978, CIBA Pharmaceutical Co.

7. Schakenbach LH: Physiologic dynamics of acquired valvular heart disease, J Cardiovasc Nurs 1:1, 1987.

8. Ohler L, Fleagle DJ, and Lee BI: Aortic valvuloplasty: medical and critical care nursing perspectives, Focus Crit Care 16:275, 1989.

9. Ventola CA: Nursing grand rounds: aortic and mitral valvuloplasty J Cardiovasc Nurs 1:70, 1987.

10. Rackley CE and others: Aortic valve disease. In Hurst JW and others, editors: The heart, ed 7, New York, 1990, McGraw-Hill.

11. Siefert PC: Surgery for acquired valvular heart disease, J Cardiovasc Nurs 1:26, 1987.

12. Rackley CE, Edwards JE, and Karp RB: Mitral valve disease. In Hurst JW and others, editors: The heart, ed 7, New York, 1990, McGraw-Hill.

13. Guyton A: Textbook of medical physiology, ed 6, Philadelphia, 1981, WB Saunders.

14. Anderson UK: Mitral valve prolapse: a diagnosis for primary nursing intervention, J Cardiovasc Nurs 1:26, 1987.

15. Rackley CE and others: Tricuspid valve disease. In Hurst JW and others, editors: The heart, ed 7, New York, 1990, McGraw-Hill.

16. Rackley CE and others: Pulmonary valve disease. In Hurst JW and others, editors: The heart, ed 7, New York, 1990, McGraw-Hill.

# CHAPTER 9

# Cardiomyopathy

Connie White-Williams

The cardiomyopathies are a group of heart muscle diseases of unknown cause that primarily affect the structural and/or functional capacity of the myocardium.[1,2] The classification and the nomenclature of the cardiomyopathies continue to create controversy among experts in the field. According to the World Health Organization (WHO), the etiology of disease is unknown. Once a cause has been identified the condition becomes a specific disease. The above definition differentiates cardiomyopathy from specific heart muscle disease such as valvular heart disease or coronary heart disease in which the myocardial involvement is part of a systemic disease process.[1,2] Others believe that the disease etiologies leading to the cardiomyopathy present the same clinical and pathologic features; thus, the cardiomyopathy can be classified according to the structural and/or functional abnormality of the disease. For example, ischemic heart disease resulting in ischemic cardiomyopathy would be considered a cardiomyopathy.[1,2]

## CLASSIFICATION

Cardiomyopathies can be classified as primary or secondary.[3] Primary cardiomyopathies are those conditions in which the etiology of the heart disease is unknown. In these instances, the myocardium is the only portion of the heart involved and the valves and other cardiac structures are unaffected. In secondary cardiomyopathy the myocardial disease is known and is secondary to another disease process. Common causes of secondary cardiomyopathy are ischemia, viral infections, high alcohol intake, and pregnancy. Please see Table 9-1 for a more comprehensive list of causes of secondary cardiomyopathy.

More commonly, cardiomyopathies are divided into three functional classifications: (1) dilated, (2) hypertrophic, and (3) restrictive.[1,3] Dilated cardiomyopathy is characterized by ventricular dilatation. Hypertrophic cardiomyopathy is associated with an increase in myocardial mass without ventricular dilatation. Restrictive cardiomyopathy is recognized by an impairment of ventricular diastolic filling and a decrease in cavity size. These three types are illustrated in Fig. 9-1.

Even though the three types of cardiomyopathies are pathophysiologically different, they do have several similarities. Primary cardiomyopathies are heart muscle disorders of unknown cause. The disease process primarily affects the myocardium and can often be associated with endocardial or pericardial involvement. All three types of cardiomyopathy can lead to cardiomegaly and congestive heart failure. Similarities and differences among the three types of cardiomyopathy are presented in Table 9-2.

---

**TABLE 9-1**   Causes of secondary cardiomyopathy

| Dilated | Hypertrophic | Restrictive |
|---|---|---|
| Ischemic | Genetic | Amyloid |
| Valvular | Hypertension | Endomyocardial fibrosis |
| Infectious | Obstructive valvular disease | Löffler's disease |
| Pregnancy | Thyroid disease | Sarcoidosis |
| Metabolic | Glycogen storage disease | Neoplastic tumor |
| Hypertension | Friedreich's ataxia | Ventricular thrombus |
| Cardiotoxic | Infants of diabetics | |
| • Alcohol | | |
| • Adriamycin | | |
| • Cobalt | | |

Modified from Wynne J and Braunwald E: The cardiomyopathies and myocarditides. In Braunwald E, editor: Heart disease: a textbook of cardiovascular medicine. Philadelphia, 1988, WB Saunders and personal notes of Robert C. Bourge.

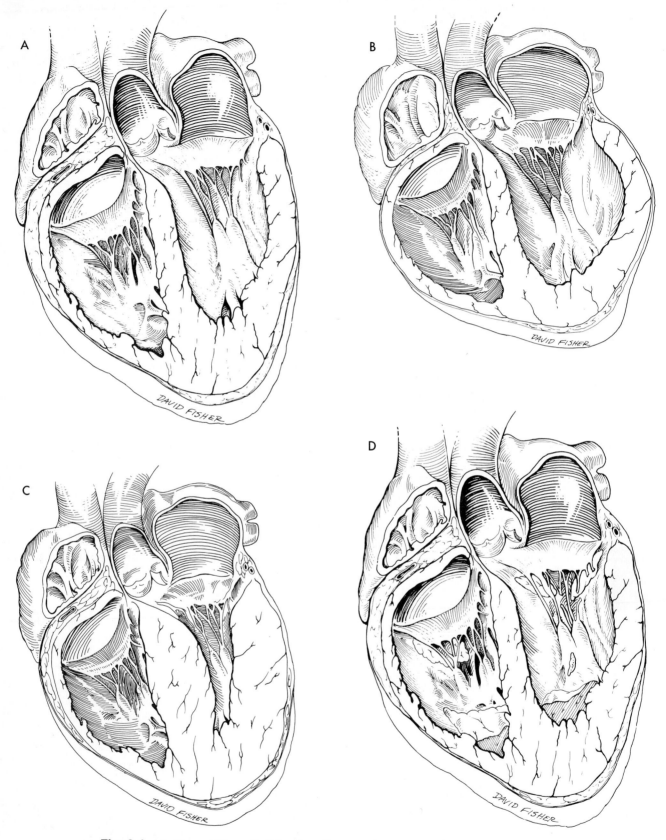

**Fig. 9-1**   **A,** Normal Heart. **B,** Dilated cardiomyopathy. **C,** Hypertrophic cardiomyopathy. **D,** Restrictive cardiomyopathy. (Illustrations by David Fisher, University of Alabama at Birmingham, Photography and Graphics.)

**TABLE 9-2** Characteristics of the three cardiomyopathies

| Characteristics | Dilated | Hypertrophic | Restrictive |
|---|---|---|---|
| Myocardial mass | ↑ > ↑↑ | ↑↑↑ | nl > ↑ |
| Ventricular cavity size | ↑↑ > ↑↑↑↑ | ↓↓ > nl | ↓ |
| Dilated atrial cavities | + | + | + |
| Asymmetric septal hypertrophy | 0 | + | 0 |
| Myocardial fiber disorientation | 0 | + | 0 |
| Contractile function | ↓↓↓ | ↑↑ > ↓ | nl > ↓ |
| Ventricular inflow resistance | 0 | + + | + |
| Ventricular outflow obstruction | 0 | 0 ⇌ + | 0 |
| Left ventricular filling pressure | ↑↑ | nl | ↑ |
| Intracardiac thrombi | + | 0 | + |

From Wenger NK, Goodwin JF, and Roberts WC: Cardiomyopathies and myocardial involvement in systemic disease. In Hurst JW and others: The heart, New York, McGraw Hill, p 1182. Reproduced with permission from the publisher.

## DILATED CARDIOMYOPATHY

Dilated cardiomyopathy is the most common form of cardiomyopathy. Although in many cases the etiology is not known, many factors appear to be associated with its etiology, for example, alcohol, inflammation, myocarditis, infiltrative disorders, metabolic disorders, and pregnancy. The course of dilated cardiomyopathy is one of progressive deterioration with three fourths of the patients dying within 5 years of diagnosis.[3,4] Dilated cardiomyopathy usually occurs between 30 and 40 years of age in the adult population.[4] In the 1989 International Heart Transplantation Registry, cardiomyopathy was implicated in over 50% of the almost 10,000 cardiac transplants performed throughout the world.[5]

### Pathophysiology

Dilated cardiomyopathy is characterized by four dominant features: (1) cardiomegaly with ventricular dilatation, (2) impairment of systolic function, (3) atrial enlargement, and (4) stasis of blood in the left ventricle.

Cardiomegaly is the result of dilatation of the heart chambers with greater dilatation occurring in the ventricles than in the atria. The comparison of the increased cavity size of dilated cardiomyopathy with a normal heart can be seen in Fig. 9-1. The second characteristic of dilated cardiomyopathy is decreased ventricular contraction, which leads to impairment of systolic function. Poor contractility results in a decreased stroke volume and, thus, a reduced ejection fraction. In dilated cardiomyopathy a 15% to 20% decrease in the ejection fraction is common.[6] The inadequacy of the systolic function leads to an elevated end-diastolic volume (EDV), which may progress to pulmonary congestion. The elevation in EDV is a compensatory mechanism (Frank-Starling law) by the heart to maintain the stroke volume in the presence of the decreased ejection fraction.

The body continues to compensate by further increasing EDV and, consequently, stroke volume, and by increasing catecholamine circulation with augmentation of contractility and heart rate.[7] Also, the kidneys begin to retain sodium and water in an effort to maintain cardiac output. Sodium and water retention may be one of the first signs of cardiac impairment.[6] Activation of the renin-angiotensin mechanism further increases ventricular filling through its vasoconstrictive properties. When these compensatory mechanisms fail, congestive heart failure progresses. In the decompensated heart, increasing venous return and systemic vascular resistance increases left ventricular stroke work, leading to left ventricular and left atrial dilatation. Left heart failure (pulmonary venous hypertension) is a common occurrence; however, biventricular failure (pulmonary and systemic venous hypertension) occurs in many patients.

Atrial enlargement also occurs in dilated cardiomyopathy. With the ventricles holding more blood (increased EDV) and the poor ventricular contractility, increased work is required of the atria to eject blood into the ventricles. This increased work results in atrial stretch and dilatation and ultimately a decrease in the rate of myofibril shortening. According to the law of Laplace, dilatation coincides with greater wall tension which, in turn, results in a greater metabolic demand and increased myocardial oxygen consumption.

Finally, because of the reduced ejection fraction, stasis of blood in the ventricle occurs, leading to an increased incidence of thrombus formation. The most frequent sites of thrombus formation are the left ventricle, the right ventricle and right atrial appendage, and the left atrial appendage.[1,2]

## Pathology

On postmortem examination, both ventricles are found to be dilated with one more dilated than the other. The atria are also dilated. The cardiac valves and coronary arteries are usually normal. Minimal left ventricular hypertrophy is present and appears to have a protective role in dilated cardiomyopathy since it may reduce wall stress and further dilatation. Intracavity thrombi are commonly seen as described above. Histologic findings reveal interstitial and perivascular fibrosis especially in the left ventricular subendocardium.[2] Dilated cardiomyopathy may be associated with loss of functioning myofibrils and contractile elements. Unfortunately, histologic findings of dilated cardiomyopathy are relatively nonspecific.[1] Please see Fig. 9-2 for a cross-sectional view of dilated cardiomyopathy.

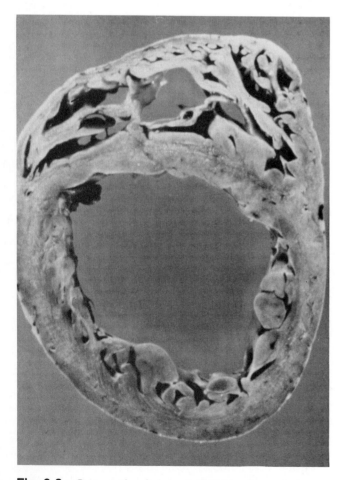

**Fig. 9-2**   Cross-sectional view of dilated cardiomyopathy. (Photographs courtesy of Shirley Smith, MD, University of Alabama at Birmingham, Department of Pathology.)

## Clinical Presentation

The signs and symptoms of dilated cardiomyopathy develop insidiously. Some patients with left ventricular dilatation may be asymptomatic for years. Symptomatic patients present with fatigue, weakness, and/or dyspnea because of low cardiac output. Over time the body has compensated for the decreased ventricular contractility and decreased stroke volume by increasing EDV and circulating catecholomines. However, as the cardiomyopathy progresses, the body may no longer be able to compensate, particularly with exertion. Consequently, early symptoms include dyspnea on exertion, changes in exercise tolerance, and palpitation. These symptoms progress to orthopnea, paroxysmal nocturnal dyspnea, and dyspnea at rest. With continued deterioration, the body will begin to decompensate and congestive heart failure (CHF) will ensue.

The precordial examination reveals a laterally displaced apical impulse caused by the ventricular dilatation. An $S_4$ may precede the development of CHF while an $S_3$ is auscultated once decompensation occurs. A summation gallop is often appreciated with tachycardia.

The systolic blood pressure is normal or low with a narrow pulse pressure. Pulsus alternans is common with severe failure. Also distended jugular neck veins, peripheral edema, and ascites with liver enlargement are present with severe failure.

## Diagnostic Tests

The chest roentgenogram shows cardiomegaly caused by left ventricular enlargement. Signs of pulmonary venous hypertension may be present. Finally, pleural effusions may also be evident because of the progressive left ventricular dysfunction. See Fig. 9-3 for an example of a chest x-ray of a patient with dilated cardiomyopathy.

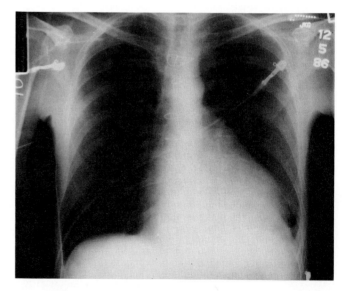

**Fig. 9-3**   Chest x-ray of dilated cardiomyopathy.

The electrocardiogram (ECG) usually reveals sinus tachycardia. Tachycardia manifests as a compensatory mechanism to compensate for the reduced cardiac output. Dysrhythmias are common manifestations of dilated cardiomyopathy.[3]

Atrial and ventricular tachydysrhythmias, conduction disturbances, and left bundle branch block may all be seen in dilated cardiomyopathy. When left ventricular fibrosis is present, Q waves may appear. It is important, however, to rule out myocardial infarction in these cases. ST-segment and T-wave abnormalities are common in patients with dilated cardiomyopathy.[3,8]

Echocardiography is a useful diagnostic test in distinguishing dilated cardiomyopathy from other abnormalities. With M-mode, two-dimensional or Doppler echocardiography, the size of the ventricular cavity can be assessed, the thickness of the heart muscle walls can be measured, and the cardiac valves can be evaluated.[9] In addition, the ventricular ejection fraction can be estimated in order to assess left ventricular impairment. See Fig. 9-4 for a comparison of dilated and hypertrophic cardiomyopathy on echocardiogram.

Invasive cardiac catheterization and coronary angiography is limited in differentiating the manifestations of dilated cardiomyopathy. The coronary arteries are usually normal. Pulmonary artery wedge, left atrial, and left ventricular end-diastolic pressures are elevated, manifesting poor contractility and diminished cardiac output.[8]

If the risk of the dye load is not present, left ventriculography can reveal abnormal wall motion, cavity size, and presence and degree of mitral regurgitation. Endomyocardial biopsy may be performed but rarely provides information that is significant for the treatment of dilated cardiomyopathy.

Holter monitoring for ventricular ectopy may be important in the prognosis of the patient. Some studies report that high-grade ectopy portends a grave prognosis or higher incidence of sudden cardiac death.[10]

## Medical and Surgical Interventions

The goal of medical intervention in dilated cardiomyopathy is to reduce the workload of the heart and improve symptoms of congestive heart failure. Thus the treatment is more palliative than curative. In patients in whom a cause has been identified, the treatment is directed toward that cause. For example, in alcoholic cardiomyopathy, abstinence from alcohol is an absolute requirement. Ceasing alcohol consumption may limit or reverse the progressive course of cardiomyopathy.[3,11] Demakis and associates[12] studied 57 patients with cardiomyopathy associated with alcohol. Patients who abstained from alcohol and had a short duration of symptoms before the initiation of therapy experienced a more favorable course; 30 of the 57 patients experienced deterioration of their disease, and 26 of these 30 patients continued to drink heavily.[12] Of the 30 patients, 24 had a mean survival time of 36 months.[12]

Corticosteroids may be used in the treatment of cardiomyopathy occurring secondary to sarcoidosis and in postviral cardiomyopathy. However, these therapies remain controversial.

In idiopathic dilated cardiomyopathy the treatment is nonspecific. Moreover, a cluster of medical interventions is directed toward the pathophysiologic manifestations. Pharmacologic treatment, nutritional instruction, and cardiac rehabilitation may help to alleviate the symptoms of CHF and improve cardiac output.

The initial therapy for treatment of CHF secondary to dilated cardiomyopathy includes agents such as digitalis

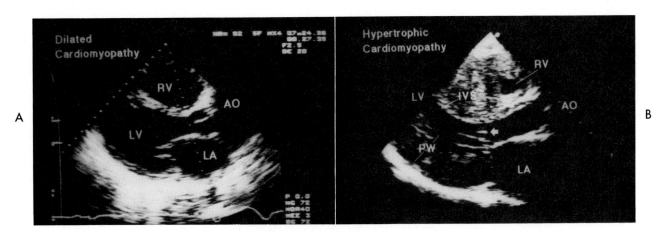

**Fig. 9-4**   **A,** Dilated cardiomyopathy echocardiogram. **B,** Hypertrophic cardiomyopathy echocardiogram. (Photographs courtesy of Po Fang, MD, University of Alabama at Birmingham, Department of Medicine.)

and diuretics.[8,13,14] Digitalis is a positive inotropic agent, increasing myocardial contractility and slowing the renin-angiotensin response in CHF.[13] Since digitalis has a relatively narrow therapeutic range, caution should be taken to avoid life-threatening dysrhythmias.[7] It should be noted that diuresis can exacerbate problems of hypokalemia and hypomagnesemia; therefore potassium or magnesium should be supplemented if indicated.

Specific vasodilator therapy consisting of nitrates, hydralazine, nitrate-hydralazine combinations, or prazosin may improve ventricular performance. Nitrates act by producing venous dilatation and arteriolar relaxation with a subsequent decrease in preload and afterload. Hydralazine works effectively to decrease afterload by producing arterial dilatation. The nitrate-hydralazine combination therapy provides a more balanced preload and afterload reduction.[13] A Veteran's Administration study of over 600 patients with congestive heart failure indicated that the nitrate-hydralazine combination improved survival by increasing the ejection fraction.

Inactivation of the renin-angiotensin system by angiotensin-converting enzyme (ACE) inhibitors such as captopril or enalapril is useful in patients with dilated cardiomyopathy and CHF. ACE inhibitors decrease vascular resistance and ventricular afterload, thus increasing cardiac output. Also, ACE inhibitors increase sodium and water excretion, which decreases venous return to the heart.

The use of beta-adrenergic antagonists has been reported as helpful in the treatment of dilated cardiomyopathy. These agents reduce myocardial oxygen demand, improve ventricular filling, and inhibit sympathetic vasoconstriction.

Antidysrhythmic agents may be used in the treatment of symptomatic dysrhythmias associated with dilated cardiomyopathy. However, caution is required since some of these drugs decrease myocardial contractility. Rhythm control may be accomplished by inserting an automatic implantable pacemaker for the appropriate candidate. Because of the high incidence of thromboemboli in patients with dilated cardiomyopathy and congestive heart failure, anticoagulation is desirable.

As a last resort, after medical therapy has failed, the patient may be considered for cardiac transplantation. The candidate for transplantation is generally less than 60 years of age, is in a New York Heart Association class III or IV, and has a life expectancy from 6 months to 1 year. See Chapter 12 for a further discussion of cardiac transplantation.

## HYPERTROPHIC CARDIOMYOPATHY

Over the years hypertrophic cardiomyopathy has also been known as *idiopathic hypertrophic subaortic stenosis* (IHSS) and *hypertrophic obstructive cardiomyopathy*. Although the etiology of hypertrophic cardiomyopathy is unknown. It is speculated that its development is genetically transmitted

as an autosomal dominant trait. Hypertrophic cardiomyopathy occurs less commonly than dilated cardiomyopathy and is more often seen in males than in females.[7,8] Hypertrophic cardiomyopathy is usually diagnosed in young adulthood and is often seen in active, athletic individuals; it is classically defined as a disease of unknown origin with a greatly hypertrophied, nondilated ventricle, which is manifested in the absence of other cardiac or systemic disease.

### Pathophysiology

Four main abnormalities are found in hypertrophic cardiomyopathy: (1) ventricular hypertrophy, (2) rapid contraction of the left ventricle, (3) impaired relaxation, and (4) intracavity systolic pressure gradients. These characteristics determine the signs, symptoms, and prognosis of the patient with this cardiomyopathy. Unlike dilated cardiomyopathy in which systolic function is impaired, the most characteristic abnormality in hypertrophic cardiomyopathy is diastolic dysfunction.[3] Ventricular hypertrophy is associated with a thickened intraventricular septum and ventricular free wall. The hypertrophy is commonly symmetrical but can have varying patterns. The hypertrophy can occur only in the anterior portion of the septum or it can affect all of the regions in the left ventricle except the basal anterior septum. The ratio of the thickness of the septum to the free wall is usually greater than 1:3 to 1:5. This ratio is in contrast to the normal heart where the ratio is usually 1:0 and always less than 1:3.[3] With the increased thickness of the free wall and septum, the ventricular cavity is decreased, leading to abnormal left ventricular stiffness during diastole. The end result is impaired ventricular filling as the ventricle becomes noncompliant and unable to relax and receive blood from the atrium. This abnormality in relaxation manifests in an elevation of the left ventricular end-diastolic pressure. This elevated pressure contributes to high atrial, pulmonary venous, and pulmonary capillary pressures, all of which lead to dyspnea. Tachycardia, a compensatory mechanism, further impedes ventricular filling time, thus reducing ventricular volume. The most controversial characteristic is the dynamic systolic pressure gradient and the etiology of this gradient. The pressure gradient is found in approximately 40% of patients with HCM.[1] Initially, the pressure gradient was thought to be caused by the hypertrophy and the powerful muscle action during ejection. In contrast, many propose that the pressure gradient is the result of the further narrowing of an already small outflow tract produced by the systolic anterior motion (SAM) of the mitral valve on the septum.[2,3] As a result of the abnormal motion, the mitral valve becomes thickened and develops plaque and may become incompetent. However, the question remains whether the pressure gradient is related to the displacement of the mitral valve or to the powerful contraction of the hypertrophied heart.

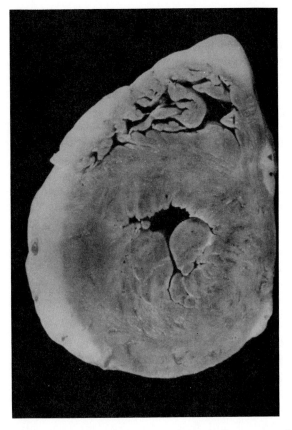

**Fig. 9-5**  Hypertrophied heart. (Photograph courtesy of Shirley Smith, MD, University of Alabama at Birmingham, Department of Pathology.)

The hypertrophic cardiomyopathic heart at necropsy (Fig. 9-5) shows (1) a normal or small left and right ventricular cavity, (2) dilated atrial cavities, (3) abnormal intramural coronary arteries, (4) greater thickening of the ventricular septum than of the ventricular free wall, (5) mural fibrous plaque, (6) a thickened mitral valve, and (7) myocardial fiber disarray.[1]

On histologic examination, disorganization of myocardial fibers and the cell-to-cell arrangement (disarray) are distinctive characteristics of hypertrophic cardiomyopathy. This disorganization and disarray have been found in other diseases; however, in hypertrophic cardiomyopathy, the abnormality is more extensive. In fact, patients with hypertrophic cardiomyopathy with large pressure gradients tend to have more myofibril disarray than those without systolic pressure gradients.

### Clinical Presentation

The most common symptom of the person with hypertrophic cardiomyopathy is dyspnea, which is largely a result of elevated left ventricular diastolic pressure. Angina pectoris, fatigue, and syncope also are reported. Angina pectoris is caused by a variety of mechanisms: (1) decreased oxygen available to supply the increased demand of the hypertrophied heart, (2) narrowing of the transmural coronary arteries, and (3) impaired diastolic relaxation with subendocardial ischemia. Syncope is caused by decreased ventricular filling and, thus, a decrease in cardiac output. Some patients may remain asymptomatic while in others the first manifestation may be sudden cardiac death. Physical exertion has been found to exacerbate the symptoms of hypertrophic cardiomyopathy. In addition, the physical signs and symptoms depend on the magnitude of the pressure gradient found in the left ventricle. With a pressure gradient, three predominant physical findings emerge. First, a typically harsh, crescendo-decrescendo systolic murmur is heard best between the apex and the left sternal border. This murmur may radiate to the axilla or base of the heart, but it rarely radiates to the neck. Also, the murmur is increased by standing and by the Valsalva maneuver, and it is decreased by squatting. This systolic murmur reflects mitral regurgitation and the late onset of the ventricular outflow gradient. Thus this murmur is more holosystolic and blowing at the apex and midsystolic and harsher at the lower sternal border.[3] Second, the arterial pulse is abrupt and ill-sustained. The jerky quality results from the powerful contraction of the left ventricle. Finally, a prominent cardiac apical impulse is formed by the interruption of ejection by the outflow gradient in the left ventricle. A presystolic apical impulse is formed by the forceful atrial contraction in an effort to eject blood into a poorly compliant ventricle.

The first heart sound is usually normal and the second heart sound is often split. Both $S_3$ and $S_4$ commonly can be auscultated.

### Diagnostic Tests

The chest roentgenogram is usually normal in hypertrophic cardiomyopathy except in patients with severe disease in which the cardiac silhouette is enlarged.

The most common abnormalities on the ECG are an increased voltage and duration of the QRS complex and T-wave inversion, which reflects hypertrophy. Other features are a short PR interval, Q waves in the inferior and precordial leads, and a P wave abnormality that is usually caused by left atrial enlargement.[1,3] Ventricular dysrhythmias are common in patients with hypertrophic cardiomyopathy with one fourth of the patients experiencing ventricular tachycardia, and one fourth to one half experiencing supraventricular tachycardia.[15] It has been reported that patients with asymptomatic ventricular tachycardia recorded on a Holter monitor have a higher incidence of sudden death than patients who do not have ventricular tachycardia[16]; 5% to 10% of the patients experience atrial fibrillation.[15,17]

The echocardiogram is the primary diagnostic tool revealing the classic feature of hypertrophic cardiomyopathy, which is left ventricular hypertrophy (Fig. 9-4). Two dimensional echocardiography can measure septal and free wall orientation and thickness. The echocardiogram can also detect the narrowing of the left ventricular outflow tract. Color Doppler nicely reveals mitral regurgitation.

Radionuclide image techniques are also used in the diagnosis of hypertrophic cardiomyopathy. Gated radionuclide ventriculography with labeling of the blood depicts the size and motion of the septum and left ventricle. Abnormal diastolic function can be observed by analysis of the blood pool scan. Thallium-201 imaging confirms the thickness of the septum and the free wall.

Cardiac catheterization can also be helpful in diagnosing hypertrophic cardiomyopathy, revealing decreased diastolic left ventricular compliance and abnormal pressure gradients, if present.

### Medical and Surgical Interventions

Interventions for hypertrophic cardiomyopathy are directed toward: (1) decreasing the force of ventricular contraction (increasing ventricular volume) and (2) decreasing the outflow obstruction.

Of the beta-adrenergic blockers, propranolol is the most commonly used in hypertrophic cardiomyopathy. Beta-adrenergic agents have both a negative inotropic and negative chronotropic effect, both of which reduce myocardial oxygen demand. Furthermore, beta-blocking agents decrease the force of contraction and increase diastolic filling time by slowing the heart rate. By decreasing contractility and increasing filling time, the outflow obstruction is reduced.[1,3]

Calcium antagonists (verapamil, diltiazem, nifedipine) are an alternative to beta-blocking agents in the treatment of hypertrophic cardiomyopathy. Verapamil, the most common agent used in hypertrophic cardiomyopathy, improves diastolic filling time by promoting relaxation, resulting in an increased exercise tolerance. Also, by decreasing myocardial contractility, verapamil can diminish the left ventricular outflow gradient. Adverse effects of verapamil include suppression of the sinus node, atrioventricular (AV) conduction inhibition, negative inotropic effects, and vasodilatation.[3,18] These side effects may manifest as hypotension, pulmonary edema, and death.[18] Nifedipine is a more potent vasodilator than verapamil, but with less AV conduction inhibition effects.[19] A combination of nifedepine and propranolol has been shown to be beneficial in the treatment of hypertrophic cardiomyopathy.[20] Diltiazem has been found to improve diastolic function by increasing relaxation and prolonging filling time.[21]

For patients who experience ventricular tachycardia, amiodarone has been used effectively to treat supraventricular and ventricular tachycardias.[22] Atrial fibrillation should be treated as an emergency and be electrically converted before hemodynamic compromise develops. Anticoagulants are recommended in patients with chronic atrial fibrillation.

Strenuous exercise shoud be avoided because of the risk of sudden cardiac death. Competitive sports are contraindicated if left ventricular hypertrophy, evidence of outflow gradient, significant ventricular dysrhythmias, or a history of sudden death are present.[23]

A variety of surgical treatments may be employed for hypertrophic cardiomyopathy. The most common surgical operation is excision of a part of the hypertrophied septum (septal myotomy-myectomy). This procedure reduces the outflow tract obstruction and mitral regurgitation.

Antibiotic prophylaxis is indicated prior to invasive procedures to protect against infective endocarditis. The infection usually develops on the mitral or aortic valve.

## RESTRICTIVE CARDIOMYOPATHY

Restrictive cardiomyopathy is a heart muscle disease in which the diastolic ventricular volume and stretch are impaired by fibrotic lesions. Systolic function remains relatively unimpaired. Of the three cardiomyopathies, restrictive cardiomyopathy is the least common.

### Pathophysiology

Although the specific etiology of restrictive cardiomyopathy is unknown, a number of pathologic processes may result in restrictive cardiomyopathy. Myocardial fibrosis, hypertrophy, and infiltration produce stiffness of the ventricular wall and decreased ventricular filling with subsequent diastolic dysfunction. Secondary causes of restrictive cardiomyopathy include amyloidosis, endocardial fibrosis, glycogen deposition, hemachromatosis, sarcoidosis, and myocardial fibrosis of diverse etiologies.[24]

The principal characteristic of restrictive cardiomyopathy is cardiac muscle stiffness, which is caused by the fibrotic or infiltrative changes in the heart muscle. These changes restrict ventricular filling and lead to a reduced cardiac output.

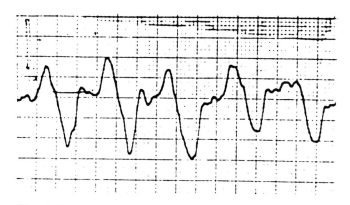

**Fig. 9-6** Square root sign of a patient with restrictive cardiomyopathy. (Courtesy of Robert C. Bourge, MD, University of Alabama at Birmingham, Department of Medicine.)

## Clinical Presentation

The patient with restrictive cardiomyopathy presents with symptoms similar to those of dilated cardiomyopathy. Angina pectoris, syncope, fatigue, and dyspnea on exertion are commonly reported. Exercise intolerance is the most frequent symptom since the heart cannot increase cardiac output by tachycardia without compromising ventricular filling.[3]

In advanced disease, peripheral edema, elevated central venous pressure, and ascites may be present.[24] On physical examination, an $S_3$, $S_4$, or both may be auscultated. Also, jugular vein distention and a palpable apical impulse may be evident.

**TABLE 9-3** Functional classification of the cardiomyopathies

| | Dilated | Restrictive | Hypertrophic |
|---|---|---|---|
| Symptoms | Congestive heart failure, particularly left-sided<br>Fatigue and weakness<br>Systemic or pulmonary emboli | Dyspnea, fatigue<br>Right-sided congestive heart failure<br>Signs and symptoms of systemic disease (e.g. amyloidosis, iron storage disease) | Dyspnea, angina pectoris<br>Fatigue, syncope, palpitations |
| Physical examination | Moderate to severe cardiomegaly; $S_3$, $S_4$<br>Atrioventricular valve regurgitation, especially mitral | Mild to moderate cardiomegaly; $S_3$, $S_4$<br>Atrioventricular valve regurgitation; inspiratory increase in venous pressure (Kussmaul's sign) | Mild cardiomegaly<br>Apical systolic thrill and heave, brisk carotid upstroke<br>$S_4$ common<br>Systolic murmur that increases with Valsalva maneuver |
| Chest roentgenogram | Moderate to marked cardiac enlargement, especially left ventricular<br>Pulmonary venous hypertension | Mild cardiac enlargement<br>Pulmonary venous hypertension | Mild to moderate cardiac enlargement<br>Left atrial enlargement |
| ECG | Sinus tachycardia<br>Atrial and ventricular dysrhythmias<br>ST-segment and T-wave abnormalities<br>Intraventricular conduction defects | Low voltage<br>Intraventricular conduction defects<br>AV conduction defects | Left ventricular hypertrophy<br>ST-segment and T-wave abnormalities<br>Abnormal Q waves<br>Atrial and ventricular dysrhythmias |
| Echocardiogram | Left ventricular dilatation and dysfunction<br>Abnormal diastolic mitral valve motion secondary to abnormal compliance and filling pressures | Increased left ventricular wall thickness and mass<br>Small or normal-sized left ventricular cavity<br>Normal systolic function<br>Pericardial effusion | Asymmetrical septal hypertrophy (ASH)<br>Narrow left ventricular outflow tract<br>Systolic anterior motion (SAM) of the mitral valve<br>Small or normal-sized left ventricle |
| Radionuclide studies | Left ventricular dilatation and dysfunction | Infiltration of myocardium<br>Small or normal-sized left ventricle<br>Normal systolic function | Small or normal-sized left ventricle<br>Vigorous systolic function<br>Asymmetrical septal hypertrophy |
| Cardiac catheterization | Left ventricular enlargement and dysfunction<br>Mitral and/or tricuspid regurgitation<br>Elevated left- and often right-sided filling pressures<br>Diminished cardiac output | Diminished left ventricular compliance<br>Square root sign in ventricular pressure recordings<br>Preserved systolic function<br>Elevated left- and right-sided filling pressures | Diminished left ventricular compliance<br>Mitral regurgitation<br>Vigorous systolic function<br>Dynamic left ventricular outflow gradient |

From Wynne J and Braunwald E: The cardiomyopathies and myocarditides. In Braunwald E, editor: Heart disease: a textbook of cardiovascular medicine, Philadelphia, WB Saunders Co, p 1412. Reproduced with permission from the publisher.

## Diagnostic Tests

The chest roentgenogram may be normal or show cardiomegaly. Pleural effusions and pulmonary congestion may be evident in those who have progressed to congestive heart failure.

The ECG shows sinus tachycardia. The most characteristic feature is the diffusely decreased voltage seen in amyloidosis. AV conduction abnormalities are also seen frequently in amyloidosis. Atrial fibrillation and complex ventricular dysrhythmias are common features of restrictive cardiomyopathy.

The clinical features of restrictive cardiomyopathy and constrictive pericarditis are similar, but not the same. The echocardiogram is helpful in distinguishing between restrictive cardiomyopathy and constrictive pericarditis. The echocardiogram reveals thickened ventricular walls, small ventricular cavities, and dilated atria in restrictive cardiomyopathy; however, these findings are not evident in constrictive pericarditis. In addition, endomyocardial biopsy, computerized tomography, and nuclear imaging are useful in differentiating between constrictive pericarditis and restrictive cardiomyopathy. A characteristic hemodynamic feature in both conditions is a deep and early decline of ventricular pressure at the onset of diastole with a rise to a plateau.[25] This dip and plateau is called the square root sign (Fig. 9-6). Both right and left filling pressures may display the dip and plateau. However, the left ventricular end-diastolic pressure is usually greater than the right in restrictive cardiomyopathy while the pressures are equal in constrictive pericarditis. Also an M or W waveform may be apparent on the pulmonary wedge tracing.

## Medical and Surgical Intervention

The treatment of restrictive cardiomyopathy is palliative and is similar to that of dilated cardiomyopathy and congestive heart failure. Medical intervention focuses on diuretic therapy, sodium and water restriction, anticoagulation, and treatment of dysrhythmias. A pacemaker is inserted to treat AV conduction blocks. Surgical intervention includes excision of the thickened endomyocardial plaque or mitral or tricuspid valve replacement, if needed.

## CONCLUSION

The cardiovascular nurse will encounter the patient with cardiomyopathy often during the course of the disease. Frequent hospitalizations and clinic visits will be required for treatment of congestive heart failure and monitoring of the disease process. Some nurses may care for patients who are awaiting cardiac transplantation.

In this chapter, the pathophysiology and clinical presentation of dilated, hypertrophic, and restrictive cardiomyopathy have been presented. A comprehensive functional classification of the cardiomyopathies is presented in Table 9-3. It is important for cardiovascular nurses to understand the pathology and manifestations of this group

of cardiac diseases. This understanding will enable the nurse to direct care toward minimizing the complications and discomforts of the cardiomyopathy. Education of the patient and family is imperative during the disease process. The ultimate goal of nursing care for patients with cardiomyopathy is an improvement in their quality of life while they live with the disease.

## REFERENCES

1. Wenger NK, Goodwin JF, and Roberts WC: Cardiomyopathy and myocardial involvement in systemic disease. In Hurst JW and others, editors: The heart, New York, 1986, McGraw Hill, Inc.
2. Goodwin JK: Overview and classification of the cardiomyopathies. In Shaver JA, editor: Cardiovascular clinics, Philadelphia, 1988, FA Davis Co.
3. Wynne J and Braunwald E: The cardiomyopathies and myocarditides. In Braunwald E, editor: Heart disease: a textbook of cardiovascular medicine, Philadelphia, 1988, WB Saunders Co.
4. O'Connell JB and Gunnar RM: Dilated-congestive cardiomyopathy: prognostic features and therapy, Heart Transplant 2:7-17, 1982.
5. Heck CF, Shumway SJ, and Kaye MP: The registry of the international society for heart transplantation: sixth official report—1989, Heart Transplant 8:271-276, 1989.
6. Gravanis MB and Ansari AA: Idiopathic cardiomyopathies, Arch Pathol Lab Med, 3:915-929, 1987.
7. Francis GS and Pierpont GL: Pathophysiology of congestive heart failure secondary to congestive and ischemic cardiomyopathy. In Shaver JA, editor: Cardiovascular clinics, Philadelphia, 1988, FA Davis Co.
8. Miller DH and Borer JS: The cardiomyopathies: a pathophysiologic approach to therapeutic management, Arch Intern Med 143:2157-2162, 1983.
9. Uretsky: BF: Diagnostic considerations in the adult patient with cardiomyopathy or congestive heart failure. In Shaver JA, editor: Cardiovascular clinics, Philadelphia, 1988, FA Davis Co.
10. Meinertz T and others: Significance of ventricular arrhythmias in idiopathic dilated cardiomyopathy, Am J Cardiol 53:902-907, 1984.
11. McHugh MJ: The patient with alcoholic cardiomyopathy, Cardiovasc Nurs 2:13-23, 1987.
12. Demakis JG and others: The natural course of alcoholic cardiomyopathy, Ann Intern Med 80:293-297, 1974.
13. Leier CV and Unverferth DV: Medical therapy of end-stage congestive and ischemic cardiomyopathy. In Shaver JA, editor: Cardiovascular clinics, Philadelphia, 1988, FA Davis Co.
14. Johnson RA and Palacios I: Dilated cardiomyopathies of the adult, N Engl J Med 307:1051-1058, 1982.
15. Maron BJ and others: Prognostic significance of 24-hour ambulatory electrocardiographic monitoring in patients with hypertrophic cardiomyopathy: a prospective study, Am J Cardiol 48:252-257, 1981.
16. McKenna WJ: Arrhythmia and prognosis of hypertrophic cardiomyopathy, Eur Heart J 4(suppl F):225-234, 1983.
17. McKenna W, Harris L, and Deanfield J: Syncope in hypertrophic cardiomyopathy, B Heart J 47:177-179, 1982.
18. Epstein SE and Rosing DR: Verapamil: its potential for causing serious complications in patients with hypertrophic cardiomyopathy, Circulation 64:437-441, 1981.
19. Lorell BH and others: Modification of abnormal left ventricular diastolic properties by nifedipine in patients with hypertrophic cardiomyopathy, Circulation 65:499-507, 1982.
20. Landmark K and others: Hemodynamic effects of nifedipine and propranolol in patients with hypertrophic cardiomyopathy, B Heart J 48:19-31, 1982.
21. Suwa M, Hirota Y, and Kawamura K: Improvement in left ventric-

ular diastolic function during intravenous and oral diltiazem treatment in patients with hypertrophic cardiomyopathy: an echocardiographic study, Am J Cardiol 54:1047-1053, 1984.

22. McKenna WJ and others: Amiodarone for long-term management of patients with hypertrophic cardiomyopathy, Am J Cardiol 54:802-810, 1984.

23. Maron BJ and others: Task force III: hypertrophic cardiomyopathy, other myopericardial diseases and mitral valve prolapse, J Am Coll Cardiol 6:1215, 1985.

24. Siegel RJ, Shah PK, and Fishbein MC: Idiopathic restrictive cardiomyopathy, Circulation 70:165-169, 1984.

25. Benotti JR, Grossman W, and Cohn PF: The clinical profile of restrictive cardiomyopathy, Circulation 61:1206-1212, 1980.

# CHAPTER 10

# Cardiovascular Drugs

Ruth Stanley

The drugs available to treat cardiovascular disease continue to increase in number and complexity. As more is learned about the physiology and pathophysiology of cardiovascular disorders, new strategies for drug therapy are developed. At present, however, few drugs are exact, precise, and specific in their action. Therefore much of drug therapy remains an art in which guidelines must be specifically tailored to meet an individual patient's needs. This chapter presents selected pharmacologic aspects of drugs used to treat cardiovascular disorders. Although some overlap is evident, the agents are grouped in general classifications according to their pharmacologic action.

## CLINICAL PHARMACOKINETICS[1]

A drug exerts its pharmacologic effects when it reaches a critical concentration at a specific site of action. Factors that determine drug concentration include the processes of drug absorption, distribution, biotransformation, and elimination. *Pharmacokinetics*, the quantitative study of these processes, provide a rational basis to determine the method of administration, dose strength, and dose timing.

*Elimination half-life* ($t_{1/2}$) is an important concept and refers to the amount of time required for the serum concentration of a given drug to decline by 50%. Elimination half-life can be altered by various disease states (e.g., congestive heart failure, renal failure, liver insufficiency) as well as concomitant drug therapy. With repeated dosing of a given drug, serum blood levels will rise until equilibrium is established between the dose administered and the amount eliminated (see Fig. 10-1). It normally takes five half-lives to reach this steady state. Steady state can be achieved more rapidly in drugs with a long half-life if loading doses are used. Because loading doses will allow a desired concentration to be achieved quickly, these large doses are preferred in acute situations when a quick onset is necessary (e.g., procainamide in ventricular tachycardia). A maintenance dose is the amount of drug administered at a given time interval to maintain a steady-state serum level.

These concepts are important when dosing and monitoring a cardiac patient receiving antidysrhythmics or digoxin. These drugs have a therapeutic range of serum levels that will produce the desired clinical effects. Concentra-

tions above this range are likely to produce toxicity, while those below will be ineffective. In Fig. 10-1, the dotted lines enclose the therapeutic range of 5 to 12 µg/ml. The trough level is 5 µg/ml or the lowest effective serum concentration, and the peak level is 12 µg/ml.

Plasma drug concentrations are often used to guide therapy, but this method must be interpreted and used according to the individual clinical situation. Plasma drug concentrations are especially useful to identify toxic concentrations and to determine an apparent drug failure caused by unexpectedly low-plasma levels. However, for a given patient, drug toxicity may occur at a drug concentration usually considered to be therapeutic, and a subtherapeutic effect of a drug may occur at a drug concentration considered to be toxic. In addition measurement of plasma drug concentration does not consider the contribution of metabolites or changes in protein binding, which may contribute to overall drug effect. Therefore plasma drug concentrations must be approached as any other laboratory test, that is, in light of the entire clinical picture of the patient.

A number of common variables modify therapy by affecting the relationship between drug dose and drug effects. These variables include age, weight, gender, nature of heart disease, route of administration of drug, patient tolerance, physiologic milieu (e.g., acid-base balance, electrolytes, hypoxia), and concurrent medications. Antihypertensive, antianginal, diuretic, and vasodilating agents cannot be dosed based on serum blood levels. As a result, these agents are monitored by both objective (e.g., hypotensive response, duration of action, and reduction in anginal attacks) and subjective (e.g., side effects and quality of life) measures. Thus the pharmacodynamic profile (effect of the drug in the body) is more important than the pharmacokinetic properties (half-life) for many classes of cardiovascular drugs. Appropriate use of these agents requires an accurate assessment of both drug effect and hemodynamic response to that effect.

## CLINICAL PHARMACOLOGY[2,3]

The parasympathetic and sympathetic divisions of the autonomic nervous system control and regulate the cardiovascular system. The major neurotransmitter of the para-

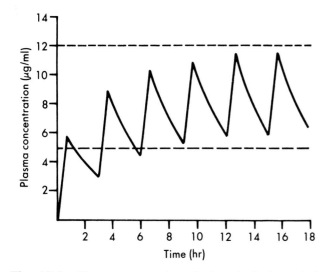

**Fig. 10-1** Plasma concentration of a hypothetic drug administered at dosage intervals equal to an elimination half-life of 3 hours. Five half-lives are required to reach a steady-state level. A hypothetic range of effective plasma concentration is illustrated by hash lines.

sympathetic system is *acetylcholine*. The vagus nerve provides dense innervation to the heart, where cholinergic tone predominates over sympathetic tone with the body at rest. Stimulation of the parasympathetic system results in a decrease in heart rate and cardiac conduction. No parasympathetic innervation to the vasculature exists, although the vessels contain receptors and respond to locally released factors.

The major end-organ neurotransmitter of the sympathetic system is *norepinephrine*. Adrenergic receptors are classified into the two major subgroups of alpha receptors and beta receptors. This classification is based on the differences in the physiologic actions and relative potency of the various catecholamines (e.g., norepinephrine, epinephrine, isoproterenol). For the cardiovascular system, stimulation of alpha receptors located in the heart and smooth muscle of arterioles results in increased myocardial contractility and arteriolar vasoconstriction. Beta receptors are located in the heart, arterioles (primarily skeletal muscle arterioles), and lungs. In the heart, stimulation of the beta receptors increases heart rate, contractility, and conduction velocity. Beta-receptor stimulation of the arterioles and lungs results in dilatation.

### Subclassification of Alpha-Adrenergic Receptors

The alpha-adrenergic receptors have also been subclassified into alpha$_1$ and alpha$_2$ receptors, but the subclassification is not analogous to that of beta receptors.

As depicted in Fig. 10-2, the adrenergic neural terminal is composed of the presynaptic sympathetic neuron, the synaptic cleft, and the postsynaptic effector cell. Alpha receptors, located in the effector cell, are termed *postsynaptic*,

or *alpha$_1$, receptors*, whereas receptors on the nerve terminal are *presynaptic*, or *alpha$_2$, receptors*.

Stimulation of the alpha$_1$ (postsynaptic) receptor mimics the effects of norepinephrine on the effector cell, whereas inhibition of the alpha$_1$ receptor antagonizes these effects. On the other hand, the alpha$_2$ receptor serves an autoregulatory function. Stimulation of the alpha$_2$ (presynaptic) receptor inhibits release of norepinephrine from the nerve terminal, thus diminishing norepinephrine's effects on the effector cell. Inhibition of the alpha$_2$ receptor stimulates release of norepinephrine.

Stimulation of central alpha$_2$ adrenoreceptors in the ventrolateral medulla results in a reduction of sympathetic outflow to the periphery. Clinically, this would result in a decrease in arterial blood pressure with concomitant bradycardia. In addition, central alpha$_2$ adrenoreceptor stimulation may enhance parasympathetic tone.

### Subclassification of Beta-Adrenergic Receptors

The response of beta-adrenergic stimulation or inhibition may be further subclassified into beta$_1$ and beta$_2$ action. This division is not complete because the activity of drugs on beta$_1$ and beta$_2$ receptors overlaps. However, differences in the relative potency of drugs to stimulate (agonist activity) or inhibit (antagonist activity) either beta-receptor subtype allows more selective use of drugs.

The postsynaptic beta$_1$ receptors are found primarily in the heart, and stimulation results in increased force and rate of contraction. In addition, atrioventricular (AV) nodal conduction time and refractoriness are decreased, which produces accelerated conduction of impulses through the myocardium. Beta$_1$ receptors can be stimulated by isoproterenol, epinephrine, or norepinephrine.

Postsynaptic beta$_2$ receptors predominate in the blood vessels and lungs. Stimulation by isoproterenol or epinephrine results in dilated arterioles and bronchioles. Presynaptic beta$_2$ receptors mediate the positive feedback mechanism and enhance sympathetic activity at that neuronal synapse. These presynaptic receptors are much more sensitive to epinephrine than to norepinephrine; thus the role of these receptors in maintaining vascular tone is unclear.

### INOTROPES[3-10]
### Digitalis Glycosides

Digitalis preparations are the oldest and most widely used drugs in the treatment of heart disease. Many forms of digitalis are available, but digoxin is the agent most often employed.

**Cardiovascular actions.** Digitalis increases myocardial contractility, a positive inotropic effect. The mechanism by which digitalis increases myocardial contractility appears to involve an increase in intracellular calcium. It is postulated that by inhibition of the sodium-potassium (Na$^+$-K$^+$) membrane pump, digitalis increases the intra-

PRESYNAPTIC                                        POSTSYNAPTIC

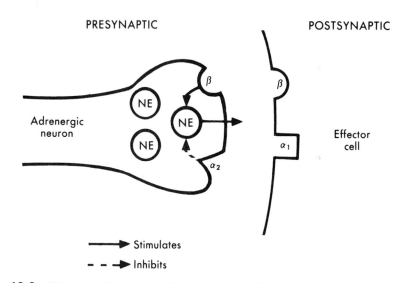

⟶ Stimulates

- - ⟶ Inhibits

**Fig. 10-2**   Diagram of the adrenergic nerve terminal illustrating alpha$_1$-, alpha$_2$-, and beta-adrenergic receptors in presynaptic and postsynaptic positions. Effector cell contains alpha$_1$- and beta-adrenergic receptors, which interact with norepinephrine to produce end-organ effects. The presynaptic alpha$_2$- and beta-adrenergic receptors interact with norepinephrine to stimulate (beta receptor) or inhibit (alpha$_2$ receptor) further norepinephrine release.

cellular pool of calcium ions available for excitation-contraction coupling. Catecholamines (epinephrine, norepinephrine) also increase myocardial contractility, but their mechanism of action is different from that of digitalis, as evidenced by the finding that the effects of digitalis on contractility are not inhibited by beta-adrenergic blocking drugs.

The positive inotropic effects of digitalis are evident in normal and failing hearts; however, the net effect on myocardial oxygen consumption differs in these two conditions. Digitalis increases oxygen consumption in the normal, nonfailing ventricle, whereas in the failing myocardium, the net effect of digitalis is to decrease ventricular size and reduce wall tension, changes that decrease myocardial oxygen consumption. An additional factor that decreases myocardial oxygen consumption is the decrease in heart rate produced by digitalis, particularly in patients with atrial fibrillation.

Digitalis produces cardiac electrophysiologic effects by direct cellular actions and indirect actions mediated by the parasympathetic nervous system. One major clinically important antidysrhythmic action of digitalis is to prolong AV nodal refractoriness and conduction time. Digitalis also shortens atrial and ventricular refractoriness, generally depresses normal automaticity in Purkinje fibers, but may produce abnormal forms of automaticity.

Digitalis has actions on the central nervous system and autonomic nervous system. Through direct vascular and sympathetic neural actions, digitalis produces vasoconstriction, but in patients treated with digitalis for heart failure, the increased cardiac output and reflex vasodilatation usually outweigh the direct effects of vasoconstriction.

### Clinical uses

1. Digoxin is the most frequently used drug in this class of agents. Although effective in patients with congestive heart failure and tachydysrhythmias, digoxin therapy has been questioned in patients with heart failure who have normal sinus rhythm. Patients more likely to have sustained improvements in cardiac function with chronic digoxin use typically exhibit the following characteristics: dilated failing hearts, impaired systolic function (ejection fraction < 35%), an S$_3$ gallop, and atrial enlargement. Patients with elevated filling pressures and preserved systolic function or with hypertrophic cardiomyopathy should receive digoxin only under careful supervision.

2. As an antidysrhythmic agent, digoxin is effective in treating paroxysmal supraventricular tachycardia and in controlling ventricular rate in atrial fibrillation or atrial flutter.

### Dosage and administration (see Tables 10-1 and 10-2, and box on p. 357.)

1. The half-life of digoxin is approximately 36 hours in patients with normal renal function. The half-life will increase as renal function declines, and patients require less frequent dosing to achieve therapeutic serum concentrations (e.g., 0.125 mg every other day rather than 0.125 mg every day). Although digoxin has a long half-

**TABLE 10-1** Digoxin elimination

| Creatinine Clearance | Approximate Half-life | Approximate Time to Reach 90% Steady State |
|---|---|---|
| ≤5 ml/min | 3.2 days | 13 days |
| 6-15 ml/min | 3.0 days | 12 days |
| 16-35 ml/min | 2.5 days | 10 days |
| 36-60 ml/min | 2.0 days | 8 days |
| ≥61 ml/min | 1.6 days | 6 days |

**TABLE 10-2** Factors that affect digoxin serum levels

| Factor | Serum Level |
|---|---|
| Renal disease | Increased |
| Hepatic disease | Increased |
| Severe congestive heart failure | Increased |
| Malabsorption | Decreased |
| **DRUG INTERACTIONS** | |
| Quinidine | Increased |
| Verapamil | Increased |
| Amiodarone | Increased |
| Spironolactone | Increased |
| Antacids | Decreased |
| Kaolin-pectin preparations | Decreased |
| Bile acid–binding resins | Decreased |

## FACTORS THAT INCREASE MYOCARDIAL SENSITIVITY TO DIGOXIN

| | |
|---|---|
| Severe congestive heart failure | Pulmonary heart disease |
| Hypothyroidism | Myocardial ischemia |
| Hypokalemia | Myocardial infarction |
| Hypomagnesemia | Myocarditis |
| Hypercalcemia | Cardiomyopathies |
| | Valvular lesions |

life, loading doses are not necessary for the inotropic response and are only indicated when treating dysrhythmias. Therapeutic serum concentrations are 0.5 to 2.0 ng/ml.

2. Loading dose: 0.25 mg intravenously (IV) slowly, then 0.25 mg IV every 6 hours up to a total loading dose of 1.0 to 1.5 mg. Loading doses may also be given orally.
3. Maintenance dose: 0.125 to 0.50 mg orally or IV daily. Adjust dose at 1- to 2-week intervals to achieve the desired serum level and therapeutic response.
4. For accurate serum levels, the patient should be at steady state if no loading dose was given. Determine the digoxin level 8 to 24 hours after drug administration or immediately before administering the next dose. If determined earlier, the serum level will be higher than the actual steady-state level.
5. The dose of digoxin should be halved when quinidine, verapamil, or amiodarone are given concurrently.
6. Generic preparations of digoxin should be discouraged. Lanoxin products have established bioavailability and absorption patterns and should be used. Lanoxin is available as tablets, caplets, elixir, and injection for parenteral use.
7. Monitor blood pressure, heart rate, electrocardiogram (ECG), signs and symptoms of disease state, renal function, electrolyte levels, and serum blood levels.

Cautions and side effects (see the box on p. 358)

1. Cardiac dysrhythmias are the first sign of digoxin toxicity in more than 50% of toxic patients. If digoxin toxicity is suspected, stop the drug, determine serum blood and electrolyte levels, and obtain an ECG. Digoxin immune Fab (Digibind) is indicated for the treatment of potentially lethal digoxin intoxication (e.g., severe ventricular dysrhythmias, progressive bradydysrhythmias). Each vial of Digibind will bind approximately 0.6 mg of digoxin. To calculate the total amount of digoxin in the body, use the following equation:

$$\text{Digoxin in body (mg)} = \frac{(\text{Serum concentration}) (5.6) (\text{Weight [kg]})}{1000}$$

To calculate the number of vials needed, use the following equation:

$$\text{Number of vials needed} = \frac{\text{Digoxin in body (mg)}}{0.6 \text{ (mg/vial)}}$$

Administer the Digibind over 30 minutes through a 0.22 μm membrane filter. The drug may be given as an IV bolus if necessary.

2. If the dysrhythmia is not life threatening, hold the digoxin dose until normal sinus rhythm is restored. If digoxin therapy is to be continued, consider using a lower dose or less frequent interval.
3. Monitor electrolyte levels closely when toxicity is suspected or documented. Serum potassium levels will fall with the use of Digibind, and supplemental potassium may be indicated. If the dysrhythmias are associated

## DIGOXIN SIDE EFFECTS

**CARDIAC (70% to 90%)***

1. Changes in rhythm (effects on cardiac automaticity and conduction)
   a. Premature ventricular contractions, coupled rhythm (bigeminy)
   b. Ventricular tachycardia; precursor of ventricular fibrillation; may be mechanism of sudden death in digitalis intoxication
   c. Nonparoxysmal AV junctional tachycardia with or without AV block
   d. Atrial tachycardia with or without block; most frequently seen in patients with associated potassium deficiency caused by concurrent use of thiazide diuretics
   e. Most dysrhythmias may be produced by digitalis excess
2. Effect on conduction system
   a. Prolonged PR interval
   b. Slow heart rates, including sinus bradycardia and first-, second- (type 1 Wenckebach), and third-degree AV block
3. Cardiac failure

**NEUROLOGIC (13% TO 25%)***

1. Mental depression and personality changes
2. Abnormal visual sensations
   a. Color (especially brown, yellow, and green)
   b. Scotoma
   c. Blurred or dimmed vision
   d. Photophobia
3. Cerebral excitation, manifested as headache, vertigo, increased irritability, convulsions
4. Peripheral neuritis
5. Generalized muscular weakness

**GASTROINTESTINAL (50% TO 75%)***

1. Anorexia
2. Nausea
3. Vomiting
4. Diarrhea

**OTHER**

1. Gynecomastia
2. Allergic manifestations such as skin rash

*Frequency of occurrence with digitalis toxicity.

with hypokalemia, potassium replacement may correct the dysrhythmia with no change in the drug concentration.

4. Central nervous system and gastrointestinal side effects are more likely to occur in the elderly population. In addition, these adverse effects may occur with serum levels in the normal range. These effects can be controlled by decreasing the drug dose or prolonging the interval between doses.

5. Digoxin-toxic patients are sensitive to electrical countershocks and may develop ventricular tachycardia or fibrillation if they receive electrical cardioversion.

### Dopamine (Intropin)

Dopamine, an endogenous catecholamine, is the immediate precursor in the synthesis of norepinephrine. The cardiovascular effects of dopamine result from actions mediated through dopamine-specific receptors and alpha- and beta-adrenergic receptors.

Cardiovascular actions (see Table 10-3). The predominant cardiovascular effects of dopamine depend on the dose administered. At doses less than 2 $\mu$g/kg/min, dopamine-specific effects predominate. As the dose is increased, the beta-adrenergic effects predominate. These effects include increases in myocardial contractility, cardiac output (CO), and renal blood flow with little or no vasoconstriction. At doses greater than 7.5 $\mu$g/kg/min, alpha-adrenergic effects dominate, leading to vasoconstriction and increased mean arterial pressure (MAP). Increases in systemic vascular resistance (SVR) at higher doses will normally offset any improvements in CO, renal blood flow, or pulmonary capillary wedge pressure (PCWP) and may

**TABLE 10-3** Dose-dependent cardiovascular effects of dopamine

| Dose (μg/kg/min) | Receptor | Clinical Effect* |
|---|---|---|
| 0.5-2.0 | Dopamine | Increased RBF, MBF<br>Diuresis |
| 2-7.5 | Dopamine/beta | Increased RBF, MBF<br>Increased CO<br>May decrease PCWP |
| 7.5-20 | Dopamine/beta | Increased SVR, PVR |
| | Alpha | Variable changes in CO, RBF, PCWP |
| >20 | Alpha (primary) | Increased PVR, SVR |
| | Beta (secondary) | Decreased CO, RBF, MBF<br>Increased PCWP |

*RBF, Renal blood flow; MBF, mesentary blood flow; CO, cardiac output; PCWP, pulmonary capillary wedge pressure; SVR, systemic vascular resistance; PVR, peripheral vascular resistance.

**TABLE 10-4** Inotropes

| Drug | Dilution* | Dose (μg/kg/min) |
|---|---|---|
| Dopamine | 400 mg/250 ml IVF | 0.5-20 |
| Dobutamine | 500 mg/250 ml IVF | 2.5-20 |
| Amrinone | 500 mg/250 ml IVF | 2.5-20 |
| Milrinone | 50 mg/250 ml IVF | 0.375-0.750 |

*IVF, Intravenous fluid.

actually worsen these parameters. As much as 50% of dopamine's hemodynamic actions may be produced by norepinephrine release. Thus dopamine has a less pronounced hemodynamic effect in patients who have myocardial norepinephrine depletion (e.g., congestive heart failure). Dopamine is usually combined with inotropes (e.g., dobutamine) or other sympathomimetic vasopressors (e.g., norepinephrine) to achieve optimum hemodynamic effects when patients appear refractory to dopamine alone. When using this agent alone or in combination, it is important to assess accurately baseline hemodynamics and altered hemodynamics secondary to drug therapy.

### Clinical uses

1. The unique hemodynamic effects of dopamine make it an important agent in the treatment of cardiogenic, septic, or traumatic shock.
2. Low-dose (0.5 to 2.0 μg/kg/min) dopamine alone or in combination with other inotropes is used to treat chronic congestive heart failure that has been refractory to treatment with diuretics and digitalis. Such therapy is temporary and used only until more definitive long-term treatment can be formulated.
3. Doses greater than 7.5 μg/kg/min are effective in hemodynamically significant hypotension but should be avoided in patients with congestive heart failure unless another selective inotrope (e.g., dobutamine) is used concomitantly.

### Dosage and administration (see Table 10-4)

1. Dopamine is administered intravenously and is compatible with all IV fluids. Dopamine can be concentrated for patients who are volume restricted, but caution should be exercised when mixing greater than 1600 mg in 250 ml IV fluid.
2. Dopamine infusions should be given through a central line if possible. If local extravasation exists, tissue necrosis will occur. Immediately treat the area with small injections of phentolamine for a total dose of 5 to 10 mg. Phentolamine is maximally effective if used within 6 hours of the extravasation and is useless if used after 24 hours.
3. Doses should be adjusted based on hemodynamic monitoring. Monitor CO, ECG, PCWP, MAP, SVR, blood pressure, heart rate, renal function, electrolyte levels, and signs and symptoms of the disease state.
4. Doses should be titrated upward according to the clinical situation (see Table 10-3). To titrate the patient off dopamine, reduce the dose by 1 to 5 μg/kg/min every 15 to 30 minutes. Allow time for the patient to react hemodynamically to the change in dose. As the dose is titrated to below 5 μg/kg/min, some patients may become hypotensive. If they are hemodynamically stable, stop the drip with no further titration. If they are hemodynamically compromised, increase the rate to the previous dose and titrate at lower increments (e.g., 1 to 2 μg/kg/min).
5. Dopamine is inactivated in alkaline solutions.
6. Dopamine is compatible with aminophylline, bretylium, calcium chloride, dobutamine, heparin, lidocaine, potassium chloride, epinephrine, isoproterenol, and verapamil.
7. Monoamine oxidase inhibitors may increase the effects of dopamine, necessitating lower doses of dopamine for production of the desired hemodynamic response.
8. If using vasopressor doses, maintain an adequate circulating blood volume when possible. If the patient is hypovolemic, vasoconstricting doses may worsen cardiac function.
9. In patients with good left ventricular function immediately following coronary artery bypass graft, low-

dose dopamine and fluid may cause less tachycardia than dobutamine alone when used to augment cardiac function.

10. Dopamine can be combined with inotropes and vasodilators to produce greater increases in cardiac output and greater reductions in PCWP.

11. Although dopamine is available in a syringe, it must be diluted before use. *Do not* administer the dose via IV push.

12. Doses of 50 μg/kg/min or more may be necessary in some patients. However, most patients will reach a plateau level at a given dose, and increments in dose will not affect blood pressure or vascular resistance. If the patient is still hypotensive, a more potent vasopressor (e.g., phenylephrine, norepinephrine) should be initiated.

### Cautions and side effects

1. The most serious adverse side effect of dopamine is the genesis or exacerbation of dysrhythmias.

2. Dopamine, especially in higher doses, may increase the demand for myocardial oxygen and cause further myocardial ischemia in the presence of coronary artery disease. Thus dopamine may precipitate angina pectoris.

3. Occasionally, low doses (e.g., 2 μg/kg/min) may produce vasodilatation and hypotension.

4. Other side effects of dopamine include nausea, vomiting, headache, restlessness, and tremor.

5. Concomitant use of other sympathomimetics increases the incidence of side effects. The smallest effective dose should always be used to reduce the risk for toxicity.

## Dobutamine (Dobutrex)

Dobutamine is a synthetic catecholamine designed to achieve positive inotropic effects without the chronotropic and peripheral vasoconstricting effects caused by other sympathomimetic agents.

**Cardiovascular actions.** Dobutamine is a selective beta$_1$ agent that directly stimulates beta receptors to increase contractility. The hemodynamic changes seen with this agent are increased cardiac output (CO), decreased pulmonary capillary wedge pressure (PCWP), and increased renal blood flow (RBF). The magnitude of change in RBF and PCWP is directly related to the magnitude of change in CO. Dobutamine produces a greater increase in left ventricular contractility (and stroke volume [SV]) with less change in myocardial oxygen demands than does dopamine, isoproterenol, norepinephrine, or epinephrine. In patients with poor left ventricular function, dobutamine will induce a reflex reduction in systemic vascular resistance (SVR) and produce little change in the heart rate. Dobutamine has no dose-dependent effects and is the preferred inotrope because of its consistent effects on CO and myocardial oxygen demand.

### Clinical uses

1. Dobutamine is the agent of choice for emergency treatment of severe heart failure resulting from various etiologies, especially in shock states caused by direct myocardial decompensation.

2. When shock is caused by vascular collapse and marked vasodilatation, as in anaphylactic shock, the absence of vasoconstrictor effects argues against the use of dobutamine. Dobutamine should be reserved for patients with combined ventricular dysfunction and elevated filling pressures.

3. In patients with poor left ventricular function following coronary artery bypass graft, dobutamine improves SV and decreases filling pressures with less positive chronotropy than dopamine.

4. Dobutamine is the preferred inotrope in patients following cardiac transplant because its action does not depend on myocardial stores of norepinephrine.

### Dosage and administration (see Table 10-4)

1. Dobutamine is administered intravenously and is compatible in all IV fluids. Dobutamine can be concentrated for patients who are volume restricted up to a maximum of 1250 mg in 250 ml IV fluid.

2. Dobutamine solutions may develop a pink discoloration that increases with time. This discoloration results from a slight oxidation of the drug, and no significant loss of drug potency occurs if diluted solutions are used within 24 hours of preparation.

3. Doses should be initiated at 2.5 to 5.0 μg/kg/min and titrated according to desired response. Doses that increase the heart rate by more than 10% over baseline values should be used cautiously because of the potential increase in myocardial oxygen demands. Doses up to 40 μg/kg/min have been used, but most patients respond at doses between 2.5 and 20 μg/kg/min.

4. Intermittent therapy may be useful in some patients with chronic congestive heart failure. Doses of 1.5 to 15 μg/kg/min for 4 to 72 hours weekly have provided sustained clinical and hemodynamic benefit in some patients. However, this therapy should be used cautiously until those patients who respond best can be clinically identified.

5. Dobutamine is compatible with atropine, dopamine, epinephrine, heparin, isoproterenol, lidocaine, norepinephrine, and procainamide.

6. Dobutamine should be titrated 2.5 to 5 μg/kg/min every 15 to 30 minutes. Allow time for the patient to react hemodynamically to the change in dose.

7. Dobutamine is inactivated in alkaline solutions.

8. Doses should be adjusted based on hemodynamic response. Monitor CO, ECG, PCWP, SVR, heart rate, blood pressure, mean arterial presure, renal function,

electrolyte levels, and signs and symptoms of the disease state.

9. Dobutamine can be combined with other inotropes and vasodilators to produce greater increases in CO and greater reductions in PCWP and SVR.

10. Most cases of extravasation produce no signs of tissue damage or necrosis. There is only one case report of dermal necrosis with extravasation.

11. Tolerance will develop in some patients after 72 hours of therapy and can be overcome by increasing the dose or altering concomitant drug therapy. When critically ill patients reach a plateau level at a given dose, another inotrope (e.g., milrinone, amrinone) may be added to augment cardiac function.

### Cautions and side effects

1. Dobutamine may increase heart rate, blood pressure, and the development of dysrhythmias. Thus constant monitoring of these parameters and prompt dosage reduction is mandatory if these effects occur.

2. Occasionally, nausea, headache, angina pectoris, and dyspnea may occur.

3. Dobutamine is contraindicated in idiopathic hypertrophic subaortic stenosis (IHSS).

## Phosphodiesterase Inhibitors

*Amrinone* (Inocor) and *milrinone* (Primacor) increase contractility by a mechanism that is distinct from digitalis, dopamine, or dobutamine.

Cardiovascular actions. Amrinone and milrinone inhibit myocardial cellular phosphodiesterase and increase the availability of calcium in the myocardium. Also, these agents are vasodilators and reduce systemic vascular resistance (SVR) by an unknown mechanism. The hemodynamic effects are decreased SVR (direct effect) and PCWP and increased CO and renal blood flow. These effects are comparable to those of dopamine and dobutamine and are additive when amrinone or milrinone are used in combination with these agents. Although amrinone and milrinone are potent inotropes with unique hemodynamic profiles, they remain second-line agents because of their toxicity and propensity to increase myocardial oxygen demand more than dobutamine. Investigational oral forms of these agents have been associated with increased mortality secondary to acute worsening of heart failure or dysrhythmias. There has been some speculation that prolonged IV use may be detrimental, but this theory has not been clinically substantiated at present. Both amrinone and milrinone are excellent short-term inotropic agents that should be used with careful monitoring.

### Clinical uses

1. Both agents are indicated for the treatment of congestive heart failure and cardiogenic shock.

2. These agents have additive inotropic effects when combined with dobutamine or dopamine.

### Dosage and administration (see Table 10-4)

1. Amrinone should be administered in one-half normal saline or normal saline at dilutions of 3 mg/ml or less. Amrinone is light sensitive and should be covered after dilution.

2. Milrinone is compatible in most IV fluids at concentrations up to 50 mg in 250 ml IV fluid.

3. Loading dose. (a) Amrinone: 0.75 mg/kg IV bolus over 5 to 30 minutes. Hemodynamic collapse secondary to vasodilatation may occur in some patients; caution should be used. The bolus may be repeated every 30 minutes based on response. (b) Milrinone: 50 µg/kg over 10 minutes.

4. Maintenance doses. (a) Amrinone: 5 to 20 µg/kg/min. (b) Milrinone: 0.375 to 0.75 µg/kg/min.

5. Milrinone is eliminated renally, and the maintenance dose should be decreased proportionately to the decrease in renal function.

6. Both agents should be adjusted for the desired hemodynamic response. Monitor CO, ECG, PCWP, SVR, heart rate, mean arterial pressure, electrolyte levels, renal function, and signs and symptoms of disease state.

7. Amrinone is incompatible with furosemide.

8. Intermittent IV amrinone therapy has been attempted in patients with end-stage congestive heart failure. At present this approach is discouraged.

9. The duration of hemodynamic effects with both amrinone and milrinone is 60 to 90 minutes with bolus dosing or discontinuation of IV drip. Therefore titration of these agents is much more difficult than with either dopamine or dobutamine. Both agents should be titrated slowly (e.g., 1 to 5 µg/kg/min for amrinone, 0.025 to 0.1 µg/kg/min for milrinone) every 60 to 90 minutes. More time may be necessary between titrations if the patient has altered renal or hepatic function or has been maintained on these agents for more than 3 days. Patients are typically more difficult to titrate if they have a low CO and a high PCWP. Never abruptly stop either of these agents; patients may decompensate rapidly and require a bolus dose of these agents to be sustained. Carefully monitor the hemodynamic changes that occur with dose reductions, and slow the process if the patient cannot maintain the desired hemodynamic response. It may take 24 to 48 hours to withdraw therapy successfully in some patients.

### Cautions and side effects

1. Amrinone causes a dose-dependent, asymptomatic thrombocytopenia in up to 4% of patients. The frequency increases with doses greater than 18 mg/kg/day. Platelet counts return to normal within 2 to 7 days

after decreasing the dose or discontinuing therapy. In most cases a reduction in dose is sufficient. Since the reaction is not secondary to an immune response, platelet transfusions can be used in patients who cannot be titrated. Milrinone induces thrombocytopenia in 1% of patients. The use of concomitant antiplatelet agents should be monitored closely.

2. Milrinone induces or exacerbates ventricular dysrhythmias in approximately 12% of patients. Of these dysrhythias, 8% are asymptomatic increases in premature ventricular contractions and 4% are increases in ventricular tachycardia. Milrinone increases AV nodal conduction and may be detrimental in some patients. The drug should be discontinued in patients who develop these side effects.

3. Other side effects common to both agents include nausea, headache, angina, hypotension, and increased liver enzymes.

## SYMPATHOMIMETICS[2,3,6,7]
### Epinephrine (Adrenalin, others)

Epinephrine is an important endogenous hormone that is produced and released by the adrenal gland in response to stress.

**Cardiovascular actions.** Epinephrine binds very strongly to both alpha and beta receptors. In the heart epinephrine stimulates beta$_1$ receptors to increase contractility, AV nodal and Purkinje fiber conduction, and sinoatrial nodal firing. Epinephrine may also accelerate firing of ectopic foci. As a result, epinephrine significantly increases myocardial oxygen demands. Beta$_2$-receptor stimulation results in prolonged vasodilatation and bronchodilatation because of the drug's strong affinity for this receptor. This action is clinically important at low doses (e.g., 0.005 to 0.02 $\mu$g/kg/min), resulting in reduced vascular resistance. The diastolic blood pressure will fall, but the systolic will be maintained if there is an adequate circulating blood volume to maintain cardiac output (CO). Epinephrine also stimulates alpha receptors, and vasoconstriction predominates with doses greater than 0.02 $\mu$g/kg/min. Alpha stimulation results in increased systemic and peripheral vascular resistance (SVR, PVR) and mean arterial pressure (MAP), all of which increase the workload of the heart.

### Clinical uses

1. Epinephrine is most often employed clinically during cardiac arrest and cardiogenic shock to stimulate cardiac pacemaker activity and increase contractility.
2. Epinephrine is often the drug of choice in the immediate treatment of anaphylaxis or reversible bronchospasm.

### Dosage and administration (see Table 10-5)

1. Prediluted syringes with 1:10,000 solution for IV bolus during cardiac arrest are to be administered every 5 minutes as needed.
2. Prediluted epinephrine in 1:1000 solution for subcutaneous injection during anaphylaxis can be repeated every 5 to 10 minutes. Use the same dose for bronchospasm, but repeat every 20 to 30 minutes.
3. Epinephrine is compatible in most IV fluids. IV drips can be mixed by adding 1 to 4 mg to 250 ml IV fluid. Solutions may be concentrated for volume-restricted patients, but caution should be used.
4. Beta-adrenergic effects predominate at doses less than 0.02 $\mu$g/kg/min. IV doses of 0.05 to 0.07 $\mu$g/kg/min are recommended for alpha-adrenergic effects. Titrate dose to desired response.
5. Epinephrine is compatible with dopamine, dobutamine, norepinephrine, and potassium.
6. If given by endotracheal administration, deliver the drug deeply into the airway and give 1 mg initially.
7. If infiltration occurs, local injections of 5 to 10 mg of phentolamine are usually effective if used within 6 hours.
8. Epinephrine is unstable in alkaline solutions.
9. Avoid using epinephrine if it is discolored or has precipitated in the IV fluid.
10. Epinephrine is useful in combination with other agents but should be discontinued as soon as possible to avoid excessive metabolic demands on the heart.
11. Monitor CO, MAP, SVR, ECG, blood pressure, heart rate, pulmonary capillary wedge pressure, and electrolyte levels.

### Cautions and side effects

1. Overdose has occurred when patients have been accidentally given 1:1000 (10 mg) solutions in an emergency situation. The blood pressure will rise acutely, leading to possible cerebral hemorrhage. The pressure will then fall abruptly after 10 to 20 minutes secondary to the effects of the drug on the beta receptors. Therefore use of a short-acting agent will control the initial hypertension, and the subsequent hypotension will respond to sympathomimetics if necessary.
2. Epinephrine may exacerbate ventricular dysrhythmias.

| TABLE 10-5 Sympathomimetics | | |
|---|---|---|
| **Drug** | **Dilution*** | **Dose** |
| Epinephrine | 4 mg/250 ml IVF | 0.05-0.07 $\mu$g/kg/min |
| Norepinephrine | 8 mg/250 ml IVF | 2.0-24 $\mu$g/min |
| Isoproterenol | 1 mg/250 ml IVF | 0.5-5 $\mu$g/min |
| Phenylephrine | 5 mg/250 ml IVF | 0.04-0.06 mg/min |

*IVF, Intravenous fluid.

3. Disturbing reactions of fear, anxiety, and tension may occur.
4. Epinephrine may precipitate myocardial ischemia because of the inability of coronary blood flow to meet increased myocardial oxygen requirements.
5. Epinephrine may produce headache, tremor, and weakness.
6. Renal blood flow, glomerular filtration rate, and sodium excretion are usually reduced after the administration of epinephrine.
7. Epinephrine drips may reduce serum potassium levels by as much as 0.8 mEq/L. ECG changes are usually apparent as well, placing the critically ill patient at risk for serious dysrhythmias.

## Norepinephrine (Levophed, others)

Norepinephrine is the biosynthetic precursor to epinephrine and the neurotransmitter of the sympathetic nervous system.

**Cardiovascular actions.** Norepinephrine stimulates primarily alpha but also beta receptors. Very low doses of norepinephrine produce mainly beta$_1$-adrenergic effects, resulting in increased contractility, chronotropy, and cardiac conduction. More often norepinephrine exerts a predominant alpha-adrenergic stimulating effect resulting in increased peripheral vascular resistance (PVR) and mean arterial pressure (MAP). Cardiac output (CO) usually remains unchanged or decreased because of the increased PVR and reflex slowed heart rate that result from vagal activation. Coronary blood flow increases, whereas renal, cerebral, visceral, and skeletal blood flow diminishes.

### Clinical uses

1. Norepinephrine is used to treat hypotension and shock, but it has largely been replaced in clinical practice by the newer agents dopamine and dobutamine.
2. Norepinephrine may be especially useful when hypotensive states are accompanied by low PVR and normal or slightly elevated CO.

### Dosage and administration (see Table 10-5)

1. Norepinephrine is compatible in most IV fluids. From 4 to 8 mg may be added to 250 ml IV fluid. More concentrated solutions can be used but may lose their potency more rapidly.
2. Do not use if a precipitate forms in the bottle or the solution is discolored.
3. Usual maintenance dose is 2 to 24 μg/min. Adjust rate to the patient's hemodynamic response, using the lowest effective dose.
4. Monitor CO, MAP, heart rate, pulmonary capillary wedge pressure, systemic vascular resistance, renal function, signs of vasoconstriction, and electrolyte levels.
5. Administer norepinephrine through a central line when possible. Extravasation with tissue necrosis can occur

rapidly in a peripheral line. If this occurs, inject 5 to 10 mg of phentolamine into the area as soon as possible. Phentolamine is most effective if used within the first 6 hours and is useless after 24 hours.
6. Typically norepinephrine is added to therapy after dopamine and should be discontinued as soon as possible. Titrate according to the patient's hemodynamic response and allow 15 to 30 minutes between adjustments in dose.
7. Norepinephrine is compatible with heparin, magnesium, dopamine, dobutamine, potassium, calcium, epinephrine, isoproterenol, and verapamil.
8. Maintain an adequate blood volume when using this agent. Hypovolemia may increase the cardiac workload and lead to ischemia.
9. Norepinephrine may be added to gastric lavage solutions in the treatment of acute gastrointestinal bleeding. The dose is 16 mg in 200 ml of iced saline.

### Cautions and side effects

1. Anxiety, respiratory difficulty, and transient headaches may result.
2. Overdose may cause severe hypertension with headache, photophobia, angina, intensive sweating, and vomiting.
3. Cardiac dysrhythmias may be produced or exacerbated.
4. Reflex bradycardia may occur in some patients, but typically the heart rate is increased.
5. Norepinephrine has additive sympathomimetic side effects when used with other catecholamines.

## Isoproterenol (Isuprel, others)

Isoproterenol is a synthetic, direct-acting, nonspecific beta-adrenergic agonist.

**Cardiovascular actions.** Isoproterenol causes almost exclusive beta-adrenergic receptor stimulation and acts on beta$_2$ (smooth muscle, bronchioles) and beta$_1$ (heart) receptors. Isoproterenol relaxes smooth muscle of bronchi, skeletal muscle vasculature, and the alimentary tract. In the heart isoproterenol increases heart rate and contractility. Isoproterenol lowers peripheral vascular resistance and decreases diastolic arterial pressures. The net hemodynamic effect is to elevate cardiac output (CO) and systolic pressure and to decrease mean and diastolic arterial pressure. In addition, myocardial oxygen consumption rises with isoproterenol administration.

### Clinical uses

1. Isoproterenol is most often used to enhance pacemaker activity and improve AV conduction during episodes of sinus bradycardia or AV block.
2. In certain cardiogenic shock states isoproterenol may be used to increase CO and decrease peripheral vasoconstriction. Isoproterenol is not indicated to treat cardiogenic shock caused by acute myocardial infarction.

3. In bronchospastic lung disease isoproterenol may be used by inhalation to produce bronchodilatation.

### Dosage and administration (see Table 10-5)

1. Isoproterenol is compatible in most IV fluids. From 1 to 4 mg can be diluted in 250 ml IV fluid. Exposure to air, light, or increased temperature may cause a pink discoloration, and the solution should be discarded. Use caution with concentrations greater than 10 mg in 250 ml IV fluid.
2. Hemodynamic effects are typically seen with doses ranging from 0.5 to 5 $\mu$g/min. However, doses exceeding 30 $\mu$g/min have been used in advanced shock. Use the lowest possible dose to achieve the therapeutic response.
3. Titrate the drug according to hemodynamic response every 15 to 30 minutes, which will allow time for the patient's response to the change in dose.
4. Isoproterenol is compatible with dopamine, dobutamine, calcium, heparin, potassium, epinephrine, norepinephrine, and verapamil.
5. Monitor ECG, CO, heart rate, blood pressure, and electrolyte levels.

### Caution and side effects

1. Isoproterenol increases myocardial oxygen consumption and may precipitate myocardial ischemia.
2. Cardiac dysrhythmias, including sinus tachycardia, premature ventricular complexes, ventricular tachycardia, or ventricular fibrillation, may result.
3. In the presence of hypovolemia the vasodilating effects of isoproterenol may produce hypotension.
4. Headache, flushing of the skin, angina, nausea, tremor, dizziness, weakness, and sweating may result.
5. Patients with symptomatic coronary artery disease, hypertrophic cardiomyopathy, and cardiac dysrhythmias are particularly susceptible to adverse cardiac effects from isoproterenol.

## Phenylephrine (Neo-Synephrine)

Phenylephrine is a synthetic agent that predominantly stimulates alpha receptors.

**Cardiovascular actions.** Phenylephrine increases total peripheral resistance and blood pressure by directly stimulating alpha receptors. Blood flow to vital organs, skin, and skeletal muscle is usually reduced. With prolonged use, circulating blood volume may decrease, which leads to increased myocardial demand. The main effect of phenylephrine on the heart is bradycardia, which results from a reflex increase in vagal tone secondary to the change in arterial pressure. The bradycardia can be blocked by atropine.

### Clinical uses

1. Phenylephrine is typically employed to treat paroxysmal supraventricular tachycardia. The hypertensive response increases vagal tone and may terminate the dysrhythmia.
2. Hypotension caused by peripheral vasodilatation, such as occurs with ganglionic blocking agents or spinal anesthesia, may be reversed by phenylephrine.
3. Phenylephrine is also useful in treating the hypotension caused by left ventricular outflow obstruction in hypertrophic cardiomyopathy.
4. This agent is not indicated in the treatment of usual forms of cardiogenic shock.

### Dosage and administration (see Table 10-5)

1. Phenylephrine is compatible in most IV fluids. From 5 to 20 mg may be diluted in 250 ml IV fluid for continuous infusion. Solutions should not be used if they are brown or contain a precipitate.
2. For continuous IV infusion in severe hypotension or shock the maintenance dose is 0.04 to 0.06 mg/min. Larger doses may be necessary to stabilize the patient (e.g., 0.1 to 0.2 mg/min). Adjust the rate to the lowest possible effective dosage for the desired hemodynamic response.
3. For supraventricular tachycardia a bolus dose of 0.5 to 1 mg IV push followed by 1 to 2 mg (if no response in 60 to 90 seconds) is sufficient to terminate the dysrhythmia.
4. Phenylephrine is compatible with lidocaine and potassium.
5. Monitor ECG, blood pressure, heart rate, cardiac output, systemic vascular resistance, mean arterial pressure, pulmonary capillary wedge pressure, urine output, peripheral vasoconstriction, renal function, and electrolyte levels
6. Titrate the dose every 15 minutes, and discontinue the drug as soon as possible to prevent hypovolemia and hypoperfusion to the extremities.
7. Phenylephrine has an additive effect when used with other vasopressors.

### Cautions and side effects

1. Excessive dosage may produce headache, excessive hypertension, severe bradycardia, and vomiting.
2. Phenylephrine may also cause restlessness, anxiety, tremor, and nervousness. These effects are additive to those of the other sympathomimetics.
3. Phenylephrine should not be administered to hypertensive patients for treatment of paroxysmal supraventricular tachycardia.

## ALPHA-ADRENERGIC BLOCKERS[2,6]

Alpha-adrenergic blocking agents directly and selectively block the stimulation of alpha-adrenergic receptors.

**Cardiovascular actions.** The effects of these agents are most prominent in peripheral vascular beds when vasoconstrictor responses are inhibited and vasodilatation results. Alpha-adrenergic blocking agents may accelerate heart rate either by reflex effects from peripheral vasodilatation or direct effects resulting from cardiac alpha$_2$-receptor inhibition, which increases norepinephrine release. The alpha-adrenergic blocking agents discussed here are *phenoxybenzamine* (Dibenzyline) and *phentolamine* (Regitine). Prazosin and terazosin are oral alpha-adrenergic blockers and are discussed under Vasodilators later in this chapter. Phenoxybenzamine inhibits alpha$_1$ receptors, and phentolamine inhibits both alpha$_1$ and alpha$_2$ receptors.

Phenoxybenzamine has a slow onset of action over several hours, and cumulative effects of daily administration appear in 7 days. Once alpha-adrenergic blockade is accomplished, it is complete and present for 3 to 4 days after discontinuation of the agent. Phenoxybenzamine reverses the pressor effect of epinephrine and competitively blocks the vasoconstrictor effects of norepinephrine. Unlike phenoxybenzamine, phentolamine has a rapid onset of action and a short duration of action. Phentolamine incompletely blocks alpha$_1$ and alpha$_2$ receptors and is more effective in blocking the effects of circulating norepinephrine or epinephrine than antagonizing responses at the adrenergic nerve ending. Blood pressure response depends on both the drug's vasodilating effect and the drug's weak beta-agonist effect.

### Clinical uses

1. Alpha-adrenergic blocking agents are indicated to inhibit excessive alpha-adrenergic stimulation that occurs either from an endogenous source, as during treatment of pheochromocytoma, or from an exogenous source, as when catecholamines are administered to treat shock.
2. Alpha-adrenergic blockers also have been used as direct vasodilators to reverse peripheral vasoconstriction that accompanies low cardiac output states, systemic hypertension, and peripheral vascular insufficiency.
3. Phentolamine is used to prevent dermal necrosis and sloughing following extravasation of norepinephrine, phenylephrine, or dopamine.

### Dosage and administration

1. Phenoxybenzamine (Dibenzyline) is available in oral form and is primarily used for the treatment of pheochromocytoma. Usual initial dose is 10 mg twice a day increased every other day until an adequate response is achieved. Normal maintenance dose is usually 20 to 40 mg two or three times daily, but some patients may require higher doses.
2. Phentolamine (Regitine) is available as an injectable powder for solution only. Phentolamine is primarily used in the diagnosis of pheochromocytoma or for prevention of dermal necrosis. The usual dose for diagnosing pheochromocytoma is 5 mg intravaneously or intramuscularly. Continuous IV drips can be given at a rate of 0.1 to 2.0 mg/min, but IV bolus doses of 5 to 10 mg are recommended by the manufacturer for the treatment of adrenergic hypertensive crisis. The dosage for dermal necrosis is 5 to 10 mg injected directly into the extravasated area. Phentolamine can be reconstituted using normal saline.
3. The use of phentolamine for essential hypertension is not recommended because most patients become refractory to the drug's antihypertensive effect.
4. Phentolamine is contraindicated in patients with myocardial infarction.
5. Monitor ECG, blood pressure, heart rate, and side effects.

### Cautions and side effects

1. As with all vasodilators, blood pressure may fall precipitously. Maintenance of adequate volume status minimizes part of this problem.
2. Other side effects of alpha-adrenergic blockers include acceleration of heart rate, miosis (constriction of the pupil), nasal stuffiness, inhibition of ejaculation, sedation, nausea, and vomiting.
3. Phentolamine and phenoxybenzamine may cause abdominal pain and exacerbate peptic ulcer disease.
4. Most of these side effects are dose-related and may be controlled by decreasing the dose. Many of the effects seen with phenoxybenzamine will decrease as therapy is continued.

### CENTRAL ALPHA AGONISTS (see Table 10-6)[3,6,8,11]

These agents stimulate central alpha$_2$ receptors in the vasomotor center of the medulla oblongata.

**Cardiovascular actions.** Alpha$_2$-receptor stimulation centrally inhibits norepinephrine release in the brain and peripheral sympathetic system. This inhibition results in decreased sympathetic activity, increased vagal stimulation, and decreased release of norepinephrine, epinephrine, and renin. When combined with beta blockers, these agents further lower heart rate by enhancing vagal activity. Central alpha agonists produce a fall in resting blood pressure, but reflex control of capacitance vessels remains intact, which helps maintain cardiac output during exercise. Renal blood flow is maintained with these agents because of a fall in renal vascular resistance. Methyldopa is slightly different from the other agents because it is a prodrug and must be metabolized to the active form. One of the metabolites acts as a false neurotransmitter, which is stored and released by the nerve terminals. Because the body stores this metabolite, the onset of methyldopa activity is delayed and the duration is prolonged.

### Clinical uses

1. These agents are used to treat chronic hypertension.
2. Clonidine can be used for hypertensive urgencies.
3. Methyldopa is typically used in toxemia.

### Dosage and administration (see Table 10-6)

1. Initial doses for these agents should be low and the dose slowly titrated up to the desired response. Sug-

**TABLE 10-6** Central alpha₂ agonists

| Agent | Trade Name | Dose | Dose Schedule* | Form | Onset (min) | Peak (hr) | Duration (hr) |
|---|---|---|---|---|---|---|---|
| Clonidine | Catapres | 0.2-1.2 mg/day | bid, tid | Oral | 30-60 | 2-4 | 6-12 |
| Guanabenz | Wytensin | 4-32 mg/day | bid | Oral | 60 | 2-4 | 6-12 |
| Guanfacine | Tenex | 1-3 mg/day | qd | Oral | 60-120 | 3-4 | 24 |
| Methyldopa | Aldomet | 1-3 g/day | bid, tid | Oral, IV | 120-180 | 3-6 | 6-12 |

*bid, Twice a day; tid, three times a day; qd, every day.

gested initial starting doses are as follows: Clonidine, 0.1 mg twice a day; guanabenz, 4 mg twice a day; guanfacine, 1 mg every day; methyldopa, 500 mg twice a day.

2. Dose of clonidine for hypertensive urgency: initially 0.2 mg orally, followed by 0.1 mg orally every hour (up to a total of 0.8 mg) until desired response. Remember that the onset of action and peak effect of this agent are gradual; thus the observed initial hypotensive effects reflect the first dose rather than the most recent dose. Hold further hourly doses until the total effect of the cumulative doses can be assessed. Most patients require a total of 0.4 mg or less for an adequate hypertensive response. Patients who are experiencing abrupt withdrawal of clonidine may require more drug and adjunct therapy to control their pressure.

3. When given intravenously for toxemia, the usual dose of methyldopa is 250 to 500 mg every 6 hours up to a maximum of 1 g every 6 hours.

4. When given in high doses, these agents may actually increase blood pressure by stimulating peripheral alpha receptors. Therefore these agents should not be given in doses higher than the recommended doses.

5. These agents should never be used in combination with one another.

6. Monitor blood pressure, heart rate, electrolyte levels and side effects.

7. Clonidine transdermal patches are useful in noncompliant patients. Patches are changed once weekly, and most patients respond to patches that deliver 0.1 to 0.2 mg/day.

8. Clonidine may also be used in alcohol, nicotine, and opiate withdrawal syndromes. Doses should be titrated to control symptoms without inducing hypotension.

9. These agents should be tapered slowly when discontinued. The tapering schedule depends on the dose and duration of therapy. Higher doses given over longer periods require more gradual tapering (e.g., reduce clonidine dose by 0.2 mg at weekly intervals). Most patients can be easily tapered off the drug in 2 weeks with no adverse effects.

10. These agents are excellent antihypertensive drugs because they do not affect most risk factors for coronary artery disease. They tend to have no effect on electrolytes or lipids and maintain exercise capacity and renal blood flow in most patients.

11. Central alpha agonists are more efficacious in the elderly population and volume-dependent hypertensive patients.

### Caution and side effects

1. All these agents may produce rebound hypertension and should not be abruptly discontinued. Patients who are concurrently taking a beta blocker are especially susceptible to severe hypertension if they stop taking the central alpha agonist. Rebound hypertension occurs more often with clonidine than with either guanabenz, guanfacine, or methyldopa, and it rarely occurs with clonidine doses of less than 0.3 mg daily. Patients who have rebound hypertension should have the drug reinstituted immediately. If necessary, IV labetalol and/or nitroprusside can be used with the oral agent if the patient has recent-onset end-organ damage. Beta blockers alone are not recommended because these agents may exaggerate the hypertensive response by providing unopposed adrenergic vasoconstriction from the increased norepinephrine release. Most patients can be easily controlled and switched to oral therapy within 24 hours.

2. Clonidine patches produce very little rebound hypertension. The patches have a gradual onset that peaks over 2 to 3 days. If a patient is to be changed from oral therapy to a patch, continue to give oral therapy and taper gradually over 2 to 3 days. This schedule prevents dramatic fluctuations in blood pressure.

3. The other major side effects associated with these agents are sedation, dry mouth, impotence, constipation, dizziness, hypotension, nasal congestion, and headache. These effects are primarily dose related and can be controlled by decreasing the dose.

4. Allergic contact dermatitis occurs frequently with the transdermal patches. If dermatitis occurs, the patch should be discontinued and oral clonidine gradually initiated.

5. A positive Coombs' test may occur in up to 25% of patients taking methyldopa, but less than 1% develop hemolytic anemia.
6. Hepatic disease has also been associated with methyldopa use. This agent should be used with caution in any patient who has a history of hepatic disease.
7. Fluid and sodium retention usually occurs over long-term therapy with these agents, especially with higher doses.

## GANGLIONIC AGENTS[2,6,8]

Ganglionic agents act directly on the adrenergic ganglionic neurons.

**Cardiovascular actions.** There are three agents in this class: guanethidine (Ismelin), guanadrel (Hylorel), and reserpine. Guanethidine and guanadrel deplete norepinephrine from presynaptic storage granules, resulting in a reduction in total peripheral resistance. These two agents also inhibit action potential–induced release of norepinephrine. Reserpine gradually depletes norepinephrine from postganglionic neurons and is considered a weak agent when used alone.

### Clinical uses

1. Guanethidine and guanadrel are used in the treatment of hypertension. They are considered last-line agents because of their toxicity.
2. Low doses of reserpine combined with diuretics are beneficial in treating elderly patients with hypertension.

### Dosage and administration

1. Guanethidine should be initiated at 10 mg/day and gradually increased in 10 to 25 mg increments at 5- to 7-day intervals. Guanadrel should be initiated at 5 mg twice a day and gradually increased to 20 to 75 mg twice a day. Reserpine should be initiated at 0.1 mg every day and increased as necessary to a dose no greater than 0.25 mg every day.
2. Patients should be titrated to the lowest possible effective dose to prevent side effects.
3. These agents are additive with other antihypertensive agents. They should be used cautiously in the presence of other agents that affect the adrenergic nervous system.
4. Monitor blood pressure, heart rate, and side effects.

### Caution and side effects

1. Guanethidine and guanadrel frequently cause orthostatic hypotension, which produces symptoms of dizziness, weakness, lassitude, or syncope. This is particularly hazardous in the elderly population.
2. Fluid retention and edema occur with guanethidine and guanadrel, which may exacerbate congestive heart failure in some patients.
3. Reserpine causes dose-related mental depression in ap-

proximately 10% of patients taking 0.25 mg/day. Patients taking doses greater than 0.25 mg/day experience significantly more depression and psychologic difficulties. Reserpine is contraindicated in any patient who has a history of mental depression or suicidal tendencies.
4. All these agents may cause diarrhea, abdominal pain, exacerbation of peptic ulcer disease, or epigastric distress. These adverse effects occur more often with reserpine.
5. Other adverse effects that may occur with these agents include impotence, bradycardia, and nasal congestion.
6. Cardiovascular collapse may occur if these agents are given with some drugs used in surgical anesthesia.

## BETA BLOCKERS (see Table 10-7)[11,12,13]

Beta-adrenergic blocking agents act by competitive inhibition of adrenergic neuronal or hormonal action at the beta receptor.

**Cardiovascular actions.** As a result of specific receptor interaction in the heart, beta-adrenergic blocking agents inhibit increases in heart rate, AV nodal conduction, and myocardial contractility that result from beta-receptor stimulation. In addition, beta-adrenergic blocking agents inhibit bronchodilatation, peripheral vasodilatation, and renin release induced by adrenergic stimulation. Although these are their most common, clinically significant effects, beta-adrenergic blocking agents act in all organs to inhibit the effects of beta-receptor stimulation.

Propranolol was the first beta-adrenergic antagonist to achieve widespread clinical use, but multiple agents are now available, all having the primary effect of blocking beta receptors. Differences in clinical pharmacologic effects of these agents may be categorized according to their relative selectivity for beta$_1$ receptors, intrinsic agonist activity, relative lipid solubility, and membrane-stabilizing effects. Each agent also has a unique pharmacokinetic profile and potency that determine dosage strength and administration schedule. These properties of the available beta-adrenergic blocking agents are listed in Table 10-7.

The term *cardioselectivity* is used to describe a beta blocker that has predominant effects on beta$_1$ receptors and therefore has its major effects on the heart. The most common clinical advantage of cardioselectivity is that there is less inhibition of bronchodilatation and vasodilatation, effects mediated primarily by beta$_2$ receptors. Therefore cardioselective agents may lower the potential for bronchospasm in patients with chronic lung disease. A theoretic disadvantage of cardioselective agents is that catecholamine-induced potassium release from skeletal muscle and excretion is not blocked, and hypokalemia may be more frequent with these agents. The clinical significance of this effect has not been firmly established. Selectivity for beta$_1$- or beta$_2$-receptor inhibition is relative, and higher doses of cardioselective agents also produce inhibition at beta$_2$-

**TABLE 10-7** Beta blockers

| Agent | Trade Name | Oral Dose* | IV Dose* | Cardio-selective[†] | Intrinsic Agonist Activity[†] | Membrane Stabilizing Effect[†] | Hydrophilic[†] |
|---|---|---|---|---|---|---|---|
| Propranolol | Inderal | 40-160 mg bid to qid | 0.1-0.15 mg/kg in 1 mg increments q 5 min | − | − | + | − |
| Metoprolol | Lopressor | 50-100 mg bid | 5 mg q 5 min × 3 doses | + | - | - | - |
| Atenolol | Tenormin | 50-100 mg qd | 5 mg q 5 min × 2 doses | + | − | − | + |
| Nadolol | Corgard | 40-160 mg qd | — | − | − | − | + |
| Timolol | Blocadren | 10-20 mg bid | | − | − | − | − |
| Pindolol | Visken | 5-30 mg bid | | − | + | + | − |
| Dilevalol | Unicard | 100-800 mg qd | | − | + | − | − |
| Acebutolol | Sectral | 200-600 mg bid | — | + | + | + | + |
| Betaxolol | Kerlone | 10-40 mg qd | — | + | − | + | + |
| Esmolol | Brevibloc | — | 500 µg/kg/min × 1 minute then 50 µg/kg/min titrated up by 50 µg/kg/min q 5 min; maximum dose: 300 µg/kg/min | + | − | − | − |
| Labetalol | Normodyne Trandate | 100-400 mg bid | 20 mg IV push, then 40-80 mg q 10-15 min; maintenance infusion: 1-2 mg/min | − | + | − | − |

*bid, Twice a day; qid, four times a day; qd, every day; q, every.
†+, Present; −, absent.

receptor sites. In addition, there is neither complete segregation nor different beta-receptor subtypes in each organ; thus, for example, about 15% to 20% of cardiac beta receptors are composed of beta$_2$ receptors.

When a drug occupies a receptor site, thereby blocking that receptor site to its usual agonist, the drug itself may possess weak agonist activity or intrinsic sympathomimetic activity. One example of the clinical effects of intrinsic agonist activity is that these agents inhibit an exercise-induced increase in heart rate with a minimum effect on resting heart rate when compared to other beta-adrenergic antagonists that do not possess this activity. This property may confer a slight advantage to these agents in some clinical situations, such as the treatment of hypertension. However, intrinsic agonist activity appears to preclude the use of these agents for the treatment of angina pectoris and in prophylaxis following myocardial infarction.

Beta-adrenergic blocking agents may be classified as primarily lipid soluble (*lipophilic*) or water soluble (*hydro-philic*). The potential importance of this property derives from the suggestion that hydrophilic compounds are less able than lipophilic compounds to cross the blood-brain barrier and thus have fewer side effects on the central nervous system. Lastly, membrane-stabilizing effects are direct effects on membrane action potentials similar to those produced by quinidine or other local anesthetics. These effects probably play a minor role in the antidysrhythmic potential of beta-adrenergic blocking agents. For example, in the case of propranolol, these effects are present only at very high drug concentrations.

### Clinical uses

1. *Angina pectoris*. The goal in treatment is to decrease myocardial oxygen demands. This goal is accomplished primarily by lowering heart rate but also by decreasing myocardial contractility. Clinical effects appear additive to those of calcium channel blockers and nitrates. The usual goal is to lower resting heart rate to 50 to 60

beats/min and to blunt the heart rate response to exercise.

2. *Dysrhythmias.* Usual indications are to control the ventricular response to atrial flutter or fibrillation and to terminate and prevent recurrences of paroxysmal supraventricular tachycardia. Beta blockers are useful in treating selected ventricular dysrhythmias, such as some dysrhythmias induced by exercise, adrenergic excess, or digitalis toxicity.

3. *Post–myocardial infarction.* Some beta-adrenergic blockers reduce mortality for up to 3 years following myocardial infarction. Agents specifically indicated for this use are timolol (Blocadren), metoprolol (Lopressor), propranolol (Inderal), and atenolol (Tenormin). IV beta blockers are also useful in the early stages of acute myocardial infarction to accompany the administration of thrombolytic agents. IV metoprolol and atenolol are specifically indicated for this purpose.

4. Additional uses include the treatment of hypertrophic cardiomyopathy, the cardiovascular manifestations of hyperthyroidism, and anxiety states.

### Dosage and administration (see Table 10-7)

1. Metoprolol and atenolol are the primary IV agents used in early acute myocardial infarction. Metoprolol can be given as a 5 mg IV bolus every 5 minutes for a total dose of 15 mg. Atenolol is given as a 5 mg IV bolus and repeated once for a total dose of 10 mg. Beta blockers are most efficacious in patients who have transmural, anterior myocardial infarctions and who are clinically tachycardic and hypertensive. These agents are excellent adjunct therapy to thrombolytics and aspirin in this patient population. Beta blockers should be used cautiously in patients with hypotension or cardiogenic shock.

2. Oral therapy should be instituted after IV loading in patients with acute myocardial infarction. Metoprolol may be given as 50 mg orally every 6 hours for 48 hours, then 100 mg twice a day. Atenolol may be given as 50 mg orally twice a day for 48 hours, followed by 100 mg orally every day. Maintenance doses should maintain the resting heart rate in the range of 50 to 60 beats/min.

3. Therapy should be initiated with low doses and slowly titrated for the desired response. Monitor blood pressure, heart rate, ECG, electrolyte levels, and side effects.

4. Nadolol and atenolol dosages should be reduced by one half in patients with creatinine clearance less than 40 ml/min. If the clearance is less than 20 ml/min, the dose may be given every other day.

5. Avoid abrupt cessation of therapy. Rebound hypertension may occur, and these agents should be gradually tapered over 2 weeks when discontinued.

6. Beta blockers may be useful in some patients with congestive heart failure, but their role has yet to be

determined. At present these agents are not recommended for such patients.

### Cautions and side effects

1. Because these agents decrease myocardial contractility, they may exacerbate or induce congestive heart failure in some patients. Beta blockers have additive negative inotropic effects with other agents that depress contractility. Nonselective agents may worsen afterload abnormalities by increasing peripheral resistance. Therapy should be discontinued in patients who develop signs and symptoms of heart failure.

2. Because these agents depress sinoatrial (SA) and AV nodal conduction, bradydysrhythmias may occur. Symptomatic bradycardia and AV block are typically seen in patients if beta blockers are administered with other drugs that may depress SA or AV nodal conduction. Many patients respond to a lower dose of beta blocker, and therapy should be discontinued if they do not.

3. Nonselective beta antagonists or high doses of cardioselective antagonists exacerbate or induce bronchospasm in some patients. Patients with a history of pulmonary disease should be monitored closely while receiving beta blockers. Selective agents with intrinsic agonist activity are generally better tolerated by these patients. If bronchospasm occurs, isoproterenol should be given by inhalation therapy.

4. Peripheral vascular disease may be worsened by the use of these agents. Many patients complain of cold extremities, pain, tingling, or burning sensations in their extremities. Doses should be reduced, or agents with intrinsic agonist activity or cardioselectivity may be used as alternatives. The drug should be discontinued if these effects continue.

5. Beta blockers mask hypoglycemic symptoms that are mediated by the adrenergic system. These agents also delay the recovery time from hypoglycemia. These effects are more prominent with the use of nonspecific agents but can be seen with all agents. Agents with intrinsic agonist activity or cardioselectivity should be used in diabetic patients if beta blockers must be employed.

6. Dizziness, weakness, fatigue, nightmares, vivid dreams, insomnia, and general lassitude may be experienced by patients receiving these agents. The dose should be reduced if possible or a hydrophilic agent used when possible.

7. Other possible side effects are diarrhea, nausea, rash, and impotence.

8. Beta blockers adversely affect the blood lipid profile by increasing serum low-density lipoproteins and reducing serum high-density lipoproteins. Agents that are cardioselective or possess intrinsic agonist activity have the least effects on serum lipids and should be

used in patients who are at risk for this side effect.

9. Beta blockers typically reduce exercise tolerance in patients.

10. Beta blockers are additive with other hypotensive agents and should be used cautiously with other agents that affect the adrenergic system.

11. Patients will often complain of excessive fatigue when initiating beta-blocker therapy. It may take days to weeks for their bodies to adjust to the change.

12. Abrupt cessation of therapy may exacerbate angina, myocardial infarction, or dysrhythmias in patients with ischemic heart disease. These patients should be monitored closely. It is unclear whether slowly reducing the dose of a beta blocker before discontinuation would prevent this effect.

## VASODILATORS[*]
### Nitrates

This category includes *nitroglycerin* and *isosorbide dinitrate*. Their pharmacologic actions are caused by the property of nitrate to relax smooth muscle, especially in vascular beds.

**Cardiovascular actions.** Nitrates are primarily venodilators but may also produce arteriolar dilatation at higher doses. Their major hemodynamic effect is to lower left and right ventricular filling pressures (preload), which improves exercise tolerance, pulmonary congestion, and dyspnea. Cardiac output may be increased in a failing ventricle if preload is elevated before administration of these agents. Nitrates are also potent coronary vasodilators and increase blood flow through normal, collateral, or occluded coronary arteries.

Nitrate therapy can be complicated by the development of tolerance to these agents. In the smooth muscle, nitrates are converted to nitrites, which actually produce vasodilatation. The successful metabolism of nitrates depends on the balance of two factors: the availability of sulfhydryl groups for the conversion and the amount of drug that is delivered to the vascular smooth muscle. Tolerance develops when the drug cannot be adequately metabolized because of a depletion of sulfhydryl groups. In patients with good cardiac output, tolerance may develop rapidly because sustained amounts of drug are present in the smooth muscle. In contrast, patients with heart failure may not develop tolerance because less drug is available for metabolism, thus preventing sulfhydryl group depletion. In patients who develop tolerance to the cardiovascular actions, drug-free intervals of 8 to 16 hours allow time for the body to replenish the sulfhydryl groups.

### Clinical uses

1. Nitroglycerin is the preferred drug in the treatment of acute episodes of angina pectoris because of the rapid

onset of its action and its ability to decrease myocardial oxygen demands and dilate coronary vessels.

2. Nitrates are effective in the treatment of stable, unstable, and variant angina. They have additive effects to reduce anginal pain when used with calcium channel blockers or beta blockers.

3. Nitrates are beneficial in the treatment of acute myocardial infarction. Nitrates improve blood flow to ischemic areas during periods of prolonged ischemia.

4. Nitrates are effective for reducing preload, thus improving pulmonary congestion in patients with congestive heart failure. They have additive effects when combined with other vasodilators.

### Dosage and administration (see Table 10-8)

1. Patients may complain of specific side effects at times when the drug is at its peak concentration. Some patients may require shorter or longer dosing intervals based on the duration of the pharmacologic effect in that patient.

2. Doses greater than those listed may be necessary and have been shown to be effective in some patients with angina and heart failure.

3. Sublingual tablets should cause a burning sensation when placed under the tongue. Nitroglycerin sublingual doses should be repeated every 5 minutes for 15 minutes in patients suffering from an acute anginal attack. If the pain persists, the patient should seek medical attention.

4. Nitroglycerin should be diluted in glass containers for IV administration. Unpredictable amounts of the drug may be lost in polyvinyl chloride plastic containers. Nitroglycerin injection is compatible in most IV fluids. Some injectable solutions contain large percentages of alcohol, and the solutions should never be concentrated more than 150 mg in 250 ml IV fluids. If a precipitate or separation of the solution is noted, it should be discarded and a more dilute solution used.

5. Transdermal patches have been associated with tolerance in a large percentage of patients. Their use should be monitored closely in patients with unstable angina.

6. If tolerance with oral dosing develops, separate the doses with a greater dosing interval. A twice-daily dosing schedule at 8 A.M. and 2 P.M. has been successfully used in many patients. This dosing scheme maintains an excellent vasodilator response with little or no tolerance in patients with angina. The sustained-release preparations are ideal for this type of dosing.

7. Doses should be gradually increased to maximize response and reduce side effects. For IV dosage, start at 5 to 10 µg/min and titrate 5 µg/min every 3 to 5 minutes to control chest pain and maintain systolic blood pressure at 90 mm Hg or greater.

8. Nitroglycerin tablets should be kept in the original glass container and closed tightly after each use. Tablets

### TABLE 10-8   Nitrates

| Agent | Onset (min) | Peak (hr) | Duration (hr) | Dose* |
|---|---|---|---|---|
| **ISOSORBIDE DINITRATE** | | | | |
| Sublingual | 5-20 | 0.5-1.0 | 1-3 | 2.5-10 mg prn |
| Oral tablets | 15-45 | 1-2 | 4-6 | 10-100 mg q 3-6 hr |
| Sustained release | 30-180 | 1-2 | 6-12 | 20-80 mg q 6-12 hr |
| **NITROGLYCERIN** | | | | |
| Sublingual | 2-5 | — | 0.25-0.5 | 0.2-0.6 mg prn |
| Buccal | 1-2 | 0.5 | 4-6 | 1-3 mg q 4-6 hr |
| Spray | 2-5 | — | 0.25-0.5 | 1 or 2 sprays prn |
| Topical paste | 30-60 | 2-3 | 3-6 | 0.5-3 inches q 3-6 hr |
| Transdermal patch | 30-60 | 2-3 | 12-24 | 2.5-15 mg daily |
| Tablet | 20-45 | 1-2 | 3-6 | 6.5-19.5 mg q 4-6 hr |
| Intravenous | <1 | — | 0.25-0.5 | 10-300 μg/min |
| Sustained release | 20-45 | 1-2 | 8-12 | 2.6-9 mg q 8-12 hr |

*prn, As necessary; q, every.

should be stored in a cool, dark place and the cotton removed from the bottle.

9. Monitor blood pressure, heart rate, pulmonary capillary wedge pressure, cardiac output, and side effects.

### Cautions and side effects

1. Nitrate therapy may cause postural hypotension, syncope, dizziness, headache, flushing, tachycardia, and nausea. The effects are dose related and can be alleviated by reducing the dose of nitrate. With continued therapy most patients become tolerant to these effects within 2 weeks of stable therapy.
2. Abrupt withdrawal of nitrate therapy may precipitate angina or pulmonary congestion in some patients.
3. Skin reactions requiring discontinuation of therapy have occurred in 40% of patients using transdermal patches.
4. Methemoglobinemia occurs rarely with the use of high-dose nitrates.
5. Rotate the placement of nitroglycerin ointment and patches to reduce local rash and irritation. Avoid coarsely haired regions and use occlusive dressings (e.g., plastic wrap over ointment) when possible to increase the absorption of the paste.

### Nitroprusside (Nipride)

Sodium nitroprusside is a vasodilating agent that acts directly on vascular smooth muscle independent of autonomic innervation.

**Cardiovascular actions.** Nitroprusside has a balanced effect to dilate arterioles and venules equivalently, thus decreasing both preload and afterload of the heart. In the failing heart afterload reduction increases the cardiac output either with a minimum decrease in mean arterial blood pressure or with none. Heart rate tends to remain unchanged or to increase slightly. Decreased preload, resulting from venodilatation, decreases pulmonary capillary wedge pressure. Beneficial hemodynamic effects are observed when the filling pressure and systemic resistance are elevated prior to therapy and cardiac output is depressed, as occurs in the failing myocardium. In normal hearts, however, or when left ventricular filling pressure is normal or low, nitroprusside produces hypotension and tachycardia with little change in cardiac output.

### Clinical uses

1. Nitroprusside is a potent, rapid-acting IV antihypertensive agent used to control hypertensive emergencies.
2. Nitroprusside is used in patients with severe left ventricular failure who have an adequate blood pressure (systolic, ≥ 90 mm Hg) and an elevated wedge pressure. The drug is an excellent adjunct to inotropes when the blood pressure can be maintained. The combination of dopamine and nitroprusside produces similar hemodynamic responses to that of dobutamine or amrinone alone.

### Dosage and administration

1. Nitroprusside is available in parenteral form only. Nitroprusside can be diluted in most IV fluids and concentrated for volume-restricted patients. The infusion bottle should be protected from light by an opaque wrapping.
2. The maintenance infusion rate is 0.5 to 10 μg/kg/min. The rate should be adjusted to the patient's hemodynamic response, and the administration rate should be

carefully controlled through the use of an infusion pump. Infusion rates should be kept at about 4 µg/kg/ min to avoid cyanide toxicity in patients receiving the drug for several days. Patients with normal renal function will usually not develop thiocyanate toxicity with prolonged use (e.g., 14 days) if the total dose is less than 70 mg/kg. Thiocyanate levels of 10 µg/ml or greater are considered toxic.

3. Rapid infusions may cause nausea, itching, diaphoresis, restlessness, palpitations, and headache.
4. Because of the agent's short duration of action (3 to 5 minutes), titration is very easy. Dosage increments can be made every 5 to 10 minutes when adjustments are necessary.
5. Monitor blood pressure, heart rate, thiocyanate levels, electrolyte levels, and side effects.

### Cautions and side effects

1. Reflex tachycardia, hypotension, abdominal pain, nausea, restlessness, and headache are dose-related side effects and can be controlled by reducing the infusion rate.
2. Thiocyanate will accumulate with long-term therapy (e.g., longer than 14 days) or earlier in patients with renal dysfunction. Toxicity is manifested initially as fatigue, anorexia, nausea, headache, mental confusion, or muscle spasms. Severe toxicity leads to tachypnea, altered consciousness, convulsions, metabolic acidosis, or coma. Fatalities have been reported.
3. Nitroprusside is contraindicated in patients with hypertension secondary to coarctation of the aorta or arteriovenous shunts.

### Direct Arteriolar Vasodilators (see Table 10-9)

These agents directly relax vascular smooth muscle more in arterioles than in veins. These agents include hydralazine, pinacidil, minoxidil, and diazoxide.

Cardiovascular actions. These agents are potent vasodilators that directly relax arteriolar smooth muscle, resulting in a reduction of total peripheral resistance. The subsequent decrease in blood pressure produces a reflex sympathetic activation, which is manifested as an increase in heart rate, cardiac output, and renin secretion with a redistribution of renal blood flow. Because these changes may attenuate the antihypertensive response, these agents should be administered with a diuretic and sympatholytic agent if used for long-term therapy. They are not recommended for initial therapy or monotherapy of hypertension or heart failure.

### Clinical uses

1. These agents are indicated for the treatment of hypertension that has not responded to previous therapy employing diuretics, beta blockers, angiotensin-converting enzyme (ACE) inhibitors, and/or calcium channel blockers.
2. These agents are indicated for cautious use in patients with low-output heart failure. Hydralazine is the primary agent in this class used for this indication because it produces less sodium and water retention when compared to the other agents.
3. These agents may be used in the treatment of hypertensive emergencies. Diazoxide is given intravenously for this indication only.
4. Hydralazine is indicated for the treatment of toxemia. Patients should be carefully monitored because many of the side effects of hydralazine resemble the clinical symptoms of eclampsia.

### Dosage and administration (see Table 10-9)

1. Monitor blood pressure, heart rate, fluid retention, electrolyte levels, and side effects.
2. Doses should be low initially and slowly titrated upward to achieve the desired response. These agents have additive effects with other hypotensive agents.
3. Minoxidil is a useful adjunct agent for controlling severe

| TABLE 10-9 Direct arteriolar vasodilators | | | | | | |
|---|---|---|---|---|---|---|
| **Agent** | **Trade Name** | **Route** | **Onset (min)** | **Peak (hr)** | **Duration (hr)** | **Dose*** |
| Hydralazine | Apresoline | Oral | 60 | 2-4 | 6-12 | 25-100 mg qid |
| | | IM | 20-40 | 1-2 | 3-8 | 5-10 mg q 6 hr |
| | | IV | 10-20 | 0.5-1 | 3-8 | 5-10 mg q 6 hr |
| Pinacidil | Pindac | Oral | 1-3 | 5-7 | 12 | 12.5-25 mg bid |
| Minoxidil | Loniten | Oral | 30 | 4-8 | 12-48 | 5-20 mg bid |
| Diazoxide | Hyperstat | IV | 1-2 | 0.03 | 4-24 | 50-150 mg q 5 min or infusion at 7.5-30 mg/min up to 5 mg/kg |

*qid, Four times a day; bid, twice a day; q, every.

hypertension, such as in dissecting aortic aneurysms. Minoxidil can be used concomitantly with nitroprusside and a beta blocker to achieve maximum reduction in blood pressure.

4. Minoxidil is also an excellent adjunct agent in patients with renal failure who have uncontrolled hypertension. It is usually more effective than the other agents in this class.

5. Hydralazine and nitrates used in combination for patients with heart failure may reduce morbidity and mortality in this population. This combination therapy is an effective alternative for patients who cannot tolerate ACE inhibitors.

### Cautions and side effects

1. Hypotension may occur with these agents and may be manifested clinically by syncope, dizziness, or palpitations. Many patients experience these effects at the time of the drug's peak concentration. These adverse effects can be eliminated by reducing the dose, separating antihypertensive agents, or giving the drug with food. If the patient remains hypotensive, the drug should be discontinued.

2. Reflex tachycardia and angina typically occur with these agents and may lead to myocardial ischemia. Use these agents cautiously in patients with a history of coronary artery disease.

3. Sodium and water retention occur frequently and often result in weight gain. Concomitant use of diuretics is necessary to alleviate this side effect.

4. Hydralazine has produced a syndrome resembling systemic lupus erythematosus or rheumatoid arthritis in about 7% of patients. Clinical manifestations include fever, arthralgia, splenomegaly, lymphadenopathy, asthenia, malaise, pleuritic chest pain, edema, and a positive antinuclear antibody reaction. Occasionally a rash appears. Patients should be discontinued from hydralazine if these symptoms are noted. This reaction occurs more frequently in women and in high-dose regimens (>200 mg/day).

5. Minoxidil may cause hair growth in some patients. A topical minoxidil product is available for male pattern baldness.

### Prazosin (Minipress), Terazosin (Hytrin)

Prazosin and terazosin are orally effective alpha-adrenergic blocking agents.

**Cardiovascular actions.** Prazosin and terazosin selectively block alpha$_1$-adrenergic receptors to reduce peripheral vascular resistance. The net effect is the dilatation of both arterioles and venules equally, which is similar to the effect of nitroprusside. The cardiac acceleration following vasodilatation with hydralazine or after nonselective alpha-receptor blockade with phentolamine does not occur with these agents. As a result of decreased systemic resistance,

cardiac output increases and blood pressure falls, both in hypertensive patients and in patients with congestive heart failure. The improvement in cardiac output, however, may not be maintained during chronic therapy, since tolerance to these agents' effects seems to develop.

### Clinical uses

1. Prazosin and terazosin are employed as oral vasodilators in the treatment of hypertension. Tolerance to the hypotensive effects usually does not develop.

2. These agents may be used for low-output states, but tolerance usually develops rapidly with chronic dosing. Thus these agents are not recommended for initial therapy.

### Dosage and administration

1. Initiate these agents with lower doses and slowly titrate to achieve the desired effect: prazosin, 1 mg orally twice a day (range, 6 to 15 mg/day); terazosin, 1 mg orally at bedtime (range, 1 to 5 mg/day).

2. The first dose should be given at bedtime to avoid first-dose syncope. Each increment in dose may precipitate syncopal episodes, and patients should be closely monitored.

3. These agents are available for oral use only.

4. Monitor blood pressure, heart rate, and side effects.

5. The full antihypertensive effect of these agents may not be achieved for 2 to 4 weeks.

6. These agents are additive with other hypotensive agents and synergistic with calcium channel blockers. The combination of these agents is especially beneficial in volume-dependent hypertensive patients who have renal insufficiency.

### Cautions and side effects

1. First-dose syncope usually occurs 30 to 90 minutes after the initial dose. The patient should be informed of this effect and avoid arising suddenly. Patients who are hypovolemic are more likely to have syncope with these agents.

2. Other adverse reactions include dizziness, headache, drowsiness, nausea, lethargy, fluid retention, urinary incontinence, and palpitations.

3. Most side effects are dose related and can be relieved by reducing the dose.

### DIURETICS (see Table 10-10)[6,8,10,11,16]

Diuretic agents increase the elimination of salt and water by the kidney.

**Cardiovascular actions.** Diuretics are classified into several different types of agents and differ primarily in their mechanism of action and potency. All agents reduce sodium and water reabsorption, which leads to a decreased circulating blood volume and left ventricular filling pressure (preload). Blood pressure is initially reduced by the

**TABLE 10-10** Commonly used diuretics

| Agent | Trade Name | Route | Onset (min) | Peak (hr) | Duration (hr) | Dose (mg/day) |
|---|---|---|---|---|---|---|
| **THIAZIDES** | | | | | | |
| Chlorothiazide | Diuril | Oral | 60-120 | 3-6 | 6-12 | 500-1000 |
| | | IV | 15 | 0.5 | 2 | 250-1000 |
| Hydrochloro-thiazide | Hydrodiuril | Oral | 60-120 | 3-6 | 6-12 | 12.5-100 |
| Metolazone | Zaroxolyn | Oral | 60-120 | 3-6 | 12-24 | 5-20 |
| **LOOP DIURETICS** | | | | | | |
| Ethacrynic acid | Edecrin | IV | 30 | 2 | 6-12 | 50-400 |
| Furosemide | Lasix | Oral | 30-60 | 1-2 | 6-8 | 40-1500 |
| | | IV | 5-10 | 0.5-1.0 | 2 | 40-1000 |
| Bumetanide | Bumex | Oral | 30-60 | 1-2 | 4-6 | 1-10 |
| | | IV | 5-10 | 0.5-1.0 | 2-3 | 1-10 |
| **POTASSIUM-SPARING DIURETICS** | | | | | | |
| Amiloride | Midamor | Oral | 120 | 10 | 24 | 5-10 |
| Spironolactone | Aldactone | Oral | Gradual | 72 | 48-72 | 25-200 |
| Triamterene | Dyrenium | Oral | 120-240 | 6 | 9-24 | 100-300 |
| **ACETAZOLAMIDE** | Diamox | Oral | 60 | 2-4 | 8 | 250-500 |

change in plasma volume and cardiac output, but long-term treatment with diuretics results in reduced total peripheral resistance, which occurs once the plasma volume has normalized. *Potassium-sparing diuretics* and *acetazolamide* are weak agents and often ineffective when used alone. *Thiazides* are moderately effective but are useless in patients with a creatinine clearance less than 30 ml/min. Metolazone, although a thiazide derivative, is effective in renally impaired patients and useful in combination therapy. The *loop diuretics* are the most potent agents and can be given alone or in combination in any patient population.

### Clinical uses

1. Diuretics are used in the chronic treatment of hypertension. These agents are especially effective in volume-dependent hypertensive patients and can be used alone or concomitantly with other antihypertensives.
2. Diuretics are indicated for the chronic and acute treatment of congestive heart failure. Although effective in reducing the symptoms of failure, diuretics have no direct effect on the failing myocardium.
3. Diuretics are also indicated for edema and chronic renal insufficiency.

### Dosage and administration

1. Thiazide diuretics are often advocated as the preferred agents for the initial diuretic treatment of hypertension,

edema, or mild heart failure. Some commonly used agents are listed in Table 10-10. Thiazides appear to have a more potent hypotensive effect initially because of the greater loss of sodium as compared to free water with diuresis. Thiazides are synergistic with angiotensin-converting enzyme inhibitors and beta blockers.
2. Loop diuretics are preferred over thiazides as initial therapy in patients with renal insufficiency or symptoms of pulmonary congestion. For acute pulmonary edema, a bolus dose of furosemide of 0.5 to 1 mg/kg can be given initially and then doubled in 2 hours if an inadequate response is obtained.
3. Doses should be low initially and slowly adjusted according to response. Doses of hydrochlorothiazide greater than 100 mg/day (or 1000 mg/day for chlorothiazide) are ineffective for further increasing diuresis. If patients are unresponsive, a loop diuretic should be initiated and the thiazide stopped. Once patients appear refractory to loop diuretics, combination therapy should be employed using both metolazone and a loop diuretic. Chlorothiazide is the only thiazide available parenterally and may be used as an alternative to metolazone.
4. Patients with poor renal function respond better to larger daily doses than to smaller, twice-daily doses.
5. Fluid removal is more difficult in patients with a low albumin level because of decreased colloid osmotic pres-

sures. Patients should have fluids removed slowly to prevent volume depletion. A good general rule is 1 kg/day in most patients and 0.5 kg/day in ascitic patients.

6. Patients unresponsive to furosemide may be switched to bumetanide, which is 40 times more potent than furosemide (e.g., 1 mg bumetanide equals 40 mg furosemide). Many patients respond well to alternating loop diuretics and maintain a better diuresis than with chronic use of one agent for an extended time.

7. Patients receiving IV diuretics should be switched to oral therapy as soon as possible. Many patients with long-term heart failure require extremely large oral doses because of renal insufficiency and poor oral absorption. Diuretic doses may be altered significantly by the concurrent use of potent vasodilators.

8. Monitor blood pressure, heart rate, urine output, pulmonary capillary wedge pressure, renal function, electrolyte levels, and side effects.

### Cautions and side effects

1. Hypokalemia is the most common and serious adverse effect of these agents (except for the potassium-sparing agents). The use of these agents typically reduces the serum potassium level by 0.5 to 1 mEq/L, depending on the preexisting level and body stores. Potassium should be carefully monitored and replaced accordingly (see Potassium monograph later in this chapter).

2. The most common adverse effect of potassium-sparing diuretics is hyperkalemia. These agents should be avoided in patients with renal insufficiency. Stopping the diuretic should return the potassium level to normal.

3. Other adverse effects of these agents include hyponatremia, hypomagnesemia, abnormalities in uric acid and calcium, fatigue, hypovolemia, and metabolic alkalosis. Most are dose related and can be minimized by reducing the diuretic dose.

4. Loop diuretics may cause ototoxicity if given parenterally in high doses over short periods. The risk is greatest with ethacrynic acid and least with bumetanide. Doses should be administered no faster than 40 mg/min for furosemide, 1.0 mg/min for bumetanide, and 2.5 mg/min for ethacrynic acid.

5. Thiazide diuretics may produce glucose intolerance in borderline diabetic patients or elderly patients. Carefully monitor the serum glucose concentration in patients receiving high doses of these agents.

6. Thiazide diuretics increase serum low-density lipoprotein cholesterol and triglyceride levels and reduce high-density lipoprotein cholesterol levels. These effects may be potentially deleterious in patients with existing coronary artery disease. A notable exception to this is indapamide, which has minimum effects on serum lipid levels.

7. Patients receiving diuretics may experience a reduction in their exercise capacity. As the plasma volume normalizes with continued therapy, this effect should lessen.

8. Patients who develop hypokalemia with these agents typically have low magnesium levels as well. If the magnesium levels are low, oral or parenteral magnesium therapy is necessary before potassium supplementation or else the potassium levels will remain low despite replacement therapy.

9. Because acetazolamide is a carbonic anhydrase inhibitor, this drug may cause metabolic acidosis and can be used to treat diuretic-induced alkalosis.

## ACE INHIBITORS (see Table 10-11)[4,5,17,18]

The angiotensin-converting enzyme (ACE) inhibitors are potent, orally active agents that block the conversion of angiotensin I to angiotensin II.

**Cardiovascular actions.** The three agents in this class are equally effective at equipotent doses. All three competitively inhibit ACE, thereby blocking the formation of angiotensin II, a potent endogenous vasopressor. Angiotensin II also stimulates the sympathetic nervous system and the release of aldosterone, a hormone that retains sodium and eliminates potassium. By lowering angiotensin production, these agents produce both acute and sustained reductions in preload and afterload. These agents reduce mean arterial pressure, right atrial pressure, and left ventricular end-diastolic volume and pressure; they increase cardiac output and stroke volume. The reduction in aldosterone results in a mild diuresis and less volume expansion with continued use.

### Clinical uses

1. These agents are indicated for the treatment of hypertension. They are synergistic with thiazide diuretics and additive with the other hypotensive agents. They are indicated as first-line therapy and are particularly efficacious in vasoconstrictive (or high-renin) forms of hypertension.

2. These agents are indicated for the treatment of congestive heart failure (CHF). They are the only form of therapy at present that significantly reduces both the morbidity and the mortality associated with CHF. ACE inhibitors can be used for initial therapy in many patients instead of diuretics or digitalis. The hemodynamic effects of these agents are additive to those of other vasodilators or inotropes. Early initiation of therapy in asymptomatic patients with left ventricular hypertrophy may delay the progression of the failing myocardium.

### Dosage and administration (see Table 10-11)

1. Dosages should be low initially and slowly titrated upward to the desired response. Patients with CHF may be especially sensitive to these agents and require

**TABLE 10-11** ACE inhibitors

| Agent | Trade Name | Onset (hr) | Peak (hr) | Duration (hr) | Dose (mg)* |
|-------|-----------|-----------|-----------|---------------|------------|
| Captopril | Capoten | 0.5 | 1-1.5 | 8-24 | 6.25-100 q 8-12 hr |
| Enalapril | Vasotec | 3-4 | 4-8 | 12-24 | 2.5-40 q 12-24 hr |
| Lisinopril | Zestril, Prinivil | 3-4 | 6-8 | 24 | 2.5-40 q 24 hr |

*q, Every.

smaller doses given at extended intervals (e.g., captopril, 6.25 mg every 12 hours). Carefully monitor the hypotensive effects of these agents in this population, especially during the peak effect.

2. Patients with renal insufficiency should be titrated carefully to avoid worsening of renal function secondary to hypotension. Diabetic nephropathy and hypertension are typically seen together, and ACE inhibitors are beneficial in reducing both the proteinuria and the blood pressure in these patients when given in appropriate doses.

3. Patients with CHF receiving these agents may need their diuretic dose adjusted when ACE inhibitors are initiated. If given while the patient is hypovolemic, these agents may worsen cardiac and renal function. Also, patients on severe salt restriction diets should be monitored closely and their diets liberalized if necessary. The manufacturer suggests holding diuretic therapy for 1 week, if possible, before initiating ACE inhibitor therapy in stable patients.

4. Monitor blood pressure, heart rate, renal function, cardiac output, pulmonary capillary wedge pressure, electrolyte levels, and side effects.

5. These agents do not adversely affect the serum lipid profile.

6. These agents maintain exercise tolerance in hypertensive patients and may improve quality of life.

7. ACE inhibitors and beta blockers should not be used concurrently for additive hypotensive effects. These agents are rarely additive and produce more adverse effects when used concomitantly.

### Cautions and side effects

1. Higher doses of these agents produce significantly more adverse effects. Patients with preexisting renal dysfunction are at higher risk to develop adverse effects than other patients.

2. Proteinuria, azotemia, and renal insufficiency rarely occur in patients with normal renal function who receive standard doses. Onset is usually after the third month of chronic therapy but may occur more rapidly if the patient is receiving diuretics or becomes hypotensive.

3. Less than 2% of patients may develop a persistent non-productive cough while receiving these agents. If a cough occurs, patients may be switched from one agent to another.

4. Other adverse effects that may occur include dizziness, eosinophilia, neutropenia, angioedema, rash, nausea, metallic taste, and headache. These agents should be stopped if the patient develops angioedema or neutropenia. The other adverse effects are usually self-limiting and disappear with continued therapy.

5. Hypotension will occur if the patient is sodium depleted, hypovolemic, hyperreninemic, or overdosed. A reduction in dose and fluid replacement will restore blood pressure in most patients.

6. Hyperkalemia may develop in some patients, especially those with renal insufficiency. Potassium supplements and potassium-sparing diuretics should be used cautiously.

## CALCIUM CHANNEL BLOCKERS
(see Table 10-12)[13,19-21]

Calcium channel blockers inhibit the transmembrane influx of extracellular calcium ions across the membranes of myocardial and smooth muscle cells.

Cardiovascular actions. Each of the calcium antagonist agents exerts its pharmacologic action by slightly different actions on the calcium channel, which results in variable hemodynamic effects (see Table 10-12). *Nifedipine, nicardipine,* and *nitrendipine* are primarily peripheral vasodilators with less of an effect on coronary or cerebral blood flow. These three agents have no direct electrophysiologic properties and alter cardiac conduction only as a reflex action to afterload reduction. *Diltiazem* moderately decreases AV nodal conduction and is a potent coronary vasodilator. Diltiazem has minimum effects on peripheral vascular tone and tends to produce vasodilatation primarily when vasoconstriction is present. *Verapamil* has the most potent effects on heart rate and conduction and vasodilates both coronary and peripheral smooth muscle. *Nimodipine* is primarily a cerebral vasodilator with no effect on peripheral, coronary, or conducting tissues. Nimodipine is only indicated for the treatment of subarachnoid hemorrhage. All these agents except nimodipine have negative inotropic effects on the myocardium; verapamil possesses the greatest and diltiazem the least.

TABLE 10-12 Calcium channel blockers

| Agent | Trade Name | Route* | Onset (min) | Peak (hr) | Duration (hr) | Dose (mg)* | Cardiovascular Actions† ||||||
|---|---|---|---|---|---|---|---|---|---|---|---|---|
| | | | | | | | Vasodilatation ||| Contractility | Heart Rate | AV Nodal Conduction |
| | | | | | | | Peripheral | Coronary | Cerebral | | | |
| Diltiazem | Cardizem | Oral | 30-90 | 0.5-1 | 6-10 | 30-120 q 6-8 hr | + | +++ | + | 0, ↓ | 0, ↓ | ↓ |
| | | SR | Gradual | 6-11 | 12-24 | 120-480 q 12-24 hr | | | | | | |
| Verapamil | Isoptin, Calan | Oral | 30 | 0.5-1 | 6-8 | 40-120 q 6-8 hr | ++ | + | + | ↓↓ | 0, ↓ | ↓↓ |
| | | SR | Gradual | 5-7 | 12-24 | 120-480 q 12-24 hr | | | | | | |
| Nifedipine | Procardia, Adalat | Oral | 30-90 | 0.5-2 | 4-8 | 10-30 q 6-8 hr | +++ | ++ | ++ | ↓, Reflex ↑ | 0, Reflex ↑ | 0 |
| | | SR | Gradual | — | 24 | 30-90 q 24 hr | | | | | | |
| Nicardipine | Cardene | SL | 10-30 | 0.5-1 | 3-4 | 10 prn | +++ | ++ | ++ | ↓, Reflex ↑ | 0, Reflex ↑ | 0 |
| | | Oral | 20-30 | 0.5-2 | 6-8 | 20-40 q 8 hr | | | | | | |
| Nitrendipine | Baypress | Oral | 30-90 | 1-2 | 8-24 | 10-40 q 12-24 hr | +++ | ++ | ++ | ↓, Reflex ↑ | 0, Reflex ↑ | 0 |
| Nimodipine | Nimotop | Oral | — | 0.5-1 | 4-6 | 60 q 4 hr for 21 days | + | + | +++ | 0 | 0 | 0 |

*SR, Sustained release; SL, sublingual; q, every; prn, as needed.
†↑, Increase; 0, no change; ↓, decrease; +, mild; ++, moderate; +++, potent.

## Clinical uses

1. All these agents except nimodipine are approved for the treatment of hypertension. All agents are equally efficacious, and choice of agent should be based on adverse effects and hemodynamic profiles of the various agents. Calcium channel blockers are useful as initial therapy and particularly beneficial in volume-dependent hypertensive patients. These agents are additive with other antihypertensives and synergistic with prazosin and terazosin.

2. All these agents except nimodipine are useful in the treatment of stable, unstable, and vasospastic angina. Calcium channel blockers are the preferred agents for vasospastic angina. These agents have additive effects when combined with nitrates or beta blockers.

3. Diltiazem is beneficial in reducing morbidity and mortality in patients with non–Q wave infarctions. The usefulness of calcium channel blockers in transmural infarctions remains to be proved.

4. Nimodipine is indicated for the prevention of cerebral vasospasm following subarachnoid hemorrhage. Therapy should be initiated within 96 hours of the cerebrovascular accident and continued for 21 days.

5. Verapamil is indicated for the treatment of supraventricular dysrhythmias. It can be used in combination with digoxin to control ventricular rate in patients with atrial flutter and/or fibrillation.

6. Verapamil is effective in treating hypertrophic cardiomyopathy.

## Dosage and administration (see Table 10-12)

1. Initiate therapy with low doses and titrate the dose according to response. For rapid, effective control, patients should be stabilized on intermittent oral dosing before switching to sustained-release preparations.

2. Elderly patients may be sensitive to the effects of these agents and should be carefully monitored at initiation of therapy.

3. These agents may worsen heart failure and should be carefully monitored in patients with a history of left ventricular dysfunction.

4. These agents do not adversely affect the serum lipid profile and may improve quality of life.

5. These agents do not affect exercise tolerance.

6. Monitor blood pressure, heart rate, ECG, electrolyte levels, and side effects.

7. Verapamil can be given intravenously for supraventricular dysrhythmias. The dose is 5 to 10 mg as an IV bolus over 2 to 3 minutes and repeated every 30 minutes as needed. If necessary, verapamil can be given by constant infusion at a rate of 1-10 mg/hour. Carefully adjust the infusion rate to the lowest possible dose that controls the dysrhythmia.

8. When mixed for continuous IV infusion, verapamil should not be concentrated more than 1 mg/ml. Verapamil is compatible for mixing in most IV fluids.

9. Verapamil is compatible with aminophylline, bretylium, calcium, digoxin, lidocaine, procainamide, atropine, dopamine, dobutamine, epinephrine, heparin, isoproterenol, nitroglycerin, norepinephrine, potassium, propranolol, and quinidine.

## Cautions and side effects

1. Verapamil is associated with the largest incidence of side effects but is usually well tolerated in most patients. Less than 6% of patients require discontinuation of the drug because of side effects. Constipation occurs in less than 9% of patients. Major hemodynamic and severe conduction abnormalities occur in less than 2% of patients; concomitant use of beta blockers increases this incidence. Hypotension may occur with parenteral use, and IV calcium before verapamil administration prevents hypotension without blocking the drug's dysrhythmic effect.

2. Nifedipine, nicardipine, and nitrendipine have major side effects related to their vasodilatory properties. Dizziness, flushing, headache, syncope, and lightheadedness may occur in up to 25% of patients and are generally dose related. A reduction in dose will alleviate these symptoms. Peripheral edema occurs less frequently than with other vasodilators.

3. All these agents may worsen heart failure or cause hypotension.

4. Rash occurs in about 1% of patients receiving diltiazem. Bradydysrhythmias rarely occur with the use of this agent alone but are more frequent when combined with another agent that slows myocardial conduction.

5. Nifedipine, nicardipine, and nitrendipine may paradoxically worsen angina pain secondary to a reflex increase in sympathetic tone. Verapamil occasionally worsens angina pain if the patient becomes hypotensive or bradycardiac and if the patient has poor left ventricular function before therapy.

6. Verapamil increases digoxin levels almost twofold in some patients. Digoxin levels should be carefully monitored with initiation of verapamil therapy, and the digoxin dose should be halved if the patient is not receiving quinidine concomitantly.

7. Other side effects common to these agents include nausea, headache, dizziness, and rash.

8. Diltiazem increases serum cyclosporine levels, necessitating careful monitoring of these patients to prevent cyclosporine toxicity.

## THROMBOLYTIC AGENTS (see Table 10-13)[6,22-24]

Thrombolytic agents act directly to lyse formed thrombi.

**Cardiovascular actions.** All these agents stimulate the conversion of plasminogen to plasmin by various mechanisms. Plasmin degrades fibrin, fibrinogen, and other procoagulant proteins, causing the breakdown of fresh thrombi. *Streptokinase, urokinase,* and *APSAC* (an anisoylated streptokinase complex) bind directly to circulating

**TABLE 10-13** Thrombolytic agents

| Agent | Trade Name | Dose (after MI)* | Dose (DVT/PTE)* | Reocclusion (%) | Reperfusion (%) | Clot specificity† | Bleeding complications† | Expense† |
|---|---|---|---|---|---|---|---|---|
| Streptokinase | Streptase, Kabikin- ase | 1.5 million IU over 1 hr | 250,000 IU over 30 min, then 100,000 IU/hr for 24-72 hr | 20 | 65 | + | + + + + | + |
| Tissue plas- minogen activator (TPA) | Activase | 60 mg over 1 hr (6-10 mg in the first 1-2 min), then 20 mg/hr for 2 hr for total dose of 100 mg | — | 20 | 70 | + + + | + + + + | + + + + |
| Urokinase | Abbokinase | — | 4400 IU/kg IV load over 10 min, then 4400 IU/kg/hr for 12 hr | <10 | 66 | + + | + + + + | + + + |
| APSAC | Eminase | 30 units IV over 3-5 min | — | <10 | 68 | + + | + + + + | + + |

*MI, Myocardial infarction; IU, International Units; DVT/PTE, deep vein thrombosis/pulmonary thromboembolism.
†+, Weakly positive; + +, positive; + + +, strongly positive; + + + +, very strongly positive.

plasminogen, prompting the conversion to plasmin. *Tissue plasminogen activator* (TPA) binds specifically to fibrin in the thrombus and converts entrapped plasminogen to plasmin, initiating local thrombolysis. Thus TPA is more clot specific than the other agents. Although these agents are distinctly different when compared regarding clot specificity, reperfusion, and potency, confusion exists over the importance of these characteristics. No one agent has proved to be superior to any other agent in reducing morbidity or mortality if used within 6 hours of the onset of chest pain in acute myocardial infarction. All these agents produce bleeding to the same extent and must be used with adjunct heparin and/or aspirin therapy to prevent reocclusion.

### Clinical uses

1. These agents are used in acute myocardial infarction to lyse obstructive thrombi in coronary arteries. These agents appear to be most efficacious in transmural, anterior myocardial infarctions. Data suggest that these agents lower the incidence of mortality by approximately 20% to 25%. This effect is additive with that of the beta blockers, antiplatelet agents, and heparin. These agents should be initiated within the first 6 hours of the onset of chest pain.
2. Streptokinase and urokinase are indicated for the treatment of deep vein thrombosis and pulmonary embolism. The effectiveness of these agents is diminished in patients with thrombosis of more than 5 days' duration.
3. Urokinase can be used to clear occluded catheters. The dose is 5000 IU injected with a tuberculin syringe into the catheter; aspirate after 20 to 30 minutes and repeat if necessary.

### Dosage and administration (see Table 10-13)

1. Heparin should be initiated immediately in patients after the completion of TPA infusions (see following Heparin monograph for dosing). Heparin should be initiated 3 to 6 hours after the completion of streptokinase infusions to minimize bleeding. The activated partial thromboplastin time (APTT) should be kept at 2 times the control value.
2. Aspirin therapy should be initiated within 24 hours of admission. The addition of aspirin, 81 mg ("baby" strength) or 325 mg (regular strength), does not significantly increase the risk of bleeding with concurrent thrombolytic therapy. Aspirin significantly reduces the incidence of reocclusion.
3. Beta blockers should be initiated within 6 hours of onset of chest pain for maximum benefit. (See Beta Blockers monograph earlier in this chapter.)
4. Contraindications to thrombolytic therapy include active internal bleeding, intracranial neoplasm, severe hypertension (systolic > 180 mm Hg or diastolic > 110 mm Hg), recent cerebrovascular event (within 2 months), recent surgery (within 10 days), organ biopsy, trauma, prolonged cardiopulmonary resuscitation, or hemostatic defects.
5. Known allergy or recent exposure (within 6 months) to streptokinase or APSAC precludes the use of either agent.
6. Relative contraindications include recent abdominal procedure (within 10 days), gastrointestinal hemorrhage, or bacterial endocarditis.
7. Older patients have a greater mortality associated with acute myocardial infarction, but the use of these agents may be limited by side effects. Elderly patients are at greater risk for hemorrhage, and thrombolytic agents should be used cautiously in patients 75 years or older.
8. When diluting these agents, do not shake the vials. These compounds are protein substances and will foam when shaken. Gently roll the vials between your hands.
9. Monitor blood pressure, heart rate, ECG, chest pain, APTT, electrolyte levels, and bleeding.

### Cautions and side effects

1. Hemorrhage is the major complication in 3% to 10% of patients receiving thrombolytic agents, and none of these agents has any clear advantage over the other. Cryoprecipitate, fresh frozen plasma, packed red blood cells, and platelets may be necessary, and the patient should be typed and cross-matched on admission. Packed red cells are useful in patients with a hematocrit less than 25%, but cryoprecipitate is the best blood product for correction of the lytic state after thrombolytic therapy. Ten units of cryoprecipitate will raise the fibrinogen level about 0.7 g/L and the factor VIII level about 30%. Maintain the fibrinogen levels greater than 1.0 g/L. Occasionally, antifibrinolytic therapy may be necessary but should not be routinely employed.
2. Intracranial hemorrhage occurs in 0.5% to 1.5% of patients.
3. Most bleeding is minor and consists of oozing around catheter or venipuncture sites. Apply pressure to these areas and avoid manipulation of arterial lines.
4. Allergic reactions may occur with APSAC or streptokinase. Patients can receive diphenhydramine (Benadryl) or steroids before thrombolytic administration to prevent this reaction.
5. Transient hypotension may occur with these agents and can be corrected by volume replacement. Hypotension associated with streptokinase infusions may be related to the infusion rate, which should be reduced if the blood pressure drops significantly.

### HEPARIN[6-8]

Anticoagulants inhibit the action or formation of one or more of the clotting factors and are used to prevent and treat a variety of thromboembolic disorders. Heparin is the agent in this class that is discussed here.

Cardiovascular actions. Heparin is a naturally occurring substance, but its physiologic role has not been completely elucidated. In pharmacologic doses heparin predominantly affects blood coagulation and blood lipids. Heparin inhibits thrombin and fibrin formation by activating antithrombin III and produces prolongation of clotting time, prothrombin time (PT), and activated partial thromboplastin time (APTT). Heparin also inhibits platelet aggregation induced by thrombin. Heparin clears plasma lipids by activating lipoprotein lipase, but the clinical significance of this action is not fully understood.

## Clinical uses

1. Heparin is indicated for the treatment of thrombophlebitis, pulmonary embolism, deep vein thrombosis, catheter maintenance, and acute myocardial infarction with or without thrombolytics.
2. Heparin should be administered after initial thrombolysis to maintain patency in acute myocardial infarctions. Heparin should be initiated after streptokinase or urokinase therapy in patients with deep vein thrombosis or pulmonary embolism.
3. Heparin may be beneficial in reducing chest pain in unstable angina, but its use is controversial.
4. The use of heparin in patients after angioplasty is controversial. Reocclusion may occur less frequently in patients who receive 24 to 72 hours of therapy after this procedure. The APTT should be kept at 2 to 2.5 times the control value.
5. Heparin is used subcutaneously (SC) to prevent deep vein thrombosis in patients who are temporarily bedridden.

## Dosage and administration

1. Heparin is administered IV or SC. Oral administration is ineffective, and intramuscular administration is usually not recommended because it may produce local hemorrhage.
2. Anticoagulant doses of heparin are determined by clotting time or APTT, both of which are maintained at 1.5 to 2.5 times the control value. Continuous infusions of heparin are associated with fewer hemorrhagic side effects than are intermittent injections because a more stable anticoagulant effect is maintained.
3. Patients should be given a loading dose before initiation of a continuous infusion. Load the patient with 5000 to 10,000 units (or 50 to 75 units/kg) as an IV bolus, and initiate the drip at a rate of 1000 units/hour (or 10 to 25 units/kg/hour). Check the APTT 6 to 8 hours after the initiation or a change in therapy. The following is a suggested guideline for adjusting the heparin rate based on the APTT:
   APTT less than 1.2 to 1.3 times control: rebolus at 50 units/kg and increase infusion rate by 200 units/hour.
   APTT 1.2 to 1.3 times control: rebolus at 25 units/kg and increase infusion rate by 100 units/hour.
   APTT 1.3 to 1.5 times control: increase infusion rate by 100 units/hour.
   APTT 1.5 to 2.5 times control: make no change.
   APTT greater than 2.5 times control: hold infusion for 1 hour and decrease rate by 100 to 200 units/hour.
4. Maintain the APTT at 1.5 to 2.5 times the control value. Wait at least 6 to 8 hours after changes in therapy before drawing another APTT. After stabilizing the patient, the APTT can be drawn daily.
5. Intermittent IV or SC doses can be given at 5000 to 10,000 units every 4 to 6 hours. SC sites should be rotated.
6. For prevention of thrombosis, the dose is 5000 units SC every 12 hours.
7. Heparin disappearance rate is proportional to the dose administered because larger doses have a longer half-life. Anticoagulant effects of a single IV dose of heparin last an average of 3 to 4 hours.
8. Heparin is the preferred anticoagulant in pregnant or lactating women because it does not cross the placenta or appear in maternal milk.
9. Monitor APTT, bleeding, hematocrit, platelet count, and infusion rate.
10. Heparin is compatible in most IV fluids, and a standard dilution is 20,000 units in 500 ml IV fluid.
11. Heparin is compatible with calcium, dopamine, dobutamine, isoproterenol, lidocaine, methylprednisolone, norepinephrine, potassium, and epinephrine.

## Cautions and side effects

1. Hemorrhage is the predominant side effect, and heparin is contraindicated in the presence of active bleeding or hemorrhagic tendencies. The occurrence of hemorrhage during heparin therapy should initiate a search for a pathologic bleeding site.
2. Anticoagulant effects of heparin are reversible by the administration of protamine sulfate. Doses of 1.0 to 1.5 mg protamine will antagonize approximately 100 units of heparin, but the dose requirements fall quickly with time after the last heparin dose. In most cases discontinuation of heparin is sufficient therapy to correct anticoagulant effects.
3. Minor bleeding and bruising are normal complications that should not preclude the use of this agent.
4. Thrombocytopenia occurs in 5% to 15% of patients receiving heparin and is seen more often with bovine-derived heparin. Thrombocytopenia usually develops within 1 to 20 days (average, 5 to 9), and heparin should be discontinued if the platelet count falls below 100,000/mm³.
5. Long-term heparin therapy has been associated with alopecia, osteoporosis, neuropathy, and priapism.

## ANTIPLATELET AGENTS[25]

Both the demonstrated and the hypothesized effects of platelets suggest that these blood elements play an important role in several cardiovascular disorders, including the genesis of atherosclerotic plaque, coronary artery thrombosis, coronary spasm, and arterial thromboembolism. Therefore drugs that interfere with platelet function are potentially valuable therapeutic agents.

Cardiovascular actions. Antiplatelet drugs prolong platelet survival and interfere with the metabolism of prostaglandins and thromboxane, agents that affect the ability of platelets to aggregate and initiate thrombosis. Effects on the prostaglandins contained in vascular endothelium may also influence the net result of antiplatelet drugs. The major antiplatelet agents in current use are aspirin and dipyridamole. *Aspirin* is an irreversible inhibitor of cyclooxygenase, and *dipyridamole* increases cyclic adenosine monophosphate (c-AMP). Both decrease the aggregation of platelets, but neither affects platelet adhesion. Dipyridamole is a weak agent and ineffective when used alone in most patients. Aspirin is the most effective antiplatelet agent in use.

### Clinical uses (see Table 10-14)

1. Aspirin can be used alone or in combination with dipyridamole in the doses shown in Table 10-14.
2. Aspirin reduces the mortality associated with acute myocardial infarction by 20%.
3. Aspirin reduces the incidence of myocardial infarction and mortality by approximately 50% in patients with existing unstable angina.
4. Aspirin has not been shown to be effective in the primary prevention of coronary artery disease. The results of several studies indicate that the risk of infarction may be less but that the risk of hemorrhagic stroke may be increased.

### Dosage and administration (see Table 10-14)

1. Dipyridamole is ineffective alone and should be given with aspirin.

2. "Baby" aspirin (81 mg) may be used if patients have difficulty tolerating the 325 mg strength.
3. Some controversy has surrounded the ideal dose of aspirin. Small doses (e.g., 81 mg) effectively inhibit cyclooxygenase without significantly affecting prostaglandins. However, low doses have been clinically ineffective in some patients. Doses greater than 1000 mg may increase the incidence of side effects, with no greater antiplatelet effects than with 325 mg. The current recommended doses for any indication vary between 325 mg every day and 325 mg three times a day. Most clinical trials have used one of these two dosing schemes, and the recommendations are based on these clinical trials.

### Cautions and side effects

1. Aspirin produces gastrointestinal disturbances in some patients. This side effect can be minimized by giving the drug with food or antacid or by using an enteric-coated preparation. Occult gastrointestinal bleeding or mucosal lesions are rare with the doses recommended for antiplatelet therapy.
2. Other dose-related side effects of aspirin are tinnitus, hearing loss, hepatotoxicity, renal insufficiency, rash, hematologic abnormalities, and anemia. These effects are rarely seen at the doses employed for antiplatelet therapy.
3. Aspirin sensitivity occurs in less than 1% of the general population but in about 20% of patients with chronic urticaria and 4% of patients with chronic asthma. Mild to moderate bronchospasm may occur 15 to 30 minutes after ingesting aspirin. Patients with known sensitivity should avoid aspirin use.
4. Adverse effects with dipyridamole are transient and dose related and will resolve with continued therapy. These effects include headache, dizziness, nausea, peripheral dilatation, flushing, weakness, rash, pruritus, and aggravation of angina.

### TABLE 10-14 Antiplatelet agents

| Indication | Aspirin Dose (mg)* | Aspirin (mg) + Dipyridamole (mg)* |
|---|---|---|
| Acute myocardial infarction | 325 qd or tid | 325 tid + 75 tid |
| Unstable angina | 325 qd, tid, or qid | — |
| AV shunts | 325 qd | — |
| Coronary artery bypass | 325 qd | 325 tid + 75 tid |
| Heart valves | 325 tid | 325 tid + 75 tid |
| CVA and TIA† | 325 qid | — |
| Angioplasty | 325 qd or tid | — |

*qd, Every day; tid, three times a day; qid, four times a day.
†CVA, Cerebrovascular accident; TIA, transient ischemic attack; AV, arteriovenous.

## ANTIDYSRHYTHMICS[6,7,8,11,26]

An increasing number of antidysrhythmic drugs have become available for general clinical use. Specific electrophysiologic and pharmacologic features of these agents are presented in Tables 10-15 and 10-16. This discussion focuses on selected clinical aspects of the use of these agents.

### Disopyramide (Norpace)

Disopyramide is a class IA antidysrhythmic similar to procainamide and quinidine.

**Cardiovascular actions.** See Table 10-15 for specific electrophysiologic effects. Disopyramide increases systemic vascular resistance and exerts a negative inotropic effect on the myocardium. The combination of these effects may lead to significant left ventricular failure in some patients. Also, disopyramide has both systemic and myocardial anticholinergic properties that modify its electrophysiologic profile. For example, these anticholinergic effects may produce acceleration of the sinus rate or enhancement of AV nodal conduction.

### Clinical uses

1. Disopyramide is used in the treatment of ventricular and supraventricular dysrhythmias. It is effective in 50% to 60% of patients.
2. The role of disopyramide in antidysrhythmic therapy remains to be defined. Many physicians believe this agent should be reserved for use when the other class IA or IB agents fail.

### Dosage and administration (see Table 10-16)

1. The dosage of disopyramide should be adjusted in patients with a creatinine clearance less than 40 ml/min. The following is a guideline for initial therapy in renally impaired patients:

| Creatinine clearance (ml/min) | Dose |
| --- | --- |
| 30 to 40 | 100 mg every 8 hours |
| 15 to 30 | 100 mg every 12 hours |
| Less than 15 | 100 mg every 24 hours |

The extended-release capsules are not recommended for patients with a creatinine clearance less than 40 ml/min.

2. Trough levels should be drawn when serum levels are indicated. Steady-state levels are achieved 48 hours after the initiation of therapy in patients with normal renal function.
3. Patients may be orally loaded with 300 mg followed by 150 mg every 6 hours. This dosing scheme is not recommended because of the higher incidence of adverse effects.
4. Adjust the dose to the ECG and the patient's response.
5. Monitor ECG, blood pressure, heart rate, and side effects.

### Cautions and side effects

1. The most common adverse effects of disopyramide are anticholinergic and may require reductions in dose or cessation of therapy. Dry mouth is usually transient and decreases with continued administration. Other anti-

---

**TABLE 10-15** Electrophysiologic effects of antidysrhythmic agents*

| Agent | Sinus Rate | PR | QRS | QT | A-H | H-V | ERP: AV node | ERP: His-Purkinje | ERP: Atrium | ERP: Ventricle |
| --- | --- | --- | --- | --- | --- | --- | --- | --- | --- | --- |
| Disopyramide | 0, ↑ | 0, ↑ | ↑ | ↑ | ↑, ↓ | 0, ↑ | ↑, ↓ | 0, ↑ | ↑ | ↑ |
| Procainamide | 0 | 0, ↑ | ↑ | ↑ | 0, ↑ | 0, ↑ | 0, ↑ | 0, ↑ | ↑ | ↑ |
| Quinidine | 0, ↑ | 0, ↑ | ↑ | ↑ | ↑, ↓ | 0, ↑ | ↑, ↓ | 0, ↑ | ↑ | ↑ |
| Lidocaine | 0 | 0 | 0 | 0 | 0, ↓ | 0 | 0, ↓ | 0, ↑ | 0 | 0 |
| Mexiletine | 0 | 0 | 0 | 0 | 0, ↑ | 0, ↑ | 0, ↑ | 0, ↑ | 0 | 0 |
| Tocainide | 0 | 0 | 0 | 0, ↓ | 0 | 0 | 0, ↓ | 0 | ↓ | ↓ |
| Phenytoin | 0 | 0 | 0 | 0, ↓ | 0 | 0 | 0, ↓ | ↓ | 0 | 0 |
| Encainide | 0 | ↑ | ↑ | ↑ | ↑ | ↑ | ↑ | ↑ | ↑ | ↑ |
| Flecainide | 0 | ↑ | ↑ | ↑ | ↑ | ↑ | 0 | 0, ↑ | 0, ↑ | ↑ |
| Propafenone | 0 | ↑ | ↑ | 0 | ↑ | ↑ | ↑ | ↑ | ↑ | ↑ |
| Indecainide | 0 | ↑ | ↑ | ↑ | ↑ | ↑ | ↑ | ↑ | ↑ | ↑ |
| Propranolol | ↓ | 0, ↑ | 0 | 0, ↓ | 0, ↑ | 0 | ↑ | 0 | 0 | 0 |
| Amiodarone | ↓ | ↑ | 0, ↑ | ↑ | ↑ | 0, ↑ | ↑ | ↑ | ↑ | ↑ |
| Bretylium | 0, ↑ | 0 | 0 | 0 | 0 | 0 | ↓ | 0 | 0, ↓ | 0, ↓ |
| Verapamil | 0, ↓ | 0, ↑ | 0 | 0 | 0, ↑ | 0 | ↑ | 0 | 0 | 0 |

*See Table 10-16 for trade names and classes of dysrhythmic agents.
↑, Increase; ↓, decrease; 0, no change; ERP, effective refractory period.

**TABLE 10-16** Antidysrhythmic agents

| Agent | Trade Name | Class | Administration and Dosage* | Plasma Elimination Half-Life (hr) | Plasma Concentration (µg/ml) |
|---|---|---|---|---|---|
| Disopyramide | Norpace | IA | Oral: 100-300 mg q 6 hr | 4-8 | 3-8 |
| | | | SR: 150-300 mg q 12 hr | 8-12 | |
| Procainamide | Procan | IA | IV load: 10-15 mg/kg at 20-50 mg/min | — | 4-8 |
| | | | Infusion: 1-4 mg/min | 3-4 | |
| | | | Oral: 250-1000 mg q 3-4 hr | 3-4 | |
| | | | SR: 500-2000 mg q 6 hr | 6-8 | |
| Quinidine | Quinaglute, Duraquin | IA | IV load: 5-8 mg/kg at 0.3 mg/kg/min | — | 2-5 |
| | | | Oral: 200-600 mg q 6-8 hr | 6-11 | |
| | | | SR: 324-648 mg q 6-12 hr | 6-12 | |
| Lidocaine | Xylocaine | IB | IV load: 1-2 mg/kg | 1.5 | 1.5-6 |
| | | | Infusion: 1-4 mg/min | | |
| Mexiletine | Mexitil | IB | Oral: 150-400 mg q 8 hr | 12 | 0.5-2 |
| Tocainide | Tonocard | IB | Oral: 400-800 mg q 8 hr | 12 | 4-10 |
| Phenytoin | Dilantin | IB | IV load: 10-15 mg/kg at 20-50 mg/min | 24 | 10-20 |
| | | | Oral: 100-200 mg q 8 hr | | |
| Encainide | Enkaid | IC | Oral: 25-50 mg q 6-8 hr | 3-4 | — |
| Flecainide | Tambocor | IC | Oral: 50-200 mg q 12 hr | 16-20 | 0.2-1.0 |
| Propafenone | Rythmol | IC | Oral: 150-300 mg q 8 hr | 3-6 | — |
| Indecainide | Decabid | IC | Oral: 50-200 mg q 12 hr | 15 | 300-900 |
| Propranolol | Inderal | II | IV load: 0.1-0.15 mg/kg in 1 mg increments q 3-5 min | 4 | — |
| | | | Oral: 40-120 mg q 6 hr | | |
| Amiodarone | Cordarone | III | Oral load: 800-1600 mg/day for 7-10 days | 1000-2000 | 1.5-3.5 |
| | | | Oral: 200-600 mg q 24 hr | | |
| Bretylium | Bretylol | III | IV load: 5-10 mg/kg | 8-10 | — |
| | | | Infusion: 1-4 mg/min | | |
| Verapamil | Isoptin, Calan | IV | IV load: 5-10 mg | 3-8 | — |
| | | | Infusion: 1-10 mg/hr | | |
| | | | Oral: 40-120 mg q 6-8 hr | | |

*SR, Sustained release; q, every.

cholinergic effects include constipation, dry nose, eyes and throat, and blurred vision. The most serious effect is urinary retention, and patients with benign prostatic hypertrophy are at particular risk.

2. Heart failure may be precipitated in some patients and is characterized by weight gain, shortness of breath, orthopnea, and edema. Heart failure will develop in approximately 15% of patients with no history of left ventricular dysfunction and in 80% of those with a positive history. The drug should be stopped if symptoms develop.

3. As with other antidysrhythmics, disopyramide is dysrhythmogenic and may precipitate AV block or ven-

tricular dysrhythmias. The drug should be discontinued if the dysrhythmia is worsened or new dysrhythmias appear.

4. Other side effects include hypoglycemia, headache, general fatigue, and rash.

### Procainamide (Procan)

Procainamide is a class IA antidysrhythmic similar to quinidine and disopyramide.

**Cardiovascular actions.** See Table 10-15 for specific electrophysiologic effects. Procainamide is a ganglionic blocker and may decrease systemic blood pressure, especially with parenteral administration. Procainamide may have a direct negative inotropic effect, but contractility is not depressed at therapeutic serum concentrations. The anticholinergic properties of procainamide are much weaker than those seen with either disopyramide or quinidine.

### Clinical uses

1. Procainamide is indicated for the treatment of atrial and ventricular dysrhythmias. The drug is efficacious in 60% to 80% of patients.
2. Procainamide is a primary agent in the treatment of both atrial and ventricular dysrhythmias. Combination therapy with agents outside of class IA may be more efficacious and less toxic for complex ventricular dysrhythmias.
3. The toxicity of this agent may limit its long-term use in some patients.

### Dosage and administration (see Table 10-16)

1. Procainamide may be given orally, IV, or intramuscularly (IM). IM doses must be given every 4 hours to maintain therapeutic serum concentrations.
2. The dose of procainamide should be adjusted in patients with renal dysfunction. The following guidelines can be used when initiating therapy:

| Creatinine clearance (ml/min) | Dose |
|---|---|
| 20 to 50 | 500 mg every 6 hours orally or 1 to 2 mg/min IV |
| Less than 20 | 250 to 500 mg every 6 hours orally or 0.5 to 1 mg/min IV |

3. Procainamide has an active metabolic, N-acetyl-procainamide (NAPA) that is eliminated renally. NAPA may accumulate in patients with renal insufficiency, and serum levels should be monitored (normal range, 10 to 20 μg/ml). NAPA has class III antidysrhythmic properties.
4. Use oral regular-release capsules when initiating therapy. Sustained-release products can be given when switching from IV, IM, or chronic oral therapy. The sustained-release dose is one quarter of the total dose given every 6 hours.
5. Blood levels can be drawn 12 to 24 hours after the initiation of parenteral therapy or oral therapy with regular-release capsules. Wait 24 to 48 hours for steady-state levels in patients receiving the sustained-release products. Draw trough levels.
6. When using an IV drip, avoid doubling or tripling the rate if possible. Reinfuse a bolus of 2 mg/kg for each 1 μg/ml increase in serum level desired, and increase the infusion rate accordingly. With bolus dosing, do not exceed a rate of 50 mg/min in order to avoid hypotension. Continuous infusions may also be adjusted according to weight (e.g., 0.02 to 0.08 mg/kg/min).

7. IM therapy may be painful and absorption variable.
8. Adjust the dose according to the ECG and the patient's response.
9. Monitor ECG, heart rate, blood pressure, serum levels, and side effects.
10. Procainamide is stable in most IV fluids; standard concentration is 2 g in 500 ml IV fluid.
11. Procainamide is compatible with atropine, dopamine, dobutamine, heparin, lidocaine, potassium, and verapamil.

### Cautions and side effects

1. Approximately 50% of patients develop a positive antinuclear antibody (ANA) reaction within 2 to 18 months of starting therapy. Patients with a positive ANA may develop a lupuslike syndrome characterized by polyarthralgia, arthritis, pleural effusions, dyspnea, fever, chills, myalgias, skin lesions, headache, fatigue, and nausea. Patients should be discontinued from therapy if symptoms develop. If symptoms are severe or persistent, corticosteroids may be beneficial.
2. Patients receiving more than 4 g daily may complain of nausea, vomiting, and anorexia. Procainamide can be given with food, snacks, or antacids. Sustained-release preparations may reduce these effects, especially in patients receiving greater than 2 g daily. It should be noted that the wax matrix for the sustained-release preparations often appears in the feces.
3. Procainamide may be prodysrhythmic in about 10% of patients. Torsade de pointes occurs more often in hypokalemic patients. If new dysrhythmias appear or dysrhythmias are worsened, procainamide should be discontinued. The risk for prodysrhythmic effects is increased with larger doses.
4. Other adverse effects include agranulocytosis, thrombocytopenia, neutropenia, rash, urticaria, headache, and dizziness.

## Quinidine (Quinaglute, Duraquin)

Quinidine is a class IA antidysrhythmic similar to disopyramide and procainamide.

**Cardiovascular actions.** See Table 10-15 for specific electrophysiologic effects. Quinidine is a ganglionic blocker, and decreases in blood pressure occur more often with high plasma concentrations and IV administration. Quinidine has myocardial anticholinergic properties similar to disopyramide but few systemic effects. At therapeutic serum levels quinidine does not depress myocardial contractility despite its direct negative inotropic effect.

### Clinical uses

1. Quinidine is used in the treatment of atrial and ventricular dysrhythmias. It is effective in 60% to 80% of patients.
2. Quinidine may be combined with agents from other

classes for more effective, less toxic treatment of complex dysrhythmias.

### Dosage and administration (see Table 10-16)

1. Intramuscular administration should be avoided because of erratic absorption and precipitation of the drug at the injection site.
2. Three different salts of quinidine are currently marketed. The sulfate salts contain 83% quinidine base, whereas the gluconate and polygluconate salts contain 60% to 65% quinidine base. It is important when switching a patient from one preparation to another to ensure the patient receives the same amount of quinidine base regardless of the salt form.
3. Patients can receive oral loads of quinidine if necessary, but this is discouraged because of the high incidence of adverse effects.
4. Maintenance dosage can be achieved by intermittent IV doses given every 6 hours. Each dose should be given over 60 minutes or at a rate no faster than 15 mg/min.
5. Quinidine has two active metabolites that accumulate with renal dysfunction. Direct assays measure quinidine and metabolites, whereas extractable assays measure only quinidine. The metabolites may exhibit activity with accumulation, but this is more prominent in renal failure rather than mild renal insufficiency. Extractable levels should be monitored in most patients.
6. Steady-state levels are achieved 24 hours or more after therapy is started. Trough levels should be drawn.
7. Dose should be adjusted according to the ECG, the patient's response, and serum levels.
8. Monitor blood pressure, heart rate, ECG, serum levels, and side effects.
9. Quinidine increases digoxin levels almost twofold when given concurrently. The digoxin dose should be halved with the initiation of quinidine and serum digoxin levels drawn after 3 days.

### Cautions and side effects

1. Adverse gastrointestinal effects occur in 50% to 85% of patients receiving quinidine salts and may necessitate cessation of therapy. The most common effects are nausea, diarrhea, anorexia, abdominal pain and cramps, colic, bitter taste, and vomiting. These effects are generally not dose related and result primarily from local irritation. Quinidine can be given with food or antacids, and loperamide may be necessary for temporary control of diarrhea. Changing from the sulfate to gluconate salt may be beneficial in a limited number of patients. If tolerance to these effects is not evident in 1 to 2 weeks, the drug may need to be discontinued.
2. Cinchonism, an idiosyncratic reaction, may occur in patients after the initiation of therapy. Clinical manifestations are tinnitus, headache, vertigo, fever, light-headedness, tremor, and altered vision. The dose should be reduced or the drug stopped if symptoms continue.
3. Quinidine may cause one-to-one conduction in patients with atrial fibrillation or flutter, secondary to the drug's anticholinergic properties. Tachycardia can be prevented by prior digitalization.
4. Quinidine is prodysrhythmic in approximately 10% of patients. Torsade de pointes may appear in hypokalemic patients. Patients who develop new dysrhythmias or worsened dysrhythmias should be discontinued from therapy.
5. Leukopenia and thrombocytopenia may develop within 3 months of therapy. The drug should be stopped; blood counts return to normal in 1 to 2 weeks.
6. Other adverse effects include fever, hepatotoxicity, rashes, and hemolytic anemia.

## Lidocaine (Xylocaine)

Lidocaine is a class IB antidysrhythmic similar to mexiletine and tocainide.

**Cardiovascular actions.** See Table 10-15 for specific electrophysiologic effects. Lidocaine has no effect on autonomic tone or cardiac contractility. It is a central nervous system depressant.

### Clinical uses

1. Lidocaine is indicated for the treatment of ventricular dysrhythmias. It is effective in 70% to 80% of patients.
2. Lidocaine is used prophylactically in acute myocardial infarction to prevent ventricular dysrhythmias.
3. Lidocaine may be beneficial in combination with other antidysrhythmics of another class for acutely treating refractory ventricular dysrhythmias.

### Dosage and administration (see Table 10-16)

1. Lidocaine is available for parenteral use only.
2. Intramuscular (IM) injections can be used if necessary, and absorption is more rapid from deltoid muscles. Repeated and frequent dosing is necessary with IM therapy.
3. The clearance of lidocaine will decrease with continued therapy. Serum levels and signs of toxicity should be closely monitored, especially in patients with poor renal function.
4. Steady-state levels are achieved 6 hours after changes in dose or initiation of therapy.
5. Lidocaine is stable in most IV fluids; a standard dilution is 2 g in 500 ml IV fluid. Drips can be concentrated for volume-restricted patients.
6. Lidocaine is compatible with aminophylline, bretylium, calcium, digoxin, dopamine, dobutamine, heparin, potassium, procainamide, and verapamil.
7. Monitor ECG, heart rate, blood pressure, serum levels, and side effects.

## Caution and side effects

1. Serious adverse effects requiring discontinuation are uncommon. Most are dose related and can be eliminated by reducing the dose.
2. Major central nervous system side effects include headache, drowsiness, dizziness, disorientation, confusion, lightheadedness, nervousness, and tremors. Muscle twitching and seizures may occur with toxicity.
3. Lidocaine is prodysrhythmic in some patients and should be discontinued if dysrhythmias are worsened.
4. Hypersensitivity reactions may occur rarely.

## Mexiletine (Mexitil)

Mexiletine is a class IB antidysrhythmic similar to lidocaine and tocainide.

**Cardiovascular actions.** See Table 10-15 for specific electrophysiologic effects. Mexiletine has no autonomic or negative inotropic effects. Mexiletine is a central nervous system depressant.

### Clinical uses

1. Mexiletine is indicated for the treatment of ventricular dysrhythmias. The efficacy of this agent alone is only about 50%. In combination with other antidysrhythmics or another class, mexiletine may be efficacious in 80% to 90% of patients.

### Dosage and administration (see Table 10-16)

1. The clearance of mexiletine is reduced in renal failure, and the dose should be halved or the interval extended.
2. Oral loads are not recommended because of intolerable side effects in most patients.
3. Steady-state levels are achieved 24 to 48 hours after the initiation of therapy or a change in therapy. Trough levels should be drawn. Serum levels are poorly correlated to therapeutic effect and are more useful for determining toxicity rather than therapeutic benefit.
4. Doses greater than 1200 mg daily are associated with a higher incidence of toxicity.
5. Monitor ECG, heart rate, blood pressure, and side effects.
6. Adjust the dose according to the patient's response, side effects, and ECG.

### Cautions and side effects

1. Central nervous system side effects occur in up to 40% of patients receiving mexiletine. Neurologic toxicities include fine hand tremor, dizziness, lightheadedness, nervousness, paresthesias, confusion, blurred vision, and memory loss. Most of these effects are dose related, and the dose should be reduced to minimize symptoms. If seizures occur, discontinue the drug.
2. Gastrointestinal side effects are common and include nausea, vomiting, abdominal pain, diarrhea, and an-

orexia. These effects may be related more to the amount of the dose (e.g., 150 mg versus 200 mg) rather than the total dose. Doses should be given with meals, antacids, or snacks. Smaller doses or shorter intervals may be necessary.
3. Mexiletine may worsen cardiac dysrhythmias or induce new dysrhythmias. The drug should be discontinued if this occurs.
4. Other rare effects include rash, hair loss, impotence, and arthralgias.

## Tocainide (Tonocard)

Tocainide is a class IB antidysrhythmic similar to lidocaine and mexiletine.

**Cardiovascular actions.** See Table 10-15 for specific electrophysiologic effects. Tocainide slightly increases systemic vascular resistance and has a small negative inotropic effect. However, the administration of tocainide has not been associated with any clinical evidence of worsening heart failure. The significance of these effects remains to be determined.

### Clinical uses

1. Tocainide is indicated for the treatment of ventricular dysrhythmias. It is 60% to 70% efficacious alone or in combination with other antidysrhythmics of another class.
2. The precise role of tocainide in antidysrhythmic therapy remains to be established. It may be most beneficial in patients who are responsive to lidocaine and unresponsive to class IA agents alone.

### Dosage and administration (see Table 10-16)

1. Patients may be orally loaded, but this is usually not necessary and causes more toxicity.
2. Steady-state levels are achieved after 3 days of therapy, and trough levels should be drawn.
3. Dosages should be halved or the dosing interval increased for patients with renal failure.
4. Adjust the dose according to the ECG, the patient's response, and side effects.
5. Monitor ECG, blood pressure, heart rate, serum levels, and side effects.
6. If tablets were halved, the exposed portion may cause tingling or numbness in the mouth. This is not serious and can be diminished by taking the tablet after swishing antacids in the mouth.
7. Adverse effects increase with dosages greater than 1200 mg daily.

### Cautions and side effects

1. From 30% to 50% of patients experience central nervous system toxicity, which includes tremors, dizziness, paresthesias, lightheadedness, slurred speech, and leth-

argy. These effects are usually dose related, and the dose should be reduced to minimize symptoms.

2. Seizures, psychosis, and hallucinations have occurred and necessitate discontinuation of the drug.
3. From 2% to 25% of patients experience gastrointestinal effects, the most frequent being nausea, anorexia, vomiting, and diarrhea. The drug should be given with food or antacids or the dose reduced if possible.
4. Dysrhythmias may occur in up to 10% of patients, and the drug should be stopped if this occurs.
5. Other adverse effects include bone marrow depression, pulmonary disease, and rash.

### Encainide (Enkaid)

Encainide is a class IC agent similar to flecainide and indecainide.

**Cardiovascular actions.** See Table 10-15 for specific electrophysiologic effects. Encainide has no substantial negative inotropic effects following chronic oral administration. The drug has no autonomic effects.

#### Clinical use

1. Encainide is beneficial in the treatment of supraventricular and ventricular dysrhythmias in approximately 80% to 90% of patients.
2. Class IC agents may adversely affect morbidity and mortality in patients with asymptomatic ventricular dysrhythmias following myocardial infarction.
3. Encainide is a very potent agent and should be used cautiously if combined with other antidysrhythmics.

#### Dosage and administration (see Table 10-16)

1. Encainide is metabolized to two active metabolites (ODE, MODE) with very long half-lives. Chronic administration of encainide is complicated by the effects of these metabolites as they accumulate. Titration of doses should be slow (e.g., every 3 to 5 days) and patients monitored carefully. The recommended starting dose is 25 mg every 8 hours. The dose should be increased until the QRS is prolonged 25% to 50%, toxicity occurs, or the dysrhythmia is terminated.
2. Serum blood levels can be monitored but are not clinically useful.
3. Monitor ECG, blood pressure, heart rate, and side effects.

#### Cautions and side effects

1. The most common adverse effects of encainide are dizziness, lightheadedness, visual disturbances, and headache. These effects are transient and dose related. Patients receiving doses greater than 200 mg daily may have intolerable central nervous system side effects.
2. Encainide is prodysrhythmic in approximately 10% of patients. The drug should be stopped if this effect occurs.
3. Other side effects include nausea, dyspepsia, diarrhea,

metallic taste, rash, and dyspnea. These effects occur in 2% to 4% of patients receiving less than 150 mg daily.

### Flecainide (Tambocor)

Flecainide is a class IC antidysrhythmic similar to encainide and indecainide.

**Cardiovascular effects.** See Table 10-15 for specific electrophysiologic effects. Flecainide has a moderate negative inotropic effect, which is more pronounced in patients with coronary heart disease or left ventricular failure. Flecainide has no autonomic effects.

#### Clinical uses

1. Flecainide is effective in the treatment of supraventricular and ventricular dysrhythmias in 80% to 90% of patients.
2. Flecainide may adversely affect morbidity and mortality in patients with asymptomatic ventricular dysrhythmias following myocardial infarction.
3. Flecainide is a potent agent and should be used cautiously when combined with other antidysrhythmics.

#### Dosage and administration (see Table 10-16)

1. The clearance of flecainide is decreased in patients with renal failure, and the dose should be decreased accordingly.
2. Doses greater than 400 mg daily are associated with significantly greater toxicity than lower doses. Dosages should be increased every 3 to 5 days; more rapid titration may result in serious toxicity.
3. Steady-state levels are achieved in 3 to 5 days; trough levels should be drawn.
4. Flecainide may increase digoxin and propranolol levels.
5. Monitor ECG, blood pressure, heart rate, and side effects.
6. Increase dose according to the patient's response, the ECG, and side effects.

#### Caution and side effects

1. From 10% to 30% of patients experience dizziness and visual difficulties. Other common central nervous system effects include headache, fatigue, tremor, paresthesias, spots before eyes, and blurred vision. These effects are usually dose-related and can be minimized by reducing the dose.
2. Flecainide is prodysrhythmic in 10% to 15% of patients, and the drug should be discontinued if these effects occur.
3. The drug's negative inotropic effects may exacerbate heart failure in patients with serum levels greater than 1.0 ng/ml, ejection fractions less than 35%, and complex ventricular dysrhythmias. Patients should be monitored closely and the drug discontinued if they become symptomatic.
4. Gastrointestinal toxicity, including anorexia, vomiting, nausea, and diarrhea, may occur in up to 10% of pa-

tients. These effects can be minimized by giving the drug with food or antacids.

5. Other less frequent side effects include rash, impotence, and blood dyscrasias.

## Propafenone (Rythmol)

Propafenone is a unique class IC agent that also has calcium channel and beta-blocking activity.

**Cardiovascular actions.** See Table 10-15 for specific electrophysiologic effects. Propafenone has beta-sympatholytic activity about ¼₀ the potency of propranolol. At very high doses, propafenone also blocks calcium channels. Propafenone has moderate negative inotropic effects.

### Clinical uses

1. Propafenone is indicated for the treatment of life-threatening ventricular dysrhythmias.
2. The use of propafenone is not indicated in patients with less severe ventricular dysrhythmias.

### Dosage and administration (see Table 10-16)

1. Therapeutic effect is poorly correlated to serum concentrations.
2. After initiating therapy at 150 mg every 8 hours, increase the dose at 3- to 4-day intervals. The safety and efficacy of doses greater than 900 mg daily have not been established.
3. Propafenone has a saturable first-pass absorption, and its bioavailability may increase with larger doses.
4. The drug increases serum digoxin concentrations.
5. Propafenone may increase the prothrombinemic effect of warfarin.
6. Monitor ECG, heart rate, blood pressure, and side effects.

### Cautions and side effects

1. 20% of patients require discontinuation secondary to side effects.
2. The most common side effects are dizziness, headache, altered taste, nausea, and constipation. Most are dose related, and reductions in dose will alleviate symptoms.
3. About 10% of patients experience prodysrhythmic effects and should be discontinued from propafenone therapy.
4. Propafenone may exacerbate heart failure in patients with preexisting left ventricular dysfunction. Patients should be monitored for signs and symptoms of failure, and the drug stopped if they occur.
5. Other adverse effects include paresthesias, vivid dreams, elevated liver enzymes, blood dyscrasias, and alopecia.

## Indecainide (Decabid)

Indecainide is a class IC agent similar to encainide and flecainide.

**Cardiovascular actions.** See Table 10-15 for specific electrophysiologic effects. Indecainide exerts a negative inotropic effect and may exacerbate heart failure in patients with existing left ventricular dysfunction. The drug has no autonomic effects.

### Clinical uses

1. Indecainide is indicated for the treatment of life-threatening ventricular dysrhythmias.
2. The use of indecainide is not recommended for patients with less severe ventricular dysrhythmias.

### Dosage and administration (see Table 10-16)

1. The dose should be adjusted in patients with a creatinine clearance less than 30 ml/min. The initial dose should be 50 mg daily and slowly increased to a dose of 150 mg or less daily. Increases in dose should be no less than 7 days apart and titrated to the patient's response, the ECG, and serum levels.
2. Steady state is achieved after 5 to 7 days of therapy, and trough levels should be drawn.
3. Monitor ECG, blood pressure, heart rate, serum levels, and side effects.

### Cautions and side effects

1. The most serious adverse effect of indecainide is worsening or provocation of ventricular dysrhythmias. The drug should be discontinued if this occurs.
2. Less than 1% of patients need to discontinue therapy secondary to exacerbation of heart failure. Patients should be carefully monitored for signs and symptoms of failure.
3. Chest pain, headache, constipation, blurred vision, and dyspnea occur in less than 10% of patients.
4. Other less common adverse effects include nausea, dry mouth, anxiety, insomnia, rhinitis, and back pain.

## Amiodarone (Cordarone)

Amiodarone is a class III antidysrhythmic.

**Cardiovascular actions.** See Table 10-15 for specific electrophysiologic actions. Amiodarone has sodium channel–blocking and beta-sympatholytic activity, but no parasympathomimetic activity. The reduction in blood pressure and coronary resistance is more pronounced with IV therapy. Amiodarone does not appear to produce substantial changes in left ventricular function even though it is a mild negative inotrope.

### Clinical uses

1. Amiodarone is indicated for the treatment of supraventricular and ventricular dysrhythmias. It is greater than 90% effective in most patients.
2. Amiodarone may be used cautiously in combination with other antidysrhythmics.

### Dosage and administration (see Table 10-16)

1. Amiodarone distributes extensively into tissue and concentrates in fat, liver, muscle, spleen, and kidney tissue.

The half-life of the drug is approximately 40 to 80 days with chronic dosing. Amiodarone can be measured in the serum for up to 50 days following the cessation of therapy.

2. Serum blood level is poorly correlated to therapeutic effect.
3. Patients should receive a loading dose over 7 to 10 days, followed by daily maintenance therapy. The goals are to use the lowest possible dose to terminate the dysrhythmia and prevent adverse effects. The dose should be adjusted according to the patient's response, the ECG, and toxicity.
4. Amiodarone increases digoxin levels, and the digoxin dose should be halved with concomitant therapy.
5. Amiodarone increases the prothrombinemic effect of warfarin; the dose of warfarin should be reduced with concomitant therapy.
6. Monitor ECG, blood pressure, heart rate, and toxicity.

### Cautions and side effects

1. Amiodarone causes side effects in 100% of the patients receiving the drug. Most effects occur at doses greater than 400 mg daily and with prolonged therapy; 25% of patients require cessation of therapy.
2. Corneal microdeposits occur in 50% to 100% of patients with chronic therapy. Vision is normally not affected, and the deposits will disappear if the drug is discontinued. Methylcellulose eye drops may be used for the discomfort.
3. Photosensitivity occurs in 1% to 50% of patients, and patients should avoid direct sunlight.
4. Dysrhythmias may be exacerbated by this agent in 10% of patients. The drug should be stopped if this occurs.
5. Up to 15% of patients develop pulmonary problems consisting of interstitial infiltrates, dyspnea, cough, and fibrosis. The drug should be stopped immediately, and steroids can be employed if necessary.
6. About 25% of patients will develop either hypothyroidism or hyperthyroidism. The patient should be treated appropriately for the condition and amiodarone continued.
7. Gastrointestinal disturbances, including nausea, vomiting, constipation, and anorexia, occur in up to 30% of patients. The drug can be given with food or antacids and at more frequent intervals during the day to minimize these effects.
8. Central nervous system disturbances may include sleep disorders, tremors, headache, and peripheral neuropathy. Reductions in dose usually minimize these effects.
9. Abnormal liver function tests occur in up to 20% of patients receiving chronic therapy. These alterations are usually benign but should be followed.

### Bretylium (Bretylol)

Bretylium is a class III antidysrhythmic.

**Cardiovascular actions.** See Table 10-15 for specific electrophysiologic effects. Bretylium causes an initial catecholamine depletion. In addition, there is a rise in blood pressure, heart rate, and contractility, which is followed by hypotension and decreased myocardial conduction.

### Clinical uses

1. Bretylium is most efficacious for ventricular fibrillation.
2. Bretylium may be used for ventricular tachycardia but is usually less effective than other antidysrhythmic agents.

### Dosage and administration (see Table 10-16)

1. Avoid rapid IV push of the loading dose because this may induce nausea and vomiting if the patient is alert.
2. Use cautiously if hypotension is present.
3. Bretylium is stable in most IV fluids and can be concentrated for fluid-restricted patients.
4. Bretylium is compatible with potassium, quinidine, verapamil, dopamine, and dobutamine.
5. Monitor ECG, blood pressure, heart rate, and side effects.

### Cautions and side effects

1. Hypotension is the most frequent adverse reaction and often occurs within the first hour of therapy. Hypotension may continue despite the cessation of therapy, and the patient should be monitored.
2. Other side effects include vertigo, lightheadedness, nausea, and diarrhea.

## ANTILIPEMIC AGENTS (see Tables 10-17 and 10-18)[2,6,8]
### Bile Acid–Binding Resins

*Cholestyramine* and *colestipol* are anion exchange resins with similar mechanisms of action.

**Cardiovascular actions.** See Table 10-17 for specific antilipemic effects. These agents bind bile acids in the intestines to form insoluble complexes, which are excreted in the feces. The loss of bile acids leads to increased production of bile acids in the liver and increased low-density lipoprotein (LDL) receptors, which increases LDL uptake. These agents reduce LDL serum concentrations by 15% to 30%. These agents have no direct cardiac effects.

### Clinical uses

1. Bile acid–binding resins are indicated primarily for the management of type IIa hyperlipidemia.
2. These agents are additive with other antilipemic agents and can be used in combination with other agents when necessary.
3. Bile acid–binding resins may increase triglyceride levels and should not be used alone in patients with combined hyperlipidemia and hypertriglyceridemia.

**TABLE 10-17** Antilipemic agents

| Agent | Trade Name | LDL* | HDL* | Triglycerides* | Daily Dose | Time Necessary for Maximal Effect (Weeks) |
|-------|-----------|------|------|----------------|------------|-------------------------------------------|
| Cholestyramine | Questran | ↓ | 0, ↑ | 0, ↑ | 12-24 g | 2-4 |
| Colestipol | Colestid | ↓ | 0, ↑ | 0, ↑ | 15-30 g | 2-4 |
| Niacin (nicotinic acid) | Various | ↓ | ↑ | ↓ | 1.5-6 g | 3-5 |
| Gemfibrozil | Lopid | ↓ | ↑ | ↓ | 600-1200 mg | 3-4 |
| Clofibrate | Atromid-S | ↓ | 0, ↑ | ↓ | 1-2 g | 3-4 |
| Probucol | Lorelco | ↓ | ↓ | 0 | 500-1000 mg | 4-12 |
| Lovastatin | Mevacor | ↓ | 0, ↑ | 0, ↓ | 20-80 mg | 2-4 |

*LDL, low-density lipoprotein; HDL, high-density lipoprotein; ↓, decrease; ↑, increase; 0, no change.

**TABLE 10-18** Hyperlipidemia: classification and treatment

| Classification | Prevalence | Lipid Abnormality* | Drug(s) of Choice | Alternative |
|----------------|-----------|--------------------|--------------------|-------------|
| I | Rare | ↑ Chylomicrons | None | None |
| IIa | Common | ↑ LDL | Cholestyramine, Colestipol | Lovastatin, niacin, combination therapy |
| IIb | Common | ↑ LDL ↑ VLDL | Niacin | Gemfibrozil, lovastatin, combination therapy |
| III | Uncommon | ↑ VLDL ↑ IDL | Niacin | Gemfibrozil, clofibrate |
| IV | Common | ↑ VLDL | Niacin | Gemfibrozil, clofibrate |
| V | Uncommon | ↑ Chylomicrons ↑ VLDL | Gemfibrozil, Niacin | Clofibrate |

*LDL, Low-density lipoprotein; VLDL, very low-density lipoprotein; IDL, intermediate-density lipoprotein; ↑, increase.

## Dosage and administration (see Tables 10-17 and 10-18)

1. Cholestyramine and colestipol should not be taken in the dry powder form. The bulk powder should be mixed with moisturized pulpy fruit (e.g., applesauce, crushed pineapple) or a minimum of 120 ml of fluid.
2. These agents are also available in flavored powders for reconstitution and chew bars.
3. These agents may alter the absorption of fat-soluble vitamins and folic acid.
4. Oral medications should be taken at least 1 hour before or 4 to 6 hours after these agents when possible. These agents are usually given in two to four divided doses before meals or at bedtime. Avoid concomitant doses of medication when possible.
5. The lipid-lowering effects of these agents are dose-related. Start with lower doses and titrate at monthly intervals.
6. Combination therapy with niacin or lovastatin may produce up to 60% reductions in baseline LDL.
7. Monitor serum LDL, high-density lipoprotein (HDL), and triglyceride levels and side effects.

## Cautions and side effects

1. The most common adverse effects involve the gastrointestinal tract, especially with the use of high doses or in patients greater than 60 years of age.
2. Constipation occurs in approximately 20% of patients receiving cholestyramine and colestipol. Constipation may become severe, especially in the elderly, and lead to impaction. These agents should be given with bran

cereal, stool softeners, or other soluble dietary fibers in patients who develop symptoms.

3. Other less common adverse gastrointestinal effects include abdominal pain and distention, gas, bloating, nausea, diarrhea, anorexia, exacerbation of hemorrhoids, indigestion, and heartburn. Many of these effects disappear with continued therapy.

4. These agents may alter fat absorption in doses larger than 24 g/day of cholestyramine and 30 g/day of colestipol. Serum electrolytes may also be affected at these doses.

5. Other adverse effects include rash, sour taste, and elevation of liver function enzymes.

### Niacin (Nicotinic Acid)

Niacin is an effective antilipemic agent in doses greater than 1 g daily.

**Cardiovascular actions.** See Table 10-17 for specific antilipemic effects. The exact antilipemic mechanism of niacin is unknown but thought to be related to increased activity of lipoprotein lipase, decreased esterification of triglycerides, or inhibition of lipolysis in adipose tissue. Niacin reduces triglycerides by 20% to 80%, reduces LDL levels by 15% to 30%, and increases HDL levels. These effects are dose related.

#### Clinical uses

1. Niacin is used alone or in combination for the treatment of types IIa, IIb, III, IV, and V hyperlipoproteinemia. It is the drug of choice for types IIb, III, IV, and V.

2. Niacin has additive effects when given concomitantly with other antilipemic agents.

#### Dosage and administration (see Tables 10-17 and 10-18)

1. Niacin is administered orally, preferably with meals.

2. Initial dose should be 500 mg three times a day, with 325 mg of aspirin given 30 minutes before each dose. Doses should be gradually increased at monthly intervals. Most patients experience transient side effects with the initiation of therapy; tolerance normally develops within 1 to 2 weeks.

3. Monitor serum LDL, HDL, and triglyceride levels and side effects.

4. Slow-release products are usually not effective in reducing the initial adverse effects of this agent and they may be hepatotoxic.

5. The dose of niacin should be maximized before employing combination therapy.

#### Cautions and side effects

1. Most side effects of niacin are dose related and are minimized with reductions in dose.

2. The most common side effects are cutaneous flushing, pruritus, burning or tingling, and dyspepsia. These effects usually occur within 30 minutes of ingestion and are present for 30 to 60 minutes. These effects are minimized by giving 325 mg of aspirin 30 minutes before each dose. Single doses of niacin greater than 500 mg are necessary to develop tolerance within 1 to 2 weeks. As the dose is titrated upward, the reaction may recur, and the patient should be treated prophylactically with aspirin.

3. Gastrointestinal effects may include nausea, vomiting, diarrhea, dyspepsia, peptic ulceration, and abdominal discomfort. These effects can be reduced by giving the drug with food or antacids.

4. Other side effects of niacin include cholestasis, hepatotoxicity, hyperglycemia, hepatic enzyme elevations, hyperpigmentation, hyperuricemia, and hypotension.

### Fibric Acid Derivatives

*Gemfibrozil* and *clofibrate* have similar mechanisms of action.

**Cardiovascular effects.** See Table 10-17 for specific antilipemic effects. These agents increase the activity of lipoprotein lipase, which increases the rate of catabolism of very low-density and intermediate-density lipoprotein (VLDL, IDL) to LDL. These drugs may also increase the rate of removal of these lipoproteins from plasma. Gemfibrozil and clofibrate produce a 5% to 15% reduction in LDL.

#### Clinical uses

1. Gemfibrozil and clofibrate are alternatives to niacin therapy in types III, IV, and V hyperlipidemia.

2. Gemfibrozil may also be used in types IIb and V hyperlipidemia for combination therapy.

3. These agents are used primarily for hyperlipidemias associated with hypertriglyceridemia.

4. These agents are effective in combination with other antilipemic agents.

#### Dosage and administration (see Tables 10-17 and 10-18)

1. Gemfibrozil has a lower incidence of adverse effects and may be preferred over clofibrate in most patients.

2. These agents are only available orally and can be given in two divided doses daily.

3. Doses should be low initially and given before the morning and evening meals. Doses should be titrated at monthly intervals.

4. Monitor serum LDL, HDL, and triglyceride levels and side effects.

#### Cautions and side effects

1. Clofibrate may increase twofold the incidence of cholelithiasis and cholecystitis in patients receiving long-term therapy. Thromboembolism, cardiac dysrhythmias, and intermittent claudication may occur as well.

Because of an increased incidence of morbidity and rate of overall mortality in clinical trials, clofibrate is not the drug of choice for any type of hyperlipidemia. This agent should be used as an alternative agent or in combination therapy only.
2. Other adverse effects associated with clofibrate include nausea, diarrhea, weight gain, skin rash, alopecia, weakness, impotence, flulike syndrome, increased hepatic enzymes, and decreased libido.
3. Clofibrate displaces highly protein-bound drugs and may precipitate toxicity when used concomitantly with warfarin, phenytoin, or tolbutamide.
4. Adverse gastrointestinal effects are most often seen with gemfibrozil use and include abdominal pain, nausea, diarrhea, flatulence, and epigastric pain.
5. Other adverse effects of gemfibrozil include headache, blurred vision, dizziness, eosinophilia, cholelithiasis, rash, musculoskeletal pain, mild anemia, hyperglycemia, and leukopenia.
6. As with clofibrate, gemfibrozil may potentiate the anticoagulant effects of warfarin.
7. Both these agents may have additive toxicity when given with lovastatin, manifested as musculoskeletal weakness or rhabdomyolysis.

### Probucol (Lorelco)

Probucol is structurally unrelated to any of the other antilipemic agents.

**Cardiovascular actions.** See Table 10-17 for specific antilipemic actions. Probucol combines with LDL cholesterol in the plasma, producing a particle that is more rapidly removed than normal LDL. Probucol may increase the activity of the reverse transport system, thereby reducing HDL concentrations in the plasma. This agent has no effect on triglyceride levels.

#### Clinical uses

1. Probucol is used as an alternative agent in the treatment of type IIa hyperlipidemia.
2. The drug may be useful in some patients with type III hyperlipidemia but is generally less effective than fibric acid derivatives.
3. Probucol is useful in combination with other antilipemics. The manufacturer recommends that probucol not be given with clofibrate or gemfibrozil because of increased toxicity and lack of additional benefits.

#### Dosage and administration (see Tables 10-17 and 10-18)

1. Probucol is administered orally and should be given in two divided doses with the morning and evening meals.
2. Increases in dosage should be at 3-month intervals to allow maximum effects from a single dose to occur.
3. Monitor serum LDL, HDL, and triglyceride levels and side effects.

#### Cautions and side effects

1. Probucol has a low incidence of side effects, and most are mild and transient.
2. About 10% of patients experience gastrointestinal side effects, including diarrhea, flatulence, nausea, abdominal pain, indigestion, and vomiting. These effects seldom require discontinuation of therapy.
3. Probucol may prolong the QT interval on the ECG, and serious dysrhythmias have been reported. ECGs should be obtained before and periodically during therapy.
4. Probucol decreases HDL serum concentrations. The significance of this effect is unclear.
5. Other adverse effects include eosinophilia, paresthesias, and rash.

### Lovastatin (Mevacor)

Lovastatin differs in structure and pharmacologic activity from the other antilipemic agents.

**Cardiovascular actions.** See Table 10-17 for specific antilipemic actions. Lovastatin competitively inhibits the 3-hydroxy-3-methyl-glutaryl-coenzyme A (HMG-CoA) reductase, thereby decreasing the endogenous synthesis of cholesterol. This agent may also increase hepatic LDL receptors, resulting in a greater uptake of LDL from the plasma. Lovastatin produces a dose-related 25% to 45% reduction in LDL.

#### Clinical uses

1. Lovastatin can be used as a single agent in type IIa or IIb hyperlipidemia. It is reserved as an alternative agent by some because of the unknown effects of long-term therapy.
2. Lovastatin is effective in combination with niacin and bile acid–binding resins. Caution should be used when combining this agent with clofibrate or gemfibrozil because of the increased risk for musculoskeletal toxicity.

#### Dosage and administration (see Tables 10-17 and 10-18)

1. Lovastatin is available orally and should be administered once or twice daily.
2. The dose should be low initially (e.g., 20 mg at bedtime) and titrated at monthly intervals.
3. Lovastatin should be used cautiously with immunosuppressants because of an increased risk for myopathy.
4. Monitor serum LDL, HDL, and triglyceride levels and side effects.

#### Cautions and side effects

1. The most frequent adverse effects of lovastatin are gastrointestinal and include flatulence, abdominal pain, diarrhea, and dyspepsia.
2. Mild elevations in liver enzyme function tests may occur within 6 weeks of therapy and usually do not necessitate

cessation of therapy. Increases of more than three times the upper limit of normal values indicate toxicity, and the drug should be stopped. Liver function tests should be monitored periodically during lovastatin therapy.

3. Creatinine kinase elevations are seen in approximately 11% of patients, but myalgias and muscle cramps have only been reported in 1% to 3% of patients. Patients should be advised to report muscle weakness, pain, or tenderness. The drug should be promptly discontinued if these symptoms are present.

4. Eye opacities have appeared in some patients, but no clinically important loss of visual acuity has occurred during drug therapy. Ophthalmic examinations should be performed periodically in patients receiving this drug.

5. Other adverse effects include blurred vision, headache, dizziness, insomnia, malaise, and rash.

6. The long-term side effects of this agent have not been clearly defined. Therefore its use should be carefully monitored.

## MISCELLANEOUS AGENTS
### Atropine

Atropine is a parasympatholytic agent.

**Cardiovascular actions.** Atropine blocks activity in portions of the parasympathetic nervous system by inhibiting the action of acetylcholine. In the heart atropine principally increases the rate of automatic discharge of the SA node and shortens the refractory period and conduction time of the AV node. A lesser effect, particularly in the atria, may be to increase contractility.

### Clinical uses

1. Atropine is indicated to block unwanted effects of vagal tone such as symptomatic sinus bradycardia, sinus bradycardia associated with increased ventricular ectopy during acute myocardial infarction, or AV block caused by increased vagal tone.

2. Atropine may be used in cardiac arrest to antagonize the parasympathetic drive.

### Dosage and administration

1. Atropine is administered intravenously, usually in an initial dose of 0.5 to 1.0 mg by rapid injection. Additional increments of 0.5 mg are administered until desired effects are obtained, unwanted side effects are controlled, or a total dose of 2.0 to 2.5 mg is reached.

2. Smaller doses or slower administration of atropine may evoke a vagomimetic effect that produces sinus node slowing and AV conduction delay.

3. Atropine administered through the endotracheal tube is slowly absorbed, and drug concentrations in the serum and at the site of action are low. Thus larger doses, usually twice the IV dose, are required to achieve therapeutic responses.

4. The cardiovascular effects of IV atropine are shortlived,

and chronic therapy is not indicated. Pacemaker placement should be considered in anyone who requires long-term control of their bradydysrhythmia.

5. Monitor ECG, blood pressure, heart rate, and side effects.

### Cautions and side effects

1. Many of the side effects of atropine are dose related and may produce systemic effects for several hours after administration.

2. Usual side effects are urinary retention, dryness of skin and mucous membranes, bronchial secretions, pupillary dilatation, acute glaucoma, tachycardia, blurred vision, and mydriasis.

3. Atropine-induced sinus node acceleration during acute myocardial infarction may precipitate further ischemia, which may lead to ventricular dysrhythmias and ventricular fibrillation following atropine administration.

4. Doses greater than 5 mg may produce speech disturbances, swallowing difficulties, ataxia, confusion, delirium, and hallucinations.

### Edrophonium (Tensilon)

Edrophonium is a parasympathomimetic agent.

**Cardiovascular actions.** Edrophonium is a cholinergic drug that acts by inhibiting the action of acetylcholinesterase, the enzyme that degrades acetylcholine. Cardiac effects of edrophonium are similar to those produced by enhanced vagal tone. Edrophonium decreases the sinus nodal discharge rate, increases refractoriness and conduction time of the AV node, and decreases myocardial contractility.

### Clinical uses

1. Edrophonium is primarily used to terminate episodes of paroxysmal supraventricular tachycardia (PSVT) when other vagal maneuvers such as cartoid sinus massage or Valsalva maneuver are ineffective.

2. Edrophonium may also be used to treat sinus tachycardia secondary to sympathomimetic use.

### Dosage and administration

1. Edrophonium is administered as a 5 or 10 mg IV bolus. A test dose of 1 to 2 mg may be given initially.

2. The effects of edrophonium begin within 30 to 60 seconds after administration and may last as long as 10 minutes.

3. A continuous infusion of 0.25 to 2.0 mg/min may be used if prolonged effects are desired.

4. Atropine will antagonize the effects of edrophonium.

5. Monitor ECG, blood pressure, heart rate, respiratory rate, and side effects.

### Cautions and side effects

1. Enhanced vagal tone may aggravate preexisting conditions of intestinal obstruction, bronchial asthma, or

urinary obstruction; edrophonium should be avoided in these circumstances.

2. Side effects are mainly secondary to vagal overactivity and may include nausea, perspiration, salivation, bronchial spasm, slow pulse, and hypotension.
3. To counteract any potential life-threatening complications, atropine should be immediately available when edrophonium is used.

## Sodium Bicarbonate

Sodium bicarbonate is a major extracellular buffer that acts to provide the physiologic control of acid-base balance. Bicarbonate metabolism is regulated primarily by the kidney, and the bicarbonate system is one of many acid-base systems.

### Clinical use

1. Sodium bicarbonate is employed to correct metabolic acidosis.

### Dosage and administration

1. Sodium bicarbonate is administered at a dosage of 1 mEq/kg every 10 minutes during cardiopulmonary resuscitation until circulation is restored. When possible, administration should be be guided by repeated measurements of arterial blood pH.
2. Sodium bicarbonate should be administered through a separate IV line because it may inactivate many agents, particularly the catecholamines.
3. Sodium bicarbonate will precipitate calcium, and the line should be thoroughly flushed if these agents are given through the same IV line during an emergency situation.

### Cautions and side effects

1. Treating acidosis with bicarbonate does not alter the underlying defect that caused the acidosis, such as cardiogenic shock or ventricular fibrillation.
2. Overdosage of bicarbonate will produce a metabolic alkalosis.
3. The large sodium load administered with sodium bicarbonate may worsen preexisting congestive heart failure.

## Potassium

Potassium is a major intracellular cation found principally in muscle, including cardiac tissue. The greatest amount of total body potassium is located within the cells, and intracellular concentration is approximately 30 times the extracellular concentration. Despite this, extracellular or serum potassium concentration usually correlates well with total body potassium in stable, steady-state conditions. Renal function provides the major regulation of body potassium. Certain metabolic diseases, kidney diseases, diarrhea, vomiting, diuretic therapy, or infusions of potassium-free fluids that increase extracellular fluid volume may all reduce serum potassium levels. Elevated serum potassium levels are caused by acidosis, renal failure, massive tissue necrosis, major catabolic states, and the inadvertent adminstration of potassium.

**Cardiovascular actions.** Potassium plays a major role in the maintenance of normal cellular excitability and conduction. Hypokalemia prolongs the recovery of excitability, manifested as a prolonged QT interval on the ECG, and slows AV and intraventricular conduction time. Premature ventricular complexes and disorders of AV conduction may occur. Hyperkalemia increases the rate of repolarization (shortened QT interval on the ECG) and at progressively high levels first increases and then decreases excitability and conduction velocity. Therefore potassium administration may initially facilitate conduction but later produce AV conduction delay and slow intraventricular conduction.

### Clinical use

1. Potassium supplements are used in the prevention or treatment of potassium depletion.

### Dosage and administration

1. Since potassium loss in the urine parallels sodium loss to some degree, the restriction of dietary sodium will help mitigate potassium loss.
2. Potassium chloride, which also replenishes chloride ions lost during diuresis and during sodium chloride restriction, is the preferred salt for oral administration.
3. Potassium can be replaced by oral or parenteral administration. The dose should be adjusted to the patient's needs. A serum potassium concentration of 3 mEq/L implies a total body deficit of approximately 300 mEq. Each subsequent 1 mEq/L decrease in serum concentration indicates an additional deficit of 200 to 400 mEq.
4. Changes in extracellular pH produce a reciprocal effect on plasma potassium concentrations. A change in pH of 0.1 unit can be accompanied by a change in the opposite direction of 0.6 mEq/L of serum potassium.
5. IV administration of potassium should be no more concentrated than 60 mEq/L and infused at a rate no greater than 20 mEq/hour. Concentrated solutions should be given through central lines only and carefully monitored.
6. For serum potassium concentrations greater than 2.5 mEq/L, a maximum dose of 200 mEq/day should not be exceeded. For serum potassium concentrations less than 2.5 mEq/L, a maximum dose of 400 mEq/day should not be exceeded.
7. The usual adult oral dosage for replacement is 40 to 100 mEq daily. Doses larger than 40 mEq should be separated if given in oral tablet form because the matrices of these tablets may form a complex that causes esophageal ulceration.
8. Oral potassium solutions should be diluted before ad-

ministration. Orange juice, apple juice, tomato juice, or carbonated drinks help mask the salty taste.

9. Peak elevation of serum potassium occurs 1 hour after administration (2 hours for sustained-release products), and the effect on the serum potassium is seen primarily in the first 3 hours.
10. Potassium supplements are also found in some salt substitutes and in bananas and citrus fruits.
11. Many forms and preparations of oral potassium are available. Care should be taken that the proper amount of potassium is administered if different products are employed.
12. IV infusions of potassium may cause pain or burning at the infusion site. The solution should be further diluted, and the patient should be carefully monitored for signs of phlebitis or local tissue necrosis. If there is any suspicion of extravasation or infiltration, move the IV access site and treat promptly.
13. Monitor renal function, serum potassium levels, ECG, and side effects.
14. The presence of second-degree AV block is generally a contraindication to potassium use. However, in the case of digitalis-induced atrial tachycardia with AV block, potassium administration may slow the atrial rate and restore sinus rhythm without worsening the AV block.
15. Potassium is contraindicated in patients who have severe renal impairment, untreated Addison's disease, acute dehydration, heat cramps, acidosis, and preexisting hyperkalemia from any cause.
16. Patients with concurrent hypomagnesemia should receive magnesium replacement as well. Serum potassium levels will not be corrected if the patient has a magnesium deficiency.

### Cautions and side effects

1. Rapid potassium infusion produces sinus bradycardia, depression of intrinsic pacemakers, and slowing of AV conduction to the point of block.
2. Adverse symptoms reported with potassium therapy are nausea, vomiting, diarrhea, and abdominal discomfort.
3. Hyperkalemia may occur following administration of potassium, especially in the presence of impaired renal function. Hyperkalemia may manifest as weakness, paresthesias, decreased blood pressure, and ECG changes. Cardiac dysrhythmias ranging from heart block to cardiac arrest caused by ventricular fibrillation or ventricular asystole may occur.
4. ECG manifestations of hyperkalemia include a peaked, narrowed T wave and shortened QT interval. As toxicity increases, the QRS complex widens, the PR interval lengthens, and the P wave may diminish in size or disappear.

## Adenosine (Adenocard)

Adenosine is an endogenous purine nucleoside.

**Cardiovascular actions.** Adenosine vasodilates coronary arteries, reduces atrial contractility, depresses SA and AV nodal activity, and inhibits the stimulating effect of catecholamines on the myocardium.

### Clinical uses

1. Adenosine is indicated for the conversion of paroxysmal supraventricular tachycardia (PSVT) to normal sinus rhythm (NSR), including PSVT associated with accessory bypass tracts. It is more than 90% effective for termination of tachycardias that involve the AV node as part of the reentry circuit.
2. The ultimate place in therapy for this agent remains to be determined. It is currently used in patients with PSVT when verapamil is contraindicated or ineffective.

### Dosage and administration

1. Adenosine is available for IV use only.
2. Adenosine is usually administered as a 6 mg rapid IV bolus given over 1 to 2 seconds. If the first dose does not result in conversion to NSR within 1 to 2 minutes, 12 mg should be given as a rapid IV bolus. An additional 12 mg may be administered a second time if necessary.
3. Caution should be used in asthmatic patients, since bronchoconstriction has been reported following inhaled adenosine.
4. Monitor ECG, blood pressure, heart rate, and side effects.

### Cautions and side effects

1. The most frequently reported side effects are facial flushing (18%), dyspnea (12%), retrosternal chest pressure (7%), and dysrhythmias preceding conversion to NSR.
2. Most side effects are transient, lasting less than 1 minute, and are reported by patients as being minor.
3. Patients receiving theophylline may be refractory to adenosine.
4. Patients receiving dipyridamole may be acutely sensitive to the effects of adenosine, necessitating lower initial doses.

## REFERENCES

1. Winter ME: Basic clinical pharmacokinetics, Spokane, WA, 1985, Applied Therapeutics, Inc.
2. Gilman AG and Goodman LS: The pharmacological basis of therapeutics, ed 7, New York, 1985, Macmillan Publishing Co.
3. Chernow B, editor: The pharmacologic approach to the critically ill, ed 2, Baltimore, 1988, Williams & Wilkins.
4. Katz AM: Changing strategies in the management of heart failure, J Am Coll Cardiol 13(3):513-523, 1989.
5. Parmley WM: Pathophysiology and current therapy of congestive heart failure, J Am Coll Cardiol 13(4):771-785, 1989.

6. American Society of Hospital Pharmacists: American hospital formulary service 1990, Bethesda, MD, 1990, ASHP, Inc.

7. Trissel LA: Handbook on injectable drugs, Bethesda, MD, 1990, American Society of Hospital Pharmacists, Inc.

8. Knoben JE and Anderson PO, editors: Handbook of clinical drug data, ed 6, Hamilton, IL, 1988, Drug Intelligence Publications, Inc.

9. Hilleman DE and Forbes WP: Role of milrinone in the management of congestive heart failure, Drug Intell Clin Pharm 23(5):357-362, 1989.

10. Stanley R: Drug therapy of heart failure, J Cardiovasc Nurs 4(3):17-34, 1990.

11. Morganroth J and others: Cardiovascular drug therapy, St Louis, 1986, Mosby–Year Book, Inc.

12. Frishman WH: Beta-adrenergic blockers, Med Clin North Am 72(1):37-81, 1988.

13. Strauss WE and Parisi AF: Combined use of calcium-channel and beta-adrenergic blockers for the treatment of chronic stable angina, Ann Intern Med 109:570-581, 1988.

14. Parker JO: Nitrate therapy in stable angina pectoris, N Engl J Med 316(26):1635-1642, 1987.

15. Carlson JE and Weston AH, editors: Symposium on pinacidil, Drugs 36(7):1-98, 1988.

16. Cohn J: Drug treatment of heart failure, New York, 1983, Advanced Therapeutics Communications.

17. Kostis JB: Angiotensin converting enzyme inhibitors. I. Pharmacology, Am Heart J 116(6):1580-1591, 1988.

18. Kostis JB: Angiotensin converting enzyme inhibitors. II. Clinical use, Am Heart J 116(6):1591-1605, 1988.

19. Yasuda SU and Tietze KJ: Nimodipine in the treatment of subarachnoid hemorrhage, Drug Intell Clin Pharm 23:451-455, 1989.

20. Gibson RS: Current status of calcium channel-blocking drugs after Q-wave and non Q-wave myocardial infarction, Circulation 80(suppl IV):107-119, 1989.

21. Weiner DA: Calcium channel blockers, Med Clin North Am 72(1):83-115, 1988.

22. Bang NU, Wilhelm OG, and Clayman MD: After coronary thrombolysis and reperfusion, what next? J Am Coll Cardiol 14(4):837-849, 1989.

23. Sane DC and others: Bleeding during thrombolytic therapy for acute myocardial infarction: mechanisms and management, Ann Intern Med 111:1010-1022, 1989.

24. Anderson JL, editor: Acute myocardial infarction: new management strategies, Rockville, MD, 1987, Aspen Publishers, Inc.

25. Stein B and others: Platelet inhibitor agents in cardiovascular disease: an update, J Am Coll Cardiol 14(4):813-836, 1989.

26. Wellens HJ and Bragadin P: Treatment of cardiac arrhythmias: when, how, and where? J Am Coll Cardiol 14(6):1417-1428, 1989.

# Artificial Cardiac Pacemakers and Implantable Cardioverter Defibrillators

Nancy L. Stephenson
William Combs

The artificial cardiac pacemaker is an electronic stimulator used in place of the natural cardiac pacemaker, the SA node, and/or the specialized AV conducting system in the diseased, congenitally malformed, or iatrogenically damaged heart. The pacemaker system is composed of a power source, usually a battery, electronic circuitry for generating appropriately timed stimuli, and an electrode/wire system ("lead") used to complete the electric connection between the circuitry and the myocardium. Pacemakers may be packaged for implantation totally within the body (permanent pacemakers), or they may be configured so that the electronics and power source remain outside the body (temporary pacemakers). The first completely implantable devices were reported in the late 1950s.[1,2] Currently there are an estimated one million patients worldwide who have implanted pacemakers. Advances in technology have been rapidly applied to pacemaker systems, providing noninvasively programmable single- and dual-chamber pacemakers typically weighing 25 to 50 g and lasting an estimated 6 to 10 years. These highly reliable devices are dramatically different from the 250 g, asynchronous, 18-month devices of the early 1960s.

Implantable cardioverter defibrillators are a much newer technologic development. Initially implanted in a human in February of 1980,[3] the first generation of these devices had been implanted in over 10,000 patients by the early 1990s.[4] They are large in comparison with modern pacemakers, weighing between 250 and 300 g; they are primarily implanted via epicardial routes; and they last between 2 and 3 years. However, the same advances in technology that have so dramatically affected modern pacemakers will be seen with implantable cardioverter defibrillators during the 1990s.

## INDICATIONS
### Permanent

The most common indications for permanent pacing in the United States, as reported by the latest U.S. survey, are sinus node dysfunction and atrioventricular node and His-Purkinje conduction disorders.[5] These indications accounted for 93% of all implants. Sick sinus syndrome may be manifested as sinus arrest or block, severe sinus bradycardia, or alternating periods of bradycardia and supraventricular tachycardia (bradycardia-tachycardia syndrome). Further indications for permanent pacing include the following[6]:

1. Mobitz type II second-degree AV block distal to the His bundle
2. Hypersensitive carotid sinus syndrome causing symptomatic severe slowing of sinus rate and/or AV block[7]
3. Chronic atrial fibrillation with a slow ventricular response that results in symptoms
4. Bifascicular block with prolonged His-ventricular (H-V) interval in patients who have syncope or presyncope and no other demonstrated cause of syncope (Bifascicular block with prolonged H-V interval in asymptomatic patients is generally accepted as not being an indication for permanent pacing, although the issue is not entirely resolved.)[6]
5. Termination or overdrive suppression of supraventricular and, less frequently, ventricular tachycardia resistant to drug therapy and not amenable to surgical correction[8-10]
6. Periods of bradycardia or asystole following abrupt termination (overdrive suppression) of supraventricular or ventricular tachycardia resistant to drug therapy and not amenable to surgical correction
7. Prophylactic implantation in patients after myocardial infarction (MI) complicated by advanced AV block during the acute stages of infarction; this indication also causes some controversy, and the issue is not completely settled
8. Prevention of tachydysrhythmia by providing rate maintenance in combination with drugs or by control of AV conduction through use of dual-chamber pacemakers

### Temporary

Indications for temporary pacing include the following[6,8,9]:

1. Maintenance of adequate heart rate and rhythm in patients during a variety of circumstances, such as

postoperatively, during cardiac catheterizations or surgery, during administration of some drugs that might inappropriately slow the rate, and prior to implantation of a permanent pacemaker

2. Prophylaxis following open heart surgery
3. Acute (generally anterior) MI with type II second-degree or third-degree AV block
4. Acute (generally anterior) MI with concurrent onset of right bundle branch block with left axis deviation or concurrent onset of left bundle branch block
5. Acute inferior MI with third-degree AV block refractory to pharmacologic intervention and producing ventricular dysrhythmias and/or hemodynamic compromise
6. Termination of AV nodal reentry or reciprocating tachycardia associated with Wolff-Parkinson-White syndrome (see p. 138), atrial flutter, or ventricular tachycardia
7. Suppression of ectopic activity, atrial or ventricular
8. Electrophysiologic studies to evaluate diagnoses, mechanisms, and therapy in patients who have a variety of bradydysrythmias and tachydysrhythmias[11]

## PACEMAKER MODALITIES
### NBG code

The North American Society for Pacing and Electrophysiology (NASPE) and the British Pacing and Electrophysiology Group (BPEG) code was designed as a shorthand notation to identify the many pacing modes (Table 11-1).[12]

This table provides a shorthand description of pacemaker operation. Symbols placed in the first two positions indicate the chambers in which the pacemaker functions; in the third position, the mode of operation of the pacemaker; in the fourth position, its programmability or rate modulation characteristics; and in the fifth position, its antitachycardia features. For example, if the pacing lead is inserted into the ventricle and the pulse generator is a demand ventricular type, then the chamber paced is the ventricle, and the first letter in the five-position code is *V*. The chamber sensed is the ventricle and therefore the second letter in the five-position code also is *V*. The mode of response of the pacemaker is to inhibit a pacing spike when spontaneous electric activity is sensed, and therefore *I* is in the third position. If the mode of pacing is rate adaptive (responsive), *R* is in the fourth position. If only the rate and/or output of the pulse generator can be programed externally, *P* is in the fourth position. If the pacemaker is used to treat tachycardias, then the tachydysrhythmia function is indicated in the fifth position.

Pulse generators that pace or sense in both the atrium and ventricle are indicated by the designation *D*, meaning dual. If the pacemaker does not have a function in one of the classifications, *O* is used. The different types of tachydysrhythmia functions are discussed in this chapter.

### Atrial and Ventricular Asynchronous Pacemakers (AOO, VOO)

The first pacemakers simply stimulated the myocardium at a constant rate independent of any underlying cardiac rhythm; these pacemakers only paced and did not sense any spontaneous activity. If connected to the atrium the pacemaker was referred to as an asynchronous atrial pacemaker (AOO), and if applied to the ventricles it was referred to as a ventricular asynchronous pacemaker (VOO). Asynchronous pacemakers are rarely used today, since it is relatively simple to provide noncompetitive pacemakers that avoid the potential risks of pacing during spontaneous rhythms.

### Atrial and Ventricular Demand Pacemakers (AAI, AAT, VVI, VVT)

In the early 1970s, sensing circuits were added to pacemakers so that they would stimulate only when there was no appropriate underlying spontaneous rhythm. These pacemakers paced and sensed spontaneous activity. This prevented competitive pacing and the attendant risk of

## TABLE 11-1 Five-position pacemaker code (NBG)

| I. Chamber Paced | II. Chamber Sensed | III. Mode of Response | IV. Programmability/Rate Modulation | V. Antitachydysrhythmia Functions |
|---|---|---|---|---|
| V = Ventricle | I = Inhibited | P = Simple programmable | P = Pacing | |
| A = Atrium | T = Triggered | M = Multiprogrammable | S = Shock | |
| D = Atrium and ventricle | D = Atrial triggered and ventricular inhibited | C = Communicating | D = Pacing and shock | |
| O = None | O = None | R = Rate modulation | O = None | |
| | | | O = None | |

From Bernstein A and others: the NASPE/BPEG pacemaker code, PACE 10(4):794, 1987.

inducing fibrillation. Demand pacemakers are supplied in two versions, inhibited and triggered. Inhibited devices withhold the stimulus and reset their timing on sensing spontaneous cardiac activity. Triggered devices are activated to deliver a stimulus just after spontaneous depolarization into the refractory tissue and reset their timing immediately on sensing spontaneous cardiac activity. Both types deliver a stimulus at the end of their timing cycle (pacemaker escape interval) if no spontaneous cardiac activity is detected. The triggered mode was invented to address concerns that unipolar inhibited devices might allow a patient to become asystolic if extracardiac signals (for

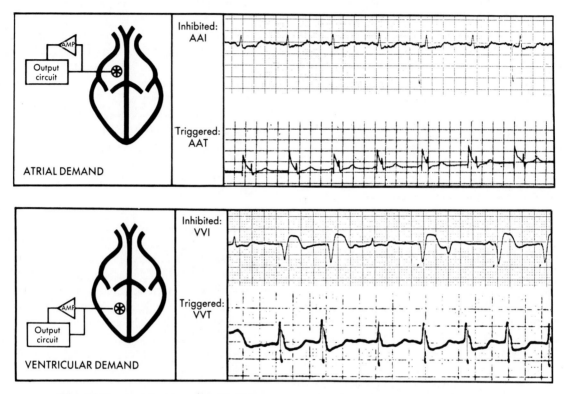

**Fig. 11-1    Atrial and ventricular demand pacemakers (AAI, AAT, VVI, VVT).** On the left are schematic diagrams of the heart; the right and left atria are in the top region of the diagrams, and the right and left ventricles are in the bottom portion. The names of the pacemakers are placed beneath the drawings of the heart, and the NBG codes are given in the middle panel. The "output" circuit (the part of the pacemaker that creates the electric stimulus), connected to the heart in the cardiac chamber marked with an *asterisk*, indicates the chamber *stimulated* by the pacemaker. The triangular element labeled *AMP* (represents the portion of the pacemaker that has an electric amplifying circuit to enable sensing of cardiac activity), connected to the heart in the cardiac chamber marked with a *circle*, indicates the cardiac chamber that is *sensed* by the pacemaker. *Circled asterisk* indicates that both *sensing and stimulation* can be accomplished at the location marked.

In the top panel a circled asterisk indicates that atrial demand pacemakers sense and pace in the atrium. In the top ECG of the upper panel the action of an atrial inhibited (AAI) pacemaker is illustrated. Note that the pacing spike is inhibited from discharging until the fifth and seventh complexes, when atrial rhythm slows slightly and allows escape of the atrial demand pacemaker. In the second ECG example each sensed P wave elicits a pacing spike delivered within the P wave (third, fourth, and fifth P waves). A pacing spike initiates the first, second, sixth, and seventh P waves. This is an example of AAT pacing.

In the lower panel a circled asterisk indicates that ventricular demand pacemakers sense and pace in the ventricle. In the upper ECG of the bottom panel the action of a ventricular demand pacemaker (VVI) is illustrated. Note that spontaneous ventricular activity inhibits pacemaker discharge, and pacing spikes are delivered only when the ventricular rate becomes slower than the escape interval of the pacemaker. In the lower ECG, pacing spikes are delivered into each of the appropriately sensed QRS complexes; this is correct operation of the VVT pacemaker.

example, pectoral muscle potentials, electric signals from radio transmitters, or power lines) were sensed, erroneously interpreted to be cardiac signals, and permitted to inhibit pacemaker output. Modern circuitry has reduced the likelihood of such occurrences, and the disadvantages of stimulating when not really necessary with a triggered mode (ECG waveform distortion, high-power requirements for the pacemaker) have resulted in relatively little usage of this form of pacing. However, it can be of value to achieve termination of some tachycardias (by externally triggering the pacemaker to deliver trains of stimuli) or to be certain diagnostically when or if the pacemaker sensed a spontaneous event; it is therefore generally available in modern pacemakers as an option. Block diagrams and typical ECGs for the ventricular demand inhibited (VVI),

ventricular demand triggered (VVT), atrial demand inhibited (AAI), and atrial demand triggered (AAT) devices are shown in Fig. 11-1.

## Atrial Synchronous Ventricular Pacemakers (VAT, VDD)

To approximate normal cardiac function more closely, sophisticated dual-chamber (atrium and ventricle) "physiologic" pacemakers were developed. The atrial synchronous ventricular pacemaker (VAT) was designed for use in patients with normal sinus function and impaired AV conduction.[13] This device senses atrial activity by means of an electrode in the atrium and, after a suitable delay, paces the ventricle, thereby providing an artificial AV node in lieu of the malfunctioning natural AV pathway. The VAT

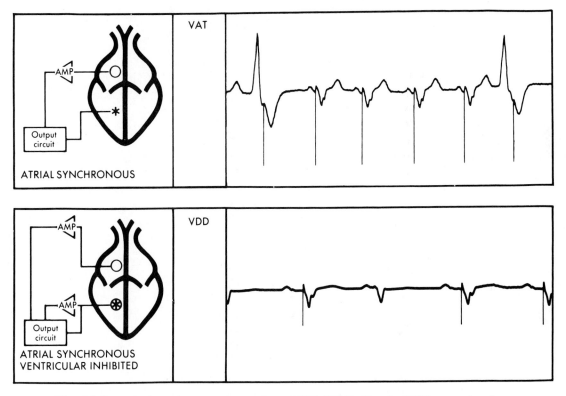

**Fig. 11-2   Atrial synchronous pacemakers (VAT, VDD).** For the VAT pacemaker *(top panel)* the circle in the atrium and the asterisk in the ventricle indicate that the pacemaker senses atrial activity and paces the ventricle. In the lower panel the circle in the atrium and the circled asterisk in the ventricle indicate that the pacemaker senses both atrial and ventricular activity and paces the ventricle (VDD).

   In the midportion of the top ECG the pacemaker delivers stimuli following each sensed P wave and produces a paced QRS complex. The first and last QRS complexes are spontaneous premature ventricular complexes (PVCs) that are *not* sensed by the pacemaker. The sinus P wave (hidden within the QRS complex) is sensed by the pacemaker and triggers it to deliver a pacing spike to the ventricle. Conceivably, such a response can deliver a stimulus into the T wave of the PVC. To avoid this problem, the VDD pacemaker has been equipped with a sensing circuit to sense spontaneous ventricular activity. Note in the lower ECG (VDD pacemaker) that the second P wave conducts to the ventricle with a PR interval shorter than the P-stimulus interval of the pacemaker. This conducted QRS complex is sensed by the pacemaker, and the pacing spike is inhibited, thus eliminating problems of pacemaker competition with spontaneous ventricular activity.

pacemaker does not pace the atrium. This method of atrial sensing and ventricular pacing preserves the atrial contribution to ventricular filling and maintains sinus control of ventricular rate. Rate limits are designed into the pacemaker so that during periods of atrial bradycardia at rates that are slower than the escape rate of the pacemaker, the unit paces as an asynchronous ventricular pacemaker at a predetermined backup rate. During atrial tachycardia the pacemaker paces no faster than its upper rate limit, yielding an AV response to sensed atrial activity that is similar to type I or type II AV block. The VAT device has been refined by the addition of circuitry that enables it to detect ventricular activity (ventricular sense amplifier). This modified pacemaker is called the atrial synchronous ventricular inhibited pacemaker (ASVIP), described in the NBG code as VDD.[14] (The VDD pacemaker, like the VAT pacemaker, does not have the ability to pace in the atrium, but it does sense in both the atrium and the ventricle and paces in the ventricle.) The VAT and VDD pacemakers are rapidly being displaced by the more flexible DDD pacemakers, which can stimulate and sense in both the atrium and the ventricle. Block diagrams and ECGs for the VAT and VDD devices are shown in Fig. 11-2.

## AV Sequential Pacemakers (DVI)

In patients who have bradycardia in addition to impaired AV conduction, the atrial contribution to ventricular filling can be preserved by using an AV sequential pacemaker (DVI).[15] This pacemaker senses only ventricular activity but is capable of pacing both the atrium and the ventricle. Following sensed or paced ventricular events the DVI pacemaker monitors the ventricle for activity. If none is detected within a prescribed pacemaker escape interval, the pacemaker stimulates the atrium. It then waits long enough to allow passage of a normal AV interval and, if no ventricular activity occurs, paces the ventricle.* Sensed ventricular activity inhibits the ventricular stimulus and resets all pacemaker timing. If the ventricular rate is sufficiently rapid, atrial stimuli are also inhibited. It is important to emphasize that the DVI pacemaker does not sense spontaneous atrial activity. A variant of the DVI pacemaker, the DDI pacemaker does sense atrial activity. This device inhibits the atrial stimulus to avoid competition between the pacemaker and an underlying atrial rhythm, but it does not provide atrial synchronous pacing. Fig. 11–3 contains the block diagram and representative ECG for the DVI pacemaker. Currently, DVI pacing is most often obtained by programming a DDD pacemaker to the DVI mode rather than by implanting a purely DVI pulse generator.

---

*Some AV sequential pacemakers are of the committed type; that is, they do not wait for normal AV conduction to occur but, instead, always deliver a stimulus to the ventricle one AV interval after delivery of an atrial stimulus.

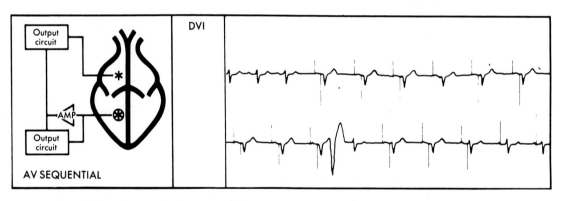

**Fig. 11-3  AV sequential pacemaker (DVI).** In the diagram the asterisk in the atrium and the circled asterisk in the ventricle indicate that the pacemaker paces the atrium, paces the ventricle, and senses spontaneous activity in the ventricle. The ECG example demonstrates this operation. The first three sinus-initiated QRS complexes occur at a rate faster than the escape rate of the pacemaker, and the pacemaker is completely inhibited. At this point, SA node discharge rate slows and the pacemaker delivers a stimulus *(upper spike)* to the atrium. Because the paced P wave does not conduct to the ventricle within the escape interval of the pacemaker, the pacemaker then paces the ventricle *(downward directed spikes)*. This occurs for three beats. Then the PR interval shortens slightly, inhibiting ventricular pacemaker discharge. The last two beats in the top strip and first three beats in the lower strip indicate pacing in the atrium and ventricle. Then a PVC occurs and is sensed, and pacemaker activity is inhibited. The pacemaker then resumes delivery of spikes to atrium and ventricle. In the terminal portion of this ECG the atrial rate speeds slightly. Since atrial activity is *not* sensed, pacemaker spikes "march" through the P wave but ventricular spikes are inhibited.

## Fully Automatic or Universal Stimulation (DDD)

In 1977 came the first clinical implants of the DDD pacemaker, a dual-chamber device that functions in the atrial synchronous mode during normal sinus activity and provides AV sequential pacing during periods of bradycardia.[16] Thus the DDD pacemaker senses and paces the atrium and the ventricle. This pacemaker operates in four modes, adapting automatically to the patient's underlying rhythm according to the schema in Table 11-2. Fig. 11-4 shows a block diagram and representative ECGs for the DDD pacemaker.

## Rate-Responsive Devices

As the benefits of rate variability associated with atrial synchronous ventricular pacing became appreciated, it was recognized that similar advantages might be available to patients with impaired atrial function.[17] However, an appropriate physiologic parameter independent of sinus nodal function is needed to set the pacemaker's rate. Substantial clinical experience exists with single and dual chamber ventricular pacemaker designs that vary pacing rate in response to changes in sensed mechanical activity of the body,[18] changes in respiratory rate or minute ventilation,[19-21] QT interval,[22-24] central venous temperature,[25] right ventricular pressure,[26-27] oxygen saturation,[28] preejection index[29] and stroke volume,[30] and ventricular depolarization gradient[31] and pH.[32] Pacing systems that use more than one sensor to minimize inappropriate pacing rates and provide more workload proportional pacing rates will be investigated in the near future. Fig. 11-5 shows a

**TABLE 11-2** Operating modes of DDD pacemakers

| Underlying Rhythm | Pacemaker Function |
| --- | --- |
| Normally conducted sinus rhythm | Totally inhibited |
| Normally conducted sinus bradycardia | Atrial pacing |
| Atrial bradycardia and prolonged or blocked AV conduction | AV sequential pacing |
| Normal sinus rhythm and prolonged or blocked AV conduction | Artrial synchronous ventricular pacing |

block diagram and representative ECGs for the VVIR and DDDR pacemakers.

The activity sensing pacemaker uses a conventional lead system for sensing and pacing and incorporates a microphone-like sensor inside the pacemaker pulse generator. This sensor responds to mechanical vibrations of the body, producing electric signals that are proportional to the patient's physical activity level. These "activity" signals are used to determine an appropriate pacing rate, an approach that affords a rapid response to patient needs, uses a sensor that is hermetically sealed within the pulse

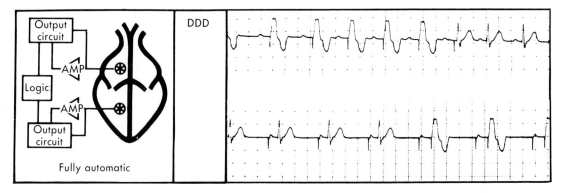

**Fig. 11-4  Fully automatic sequential pacemaker (DDD).** The diagram on the left indicates that the DDD pacemaker both senses and paces in the atrium and ventricle. The ECG on the right illustrates this feature. In the first five complete complexes, spontaneous atrial activity (P waves) is not followed by a spontaneous QRS complex within an appropriate PR interval. Therefore a pacemaker spike is delivered to the ventricle following each sensed P wave. The third QRS complex from the end occurs in time to be normally conducted from the P wave but not quite early enough to inhibit the pacemaker spike. The next QRS complexes follow a normal PR interval and thus inhibit pacemaker output. In the lower strip the development of sinus bradycardia triggers atrial pacemaker discharge, and pacemaker spikes precede the onset of P waves. Finally, in the bottom right portion, an atrial stimulus paces the atrium, and a ventricular stimulus paces the ventricle.

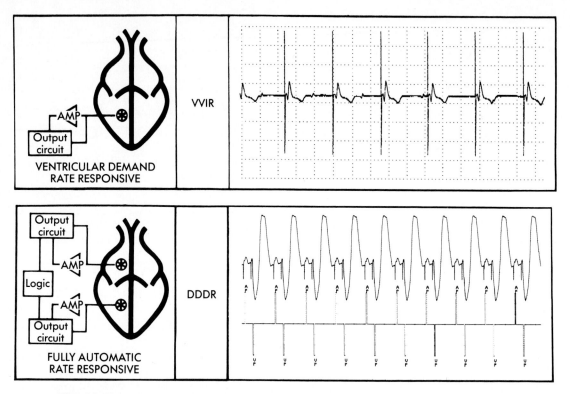

**Fig. 11-5** **Ventricular (VVIR) and fully automatic sequential (DDDR) rate-responsive pacemakers.** For the VVIR pacemaker, the circled asterisk indicates both sensing and pacing in the ventricle. The *R* in the fourth position of the NBG code indicates that the pacemaker escape interval is modulated by a sensor. In the lower panel, the diagram indicates that the DDDR pacemaker senses and paces in the atrium and ventricle. The *R* in the fourth position of the NBG code also indicates rate modulation by a sensor. The ECG illustrates rapid sensor-driven sequential pacing in the atrium and ventricle. Below the ECG is an example of a marker channel, which, when received by a pacemaker programer, indicates in this case both atrial and ventricular paced events.

generator for reliable long-term service, and requires no change in implant technique. Its disadvantages are an inability to respond to nonexercise-induced metabolic demands and the potential for minor rate increases in the presence of infrasonic environmental noises.

The respiratory-dependent pacemaker currently requires placement of two leads, a conventional cardiac pacing lead in the ventricle and an auxiliary lead in the subcutaneous tissue of the thorax. Variations in the electric impedance between the thoracic electrode and the pacemaker's indifferent electrode (generator case) reflect the patient's respiratory rate, which is processed to control the pacemaker rate. This approach uses a simple reliable sensor and is responsive to exercise and metabolic needs. It does require placement of an extra lead. The minute ventilation pacemaker measures impedance by injecting current between the ring of a standard bipolar pacing lead and the pacemaker case. Advantages of this system include proportional pacemaker rate increase to varying work load and no special lead requirements. Disadvantages include

contraindication for use in patients with high breathing rates, rate increases caused by certain maneuvers such as arm waving and rate changes caused by talking during exercise.

The QT sensing pacemaker uses a conventional electrode system to sense and pace, but it has circuitry designed to determine the interval between stimulation and the peak of the intracardiac T wave. Its operation is based on the physiologic concept that sympathetic tone increases in response to the body's need for an increased heart rate. Heightened sympathetic tone shortens the QT interval and the shortening of this QT interval produces an increase in the pacemaker rate. Advantages of this pacemaker include use of a stable rugged sensor (the standard pacing lead) that requires no change in implant technique, and the device responds to a parameter reflecting metabolic demand. Disadvantages include relatively slow response time, changes in QT interval caused by drug interactions and unreliable sensing of the T wave.

The temperature sensing pacemaker measures the tem-

**TABLE 11-3**  Summary of pacemaker modalities

| Pacemaker Type | NBG Code | Atrium | Ventricle |
|---|---|---|---|
| Atrial asynchronous | AAO | PACE | |
| Ventricular asynchronous | VOO | | PACE |
| Atrial demand | AAI/AAT/AAIR | PACE/SENSE | |
| Ventricular demand | VVI/VVT/VVIR | | PACE/SENSE |
| Atrial synchronous | VAT | SENSE | PACE |
| Atrial synchronous ventricular inhibited | VDD | SENSE | PACE/SENSE |
| AV sequential | DVI/DVIR | PACE | PACE/SENSE |
| Fully automatic | DDD/DDDR | PACE/SENSE | PACE/SENSE |

perature in the right ventricle using a thermistor in a dedicated lead. The temperature in the right ventricle falls slightly at the beginning of exercise and gradually increases as exercise continues. Temperature sensing allows pacemaker rate changes to be proportional to work load. Disadvantages of the system include use of a complicated dedicated lead, response of the system to short-duration low-level exercise, and rate responses resulting from temperature changes not initiated by exercise.

Additional, but not as extensive clinical experience exists with pacemakers that vary pacing rate in response to the ventricular depolarization gradient. This gradient is derived from the evoked potential, the derivative of the right ventricular pulse pressure waveform measured with a dedicated pressure sensor on the lead, and preejection interval and stroke volume as derived from intracavitary impedance measurements.

A summary of each of the pacemaker modes described is presented in Table 11-3.

## Mode Selection

Selection of the optimum pacemaker modality for a given patient can be rather complex, requiring knowledge of the electrophysiologic performance of the SA node, AV conduction pathways, and hemodynamic status. A reasonable, though less rigorous, mode selection can be made by considering the patient's atrial rhythm and AV conduction status, as indicated in Table 11-4.

Patients who have normal atrial rhythms do not require a pacemaker if AV conduction is also normal. If AV function is interrupted, then atrial synchronous ventricular pacing (VDD, DDD) provides a means for maintaining sinus control of ventricular rate. If the patient additionally has sinus node chronotropic incompetence, a device that provides rate variability via another sensor (DDDR) adds a means of compensating for a slow sinus mode. However, in patients who have prolonged retrograde conduction time, atrial activation following ventricular stimulation may trigger an atrial synchronous device, producing a pacemaker-mediated tachycardia. If this cannot be prevented (e.g., by use of a long atrial refractory period in the pacemaker), then DVI or DDI pacing may be used. DVI pacemakers are not triggered by atrial signals; hence they cannot induce pacemaker-mediated tachycardias. DDI pacemakers inhibit atrial pacing when an atrial signal is present, but do not track atrial signals. However, rate-responsive

**TABLE 11-4**  A guide to pacemaker mode selection*

| AV Conduction | Atrial Rhythm | | |
| | Normal | Bradycardia | Brady/Tachy |
|---|---|---|---|
| Normal, no hypersensitive carotid sinus syndrome | None | AAIR/AATR | AAIR/AATR |
| Antegrade and retrograde block | VBD<br>DDD | DDDR | DVIR/DDIR<br>VVIR/VVTR |
| Antegrade block, prolonged retrograde conduction | DDVI/DVIR<br>VVIR/VVTR | DDIR<br>VVIR/VVTR | DVIR/DDIR<br>VVIR/VVTR |

*By matching the patient's AV conduction and atrial rhythm to those in this table, an appropriate pacemaker mode can be determined. R after an NBG code indicates rate-responsive pacing.

VVIR, VVTR, DVIR, or DDIR pacemakers may be preferred to the DVI device because such pacemakers provide a varying ventricular rate as the patient's needs change.

Atrial pacing (AAI or AAT) is appropriate in patients who have atrial bradycardia and normal AV function, since it ensures the atrial contribution to ventricular filling. Rate-responsive atrial pacing (AAIR or AATR) is advantageous, since it provides additional compensation during exercise.

Atrial pacing alone is not acceptable in patients who have impaired AV conduction. In these patients dual chamber-pacing (DDD or DVI) provides atrial pacing for benefits already cited and ventricular stimulation to compensate for the lack of AV conduction.

Rate-responsive dual chamber pacing (DDDR, DVIR, or DDIR) may be preferred, since additional compensation during exercise is provided.

Finally, in patients who have atrial bradycardia and tachycardia (bradycardia-tachycardia syndrome), atrial synchronous devices (other than those incorporating specific antitachycardia features) are inappropriate because they will accelerate ventricular rhythm during periods of atrial tachycardia. In all other respects mode selection factors are comparable to those cited for patients who have only atrial bradydysrhythmias.

Ultimately, selection from among the several possible modes depends on additional factors, such as pulse generator size and patient physique, availability and unique traits of specific devices, follow-up capabilities, patient age and hemodynamic needs, and economics (dual-chamber pacemaker/lead systems typically cost 35% more than comparably advanced single-chamber systems, which in turn may cost 60% more than single nonprogrammable single-chamber devices).

## Antitachycardia Pacing[8-10,33-39]

Tachydysrhythmia control is achieved with pacemakers using one or more of three broad approaches: rate maintenance, termination of tachydysrhythmias, and prevention of onset of tachydysrhythmias.

Some therapeutic approaches to control tachydysrhythmias result in symptom-producing bradydysrhythmias. Pacing can be combined with drug therapy in such situations to prevent the bradycardia. For example, digitalis or propranolol, given to treat the tachycardia component of the tachycardia-bradycardia syndrome, may aggravate the bradycardia, establishing the need for pacemaker implantation. Similarly, surgery to interrupt the AV conducting system in a patient who has drug-refractory supraventricular tachycardia with a rapid ventricular rate results in a bradycardia (caused by the AV block) that needs to be treated by pacing.

Certain drug-refractory tachycardias, not amenable to surgical therapy, can sometimes be terminated by a pacemaker designed to produce an appropriate sequence of electric stimuli. Some of the pacemakers are activated by the patient when perceiving the presence of a tachydysrhythmia, whereas others automatically discharge when the pacemaker senses that a tachycardia is present. Various cadences of stimuli can be delivered, including short bursts at high rates, stimuli that scan the cardiac cycle and automatically change rate or shift the timing of one or more premature stimuli, and coupled or paired stimuli. A *dual-demand* pacemaker is one that automatically delivers stimuli at a fixed, but relatively slow, rate (for example, 70 beats/min) when it senses the presence of a bradycardia (for example, rates less than 70 beats/min) or a tachycardia (for example, rates greater than 150 beats/min). The tachycardia is terminated when an appropriately timed stimulus occurs during a particular part of the tachycardia cycle; this is called *underdrive termination*. Dual-chamber (DVI) pacemakers can be made to operate in the dual-demand mode and pace with short AV intervals for patients who have accessory bypass tracts. Unique custom-built devices with characteristics tailored for specific patients can also be applied.

Devices that operate automatically are being used with increasing frequency, but they must be used with extreme caution in patients with ventricular dysrhythmias. Acceleration of the tachydysrhythmia into a faster rate or an unstable rhythm such as ventricular fibrillation can occur with any pacing therapy. Therefore, repeated inductions of the tachydysrhythmia in the electrophysiology laboratory must be performed with consistently successful termination by the pacing therapy that has been selected. Most automatic devices are now used in patients with supraventricular dysrhythmias because of these concerns about patient safety.

The preferred therapeutic approach to tachydysrhythmias is prevention. In some cases simply improving the patient's hemodynamic status or restoring normal AV synchrony by means of an appropriate standard pacemaker prevents the development of tachycardia. Some patients have bradycardia-dependent tachycardias (for example, ventricular tachycardia associated with complete AV block), and pacing at normal rates eliminates the ventricular tachycardia. In others pacing at moderately elevated rates suppresses ectopy that might otherwise precipitate tachycardias. In patients with accessory AV pathways, use of an atrial synchronous or DDD pacemaker with a suitably short AV interval may preclude development of a reciprocating tachycardia while preserving normal sinus control of ventricular rate.

New options will also be available for patients with complex and life-threatening ventricular dysrhythmias. Many implantable cardioverter defibrillators entering clinical trials in the early 1990s will offer pacing therapies combined with low-energy cardioversion and backup defibrillation as well. These staged therapy devices will permit application of painless pacing therapies while protecting patients from the dangers associated with acceleration of their ventricular dysrhythmias or conversion of these rhythms into ventricular fibrillation.

## PACEMAKER PROGRAMMABILITY[40-43]

The vast majority of permanent pacemaker implants today employ a programmable pacemaker. *Programmability* can be defined as noninvasive, reversible alteration of the electronically controlled performance of an implantable device such as a pacemaker. Use of a simple magnet to convert a demand pacemaker to its asynchronous mode generally is excluded from this definition, although it is in reality a simple form of programing. In the most advanced pacemakers many performance characteristics are programmable, including rate, stimulus output amplitude or duration, amplifier sensitivity, amplifier refractory period, hysteresis, pacing mode (for example, unipolar/bipolar, VVIR/VVI/VVT/VOO), and operation of special information transfer channels (telemetry of intracardiac electrograms, sensor output waveforms, programed settings, and device operation indicators, such as "marker channel," battery status, lead impedance, and event counters). Furthermore, in dual-chamber pacemakers it is frequently possible to program AV intervals, atrial rate tracking limits, and the pacing mode (for example, DDD to DVI or VVI).

Programmability is of benefit to the clinician and patient in that it allows optimizing pacemaker function for specific patient needs, minimizes the need for invasive procedures to correct malfunctions or to revise the system to meet changing patient needs, and facilitates troubleshooting procedures. Some pacemakers have the ability to tabulate the past pacemaker operation in terms of number of paced and sensed events (e.g., rate). These types of data are commonly displayed in a histogram format. Interrogation of this information provides documentation of pacemaker operation. This information may aid in troubleshooting and in optimizing pacemaker performance. Table 11-5 indicates applications for many of the commonly available programmable parameters. It should be emphasized that programmability must be used with care, since it presents the risk of establishing inappropriate parameter settings (for example, insufficient output energy to maintain capture, dangerously high or low rates) and imposes a greater need for maintaining accurate records to prevent erroneous decisions based on lack of knowledge about the rationale for the current status of the programed settings in a given patient. Thus it is essential to document the rationale for program changes at the time at which they are made.

Many programing devices available today produce printed records of the parameter settings of the implanted pacemaker. Some printers are activated automatically when the programers are turned on, although others require specific activation. Whenever possible, it is advisable to include the printouts in the patient's records. It is also advisable to routinely determine and record all programed parameters as a first step in each patient follow-up session and as a final step. This ensures that spontaneous reprograming of the implanted device, a rare phenomenon, can be correctly identified if it should occur.

## IMPLANTABLE CARDIOVERTER DEFIBRILLATOR PROGRAMMABILITY[44-47]

Early models of implantable cardioverter defibrillators were not programmable. Their detection mechanism consisted of rate only or rate plus a morphology criterion referred to as PDF (probability density function). The type of detection mechanism as well as the specific rate cutoff was fixed at manufacture. These devices, while effective, could not accommodate changing patient characteristics, such as the addition of a new antidysrhythmic drug to the patient's therapy. Therefore, certain kinds of ventricular tachycardia were not detected because their waveforms were not consistent with the PDF morphology criterion. In addition, tachycardia rates that fell below the rate cutoff were also not detected, and some episodes of a supraventricular tachycardia were mistakenly detected and treated as if they were ventricular in origin. The addition of rate programmability to these early models, in the late 1980s, helped to address some of these limitations.

Devices in the 1990s will be extensively programmable. In addition to rate programmable features they will include a variety of tachycardia detection criteria, many types of pacing therapies, selection of waveforms, and selection of shock energy to be delivered, to name a few. They will therefore offer extensive options for a variety of patient needs.

## POWER SOURCES[48-50]

Nearly all pacemakers and defibrillators are battery-powered. External devices, especially pacemakers, typically use standard alkaline or mercury batteries of the type found in common household appliances (such as transistor radios and flashlights), although an occasional external device uses a rechargeable or lithium battery.

Virtually all current implantable devices are powered by one of the many varieties of lithium batteries. These batteries share certain characteristics that make them especially suitable for implantation, yet they are also significantly different. Each of the lithium systems offers high-energy density and a low self-discharge characteristic that ensures the delivery of maximum energy where it is needed and minimizes wasted energy. Most of the systems can be hermetically sealed to prevent ingress of body fluids and egress of tissue-damaging battery materials. Each system offers unique electric characteristics and varying degrees of reliability.[34,35] The most commonly used lithium batteries are the lithium iodide and lithium cupric sulfide batteries.

Reported performances of the major power sources clearly show the substantial progress made toward creating a pacemaker that will have sufficient longevity to curtail the need for replacement in the majority of patients. In

**TABLE 11-5** Applications of programmable pacemaker parameters

| Parameter | Patient/Pacemaker Optimization | Diagnostic Applications | Correction of Malfunctions |
|---|---|---|---|
| Rate | Improve cardiac output by allowing greater range of conducted sinus activity. Minimize angina by keeping the rate below that which produces pain. Suppress dysrhythmias. Adapte pulse generator to pediatric needs (faster rates). Terminate tachycardias with short rapid bursts. Minimize "pacemaker syndrome" (caused by AV dissociation) by selecting low rate. | Suppress pacing to access underlying rhythm by ECG. Test AV conduction with an atrial pacemaker by determining rates at which AV nodal Wenckebach behavior occurs. Test sinus function with an atrial pacemaker by using bursts of rapid pacing to determine SA node recovery times. Confirm atrial capture by altering pacemaker rate and observing concomitant ventricular rate change. | |
| Output, amplitude, or duration | Maximize pulse generator longevity by selecting output energy that provides the minimum level of stimulation consistent with reliable maintenance of pacing. Provide increased energy for high-threshold patients. Avoid extracardiac stimulation (pectoral muscle, phrenic nerve). | Evaluate pacing threshold. | Regain capture following threshold increases caused by infarcts, electrolyte disturbances, drugs. Eliminate diaphragmatic or pectoral muscle stimulation. |
| Amplifier sensitivity | Establish appropriate sensitivity to detect intracardiac electrogram while avoiding sensing of extraneous signals (pectoral muscle potentials, electromagnetic interference). Increase sensitivity for atrial sensing applications. | Alter sensitivity to evaluate possible sources of oversensing or undersensing. | Compensate for changes in intracardiac electrogram amplitude. Resolve oversensing of T waves, muscle potentials, electromagnetic interference. |
| Refractory period* | Extend duration for atrial applications to avoid sensing conducted R waves. Shorten duration in ventricular applications to detect closely coupled ectopic events. | Alter duration to evaluate possible causes of oversensing or undersensing. | Lengthen duration to avoid T wave sensing. Shorten duration to eliminate failure to sense closely coupled ectopic events. |
| Hysteresis | Minimize pacemaker syndrome by allowing sinus rhythm over widest possible rate range while establishing adequately high pacing rate when needed. | | |

*Refractory period: that portion of a pacemaker's timing cycle during which intrinsic cardiac activity will not be allowed to reset the pacemaker's lower rate escape. Upper rate limits, noise reversion timing, and other pacemaker timing sequences may or may not be reset during the refractory period depending on the specific design.

**TABLE 11-5**    Applications of programmable pacemaker parameters—cont'd

| Parameter | Patient/Pacemaker Optimization | Diagnostic Applications | Correction of Malfunctions |
|---|---|---|---|
| Unipolar/bipolar | | Evaluate lead fracture (bipolar → unipolar). Enhance stimulus artifact visibility on ECG (bipolar → unipolar). Evaluate oversensing (unipolar → bipolar). | Convert to unipolar operation to regain capture in case of lead fracture. Change mode to adapt to altered electrogram causing sensing failure. Convert to bipolar to eliminate sensing of myopotentials. Convert to bipolar to avoid extracardiac stimulation. |
| Mode | Select optimum mode (e.g., VDD for patients who have normal sinus function and impaired AV conduction). Alter mode if patient's needs change (e.g., VDD → DVI if patient develops sinus bradycardia). | Establish triggered mode to enable external control of pacemaker from chest electrodes and external stimulator to perform noninvasive electrophysiologic studies of sinus function, AV conduction, efficacy of antidysrhythmic agents. Confirm oversensing signal source by selecting triggered mode. | Change to backup mode (e.g., VVIR) if atrial portion of dual-chamber system is nonfunctional (e.g., lead displacement). Prevent oversensing by selecting asynchronous mode. |
| AV delay | Maximize hemodynamic efficacy. Control or prevent tachydysrhythmias. | | |
| Atrial-rate-tracking limit | Maintain widest range of sinus rate control without incurring angina. Control ventricular response to atrial dysrhythmias. Prevent rapid synchronization to dissociated atrial activity during ventricular escape pacing in VDD mode. Prevent occurrence of retrograde atrial activity that would result from a long delay between the triggering event in the atrium and the resultant stimulus in the ventricle. This retrograde activity can continuously trigger the pacemaker causing "pacemaker tachycardia." | Selects high rate limit for stress testing. | Reduce tracking rate limit if pectoral muscle activity triggers rapid pacing. |

*Continued.*

---

**TABLE 11-5** Applications of programmable pacemaker parameters—cont'd

| Parameter | Patient/Pacemaker Optimization | Diagnostic Applications | Correction of Malfunctions |
|---|---|---|---|
| Telemetry | | Compare programed settings to actual device operation. Use marker channel indicators to determine which events pacemaker is causing and which events are being sensed. Use electrogram to evaluate causes of undersensing or oversensing. Use electrogram to evaluate drug effect on myocardium. Use measurement of lead impedance to evaluate lead integrity. Use event counters to evaluate undersensing or oversensing. Use event counters to evaluate attainment of proper rates in rate response modes. | |

---

1988 survival probabilities were reported for large groups of pacemakers using lithium power sources.[35] A total of 9455 lithium *iodide* powered pacemakers showed a cumulative survival probability of 76% at an 8-year longevity; 3351 lithium *cupric sulfide* powered pacemakers showed a survival probability of 78% at a longevity of 8 years. These data reflect actual clinical results and clearly demonstrate the success of lithium power sources.

A very small group of special-purpose antitachycardia pacemakers is powered by radio frequency energy transmitted through the body to the implanted pulse generator. This is practical because these pacemakers are not required to pace constantly but are used to generate short bursts of rapid asynchronous stimuli to terminate episodes of tachycardia.

## PACEMAKER ELECTRODE SYSTEMS ("LEADS")[51,52]

The pulse generator is electrically connected to the heart by means of a wire and electrode system referred to as a *lead*. The electrodes may be unipolar or bipolar. In bipolar systems the positive and negative electrodes both are located within the cardiac chamber and are in contact with the endocardium or are on the heart. Unipolar systems place only the negative electrode at the heart and use a large area anode electrode, usually the metallic housing of the pulse generator, at a remote location. Either approach is clinically acceptable. Bipolar systems are less susceptible to extraneous electromagnetic interference (such as electric signals generated by nearby power lines, automobile spark plugs, and radio transmitters), extracardiac myopotential interference, unwanted extracardiac stimulation, or threshold changes caused by defibrillatory currents.

At the time of initial implantation of a pacemaker system, and at the time of each replacement of a pacemaker or a lead, electric measurements must be made to ensure that the system will function correctly. The *stimulation threshold* is the minimum amount of energy necessary to capture the chamber of the heart to be paced; output of the pacing device must therefore be higher than this amount. Measurement of *cardiac signal amplitudes* (intracardiac electrogram) ensures that these signals are large enough to be sensed by the pacing device to enable it to respond appropriately to spontaneous cardiac electric activity. These measurements are typically made using a pacing system analyzer (PSA).

## Transvenous

Permanent pacing leads are designed for either transvenous or epicardial placement. Transvenous leads are usually implanted within the right ventricular apex for ventricular pacing and in the right atrial appendage or coronary sinus for atrial applications. The leads are typically inserted via the cephalic, subclavian, or external jugular veins, using fluoroscopy for visualization and stiff wires (stylets) inserted within the lumen of the lead for control during positioning. (The stylets must be removed following lead placement to avoid damaging the lead.) A rapid technique for lead placement in the subclavian vein with minimal trauma employs a simple venipuncture using a special percutaneous lead introducer.[53] This approach has gained favor and involves minimal risk in skilled hands, although there is the possibility of inadvertently entering the pleural cavity or the arterial system. The urethane-insulated leads have reduced diameters and a decreased coefficient of friction, making it possible to pass an atrial and a ventricular lead through a single vein, and facilitating use of dual-chamber pacemakers.[54,55]

Transvenous leads come in a variety of designs, each purporting to ensure stable permanent positioning of the electrodes. Fig. 11-6 includes examples of ventricular and atrial leads with a variety of fixation mechanisms. Many atrial leads also incorporate a J shape to aid in proper positioning within the atrial appendage. The transvenous approach is associated with very low morbidity and with current lead designs, a very low rate of displacement.[56-58]

New designs in transvenous leads offer improvements in electric efficiency. Electrodes made of carbon have been shown to result in improved stimulation thresholds.[59] In another design, grooves were cut in a standard ring electrode, and the surface was then coated with small particles of platinum. Again, improvements in stimulation thresholds were noted.[60] Also available for clinical use are atrial and ventricular leads that incorporate a steroid-containing pellet behind a porous electrode, permitting minute amounts of the steroid to be dissolved by body fluids and deposited into the tissues immediately surrounding the electrode. This design decreases stimulation thresholds and increases cardiac signal amplitudes both acutely and chronically.[61-64] This approach may offer significant benefits, particularly to those patients in whom high stimulation thresholds and low cardiac signal amplitudes have resulted in repeated clinical problems with their pacemaker systems,

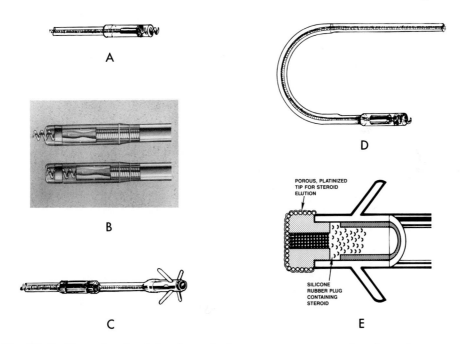

**Fig. 11-6** **Example of atrial and ventricular transvenous pacemaker electrodes.**
**A,** Unipolar endocardial urethane lead with screw-in tip electrode for active fixation to atrial or ventricular endocardial surface (Medtronic model 6957). **B,** Same lead showing the electrode in both its extended and retracted positions. **C,** Bipolar urethane ventricular electrode with flexible tines adjacent to the Target Tip electrode. The tines provide passive lead fixation by lodging within the trabecular structure of the ventricle (Medtronic model 4012). **D,** Unipolar urethane lead with J shape and screw-in tip electrode for active fixation to the atrial endocardial surface (Medtronic model 6957J). **E,** Cross section of steroid eluting electrode (Medtronic model 5023).

often necessitating use of short-lived high-output pulse generators.

## Epicardial

Epicardial leads are used far less frequently than transvenous systems, but they are of particular benefit in problem patients who have smooth, dilated right ventricles and in patients who have truncated right atrial appendages. The placement approach depends on the type of epicardial electrode used. A transthoracic approach (thoracotomy) is used to apply electrodes that are sutured to the myocardium. More commonly, for ventricular applications a sutureless corkscrew electrode is used, since this device can be applied with a transmediastinal approach avoiding entrance into the pleural cavity and reducing morbidity and discomfort.[65] Fig. 11-7 shows examples of myocardial electrodes.

## Temporary

Temporary pacing leads include transvenous catheter electrodes, wire electrodes, and, in extreme circumstances, precordial surface electrodes. Temporary transvenous catheter electrodes can be placed in a fashion similar to that used for permanent leads. Placement is facilitated by designing the catheters to be stiffer than would be acceptable for permanent use, and by sometimes incorporating additional aids such as inflatable balloons or cuffs that "float" the catheter in the bloodstream to the right ventricle. In the absence of fluoroscopy, ECG recordings from the catheter

enable the user to determine the location of the electrodes (Fig. 11-8).

Heart wires are frequently placed in the atria and ventricles of patients at the time of open heart surgery. These stainless steel wires are used during the surgical procedure and during the postoperative recovery phase. In emergency situations wire electrodes can be inserted percutaneously into the heart by a pericardiocentesis (or similar) needle.

Similarly, during emergencies surface skin electrodes placed on the chest wall can be stimulated with very high voltages to achieve cardiac pacing transthoracically. Such an approach should be used only until a transvenous catheter electrode can be positioned. One technique for noninvasive pacing has been reported to be of minimal discomfort and suitable for prolonged use. Special, large surface area electrodes and external pulse generators with very wide (about 40 msec) stimulus pulse widths are required.[66]

For temporary and permanent pacing it is important to place the electrodes in a position that provides acceptably low stimulation thresholds and sufficiently large intracardiac signals to be sensed by the pulse generator. Generally this implies acute thresholds of less than 2 mA and 1.25 V, with ventricular electrograms greater than 4 mV or atrial electrograms in excess of 2 mV. These values are often lower with steroid-eluting permanent transvenous leads. Thresholds generally rise following acute positioning, reaching a peak 2 to 4 times the acute values within the first 2 to 6 weeks and then falling to intermediate values.[67] The electrogram typically decreases in amplitude

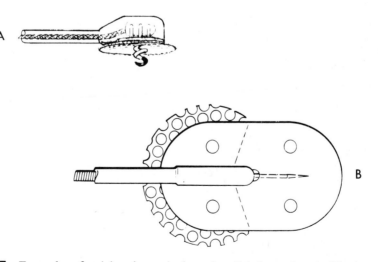

**Fig. 11-7**  **Examples of atrial and ventricular epicardial electrodes. A,** Silastic sutureless unipolar ventricular electrode with corkscrew tip. Positive fixation is achieved by screwing the electrode into the myocardium (Medtronic model 6917A). **B,** Urethane unipolar epicardial barbed-hook electrode providing positive fixation (without sutures) to either the atrial or ventricular myocardium (Medtronic model 4951).

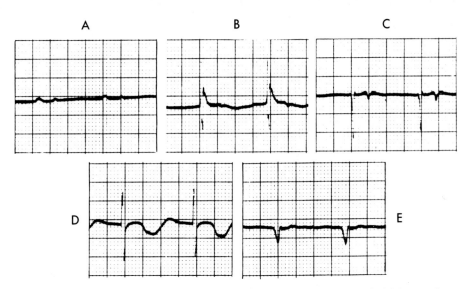

**Fig. 11-8**    Electrograms obtained when bipolar electrode is located in **A,** high superior vena cava; **B,** superior vena cava/right atrium; **C,** right atrium; **D,** right ventricle; and **E,** pulmonary artery. All tracings calibrated at 1 mV/cm except D, which is recorded at half standard.

by 15%; its rate of rise with respect to time (slew rate) decreases as much as 50% with maturation of the implant.[68] These factors must be considered when evaluating the appropriateness of a given lead position. Again, however, these changes may not be observed when steroid-eluting permanent transvenous leads are used.

## IMPLANTABLE CARDIOVERTER DEFIBRILLATOR ELECTRODE SYSTEMS[69-73]

Implantable cardioverter defibrillator systems of the early 1980s used a transvenous spring coil electrode and a ventricular patch electrode. The coil was positioned at the junction of the superior vena cava and the right atrium and the patch was placed over the apex of the left ventricle. These early systems were designed for defibrillation only. The systems were subsequently modified to include two patch electrodes and an endocardial bipolar ventricular lead or two epimyocardial unipolar leads for rate sensing and R wave synchronization when cardioversion capabilities were added to the pulse generator.

Totally nonepicardial lead systems are now undergoing clinical trials and will become commercially available in the early 1990s. These systems will eliminate the need for transthoracic implantation techniques and the resulting morbidity and longer recovery time that can accompany their use.

## POSTIMPLANTATION FOLLOW-UP OF IMPLANTABLE PACEMAKERS

Despite the reliability demonstrated by current pacemakers, it is important to monitor the patient and the pacemaker system regularly after implantation. Such monitoring has four major goals: evaluate electric function of the

pacing system to detect malfunctions or imminent power-source depletion; evaluate the implant site for possible mechanical difficulties such as erosion or infection; detect progression of the patient's cardiac problems, which may necessitate reprograming or revising the pacing system or accompanying drug regimen; and reassure patients that due concern and attention is being given their progress and offer opportunities to discuss concerns that may arise.

The follow-up schedule should be arranged to provide close monitoring during the immediate postimplantation period, moderately frequent observation during the routine service life of the system, and increased surveillance as the system nears completion of its service life. A suggested schedule is 6 weeks after implantation, annually beginning 6 months after implantation, and monthly once initial signs of power-source depletion are observed (in almost all pacemakers this appears as a rate decrease when monitored with a magnet over the pulse generator). Given the longevity of modern systems, it may be counter-productive to attempt to stretch out the last few months of service by frequent monitoring since this will probably add but 5% to 10% to the total service life while increasing monitoring costs by 30% to 40%.

Follow-up visits should be scheduled in the physician's office or in a special pacemaker clinic where the patient can be seen in person. (Telephone monitoring of the patient's ECG, pacing rate, and pulse generator stimulus duration can be of value as a supplement between personal evaluations but should not replace office visits.) Each visit should include a recording of a 12-lead ECG with a rhythm strip showing that the pacemaker appropriately captures and senses, a measurement of pacemaker parameters with appropriate rate and pulse width measurement equipment, and a general physical examination including careful scrutiny of the pacemaker pocket. If a problem is evident or if the patient reports symptoms, an x-ray film may be obtained to evaluate the lead and its position, blood tests may help uncover threshold problems related to electrolyte imbalances, and long-term ambulatory monitoring may be indicated if intermittent failures are suspected. The results of the follow-up procedure should be carefully recorded,[74] since much of the required analysis depends on changes in operation rather than on absolute values of measured parameters. This record is especially important when following patients who have programmable pacemakers and for whom changes may be totally innocuous if intentional (such as a rate change programed to improve cardiac output) or may signify device-performance problems (such as a rate decrease caused by battery depletion).

Care should be exercised in selecting follow-up equipment, and data must be analyzed with full understanding and knowledge of the idiosyncrasies of the equipment used. For example, digital monitoring and recording systems frequently do not register the pacemaker stimulus artifact reliably and reproducibly because of its extremely short duration. As a result, the pacemaker artifact may not always be recorded even if present, or its polarity and amplitude may vary markedly throughout the recording. On the other hand, such systems may substitute a standardized artifact for the real signal, eliminating diagnostic information in the process. As another example, some follow-up clinics perform waveform analysis using an oscilloscope or special ECG machine to display the waveshape of the pacemaker stimulus. One must be fully aware of the correct waveshape for each pacemaker to be evaluated. Modern pacemakers frequently produce much more complex stimulus pulse shapes than the traditional "square wave," and it is not unusual for such waveforms to be misread as signs of malfunction.

An often underestimated benefit of follow-up is a reduction in patient anxiety. A clear answer to a simple question can be extremely important to a patient's well-being. In recognition of this, some clinics have formed pacemaker clubs that allow patients to meet periodically to compare notes and provide mutual support.

## POSTIMPLANTATION FOLLOW-UP OF IMPLANTABLE CARDIOVERTER DEFIBRILLATORS[75]

Patients with implantable cardioverter defibrillators may be requested to undergo repeat induction of ventricular tachycardia and/or fibrillation in the electrophysiology laboratory prior to discharge from the hospital. The purpose is to ensure that the device continues to appropriately sense and reliably terminate the patient's dysrhythmia. Repeat testing of this type may also be needed if the patient's antidysrhythmic medications are significantly changed or if the patient is receiving shocks not believed to be associated with ventricular tachycardia or fibrillation.

Other procedures included in routine follow-up visits for currently available devices include regular discharging of the devices' capacitors into an internal test load with the device, determination of capacitor change time, determination of number of shocks delivered since the last follow-up, and status of the elective replacement indicator.

New devices with extensive memory and telemetry will offer a host of other information, including data concerning the number and type of dysrhythmias detected, the treatment delivered by the device for each dysrhythmia, and the success or failure of each treatment used. Actual stored electrocardiograms of these sequences of events will also be able to be retrieved by some devices. Adjustments can then be made to the various programmable parameters to optimize device function.

For the foreseeable future, patients with implantable cardioverter defibrillators will probably need careful and fairly frequent follow-up, so the rapid technologic advance in these devices can be both better understood and more optimally applied.

## TROUBLESHOOTING OF IMPLANTABLE PACEMAKERS[76-79]

Complex systems involving electric, mechanical, and physiologic interactions will inevitably develop malfunctions, and pacemakers are no exception. Fortunately, the detection and correction of such problems are relatively straightforward for the knowledgeable user if appropriate equipment is available.

### Equipment

The most useful troubleshooting tool is a *12-lead analog ECG machine*. This permits evaluation of pacemaker sensing, capture, and approximate rate, evaluation of electrode positioning (by vector analysis of ventricular activity), and confirmation of appropriate function for the mode of pacing employed. Multiple ECG leads are necessary for vector analysis of lead positioning and are frequently helpful in increasing visibility of small artifacts produced by bipolar systems or in evaluating atrial activity when dealing with dual-chamber or atrial demand pacemakers.

A *digital counter* is useful in obtaining accurate rate and pulse width information. These counters may be supplied as specialized patient monitors, built into pacemaker programers, or purchased alone. Such devices are necessary when evaluating pacing rate and pulse width changes caused by battery depletion, component failure, or reprograming.

A *magnet* should always be available for troubleshooting sessions. Nearly all pacemakers can be converted to asynchronous operation by the placement of a magnet over the generator site. This enables evaluation of capture when the patient's intrinsic rhythm inhibits the pacemaker and can be useful in diagnosing oversensing by disabling all sensing function. Magnet application should be used with care, since some pacemakers can be programmed by application of a suitable magnet, and there is always a definite but slight risk of inducing tachyarrhythmias when pacing asynchronously.

*Carotid sinus massage or Valsalva maneuver* may slow a patient's intrinsic rhythm and induce pacing. Such a procedure may be used to evaluate capture if a pacemaker fails to respond to magnet application because of either a component failure or a unique design having no asynchronous magnet mode.

*Exercise* may be used to speed the patient's spontaneous rate in the evaluation of sensing capability or in the evaluation of pacemaker rate increase in response to exercise in rate-responsive pacemakers.

*Chest wall stimulation* with an external stimulator connected to precordial surface electrodes can be used to test sensing function and to determine rate tracking limits for atrial tracking pacemakers (VAT, VDD, DDD).

*Manipulation* of the pulse generator in its pocket can sometimes elicit electrocardiographic signs of a loose connection or damaged lead close to the generator site.

*X-ray examination or fluoroscopy* of the chest and pacemaker system in multiple views helps determine lead position, gross lead fractures, and disconnections at the generator. A baseline x-ray film should be obtained before the patient is discharged, following implantation of the system.

An *oscilloscope* or special ECG recorder designed to display the waveshape of the pacemaker stimulus is used by some centers to evaluate lead problems or unusual component failures.

A pacemaker *programer* is an extremely useful troubleshooting tool in dealing with a programmable pacemaker, allowing the user to vary stimulus strength, amplifier sensitivity, rates, refractory periods, and pacing modes. This permits noninvasive threshold evaluation and, in some of the new systems, permits the user to obtain noninvasive intracardiac electrograms to evaluate sensing operation. Many systems include digital telemetry of the programed settings of the pacemakers allowing actual performance to be compared with expected performance. Some systems provide a *marker channel,* a noninvasively telemetered signal indicating pacemaker sensing and pacing, which in conjunction with a surface ECG clearly identifies pacemaker operation (Fig. 11-9). Other systems provide telemetered event counter data that display the number of paced and sensed events for various rate ranges (Fig. 11-10).

Invasive procedures are necessary if noninvasive approaches fail. A *pacing system analyzer* is the primary tool for invasive troubleshooting. This instrument typically can analyze the implantable pulse generator function (sensitivities, refractory periods, rates, pulse widths, and amplitudes), evaluate lead integrity and positioning, and provide electrophysiologic patient data (stimulation thresholds, electrogram amplitudes, AV conduction, sinus function).

In addition to the troubleshooting hardware, it is equally important to have detailed patient records, including prior ECGs and x-ray films, and full information on the characteristics of the implanted system. Unfortunately, it is common for a normally functioning pacemaker to be diagnosed as malfunctioning simply because of inadequate understanding of proper device operation. Systems with hysteresis,* special antitachycardia pacemakers, and synchronous pacemakers are especially vulnerable to misdiagnosis.

Pacemaker-related problems fall into five broad categories: failure to pace, loss of sensing, oversensing, pacing at an altered rate, and undesirable patient/pacemaker interactions.

## Failure to Pace

Failure to pace implies nondelivery of a stimulus or loss of capture (delivery of an ineffective stimulus that fails to depolarize the myocardium).

Failure to deliver a stimulus can result from various factors: improper connection of the lead to the generator (as when set screws are not tightened); broken lead wires with no insulation defect; "crosstalk" between atrial and ventricular portions of dual-chamber pacemakers so that the atrial stimulus is sensed by the ventricular amplifier, inhibiting the ventricular stimulus (caused by improper electrode placement or incorrect electrode types); pulse generator component failure; or power source depletion. Occasionally, a misdiagnosis of failure to pace is made when a normally functioning pacemaker is merely inhibited by the patient's intrinsic rhythm. This is especially common with programmable pacemakers set at relatively low rates. (Inappropriate nondelivery of a stimulus also may be caused by oversensing, which is discussed later.)

Loss of capture may be caused by lead dislodgement (the most common cause), myocardial perforation with lead migration to an extracardiac position, failure of lead insulation and/or wire fracture; increased stimulation threshold caused by infarction, drug effects, electrolyte imbalances, or fibrosis at the electrode site, or inappropriate programing of pacemaker stimulus strength. Lack of capture when a stimulus is delivered during the myocardial refractory period is a frequent source of misdiagnosis.

## Loss of Sensing

A pacemaker may fail to sense intracardiac signals, resulting in competitive pacing or, in the case of atrial synchronous units, loss of AV synchrony. This may be caused by the following: lead dislodgement (the most common cause); inadequate amplitude or waveshape of the intracardiac electrogram caused by inappropriate lead placement, fibrosis, infarct, drugs, or electrolyte disturbances; inappro-

---

*Pacemakers with hysteresis are designed to work as follows: the escape interval (before pacing) following the last sensed spontaneous activity exceeds the interval between subsequent consecutive pacing artifacts. This allows maintenance of normal sinus rhythm over a wide range of rates (pacemaker-inhibited) while ensuring an adequate pacing rate when needed. This type of operation is diagrammed in Fig. 11-11.

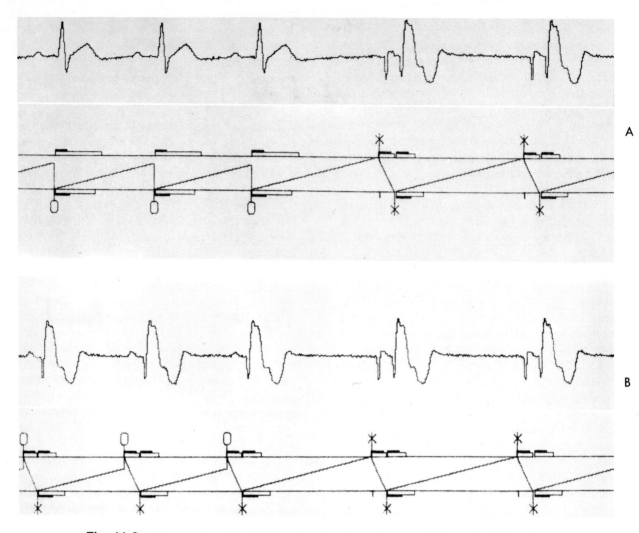

**Fig. 11-9** *Upper panel;* surface ECG and marker channel generated diagnostic ladder diagram beneath, taken from a patient with an implanted DDD pacemaker. The surface ECG may appear to show normal inhibition of the pacemaker by three cycles of sinus rhythm after which a sinus pause elicits AV sequential pacing for two cycles. The diagram, however, reveals that the pacemaker is malfunctioning and is not sensing atrial activity. In the diagram *O* represents sensing; *, pacing; *white rectangular area,* pacemaker refractory periods; *solid rectangular area,* absolute refractory periods (blanking); sloping lines between the horizontal parallel lines indicate timing of AV (\) and VA (/) escape intervals. Atrial sensing, pacing, and refractory periods are marked above the top horizontal line, and ventricular events are marked beneath the lower line. The diagram in this upper panel shows *O* beneath the first three QRS complexes, indicating that the pacemaker correctly senses ventricular depolarization, and the upward sloping line following each O shows that the pacemaker is timing VA intervals appropriately. However, there is no O on the upper rung of the diagram beneath the sinus P waves. This indicates that the pacemaker is failing to sense atrial activity. During the last two complexes the diagram shows proper AV sequential pacing with asterisks beneath the paced P and QRS complexes to indicate stimulation.

*Lower panel,* same format as above. Records obtained after the atrial amplifier of the implanted pacemaker was programed to increase its sensitivity. The pacemaker now clearly senses atrial activity during the first three cycles as evidenced by the sensing symbols *(O)* seen in the upper rung of the left portion of the ladder diagram and by the ventricular stimuli (indicated with * on the diagram) following the P waves one AV interval later. Pacemaker operation is now normal, with each P wave sensed, causing the pacemaker to deliver a ventricular stimulus one AV interval later.

```
EVENT COUNTERS AT    08:33:48

TELEMETRY VALUES:
SOURCE: HEART RATE
FORMAT: HISTOGRAM
TERM:   SHORT
BINS:   STANDARD
  RATE    TOTAL    %
  BINS   EVENTS  TOTAL      :: PACED
 (PPM)  / TERM  EVENTS  :0-25-50-75-100
  <61      0       0    : *
 61-70    179     70    : *
 71-80    12       5    :    *
 81-90     3       1    :       *
 91-100    6       2    :       *
101-110    8       3    :           *
111-120   17       7    :           *
 >120     32      12    :           *
TOTAL    257
```

**Fig. 11-10  Pacemaker event counter data.** The number of sensed and paced intervals are stored as events in eight rate ranges and presented in tabular form. The percentage of paced events in each bin are presented as between 0 and 25%, 25% and 50%, 50% and 75%, or 75% and 100%.

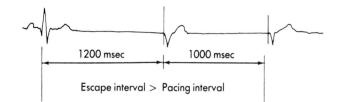

**Fig. 11-11  Diagrammatic representation of operation of a VVI pacemaker incorporating hysteresis.** The last beat of the patient's sinus rhythm is shown as the first complex on the left. Spontaneous sinus bradycardia results, and the pacemaker "escapes" at an interval of 1200 msec. The subsequent pacing interval is 1000 msec, however; thus the escape interval of the pacemaker exceeds the pacing interval (in other words, the initial escape rate of pacemaker discharge is *slower* than the subsequent rate of pacing) to allow the patient to remain in a normally conducted rhythm for as much of the time as possible.

priate programming of amplifier sensitivity, refractory periods, or mode (for example, AOO, VOO); lead fracture or insulation defect; connector defect; or component failure (such as a stuck magnetic reed switch).

Occasionally, a misdiagnosis of sensing failure is made when spontaneous activity occurs simultaneously with delivery of the pacemaker stimulus and results in fusion beats. This is because electric activity may occur within the myocardium and be visible on the surface ECG record before it reaches the pacemaker electrode site. Concurrently, the pacemaker escape interval may elapse with resultant stimulation just before arrival of the spontaneous depolarization. This apparent failure to sense is, in fact, perfectly normal operation. Another cause of apparent sensing failure is reversion to asynchronous operation in the presence of electromagnetic interference—also a normal mode of operation for many pacemakers. Finally, closely coupled intracardiac signals may occur within the voltage changes produced when a lead with a hairline fracture or loose connection makes intermittent contact or when two endocardial leads come into contact. Electromagnetic interference from power lines, radio or television transmitters, and other electric noise sources may occasionally be sensed, especially by unipolar pacemakers. Sometimes this may result in inhibition or triggering, but it more commonly produces reversion to the asynchronous mode that provides the patient with continued pacing support. Very rarely, a pacemaker may sense the afterpotentials remaining on a lead following delivery of a stimulus. This is most commonly the result of using very wide pulse widths or excessively short refractory periods.

In all cases of suspected oversensing, placing the pacemaker in an asynchronous mode (with application of a magnet if it is a permanent pacemaker, or turning off the sensitivity if it is an external pacemaker) will abolish the symptoms caused by the pacemaker malfunction and confirm the diagnosis.

### Pacing at an Altered Rate

A fairly common cause for concern is apparent operation of a pacemaker at an unexpected rate. This can be an indication of a real problem with the pacemaker system but more frequently reflects a diagnostic error.

The possible true causes of unexpected pacing at an altered rate include the following: oversensing that induces rate slowing caused by inhibition, or rate acceleration caused by triggering; rate drift, a gradual benign shift of the pacing rate caused by component aging or temperature effects (most commonly found in older pacemakers that do not use digital timing circuits); rate slowdown built into most pacemakers to indicate approaching power source depletion; and component failure (usually causing either no stimulus output or a rapid stimulation rate typically limited to less than 150 beats/min by "runaway" protection circuits).

Frequent causes of pacing at an altered rate when there is no system failure include the following: presence of a rate hysteresis that produces a long escape interval following sensed activity; reprograming of a programmable pacemaker without proper recording of the change in the patient records; tracking of spontaneous intrinsic cardiac rate accelerations with VVT, AAT, VAT, VDD, or DDD pacemakers; failure of the reader to note a nearly isoelectric atrial or ventricular complex in a single-lead ECG tracing so that the pacemaker appears to have a prolonged stimulus-to-stimulus interval; misinterpretation of nonpace-

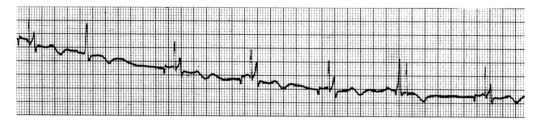

**Fig. 11-12**  Surface ECG (monitor lead) demonstrating an example of a "committed" mode DVI pacemaker. Note that the first, third, fourth, fifth, and seventh complexes are initiated by an atrial spike (small negative deflection) that paces the atrium and then a ventricular spike (large upright deflection) that paces the ventricle. The second QRS complex occurs sufficiently early to inhibit pacemaker discharge. However, the sixth QRS complex occurs early, but not early enough to inhibit the atrial discharge. Following the atrial spike (seen as the initial negative deflection preceding the onset of the QRS complex, after the P wave) a conducted QRS occurs. However, this QRS complex is not sensed by the pacemaker, which is committed to delivering a pacemaker spike (large upright spike following the QRS complex in the ST segment) regardless of spontaneous ventricular activity.

maker artifacts such as rapid spike potentials generated by muscle fasciculation or electric noise in the ECG recording system; lack of familiarity with device operation (such as a DVI pacemaker perceived to be pacing the ventricles at a rate equivalent to its VA interval when it is, in fact, pacing atrially and appropriately inhibiting the ventricular stimulus in response to conducted ventricular activity or rate responsive pacemakers in which pacing occurs at varying rates (Fig. 11-12).

### Undesirable Patient-Pacemaker Interactions

Occasionally, undesirable patient-pacemaker system interactions can develop. The pacemaker pocket may become infected or develop hematomas, or the generator may erode through the pocket site. These problems occur less frequently with the current small, lightweight generators. Some patients exhibit "twiddler's syndrome," playing with their pulse generators and rotating them in their pockets, retracting the lead and producing total system failure.

Extracardiac stimulation of the pectoralis muscles or diaphragm may be observed. These problems are generally restricted to unipolar pacemakers, although they have been reported, in rare instances, with bipolar systems. Decreasing the pulse width, voltage, or current of the stimulus can be useful in eliminating or reducing such extracardiac stimulation.

Incorrect pacing mode selection for a given patient or changes in a patient's postimplantation status can have serious consequences. For example, atrial tracking pacemakers (VAT, VDD, DDD) may detect slowly conducted retrograde atrial activity (long RP interval) following ventricular stimulation, inducing "pacemaker tachycardia" with a rate equal to the pacemaker's upper rate limit. Patients may respond poorly to other specific pacing modes depending on their underlying hemodynamic and electro-

physiologic substrates. In many such cases, the use of multiprogrammable pacemakers allows the clinician to alter the pacing system characteristics without resorting to invasive procedures.

Table 11-6 summarizes various pacemaker problems and their likely causes.

### An Illustrative Approach

The following hypothetical example demonstrates how one troubleshoots a pacemaker malfunction, in this case intermittent loss of capture and failure to sense spontaneous ventricular activity (Fig. 11-13). The patient has a ventricular demand (VVI) pacemaker implanted 1 year ago.

The first step in troubleshooting is to list the likely causes of the symptoms. Since there are two malfunctions in this example, it is highly probable, although not absolutely certain, that there is a common cause. The most likely causes are:

| Lack of capture | Lack of sensing |
|---|---|
| Lead dislodgement, perforation | Lead dislodgement, perforation |
| Lead wire fracture | Lead wire fracture |
| Lead insulation failure | Lead insulation failure |
| Pulse generator failure | Pulse generator failure |
| Inappropriate programing of output energy | Inappropriate programing of amplifier sensitivity or refractory period |
| High threshold | Inadequate electrogram amplitude (caused by infarct, electrolyte disturbance, myocardial disease) |
| Misread ECG ("loss of capture" seen only when stimulus occurs during cardiac refractory period) | Electromagnetic interference-induced (EMI) reversion to asynchronous mode |
| | Stuck reed switch |
| | Misread ECG (fusion beats) |

Analysis should begin by comparing a current 12-lead ECG with a baseline tracing predating occurrence of the problem. The current tracing should be carefully reviewed

TABLE 11-6  Pacemaker system problems and causes*

| | Nonpacing (NP) Noncapture (NC) | Non-sensing | Over-sensing | Altered Rate | Undesirable Patient/ IPG Interactions |
|---|---|---|---|---|---|
| **ACTUAL MALFUNCTIONS** | | | | | |
| Lead dislodged or perforated myocardium (possibly caused by twiddler's syndrome) | NC | X | X | X | X |
| Lead insulation failure | NC | X | X | X | X |
| Lead fracture with fluid in lumen | NC | X | X | X | |
| Skeletal muscle potentials, EMI, hairline lead fractures | NP | X | X | X | |
| Pulse generator failure | NP, NC | X | X | X | |
| Poor lead/IPG connection | NP | X | X | X | |
| Power source depletion | NC, NP | X | X | | |
| Lead fracture with dry lumen | NP | X | | | |
| Electric interference resulting in asynchronous pacing | | X | | X | |
| Cross-talk between atrial and ventricular channels | | | X | X | |
| Sensitivity too high | | | X | X | |
| Refractory period too short | | | X | X | |
| High threshold: fibrosis, infarct, drugs, electrolyte imbalance, lead position | NC | | | | |
| Low-output energy setting | NC | | | | |
| Poor electrogram: fibrosis, infarct, drugs, electrolyte imbalance, lead position | | X | | | |
| Sensitivity too low | | X | | | |
| Refractory period too long | | X | | | |
| Asynchronous mode: magnet or programed | | X | | | |
| End of service life indicator activated | | | | X | |
| High-output energy setting: extracardiac stimulation | | | | | X |
| Infection, hematoma, erosion | | | | | X |
| Sensor malfunction | | | | X | |
| **POTENTIAL MISDIAGNOSES** | | | | | |
| Recording system masks ECG signal (e.g., lead switching) | NP, NC | | X | X | |
| Recorder malfunction (e.g., paper speed error) | | X | X | X | |
| Hysteresis mode | | | X | X | X |
| Fusion of activity from pacemaker and cardiac source | NC | X | | | |
| Artifacts from source other than IPG (e.g., muscle fasciculation) | NC | | | X | |
| Stimulus falls in tissue refractory period | NC | | | | |
| Atrial stimulus misread as ventricular without capture or vice versa | NC | | | | |
| Cardiac activity is within IPG refractory period (e.g., QRS within AV interval of committed DVI pacemaker) | | X | | | |
| Rate-responsive pacemaker changing rate in response to parameter not reflected in ECG record (e.g., activity) | | | | X | |

*The column headings are symptoms of a malfunctioning pacemaker system. The leftmost entries in each row are specific mechanisms that can produce those symptoms marked with an X, NC (noncapture = ineffective stimulus), or NP (nonpacing = no stimulus artifact). After determining the type and number of symptoms exhibited by a system, one can find a match to entries in this table, thereby determining the most probable cause of the malfunction. The lower half of the table links apparent symptoms with mechanisms that do not result from pacemaker malfunction.

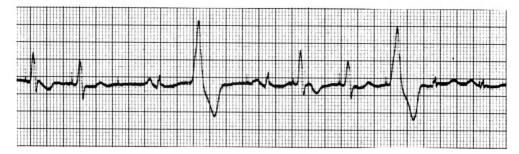

**Fig. 11-13** **Failure of a VVI pacemaker.** Note that pacing stimuli occasionally fail to elicit a paced QRS complex and also occasionally fail to sense spontaneous electric activity. Lead II.

to prevent misinterpretation of fusion beats as sensing failure or pacing artifacts during the cardiac refractory period as lack of capture. EMI-induced reversion to the asynchronous mode can usually be eliminated as a cause if the problem of nonsensing persists in a 12-lead ECG that shows no signs of electric interference. Comparison of the current and baseline ECGs establishes the presence or absence of lead position changes, including perforation, as evidenced by shifts in the paced QRS vector and pacing artifact vector.* An x-ray examination provides confirmation of significant dislodgements. Insulation defects in the lead will result in vector changes in the pacing artifact but usually not in the paced QRS complex.

Application of a magnet should result in pacing without sensing. In most pacemakers magnet application alters the pacing rate (sometimes by only a few milliseconds), confirming that the reed switch is functioning and allowing one to eliminate the possibility of non-sensing caused by a stuck reed switch.

If inappropriate programing is thought to be the problem, it is a simple matter to reprogram the amplifier sensitivity and refractory period to restore sensing and to increase the stimulus intensity to restore capture. If such reprograming fails to resolve the problem or if the parameter settings required are not within normally accepted bounds, then inappropriate programing can be excluded.

Wire fracture can produce non-sensing and lack of capture, but it is generally accompanied by random resetting of the escape interval as the broken wire ends touch intermittently. An x-ray examination can sometimes be helpful in confirming wire fracture, but not all fractures are visible on the x-ray film. In this example the regularity of the escape intervals probably eliminates wire fracture as the cause of the problem.

At this point noninvasive procedures have been explored to evaluate the majority of potential causes for the reported

malfunctions. Threshold elevation, inadequate electrogram characteristics, and pulse generator failure all require invasive evaluation, although some noninvasive determinations can be obtained if the patient has a sophisticated multiprogrammable pulse generator. Some of these devices can telemeter the intracardiac electrogram, facilitating evaluation of sensing problems. In addition, some devices allow noninvasive measurement of lead impedance. They also allow the user to obtain noninvasive threshold measurements. Nevertheless, correction of sensing and pacing failure caused by any of these factors will require invasive procedures.

In the example cited, ECG evidence, shown in Fig. 11-14, indicates a lead dislodgement. Note the axis shift in the pacemaker stimulus artifact and in the paced QRS complexes. Lead placement is the most common cause of sensing and capture failures.

## TROUBLESHOOTING OF IMPLANTABLE CARDIOVERTER DEFIBRILLATORS[80-82]

Devices of the 1980s, with minimum programmability and telemetry, primarily required evaluation for early battery depletion and for discharges of the device when sustained ventricular tachycardia or fibrillation were thought not to have occurred. This proved difficult at times, since device discharges could be triggered by many things, including supraventricular dysrhythmias, lead system problems, myopotentials, interaction with an implanted pacemaker, or actual device malfunction.

Minimizing or preventing unnecessary discharges was important, however, since these shocks caused both physical discomfort and psychologic stress in some patients.

With their extensive programmability, devices of the 1990s will probably add a new dimension in this area, since detection of the desired dysrhythmia may be affected by the programmable parameters that are selected. Knowledgeable and skilled physicians, technicians, and nurses will be required to appropriately manage these devices and the patients in whom they are implanted.

*Digital ECG systems with low sampling rates cannot be used to determine the reliability of the vector of the pacemaker artifact.

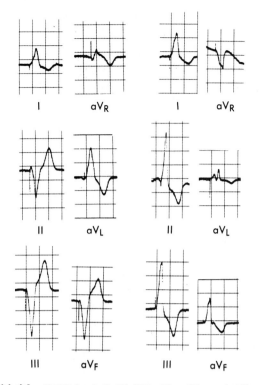

**Fig. 11-14** ECG leads I, II, III, aV_R, aV_L, and aV_F were recorded before *(left panel)* and after *(right panel)* pacemaker malfunction. VVI pacemaker developed sensing and capture problems. Note that the vector and amplitude of the spikes are different in the two 12-lead ECGs and that the generated QRS complexes also are different. This ECG example is most consistent with migration of the pacing electrode from its initial appropriate location in the right ventricular apex to a different position in the ventricle. This was the case, and the lead was repositioned.

## NURSING CARE OF PATIENTS WITH PERMANENT IMPLANTABLE PACEMAKERS AND IMPLANTABLE CARDIOVERTER DEFIBRILLATORS[83-88]

Nursing care of patients needing implantable pacemakers or cardioverter defibrillators encompasses both patients and their families and begins the moment the need for such a device is identified. Patients may have vastly different prior knowledge of these devices, ranging from having no knowledge at all to having a reasonably accurate understanding. But whatever their level of knowledge, thorough and accurate information presented in a clear and logical manner will help reassure the patient and family and stimulate acceptance of the need for the device, while letting the patient understand what life with it will be like.

Before the implant, the use of charts, drawings or models helps patients understand the parts of the implanted system and where they will be placed. Such visual aids also help patients understand how the heart functions and why the device chosen for them is necessary. Showing patients

a model of the actual device and leads to be implanted is often helpful, since patients may have very vague ideas regarding the size of the devices. These models, as well as the visual aids, are often available from various device manufacturers, sometimes at a nominal charge. Additional teaching aids such as slide series and materials written specifically for children are also usually available.

A patient booklet is usually packaged with each device, and extra copies can be obtained. Patients should be encouraged to read the booklet and to ask any questions they may have.

During any implantation procedure in which patients are fully conscious or only minimally sedated, the implant team should be careful of what they are saying, since their words can be heard and perhaps misinterpreted. Patients should be told ahead of time if there are specific things they will be asked to do during the procedure, such as coughing or deep breathing to help ensure that the lead has been securely stabilized. The absence of general anesthesia also means that patients should be told that they will be covered with surgical drapes, that their arms and legs will be secured, and that they should not move unless asked to do so. They should be told to indicate if they are in pain, such as when the device pocket is being created, so that additional local anesthesia can be given if necessary. In general, patients should be prepared for what they will see, feel, and hear, and medical and nursing personnel should be constantly attentive to minimize anxiety, to answer questions, and to reassure patients regarding the progress of the procedure.

Patients undergoing implantable cardioverter defibrillator placement are likely to be more heavily sedated or fully anesthetized, because in almost all cases it will be necessary to induce ventricular tachycardia and/or fibrillation to ensure that the device appropriately detects and terminates these rhythms. These patients may experience more stress than other patients in the preimplant period, as well as during the implant itself if they are partially awake. They may require extensive reassurance that these procedures are both safe and necessary, and that highly skilled people and equipment are available as needed to restore the normal functioning of their heart. In addition, the length of the procedure, normally considerably longer than that of a pacemaker implant, may cause additional stress and discomfort.

Postimplant nursing care is specific to the type of implant, the device system involved, the area where the patient is cared for, and the policies and procedures of the institution. Continuous ECG monitoring for a period of time helps ensure that the newly implanted device is functioning appropriately. In addition, a postoperative chest x-ray confirms proper positioning of the lead(s). The implant sites should also be checked to ensure that sutures are intact and drainage is not excessive. In some institutions restrictions are placed on body movement during the first several hours or days after implantation of a new lead system, and practices concerning length of hospitalization differ. Resumption of normal activities after device implantation varies from patient to patient, and depends to a large degree on the patient's state of health before the implant and the reason(s) a device was felt to be necessary. Patients should be encouraged to resume normal daily activities and recreational pursuits, gradually increasing the levels as their state of health permits.

Lifestyle adaptation, the most important aspect of which is regular follow-up care, should also be emphasized. Patients should have a thorough knowledge of why they now need to be seen or heard from regularly, and the type of follow-up chosen for them (clinic visits, transtelephonic monitoring, or a combination of both) should be fully explained to them. This is also the time to discuss the safe use of common electric devices such as microwave ovens, razors, electric toothbrushes, and hair dryers (all properly functioning household electric devices are generally considered safe to use), symptoms they might experience in the presence of strong continuous electric interference (commonly a return of their preimplant symptoms or an unexpected discharge of an implantable defibrillator), and what should be done if this occurs (move away from or stop using the device in question and then telephone their medical contact person). Patients who have previously been using or working with more complex electric devices on the job or for leisure activities may need special information. Such devices might include welding equipment, automobile engines, or power tools. If a patient must continue using such equipment, the manufacturer of the patient's device can be asked to assess specific situations, determine if continued use of the equipment in question is safe or if it can be modified to ensure its safe use. In general, use of electric devices by patients with implanted pacemakers or cardioverter defibrillators does not present problems unless the electric signals generated by the equipment are interpreted by the device's sensing circuits as being generated by the heart. Depending on the type of device implanted, this could then result in inappropriate inhibition of the implanted device or inappropriate triggering, especially in antitachycardia pacemakers and implantable defibrillators. But since devices differ from one manufacturer to another, and since various electric devices generate different signals, individual assessment of specific situations is essential, and it is important not to assume that patients with implanted pacemakers or defibrillators are automatically restricted in their use of certain electric devices.

Some patients may enjoy participating in clubs specifically designed for pacemaker or implantable cardioverter defibrillator recipients, or receiving newsletters and magazines designed for them. Medical and nursing personnel involved in caring for patients with these devices should therefore become familiar with what is available in their communities. Information can be obtained from local heart associations and from device manufacturers. Patients should also be encouraged to carry with them at all times the identification card issued by the manufacturer of their devices, and other medical identification information if appropriate. This is particularly important when traveling, since implanted electric devices can sometimes trigger airport security systems. In addition, should adjustment of device parameters become necessary for any reason, the device identification card will enable medical and nursing personnel to accurately identify the implanted device and quickly locate the appropriate equipment needed to reprogram it. If external defibrillation is required, it is essential that defibrillation paddles not be placed directly over an implanted device, and that assessment of the device be made as soon as possible after external defibrillation has occurred. This includes verification of the device's programed parameters, as well as verification of appropriate pacing and sensing, which in most cases should not be affected by the external defibrillation.

## SUMMARY

Implantable pacemakers of the 1990s are highly reliable and sophisticated devices that have been modified and perfected in over three decades of use. They now offer most patients in whom they are implanted the opportunity for a completely normal lifestyle, with minimum requirements for follow-up by medical personnel. Over one million people worldwide now benefit from these remarkable devices.

Implantable cardioverter defibrillators, on the other hand, are just beginning to enter widespread use, and the decade of the 1990s will offer major improvements in these devices, resulting in smaller, more easily implantable systems and more widely applicable indications for use. Major issues remain, including cost-effectiveness, complexity, and the training of personnel in appropriate management of patients. However, these services offer the hope of prolonging life in a group of patients for whom there have been few options in the past.

## REFERENCES

1. Elmquist R and Senning A: An implantable pacemaker for the heart, proceedings of the second international conference of medical-electrical engineers, London, 1959, Iliffe & Sons, Ltd.
2. Zoll P and Linenthal A: Long-term electrical pacemakers for Stokes-Adams disease, Circulation 22:341, 1960.
3. Mirowski M and others: Termination of malignant ventricular arrhythmias with an implanted automatic defibrillator in human beings, N Engl J Med 303:322, 1980.
4. Nisam S and others: AICD clinical update: first decade, initial 10,000 patients (Abstract), Rev Europ Technol Biomed 12:3, 1990.
5. Parsonnet V, Bernstein A, and Galasso D: Cardiac pacing practices in the United States in 1985, Am J Cardiol 62(1):71, 1988.
6. Zipes DP and Duffin E: Cardiac pacemakers. In Braunwald E, editor: Heart disease: a textbook of cardiovascular medicine, ed 3, Philadelphia, 1988, WB Saunders Co.
7. Sutton R, Perrins J, and Citron P: Physiological cardiac pacing, PACE 3(2):207, 1980.

8. Osborn MJ and Holmes DR: Antitachycardia pacing, Clin Prog Electrophysiol Pacing 3(4):239, 1985.

9. Duffin E and Zipes DP: Chronic electrical control of tachyarrhythmia. In Mandel WJ: Cardiac arrhythmias, their mechanisms, diagnosis and management, Philadelphia, 1987, JB Lippincott.

10. Zipes DP: Electrical therapy of cardiac arrhythmias (editorial), N Engl J Med 309:1179, 1983.

11. Akhtar M and others: NASPE ad hoc committee on guidelines for cardiac electrophysiological studies, PACE 8(4):611, 1985.

12. Bernstein A and others: The NASPE/BPEG generic pacemaker code for antibradyarrhythmia and adaptive-rate pacing and antitachyarrhythmia devices, PACE 10(4):794, 1987.

13. Nathan D, Center S, and Wu C: An implantable synchronous pacemaker for the long-term correction of complete heart block, Am J Cardiol 11:362, 1963.

14. Kruse I, Ryden L, and Duffin E: Clinical evaluation of atrial synchronous ventricular inhibited pacemakers, PACE 3(6):641, 1980.

15. Berkovits B, Castellanos A, and Lemberg L: Bifocal demand pacing, Circulation 39:44, 1969.

16. Funke HD: Three years experience in optimized sequential cardiac pacing, Stimucoeur 9(1):26, 1981.

17. Fananapazir L and others: Atrial synchronized ventricular pacing: contribution of the chronotropic response to improved exercise performance, PACE 6(3):601, 1983.

18. Humen D and others: Activity-sensing, rate-responsive pacing: improvement in myocardial performance with exercise, PACE 8(1):52, 1985.

19. Rossi P and others: Physiological sensitivity of respiratory dependent cardiac pacing: 4-year follow up, PACE 11(9):1267, 1988.

20. Lau CP and others: Rate responsive pacing with a pacemaker that detects respiratory rate (biorate), Clin Cardiol 11:318, 1988.

21. Lau CP and others: Initial clinical experience with a minute ventilation sensing rate modulated pacemaker: improvements in exercise capacity and symptomatology, PACE 11(11):1815, 1988.

22. Rickards AF, and Norman J: Relation between QT interval and heart rate: new design of physiological adaptive cardiac pacemaker, Br Heart J 45:56, 1981.

23. Fananapazir L and others: Reliability of the evoked response in determining the paced ventricular rate and performance of the QT or rate responsive (TX) pacemaker, PACE 8(5):701, 1985.

24. Goicolea de Ore A and others: Rate responsive pacing: clinical experience, PACE 8(3):322, 1985.

25. Fearnot NE and others: Increasing cardiac rate by measurement of right ventricular temperature, PACE 7(6):1240, 1984.

26. Sharma AD and others: Physiological pacing based on beat to beat of right ventricular dp/dt initial feasibility studies in man (abstract), J Am Coll Cardiol 7:3A, 1986.

27. Sutton R and others: Ventricular rate responsive pacing using the first derivative of right ventricular pressure on a sensor (abstract), J Am Coll Cardiol 11:167, 1988.

28. Wirtzfeld A and others: Regulation of pacing rate by variations of mixed venous oxygen saturation, PACE 7(6):1257, 1984.

29. Chirife R: Physiological principles of a new method for rate responsive pacing using the preejection interval, PACE 11(11):1545, 1988.

30. Salo RW and others: Continuous ventricular volume assessment for diagnosis and pacemaker control, PACE 7(7):1267, 1984.

31. Paul V and others: Closed loop control of rate adaptive pacing: clinical assessment of a system analyzing the ventricular depolarization gradient, PACE 12(12):1896, 1989.

32. Cannilli L and others: Preliminary experience with the pH-triggered pacemaker, PACE 1(4):448, 1978.

33. Fisher JD and others: Long-term efficacy of antitachycardia pacing for supra-ventricular and ventricular tachycardia, Am J Cardiol 60:1311, 1987.

34. Fisher JD, Kim SD, Mercando AD: Electrical devices for treatment of arrhythmias, Am J Cardiol 61:45A, 1988.

35. Waldecker B and others: Importance of modes of electrical termination of ventricular tachycardia for the selection of implantable antitachycardia devices, Am J Cardiol 57:150, 1986.

36. Camm AJ and Ward DE: Pacemaker treatment of tachyarrhythmias. In Iwa T and Fontaine G, editors: Cardiac arrhythmias: recent progress in investigation and management, Amsterdam, 1988, Elsevier Science Publishers B.V. (Biomedical Division).

37. Fisher JD and others: Implantable pacers for tachycardia termination: stimulation techniques and long-term efficacy, PACE 9:1325, 1986.

38. Fisher JD and others: Long-term efficacy of antitachycardia pacing for supraventricular and ventricular tachycardias, Am J Cardiol 60:1311, 1987.

39. de Belder MA and Camm AJ: Implantable cardioverter-defibrillators (ICDs) 1989: how close are we to the ideal device? Clin Cardiol 12:339, 1989.

40. Parsonnet V and Rodgers T: The present status of programmable pacemakers, Prog Cardiovasc Dis 23(6):401, 1981.

41. Furman S and Pannizzo F: Output programmability and reduction of secondary intervention after pacemaker implantation, J Thorac Cardiovasc Surg 81(5):713, 1981.

42. Hayes DI and others: Initial and early follow-up assessment of the clinical efficacy of a multiparameter-programmable pulse generator, PACE 4(4):417, 1981.

43. Billhardt RA and others: Successful management of pacing system malfunctions without surgery: the role of programmable pulse generators, PACE 5(5):675, 1982.

44. Mirowski M and others: Clinical treatment of life-threatening ventricular tachyarrhythmias with the automatic implantable defibrillator, Am Heart J 102:265, 1981.

45. Watkins L Jr, and others: Trials of the automatic implantable defibrillator in man, J Thorac Cardiovasc Surg 86:381, 1983.

46. Manz M, Gerckens U, and Luderitz B: Erroneous discharge from an implanted automatic defibrillator during supraventricular tachyarrhythmia induced ventricular fibrillation, Am J Cardiol 57:343, 1986.

47. Kelly PA and others: The automatic implantable cardioverterdefibrillator: efficacy, complications and survival in patients with malignant ventricular arrhythmias, J Am Coll Cardiol 11:1278, 1988.

48. Parsonnet V: Cardiac pacing and pacemakers, VVI, power sources for implantable pacemakers, Part I, Am Heart J 94(4):517, 1977.

49. Brennen KR and others: A capacity rating system for cardiac pacemaker batteries, J Power sources 5:25, 1980.

50. Bilitch M and others: Performance of cardiac pacemaker pulse generators, PACE 11(3):371, 1988.

51. Greatbach W: Metal electrodes in bioengineering, CRC Crit Rev Bioeng 5(1):1, 1981.

52. Smyth NPD: Techniques of implantation: atrial and ventricular, thoracotomy and transvenous, Prog Cardiovasc Dis 23(6):435, 1981.

53. Littleford P, Parsonnet V, and Spector S: Method for the rapid and atraumatic insertion of permanent endocardial pacemaker electrodes through the subclavian vein, Am J Cardiol 43:980, 1979.

54. Parsonnet V and others: Transvenous insertion of double sets of permanent electrodes, JAMA 243(1):62, 1980.

55. Parsonnet V: Routine implantation of permanent transvenous pacemaker electrodes in both chambers: a technique whose time has come, PACE 4(1):109, 1981.

56. Furman S, Pannizzo F, and Campo I: Comparison of active and passive adhering leads for endocardial pacing, PACE 2(4):417, 1979.

57. Furman S, Pannizzo F, and Campo I: Comparison of active and passive adhering leads for endocardial pacing. Part 2, PACE 4(1):78, 1981.

58. Kertes P and others: Comparison of lead complications with poly-

urethane tines, silicone rubber tined and wedge tip leads: clinical experience with 822 ventricular endocardial leads, PACE 6(5):957, 1983.

59. Timmis GC and others: The evolution of low threshold leads, Clin Prog Pacing Electrophysiol 1:313, 1983.

60. Heineman F, David M, and Helland J: Clinical performance of a pacing lead with a platinized "target tip" electrode (abstract), PACE 7:471, 1984.

61. Timmis GC and others: A new steroid-eluting low threshold pacemaker lead. In Steinbeck K, Editor: Proceedings of the seventh world symposium on cardiac pacing, Vienna, 1983.

62. Kruse IM, and Terpstra B: Acute and long-term atrial and ventricular stimulation thresholds with a steroid-eluting electrode, PACE 8:45, 1985.

63. Timmis GC and others: Late effects of a steroid-eluting porous titanium pacemaker lead electrode in man (abstract), PACE 7:479, 1984.

64. King KH and others: A steroid-eluting endocardial pacing lead for treatment of exit block, Am Heart J 106:1438, 1983.

65. deFeyter P and others: Permanent cardiac pacing with sutureless myocardial electrodes: experience in the first one hundred patients, PACE 3(2):144, 1980.

66. Zoll P, Zoll R, and Belgard A: External noninvasive electric stimulation of the heart, Crit Care Med 9(5):393, 1981.

67. Furman S, Hurzeler P, and Mehra R: Cardiac pacing and pacemakers. IV. Threshold of cardiac stimulation, Am Heart J 94(1):115, 1977.

68. Furman S, Hurzeler P, and DeCaprio V: Cardiac pacing and pacemakers. III. Sensing the cardiac electrogram, Am Heart J 93(6):794, 1977.

69. Reid PR and others: Clinical evaluation of the internal automatic cardioverter-defibrillator in survivors of sudden cardiac death, Am J Cardiol 51:1608, 1983.

70. Mirowski M: The automatic implantable cardioverter-defibrillator: an overview, J Am Coll Cardiol 6:461, 1985.

71. Mirowski M and others: Recent clinical experience with the automatic implantable cardioverter-defibrillator, Med Instrum 20:285, 1986.

72. Saksena AS and Parsonnet V: Implantation of a cardioverter defibrillator without thoracotomy using a triple electrode system, JAMA 259:69, 1988.

73. Saksena S and Calvo R: Transvenous cardioversion and defibrillation of ventricular tachyarrythmias: Current status and future directions, PACE 8:715, 1985.

74. MacGregor D and others: Computer assisted reporting system for the follow-up of patients with cardiac pacemakers, PACE 3(5):568, 1980.

75. Winkle RA and Thomas A: The automatic implantable cardioverter defibrillator: the US experience. In Brugada P and Wellens HJJ, editors: Cardiac arrhythmias: where to go from here? Mount Kisco, NY, 1987, Futura Publishing Co Inc.

76. Furman S: Cardiac pacing and pacemakers. VI. Analysis of pacemaker malfunction, Am Heart J 94(3):378, 1977.

77. Barold S: Modern cardiac pacing, Mt. Kisco, NY, 1985, Futura Publishing Co, Inc.

78. Mond HG: The cardiac pacemaker: function and malfunction, New York, 1983, Grune & Stratton.

79. Adler S and others: Advances in single-chamber pacemaker diagnostic data, PACE 9:1141, 1986.

80. Echt DS: Potential hazards of implanted devices for the electrical control of tachyarrhythmias, PACE 7(II):580, 1984.

81. Echt DS and others: Clinical experience, complications, and survival in 70 patients with the automatic implantable cardioverter/defibrillator, Circulation 71:289, 1985.

82. Yee R, Sharma A, and Klein G: Therapeutic electrical devices in the management of sudden cardiac death. In Kostis J and Sanders M: The prevention of sudden cardiac death, New York, 1990, John Wiley & Sons, Inc.

83. Moak E: Perioperative implications of pacemaker implantation, Today's OR Nurse 12(5):19, 1990.

84. Andrews CA: Cardiac pacing: state of the art, J Am Acad Physician Assist 1(6):420, 1988.

85. Porterfield LM, Porterfield JG, and DuVall C: Insertion of a permanent pacemaker, Crit Care Nurse 7(4):30, 1987.

86. Porterfield L and Porterfield JG: What you need to know about today's pacemakers, RN 50(3):44, 1987.

87. Cooper DK, Valladares BK, and Putterman LG: Care of the patient with the automatic implantable cardioverter defibrillator: a guide for nurses, Heart Lung 16(6, part 1):640, 1987.

88. Veseth-Rogers J: A practical approach to teaching the automatic implantable cardioverter-defibrillator patient, J Cardiovasc Nurs 4(2):7, 1990.

# CHAPTER 12

# Surgical Management of Coronary Heart Disease

Janine M. Neeley
Mary Sue Craft
Martha Branyon

When medical management no longer controls the pain and related sequelae of coronary heart disease, additional intervention may be necessary. This chapter will describe the care of patients requiring open heart surgery, cardiac transplantation, and the use of ventricular assist devices in these settings.

Recent medical advances have increased the options available to individuals with coronary heart disease. The focus of therapy has changed from observation of symptoms and reaction to complications, to immediate aggressive invasive intervention. The recently developed major medical therapies that have caused this change in focus include percutaneous transluminal coronary angioplasty (PTCA), vascular stenting, atherectomy, laser, and thrombolytic agents.

## CORONARY ARTERY BYPASS SURGERY
### Indications for Surgery

The decision to perform coronary artery bypass graft (CABG) surgery is based on what is possible and desirable to achieve, as opposed to what can be accomplished by medical therapy alone. When improvement in the patient's quality of life is foreseeable with surgical intervention, then coronary artery surgery is an effective alternative to medical management.

Coronary artery bypass graft surgery remains a major intervention in the treatment of individuals with coronary heart disease, with approximately 332,000 procedures performed in 1987. More than 2,000,000 Americans who have had CABG surgery are alive.[1] The desired outcomes of surgery are decreased symptomatology, improved quality of life, and increased longevity. These outcomes are accomplished by returning as near normal perfusion as possible to the myocardium.

Selection criteria remain controversial. In general, the decision for surgical intervention is based on hemodynamic and clinical parameters as well as location and severity of the lesion. Seventy-five percent occlusion of the cross-sectional area in the left coronary artery, or of all three main coronary arteries, will jeopardize a large area of the myocardium. The more proximal the lesion in the artery,

the greater the chance of massive infarction. The least disputed indication for surgery is angiographic confirmation of greater than 50% stenosis of the left main coronary artery.[2]

A principal indication for CABG is symptom severity, such as chronic disabling angina nonresponsive to vigorous medical management. Debate continues over angina as an indication for surgery. The amount of angina that is disabling is subjective and depends on the individual and his or her lifestyle. For example, most individuals in their 80s can accept activity restrictions better than those in their 30s and 40s. Additionally, noncompliance or varying physician protocols can prevent maximum medical management for the ischemic patient.

Unstable angina is also an indication for CABG. Patients with this syndrome have pain at rest, increased severity of a previously stable angina pattern, and/or a new onset angina that progresses rapidly in severity. These individuals are candidates for surgical intervention since they have low mortality at surgery and experience excellent symptom relief.[3]

Thrombolytic therapy is available at most hospitals for immediate treatment of acute myocardial infarction (MI). This medical therapy, coupled with relatively high operative mortality risks for patients with evolving infarctions, has allowed the emergent CABG surgery to be reserved for the patient with life-threatening complications. Acute congestive heart failure secondary to papillary muscle or ventricular septal rupture and ventricular aneurysm will necessitate emergency CABG.[4]

The operative mortality for the majority of patients requiring CABG is less than 1% in most centers. Factors such as advanced age, left ventricular dysfunction, number of arteries affected, location of the lesions, and incomplete revascularization are associated with higher surgical mortality.[5]

Occlusion rates in patients revascularized with saphenous vein grafts are approximately 25% the first year and over 50% 10 years after surgery.[6] These alarmingly high occlusion rates have resulted in use of the internal mammary artery (IMA) for revascularization when possible.

The IMA graft patency rate has been reported to be 88% at 1 year and 84% at 10 years.[2] In addition to superior short- and long-term patency, the patient is spared a leg incision. There are limitations to the use of the IMA graft. These include small size in some patients (especially females), vulnerability to atherosclerosis, greater operative time compared with a saphenous graft, limited access area, and increased postoperative bleeding.

The majority of patients undergo revascularization using both the saphenous vein and IMA grafts. The IMA is preferentially used to bypass left main coronary artery occlusions. The saphenous veins are then used to bypass occlusions to the remaining coronary arteries.

### Diagnosis

History and physical examination. Successful cardiac surgery is predicated on a comprehensive, organized preoperative medical history and examination. This information helps in the formation of tentative diagnoses as well as in the definition of therapeutic goals. Components of the medical history include identifying data, source of referral, present illness, past medical history, family history, psychosocial history, and reviewing all body systems.

During the history-taking, particular attention should be paid to medication usage because the patient with coronary artery disease frequently has been taking many types of medication to control symptoms, prevent complications, and improve cardiac function. Whether diuretics, cardiotonics, antidysrhythmics, antibiotics, antihypertensives, steroids, or anticoagulants are being used or not is information that is critical to include in the patient record. Drug sensitivities or allergic reactions should be noted and fully described.

A thorough, systematic physical examination will establish the patient's baseline as well as identify any factors capable of affecting the outcome of the surgery. For each body system assessed, detailed documentation describing any anatomic or physiologic abnormality must follow. Not only is it of paramount importance to evaluate the patient's cardiac function, it is also essential to evaluate the patient's respiratory, neurologic, gastrointestinal, and renal status. The skin and musculoskeletal systems offer important clues about the general health and nutrition of such a patient.

Nothing in the physical examination should be overlooked as unimportant. Most practitioners can recall situations when what was considered "insignificant" before surgery became of "critical" importance in the postoperative management of the patient. Assessment of oral hygiene, for example, may lead to the discovery of recent major dental repairs and the potential for oral infections. Incomplete wound healing or skin abrasions may be deemed risky enough to warrant postponing elective surgery until healing is complete. The use of illicit drugs, if undetected, can present major problems in postoperative pain control.

---

## COMMON LABORATORY STUDIES

**GENERAL**

Blood typing and crossmatch

**PULMONARY**

Arterial blood gases
Pulmonary function tests

**CARDIAC**

Serum enzymes (SGOT, LDH, CK isoenzymes)

**RENAL-METABOLIC**

Urinalysis
BUN
Creatinine
Urine electrolytes
Serum electrolytes
Serum lipids
Serum cholesterol
FBS

**LIVER**

Serum bilirubin
Serum proteins
Alkaline phosphatase
SGOT
LDH
SGPT

**HEMATOLOGIC**

CBC (RBC, WBC, Hgb, Hct)
Platelet count
PT
PTT
Fibrinogin

---

Laboratory studies. The box at right lists commonly performed laboratory studies for an adult patient admitted for cardiac surgery. The schedule of tests should be modified according to specific needs. Not every test should be performed on each patient and additional tests may be required for some. In general, preoperative blood studies assess formed elements, oxygen-carrying capacity, and coagulation tendencies.

Specific tests for hepatic, renal, pulmonary, metabolic, and cardiac function provide information about organ physiology for postoperative comparison.[7] A general pattern of improvement in hepatic and renal function, for example, is anticipated following cardiac surgery because congestive heart failure is reduced and cardiac output is improved. Cardiac enzymes, which indicate injured myocardial cells, assist in determining the significance of any postoperative angina and the need for further diagnostic tests. Pulmonary pathology requires careful follow-up, since normal pulmonary functioning is interrupted during surgery and residual effects of cardiopulmonary bypass may persist to some degree in the immediate postoperative period.

Chest x-ray examination. A baseline chest x-ray (CXR) examination is requested immediately before surgery whether or not previous films exist. Visualization of the heart yields valuable information about overall cardiac size and function. Analysis of the lung fields and pulmonary vessels can detect changes in pulmonary vasculature indicative of venous or arterial hypertension and increased or decreased blood flow.[7] Identification of a pneumothorax, pleural effusion, or atelectasis is very significant in preoperative management and, if necessary, should be treated before proceeding with surgery. Many patients having coronary bypass surgery have had a history of cigarette-smoking, and the CXR examination is vital in assessing pulmonary changes that would lead to inadequate ventilation and $CO_2$ retention postoperatively.

Electrocardiography. An ECG is performed on all patients before cardiac surgery because any disturbances in rate, rhythm, and conduction are noteworthy, as are changes indicative of ischemia. An ECG may also reveal any evidence of digitalis or other cardiotonic drug toxicity (that is, atrial or ventricular dysrhythmias, varying degrees of heart block), which should be remedied before surgical intervention. A baseline ECG is of particular value during postoperative management as a comparison for evaluating the electrophysiologic state of the heart.

Echocardiography. Echocardiography (echo) is used to study cardiac function noninvasively. Complications as a result of an MI, functional effects of ischemia, presence of a pericardial effusion, and congenital defects are examples of conditions that can be assessed in the preoperative patient.

Arteriography. Coronary arteriography provides a means of accurately determining the presence and extent of coronary artery disease. Arteriography provides visualization of the coronary arteries including the site and severity of stenotic lesions; characteristics of the distal coronary vessels in terms of size, disease state, and the amount of viable myocardium; an estimate of coronary blood flow; and information about collateral vessels and their functional importance.[8] Measurement of left ventricular pressure at rest or after introduction of pharmacologic agents is made possible with left ventricular catheterization, which also provides a visual analysis of wall motion, ventricular volume, and ejection fraction.

Wall motion can be further evaluated by the addition of stress (such as with atrial pacing). Left ventricular contraction can be augmented by nitrates or catecholamines to enhance identification of wall segments having potential for improved function following revascularization. Correlation of the coronary arteriogram and left ventriculogram permits delineation of bypassable coronary arteries.[8]

The information is necessary in determining operability, operative risk, and probability of operative success.

## Preoperative Management

Preoperative teaching. Preoperative teaching is done by the members of the surgical and nursing staff involved in the patient's care. Each covers information from his or her area of expertise: the surgeon reviews the patient's condition, operative plans, potential risks, and expected outcomes; the anesthesiologist discusses the type of anesthetic and the events that will take place during induction and immediately after surgery; the nurse describes postoperative nursing care, procedures, and monitoring devices.

Patient and family teaching begins on admission and continues throughout hospitalization and discharge. Effective teaching must be geared to the patient's level of understanding; teaching must be designed to alleviate anxiety rather than induce it. Teaching cardiac surgery patients is highly individualized and should be timed according to when the patient is ready to listen and learn. Family members or others who play an important part in the patient's life need to be included in the teaching sessions, since they will provide psychologic and emotional support during the recovery phase. Teaching sessions can be complemented by the use of audiovisual aids such as models of the heart, slide presentations, and visits to the intensive care unit.

Preparation for surgery. Skin preparation for surgery starts with a shower using a germicidal agent (such as chlorhexidine gluconate [Hibiclens]) to decrease skin bacteria. On the evening before surgery, the patient is shaved from chin to toes to decrease contaminaton from hair. Care is taken to avoid nicks or skin abrasions because these serve as potential sites of infection.

The night before surgery the patient is kept NPO. A laxative or enema is used to empty the lower bowel and prevent a bowel movement during the immediate postoperative phase. A mild sedative is made available to the patient the night before surgery to reduce anxiety and promote sleep.

Medications. All patient medications should be evaluated before surgery. There are varying opinions regarding when and if preoperative medication should be discontinued. The practice of administering most medicines up to the time of surgery is gaining popularity; therefore the following suggestions should be considered while the needs of each patient are determined individually.

Antibiotics. Although the value of prophylactic antibiotics is debatable and their effectiveness is difficult to establish, physicians at many centers believe that their use is warranted in cardiac surgery.[8] Administration of a broad-spectrum agent such as cephalosporin is begun the night before surgery, when the patient is on call to the OR and then continued postoperatively until invasive lines and tubes are discontinued. This protocol ensures that the antibiotic reaches the required blood level during the period when the patient is most vulnerable to infection.

**Digoxin.** Digoxin is commonly administered up to the time of surgery. There is little consensus in the medical literature about prophylactic digitalization of preoperative patients, but the drug is advantageous to patients who suffer heart failure or experience atrial fibrillation. A short-acting preparation such as digoxin permits more readily controllable drug levels than other preparations and is not washed out or removed from the tissues during cardiopulmonary bypass.

**Diuretics.** Fluid restriction is preferable to diuretic therapy in the preoperative treatment of milder forms of fluid retention because of the tendency for diuretics to produce electrolyte abnormalities. If fluid restriction alone is inadequate, then a diuretic is administered, furosemide (Lasix) being the drug of choice.

**Propranolol.** Beta-blocking agents such as propranolol (Inderal) are usually continued up to the time of surgery.

**Calcium channel blockers.** Because the therapeutic potential for verapamil and nifedipine extends to the management of cardiac dysrhythmias, angina, hypertension, cardiomyopathy, and MI, its continuation until surgery may be indicated, but the decision is made on an individual basis.

**Warfarin.** Anticoagulants are discontinued several days before surgery to allow time for clotting mechanisms to return to normal.

**Aspirin.** Aspirin can interfere with coagulation by preventing normal platelet aggregation, which is responsible for the formation of a platelet plug. The effect of aspirin persists for the life of the platelet, so it is desirable to withhold aspirin administration for at least 1 week before surgery.

## Intraoperative Management

**Anesthesia and monitoring.** The health status of the patient and type of cardiac surgery to be performed determine the anesthetic needs of a patient. Anesthesia for cardiovascular surgical procedures must provide analgesia, unconsciousness, muscular relaxation, suppression of autonomic and endocrine responses, hemodynamic stability, and support of vital organ functions.[9] A combination of inhalation and intravenous agents is used to achieve these effects. Side effects of these agents are mostly dose dependent. Severity of the side effects is lessened when agents are used in combination.[9] The reader is referred to current cardiovascular anesthesia journals and texts for a detailed list of the following agents, their advantages and disadvantages: inhalation agents (e.g., halothane, enflurane, and isoflurane ) and intravenous preparations (e.g., morphine sulfate, fentanyl, diazepam, pancuronium, and vecuronium).

Continuous ECG monitoring is required to detect myocardial ischemia and dysrhythmias during surgery. Intra-arterial, intraatrial, central venous, and pulmonary artery pressures are used to guide intraoperative management. Intravenous access is required for administration of fluids and medications. To alleviate gastric distention, a nasogastric tube is inserted and the patient's urine output is monitored via a Foley catheter. Once the patient is intubated, arterial blood gases and serum electrolytes are measured frequently. The monitoring devices and the information they provide are constantly evaluated to detect complications and identify potential trends.

**Cardiopulmonary bypass.** Perioperative MI remains the most common cause of morbidity and mortality following technically successful cardiac operations.[10] At present, the incidence of infarction ranges from 2% to 4%. The incidence has decreased over time because of advances in preoperative medical management, cardiac anesthesia techniques, and myocardial protection techniques.[11] Myocardial protection is accomplished by the use of cardioplegia and cardiopulmonary bypass.[12]

Cardioplegic fluids are used throughout the period of cardiopulmonary bypass. The fluids may vary in composition. Electrolytes (e.g., potassium, calcium, magnesium, and sodium), albumin, blood, and oxygenated crystalloids are a few elements incorporated.[12] The objectives of cardioplegia are to arrest the heart quickly and safely, create an environment of continued energy production, and counteract ischemia. The cardioplegic fluids accomplish these objectives by temperature (0° to 4° C), potassium level, and presence of buffers for neutralization of ischemic acidosis.

Cardiopulmonary bypass (CPB) is employed during intracardiac surgical procedures. CPB has three main structural elements: (1) a pump, (2) an oxygenator with reservoir function, and (3) plastic circuitry[12] (Fig. 12-1). Venous blood is drained into the oxygenator by one to two cannulae placed in the venae cavae or right atrium. Arterial blood is returned to the patient through a single cannula inserted into the ascending aorta or the femoral artery (Fig. 12-2). During bypass, blood is circulated continuously through the pump where it is filtered, temperature regulated, and oxygenated.

The purposes of CPB are to provide adequate tissue perfusion, oxygenation, and a dry, quiet operative field.[12] These purposes are accomplished by three methods: hemodilution, hypothermia, and anticoagulation.[12] Hemodilution decreases blood viscosity, systemic vascular resistance, hemolysis, and use of blood products, and it promotes postoperative diuresis.[13] Hemodilution can potentially increase extracellular water and interstitial fluid.[14] Shifting of the fluids between the interstitial and intravascular spaces occurs, particularly in the immediate postoperative period.

Hypothermia is achieved by decreasing the patient's core body temperature. Lowering of the body temperature also decreases myocardial and body metabolic needs.[12]

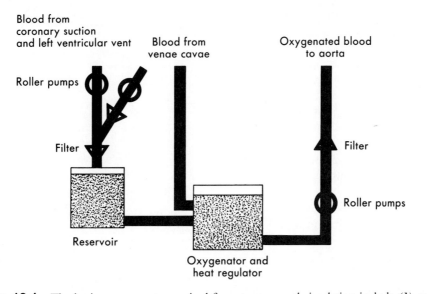

Blood from
coronary suction
and left ventricular vent

Blood from
venae cavae

Oxygenated blood
to aorta

Roller pumps

Filter

Filter

Roller pumps

Reservoir

Oxygenator and
heat regulator

**Fig. 12-1**   The basic components required for extracorporeal circulation include *(1)* connecting tubing and roller pumps for venous blood flow from the patient; *(2)* an aspirating system for retrieving blood from the surgical field; *(3)* filters within the system to remove particulate material, lipids, and gaseous emboli; *(4)* a reservoir; *(5)* an oxygenator for gas exchange; *(6)* a heat exchanger for controlling blood temperature; and *(7)* connecting tubing and roller pumps to return oxygenated blood to the patient. This system delivers a nonpulsatile blood flow with an ideal mean pressure between 50 and 85 mm Hg.

Anticoagulation reduces the sludging of blood in the capillaries, blood cell trauma, and the incidence of thromboemboli.[15] The plastic circuitry of the CPB is composed of antithromboembolic materials and is fully heparinized prior to surgery. Before the initiation of CPB, the patient receives 300 units/kg of heparin to maintain anticoagulation. Reversal is achieved with protamine sulfate. Anaphylactic reactions to administration of protamine sulfate have been noted intraoperatively and postoperatively and are sometimes fatal.[16]

There are a multitude of clinical sequelae of CPB.[12,15,17,18] Hypertension can occur because of the rise in intrinsic catecholamine levels. Myocardial depression, transient sinus bradycardia, shifts in serum electrolytes, and acidosis can result from prolonged CPB. Hemolysis of blood cells can lead to anemia and bleeding. Bleeding can result from inadequate reversal of anticoagulation, heparin rebound, destruction of platelets, and platelet dysfunction. Respiratory function may be compromised when the patient is on CPB. The reduction in pulmonary activity leads to alveolar collapse, retention of secretions, sequestration of blood in the pulmonary capillaries, pulmonary edema, and anoxia. High serum glucose levels may be noted postoperatively because of the initial suppression of insulin release.

General cerebral dysfunction secondary to CPB is related to two factors: inadequate perfusion and air embolism. Cerebral dysfunction such as severe focal strokes or

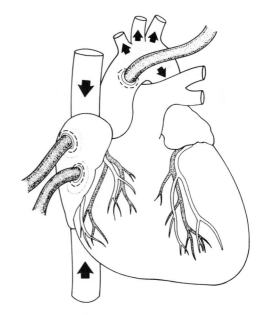

**Fig. 12-2**   Venous connections remove blood from the right heart; arterial connections return oxygenated blood via the ascending aorta while on cardiopulmonary bypass.

coma occurs in 1% of patients. Elderly patients who may have coexistent carotid artery disease are at greater risk.

**Revascularization.** As the median sternal incision is made, the saphenous vein is visualized, ligated, and tested for leakage.[11,12] The decision regarding use of the saphenous vein or the IMA for the grafts will be based on the availability and adequacy of the saphenous veins, prior cardiac surgical procedures, and vessel durability.[12] Use of saphenous vein grafts requires anastomosis to the distal vessel and to the aorta. The IMA is anastomosed directly to any of the anterior or lateral ventricular coronary vessels.[12]

On completion of the grafting, CPB is gradually discontinued. Care is taken to evacuate all air from the aorta and vessels prior to elimination of CPB. An anterior and a posterior mediastinal chest tube, a pleural chest tube (i.e., IMA graft used), along with intraatrial pressure lines, and epicardial pacing wires are inserted. On completion of these procedures, the sternum is wired together with stainless steel sutures, the skin is approximated, and a sterile occlusive dressing is applied.

## Postoperative Management

The surgeon and anesthesiologist transport patients from the operating room directly to the recovery room or intensive care unit. There patients are made hemodynamically stable, extubated, and freed from invasive monitoring lines.[19-21] During the immediate postoperative period, a subsystems approach is used to achieve the primary goal: maintenance of adequate cardiac output.[20]

On admission, the patient is connected to the ventilator. A continuous ECG, preferably lead II, is displayed on the monitor. All arterial and atrial pressure lines are assessed for patency, calibrated, and zeroed to the transducer system and monitors. Breath sounds are auscultated, and arterial blood gases are obtained to assess the adequacy of ventilation.

Mediastinal and pleural chest tubes are connected to continuous suction at $-25$ cm $H_2O$ pressure. Bleeding from the chest tubes is closely observed and measured via a marked drainage receptacle. Patency of tubes can be achieved through correct suction pressure and milking. Because of the increase in negative pressure caused by stripping, it is done only in times of emergency.[19,22] Urinary output is assessed via a Foley catheter. A nasogastric tube is assessed for placement and connected to low suction or to gravity.

All intravenous lines are assessed for patency and location. Fluids and medication infusions are checked and regulated as prescribed.[19] Atrial and ventricular pacing wires are insulated and connected to a temporary pacemaker.[23] Blood is drawn for laboratory work including cardiac enzymes, complete blood count, clotting studies, and electrolyte levels. A thorough head-to-toe assessment is performed by the admitting nurse to establish the pa-

---

## POTENTIAL NURSING DIAGNOSES

- Alteration in circulation related to decreased cardiac output
- Alteration in circulation related to an excess/deficit of fluid volume
- Alteration in oxygenation related to impaired gas exchange
- Alteration in body temperature related to hypothermia
- Infection related to invasive monitoring lines
- Alteration of skin integrity related to immobility
- Alteration in vocal communication related to presence of endotracheal tube
- Alteration in comfort related to acute pain after surgery

tient's baseline condition and identify potential nursing diagnoses (see the box above).

**Cardiovascular subsystem.** Optimum cardiovascular performance provides adequate cardiac output to meet the metabolic demands of the body. Cardiac output is assessed by both direct and indirect methods. Manipulation of the determinants of cardiac output (heart rate, preload, afterload, and contractility) improves the patient's status postoperatively.[20,24]

**Indirect methods.** The evaluation of pedal pulses is the simplest method for estimating the adequacy of cardiac output. Temperature, color, and capillary refill of the extremities also are indicators of cardiac output. Mixed venous oxygen levels ($PvO_2$ and/or $SvO_2$) provide an index of mean tissue oxygen perfusion. This value reflects the adequacy of cardiac output in the periphery. Oliguria, hyperkalemia, and base deficits are a result of metabolic acidosis secondary to low cardiac output. When these indicators are present, cardiac output is directly measured.[20]

**Direct methods.** Either thermodilution or indocyanine green dye methods are used for direct measurement of cardiac output. The values obtained are the cardiac output and cardiac index. The cardiac index is determined by dividing the cardiac output by the body surface area. A cardiac index greater than 2.0 L/min/$m^2$ reflects an adequate cardiac output postoperatively. If the cardiac index is lower than 2.0 L/min/$m^2$, then the following determinants of cardiac output must be assessed and optimized.[20]

**Heart rate and rhythm.** Normal sinus rhythm is desired, as it maximizes cardiac output by 15% because of synchronized atrial-ventricular contraction. Dysrhythmias usually occur within the first 48 hours after surgery.[20,24]

Premature ventricular contractions (PVCs) are the most common dysrhythmia and may degenerate to ventricular fibrillation. If the PVCs are greater than 6 per minute, multifocal, or near the T wave, a lidocaine bolus and continuous infusion are administered to prevent ventricular tachycardia or fibrillation. Serum potassium levels are measured and, if below 4.0 mEq/L, supplemental potassium is given. If pacing wires are present, then atrial pacing may suppress the dysrhythmias.

Premature atrial contractions also occur frequently after surgery. These beats may lead to atrial fibrillation. Atrial pacing may suppress their formation. If atrial fibrillation or atrial flutter occur, an atrial electrogram is obtained from the atrial pacing wire (Fig. 12-3). Digitalization or synchronized cardioversion are used to control or convert atrial fibrillation. Rapid atrial pacing is used to terminate atrial flutter. Other antidysrhythmic drugs (e.g., procainamide, quinidine, verapamil) may be used if these dysrhythmias persist.[20,24,25]

If ventricular tachycardia occurs and the patient remains hemodynamically stable, a lidocaine bolus is given and an infusion is initiated. If the patient is not hemodynamically stable, then cardioversion is performed according to ACLS standards.[20,26]

**Preload.** Preload is defined as the length of the sarcomeres at the end of diastole, and it is dependent on the change in volume in the ventricle from the end of systole to the end of diastole.[24] Preload is measured by the mean right atrial, mean left atrial, pulmonary artery end-diastolic, or pulmonary capillary wedge pressure. When these filling pressures are low, indicating inadequate preload, volume expanders are infused (e.g., albumin 5%, whole blood, and/or packed red blood cells). The amount and type of volume infused is determined by hematocrit, coagulation values, and renal and pulmonary status.

Autotransfusion can also be used to augment preload. The blood is collected from the chest tubes, filtered, and reinfused to the patient. The major problem with autotransfusion is the loss of clotting factors during the filtering process. The rate and adequacy of volume infusion depends on the myocardial response as reflected by the atrial filling pressures.

There is a distinct possibility that patients may develop hypovolemia and low cardiac output after coronary artery surgery. Factors contributing to this tendency include fluid shifts from the vascular spaces, changes in arterial and venous capacitance, excessive bleeding, and inadequate volume replacement. The possibility of cardiac tamponade must always be a major consideration while managing a patient with low cardiac output. The collection of fluid in the posterior portion of the pericardial sac or in the mediastinal space interferes with cardiac filling by obstructing the ability of the ventricles to eject blood. In addition to decreased cardiac output, classic indicators of cardiac tamponade include (1) increasing atrial filling pressures, (2) decreasing arterial pressure, (3) marked decrease in chest drainage, (4) widened mediastinum on chest x-ray examination, (5) distant heart sounds, (6) narrowing pulse pressure, and (7) pulsus paradoxus. Tamponade is an emergency situation requiring rapid surgical reexploration and evacuation of excess fluid.[20,27]

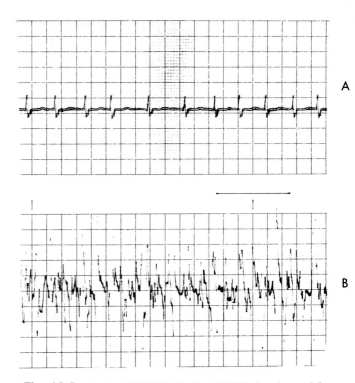

**Fig. 12-3**  **A,** Lead II ECG. **B,** Atrial ECG showing atrial fibrillation.

**Afterload.** Afterload is defined as systolic wall stress. When afterload increases, impedance to left ventricular ejection increases and cardiac output decreases. Afterload is measured by the arterial systolic blood pressure.

Systemic vascular resistance is increased after cardiac surgery, causing an increase in the systolic wall stress of the left ventricle. Thus afterload is increased, resulting in an elevated systemic blood pressure. Lowering the systemic blood pressure will improve myocardial performance, increase cardiac output, reduce left ventricular end-diastolic pressure, lower myocardial oxygen requirements, and reduce the potential for bleeding. Two modalities are commonly used for reducing afterload: vasodilating agents and intraaortic balloon pumping.

Sodium nitroprusside is the vasodilator of choice. It dilates arterial smooth muscle and, to a lesser extent, venous smooth muscle. Dilatation lowers the systemic vascular resistance, thereby decreasing afterload. These drug effects occur immediately as the infusion is begun. Arterial blood pressure must be continuously monitored while this drug is used.

Nitroglycerin can be used to decrease venous tone and coronary resistance, resulting in afterload reduction. Hydralazine, phentolamine, and chlorpromazine can also be used as afterload reducing agents. Intraaortic balloon pumping decreases afterload and increases myocardial blood flow. It is used when pharmacologic therapy fails and is discussed later in this chapter.

**Contractility.** Contractility is defined as the velocity of shortening of the myocardial muscle. The only means of augmenting the contractility of the heart is by using catecholamines such as dopamine, dobutamine, epinephrine, and norepinephrine. Each drug has unique effects on heart rate, contractility, myocardial oxygen requirements, renal perfusion, and systemic vascular resistance. Because of the variety of side effects encountered with infusion of these drugs, they are used only after the other determinants of cardiac output have been maximized.

**Pulmonary subsystem.** Most patients experience some degree of transient respiratory dysfunction in the immediate postoperative period. This dysfunction generally takes the form of decreased oxygenation and ventilatory depression, which appears as hypoxemia, alveolar hypoventilation, and reduced ventilatory reserve.

The basic components of postoperative respiratory care are (1) optimizing ventilation and pulmonary mechanics; (2) improving blood gas exchange; (3) reducing metabolic needs and oxygen consumption; and (4) assessing cardiovascular performance as it affects perfusion and oxygenation.[19,20,28]

Patients are mechanically ventilated during the first 12 to 24 hours following surgery. The level of surveillance and support is related to preexisting pulmonary disease, the patient's response to the cardiac repair, duration of cardiopulmonary bypass, and any coexisting system disorders, for example, liver or kidney disease.

Ventilator management during the postoperative period includes regulation of oxygen concentration, providing a tidal volume of 10 to 15 ml/kg, controlling respiratory rate to maintain an acceptable $PaCO_2$, and adding positive-end-expiratory-pressure (PEEP) when needed. Arterial blood gases and chest x-ray films are frequently examined while the patient remains intubated. In addition, tissue perfusion and sensorium are carefully monitored. Since it is undesirable for these patients to struggle, shiver, cough, gag, or fight the ventilator, appropriate sedation and comfort measures are provided.[20,28]

Criteria for extubation differ from patient to patient. Extubation is favored when the patient is alert and responsive, when arterial blood gases are stable with good pulmonary mechanics, and when the patient's cardiac, pulmonary, and renal systems are performing satisfactorily. Following extubation, patients are supplemented with humidified oxygen via a face mask or nasal cannula for 24 to 48 hours. A program of vigorous pulmonary toilette, which includes frequent deep breathing and coughing, chest physiotherapy, turning in bed, and ambulating as soon as possible, is employed.[28,29]

Although most patients experience acceptable spontaneous respirations by 12 to 24 hours postoperatively, some require prolonged ventilation. Often these patients have experienced respiratory complications or pulmonary disease that necessitate further support to sustain life. Excessive secretions, pneumonia, atelectasis, pleural effusions, pulmonary edema, and acute respiratory failure require highly specialized, comprehensive management.

**Renal subsystem.** Postoperative treatment centers around maintaining intravascular volume and cardiac output to ensure adequate renal perfusion. Adequacy of renal perfusion is assessed by monitoring urinary output, specific gravity, BUN, and creatinine. Other indications are daily weights, skin turgor, edema, sensorium, serum chemistries, and intravascular pressure measurements.

Electrolyte disturbances are common after cardiac surgery, but with proper management their detrimental effects can be avoided. Retention of sodium and excretion of potassium can be expected. Sodium supplements are usually not necessary, but potassium is lost in sufficient quantities to require replacement therapy. Metabolic acidosis and alkalosis may also be encountered along with occasional disturbances in calcium and magnesium concentrations.

A measurable alteration of renal function accompanies cardiac surgery. Preoperative apprehension, fluid restrictions, and surgical trauma promote increased secretion of antidiuretic hormone (ADH) and aldosterone. During the immediate postoperative period, the renal tubules must also handle products of tissue breakdown from surgery and free hemoglobin from bypass perfusion. The combined effect of these variables is responsible for the oliguria that commonly occurs after surgery. Treatment of oliguria usually consists of volume administration and, if the patient is well hydrated, a diuretic such as furosemide (Lasix).

Acute renal failure is a serious complication following surgery. A low urinary output, high urinary sodium level, rising serum potassium levels, and the failure to respond to diuretics are early signs of acute renal failure. The most frequent contributing factor to acute renal failure is low cardiac output and accompanying reduction in renal blood flow. It is therefore important to ensure hydration that promotes a urinary output of at least 30 ml/hour in adults. Other factors that seem to render patients vulnerable to acute renal failure are severe cardiac dysfunction, renal disease, and advanced age.

If acute renal failure does occur, the administration of fluids must be restricted, potassium administration must be curtailed, clearance of medications must be carefully considered, blood and urine studies must be frequently monitored, and hypertension must be controlled. An infusion of dopamine at low doses may be started. Peritoneal dialysis may also be necessary during the oliguric phase of acute renal failure to reduce fluid overload, hyperkalemia, and uremic symptoms. Diuresis may occur after the oliguric phase. Patients who are supported well and survive the oliguric and polyuric phases will ultimately regain function, although it may be months before recovery is complete.

**Neurologic subsystem.** Major neurologic complications have significantly declined because of the modern advances in cardiac surgery and cardiopulmonary bypass. Nevertheless, level of consciousness is continually assessed until the patient recovers from the anesthetic and is awake. Neurologic checks include pupillary size and reaction, gross motor movement and sensation, and orientation to person, place, and time. Any noted disorders such as failure to respond, seizures, or unilateral weakness warrant a neurologic consultation and full work-up. Management of any complication is directed toward relief of symptoms, prevention of further injury, and restoration to maximum function.

It is estimated that a large majority of adults who have open heart surgery experience some form of transient sensory disturbance postoperatively. These disturbances can be as minor as anxiety or as severe as hallucinations and delusions. If the sensory distortions are severe, the patient may cause self-harm by disrupting monitoring cables, pulling out tubes, and disturbing life-support lines. Sensory alterations in postcardiotomy patients are difficult to deal with because there are so many factors that seem to render patients vulnerable. Some of these are anesthetic agents, cardiopulmonary bypass, the ICU environment, sleep deprivation, surgical stress, advanced age, and degree of morbidity. Because of this tendency toward sensory disturbances, postoperative care must include attention to safety factors (that is, close attendance, side rails, wrist restraints prn), reorientation techniques (verbal information to patient, clocks, calendars), and normalizing the ICU environment as much as possible (family visits, day/night cycles).

**Gastrointestinal subsystem.** Gastric distention, which can place undue pressure on the lungs and heart, is avoided postoperatively by the use of a nasogastric tube connected to low intermittent suction or left to gravity. All patients, particularly those with a history of gastric bleeding, should have their gastric pH checked routinely and antacids should be administered accordingly. The abdomen is assessed for distention, pain, ascites, and bowel sounds. When normal peristalsis returns and the patient is able to take liquids by mouth, a diet is resumed and advanced as tolerated (usually a regular diet with no added salt or a 2 g low-sodium diet). Most patients eat without difficulty by 24 hours after surgery.

## Complications

**Bleeding.** Some bleeding is normal in every patient following cardiac surgery, but persistent bleeding requires special attention. The amount of bleeding that warrants concern is contingent on hemodynamic response, patient size, clotting studies, and the nature and extent of surgery. Generally more than 100 to 200 ml of blood every hour from the mediastinal tubes for the first 3 to 4 hours is considered excessive. In such a case the primary strategy in patient management is to determine the cause: is the bleeding caused by a coagulation disorder or by a surgical bleed?

All clotting parameters are evaluated. If clotting factors, such as platelets, are deficient, they are replaced. An activated clotting time (ACT) helps to determine if additional protamine is needed. If the ACT is normal, fresh frozen plasma may be administered to provide additional clotting factors. Aminocaproic acid (Amicar), which causes diffuse clotting, may also be considered a pharmacologic modality. As therapy is initiated to control the bleeding, clotting studies are repeated to determine the success of treatment. Any oozing from incision sites is carefully watched, marked, and possibly treated with Surgicel.

If bleeding continues despite normal coagulation studies, a surgical bleed is probable. Some bleeders seal themselves off without major intervention. Excessive bleeding, however, must be treated promptly. Rapid infusion of blood, plasma, and plasma expanders may be required to prevent severe depletion of circulatory volume until the patient is returned to surgery for exploration and repair.

**Infection.** Infections following coronary artery surgery can be systemic, operative, or involve any body system. A variety of organisms—bacterial, fungal, viral, and protozoal—have been found to be responsible for these infections. It is crucial that meticulous attention be paid to aseptic technique while performing all care routines, especially wound care, suctioning, and maintenance of invasive lines.[30,31]

A low-grade fever is common following surgery, but a temperature elevation beyond 24 to 48 hours after surgery is unusual and requires specific attention. Antipyretics, steroids, tepid baths, and cooling blankets may be used in addition to culturing blood, urine, and sputum for potential infectious agents.

A serious complication requiring aggressive treatment is a sternal wound infection and mediastinitis. This is a potentially life-threatening complication because of the possibility of extension to the heart, aorta, and suture lines. Initial signs and symptoms of infection may be mild but progress to purulent drainage and dehiscence. When this condition occurs, drainage, debridement, and antibiotic therapy are required. Following debridement, wound care is usually extensive and sterile technique when redressing the wound is crucial.[32,33]

## MECHANICAL DEVICES

Advancements in surgical techniques and myocardial protection have improved the results of cardiac surgery. However, the elderly and patients requiring surgical reoperation are being referred for cardiac surgery more frequently. An increasing number of these patients are requiring more advanced technology to survive cardiopulmonary bypass.[34,35] Mechanical assist devices such as the intraaortic balloon pump (IABP), ventricular assist devices (VAD), and the total artificial heart (TAH) are available for these situations.

## Intraaortic Balloon Pump

**Indications.** The primary goals of treatment with an IABP include (1) decreasing left ventricular afterload, (2) increasing coronary artery perfusion, and (3) reducing myocardial oxygen demand.[36] Patient conditions warranting use of an IABP include the following:

1. MI leading to cardiogenic shock
2. Medically refractory left ventricular pump failure
3. Papillary muscle dysfunction resulting in mitral valve regurgitation
4. Unstable angina unresponsive to medical therapy, and/or in the presence of significant coronary artery disease, or postinfarction angina
5. Recurrent ventricular dysrhythmias
6. Ventricular aneurysm
7. Left main coronary artery disease
8. Septic shock
9. Preoperative treatment of ventricular septal defect
10. Intraoperative treatment during cardiac surgery to provide pulsatile blood flow and to allow the patient to be weaned off cardiopulmonary bypass
11. Prophylaxis for cardiac surgery in high-risk patients[36,37]

**Contraindications.** There are absolute and relative contraindications for the use of an IABP.[36,37] Absolute contraindications are those conditions for which the IABP is not to be used. Relative contraindications are those conditions in which the use of IABP is occasionally appropriate. The absolute contraindications include (1) irreversible brain damage, (2) aortic valve insufficiency, and (3) aortic aneurysm. The relative contraindications include (1) peripheral vascular atherosclerosis and (2) chronic end-stage heart disease.

**Physiologic principles.** The IABP is a temporary ventricular assist device. It augments systemic and coronary circulation through the displacement of aortic blood volume in diastole (inflation). Workload of ventricular ejection is reduced in systole (deflation). Ultimately, myocardial oxygen consumption is decreased.[36] These effects are accomplished by utilizing the principles of counterpulsation.

Counterpulsation is the augmentation of diastolic pressure by inflation and deflation of a balloon. The rapid withdrawal of carbon dioxide or helium from the balloon deflates it just prior to systole.[36] The balloon is timed, automatically or manually, to inflate immediately after the closure of the aortic valve, displacing the blood retrograde toward the aortic root. With the opening of the aortic valve, the balloon deflates. Cardiac output increases as aortic root pressure is lowered and left ventricular afterload and myocardial oxygen demands are reduced.[37]

**Insertion.** Insertion methods are individualized, de-

pending on the institution and the patient's diagnoses and present condition. Typically, the IABP is placed percutaneously via the right or left femoral artery.[37] The artery is punctured with an 18-gauge angiographic needle, then a guide wire is inserted through the needle, and the needle is removed. The puncture site is enlarged with a #8Fr Teflon dilator and a #12Fr dilator sheath is inserted. The tightly wrapped balloon is inserted through the sheath, its placement verified by fluoroscopy or chest x-ray, and counterpulsation therapy is initiated.[37]

**Intraaortic balloon pump timing and weaning.** Timing of the IABP involves using the arterial pressure or ECG waveform as a guide for the inflation and deflation of the balloon.[36,37] The R wave of the ECG is the more common reference point for timing of the IABP. Verifying adequacy of counterpulsation requires observing both the augmented and nonaugmented arterial pressure waveform. The inflation of the balloon should occur at the dicrotic notch.[36] Augmentation is optimum when the assisted systolic arterial pressure exceeds the patient's unassisted systolic arterial pressure and when the assisted aortic end-diastolic pressure is 5 to 15 mm Hg lower than the patient's unassisted end-diastolic pressure. Timing of the IABP may need to be adjusted for changes in heart rate more than 10 beats/min, or for changes in cardiac rhythm.[37]

Weaning from the IABP is governed by the hemodynamic status of the patient and can be accomplished by one or both of the following methods: (1) reducing the frequency of augmentation from 1:1, to 1:2, to 1:3 at set intervals; or (2) reducing the actual augmentation from maximum to minimum.[37] Observations to be made during the therapy include vital signs, presence or absence of angina, quality and quantity of urine output, skin temperature and color, peripheral pulses, neurologic status, and cardiopulmonary status.[36,37] A patient is considered balloon dependent when one or more of the following conditions prevail:

1. Lethal dysrhythmias develop during the weaning process
2. Vasoactive medications must be increased to maintain a systolic blood pressure of 90 mm Hg or greater
3. Signs and symptoms of shock develop
4. Cardiac index is equal to or less than 2.0 L/min/m²
5. Intracardiac pressures increase during the weaning process
6. Changes in ECG (e.g., ST elevation) occur

**Complications.** Complications of IABP therapy are associated with balloon insertion, balloon pumping, and balloon removal.[37] During balloon insertion, there is a significant risk of developing ischemic extremities.[38] A reduction of blood flow to the catheterized extremity is evident by poor or absent distal pulses and a cool, pale leg. Limb ischemia occurs more frequently in patients greater than 70 years, and in female patients. Preventive measures include anticoagulation, maintenance of adequate arterial pressures, and changing the balloon insertion site at the earliest signs of ischemia. Removal of the balloon, continuous IV heparin therapy, thrombectomy, embolectomy, or, in an extreme situation, amputation may be required if the situation persists. The IABP catheter may be difficult to advance in patients with tortuous vessels or severe occlusive disease. Again, the incidence is greater for elderly patients. Use of a percutaneous balloon catheter with a J-tip guidewire or a longer sheath may reduce the occurrence of this problem.

Inability to unwrap the balloon catheter can occur. Causes include a defective balloon or a portion of the balloon remaining in the sheath. This situation may be evident by the absence or severely reduced appearance of an augmented pressure waveform. Balloon unwrapping can be ensured after verification of position by manually inflating the balloon with a 50 ml syringe of air or gas. The injected air should then be immediately aspirated.

Arterial perforation or damage can occur and may not be immediately evident. Often, it is discovered at autopsy when perforated common iliac arteries and a massive retroperitoneal bleed are noted. This complication is more common with the percutaneous method of insertion. Aortic dissection can also occur. Signs and symptoms may be vague and include back pain, inequality of pulses and/or blood pressures between left and right extremities, decreased renal function, increased angina, and neurologic deficits.

Thromboemboli can occur as a direct result of the propagation of clots from the catheter. Adequate heparinization may minimize the incidence of this complication. Treatment depends on the site and clinical manifestations. Infection tends to occur in 2% to 4% of patients and may be local or systemic. Aseptic insertion and maintenance techniques are imperative to minimize this problem. Bleeding and hematomas occur in only 1% of patients. Bleeding around the catheter insertion site and hematoma formation can occur as a result of anticoagulation therapy and thrombocytopenia. Persistent bleeding can sometimes be managed by direct pressure but may require removal of the catheter. Thrombocytopenia occurs as a direct result of the duration of counterpulsation. Platelet counts usually return to normal after cessation of IABP therapy. Platelet and packed red blood cell administration may be necessary.

During and after IABP removal, bleeding and thromboembolism can occur. Bleeding from the catheter site occurs more frequently with the percutaneous method of insertion because of the large size of the catheter and the anticoagulation therapy. Management consists of firm manual pressure until hemostasis occurs. A 5- to 10-pound sandbag should be placed over the site for several hours and the patient should remain on bedrest for 8 hours. If bleeding persists, surgical repair may be necessary. Thrombosis or emboli can occur as a result of shearing of clots during catheter removal.

## Ventricular Assist Devices

**Goals of treatment.** Ventricular assist devices (VADs) are flow assistance devices that provide temporary circulatory support for single or biventricular failure.[35] The two primary goals for utilization of a ventricular assist device are (1) to provide sufficient myocardial tissue recovery and (2) patient survival.[39]

**Indications for use of a ventricular assist device.** Patient conditions warranting the use of a VAD are divided into two categories acute and chronic ventricular failure.[34,40-43] Acute ventricular failure necessitating use of a VAD can occur from postcardiotomy ventricular failure, acute myocarditis, acute MI, and right ventricular failure.

Postcardiotomy ventricular failure is noted in patients with preoperative and intraoperative low cardiac outputs, and in patients unable to be weaned from cardiopulmonary bypass.[39] Cardiogenic shock secondary to acute MI may require ventricular assistance. Right ventricular failure secondary to left ventricular failure, acute pulmonary hypertension, or use of a left ventricular assist device (LVAD) may also require a right ventricular assist device (RVAD) or a bilateral ventricular assist device (Bi-VAD).[44]

Indications for use of a VAD in chronic ventricular failure can be noted in those patients suffering from cardiomyopathies, end-stage coronary heart disease, chronic pulmonary artery hypertension, or congenital heart disease.[44] In addition, deterioration of a patient awaiting cardiac transplantation or retransplantation may necessitate the use of a VAD.[44-47]

Patients with traumatic tears of the thoracic aorta may require a VAD. Traumatic blunt thoracic aortic injuries are commonly seen at major trauma centers and are often a result of high-speed deceleration auto accidents, airplane accidents, or falls.[48] The VAD can be used in these patients to provide a partial left heart bypass with a reduction of afterload and perfusion of the intraabdominal viscera, kidneys, and distal spinal cord during the repair of the aorta.

**Contraindications.** Contraindications to the institution of a VAD include the following[40,49]:

1. A body surface area less than 1.0 m² is a contraindication for most VAD types because of the size of the cannula
2. Bacterial endocarditis
3. Coagulopathies, including transfusion reactions
4. Massive, irreversible myocardial damage (unless utilized as a bridge to cardiac transplantation)
5. Chronic disease states such as renal failure, cancer or hepatic failure
6. Prolonged cardiac arrest with resultant neurologic damage
7. Congenital heart disease
8. Cardiac surgical procedures with technically insufficient repairs
9. Uncontrollable hemorrhage from the heart, great vessels, or other organs
10. Postoperative renal failure

**Physiologic principles.** The VAD is indicated for use in patients suffering from acute or chronic ventricular failure.[50] In these patients, the mechanical circulatory assist device can interrupt the cycle of cardiac failure, including the progression of myocardial ischemia.[51]

VADs divert the blood from the natural ventricle to an artificial pump that maintains systemic circulation. Partial bypass of either the left or right ventricle over a period of hours to days may allow the myocardium time to recover. As much as a 50% reduction in myocardial oxygen consumption has been demonstrated by use of VADs.[52] Essentially, the VAD reduces preload and afterload, provides adequate circulatory support, reduces myocardial edema and oxygen demand, and allows for the restoration of high-energy substrates like ATP.[51] Typically, the flow rate of blood is adjusted to maintain a left atrial pressure (LAP) between 4 and 12 mm Hg.

In contrast to the total artificial heart, VADs are used in parallel with the patient's own heart. Unlike IABPs, VADs are not as dependent on a certain level of left ventricular function.[45] Thus the VAD can be utilized in patients with either left, right, or biventricular failure, or in those suffering from lethal dysrhythmias.

VADs have primarily been implanted intraoperatively and postoperatively in patients who develop ventricular failure refractory to maximum pharmacologic support, IABP therapy, fluid administration, and temporary pacing.[39] There has been considerable biochemical and morphologic evidence that, on cessation of cardiopulmonary bypass, left ventricular function is depressed secondary to the development of a "stunned" myocardium.[40,41] In addition, cardiopulmonary bypass causes significant myocardial intracellular edema.[53] The exact pathogenesis of these abnormalities is unknown at present.[54] Right ventricular failure during and after cardiopulmonary bypass can be caused by left ventricular failure, inadequate cardioplegia, or rapid rewarming of the right ventricle because of its anterior location within the pericardium.[55]

**Insertion criteria.** Although cardiogenic shock and severe cardiac failure may have different etiologies, the hemodynamic criteria for the use of VADs are fairly uniform.[39,41,45,55] Specific criteria for insertion of a left ventricular assist device (LVAD) include the following:

1. Cardiac index of less than 1.8 L/min/m² despite maximum use of conventional therapy
2. Systolic aortic blood pressure of less than 90 mm Hg
3. Left atrial pressure greater than 25 mm Hg after conventional therapy
4. Urine output less than 30 ml/hour
5. Systemic vascular resistance greater than 2100 dynes/sec/cm⁵

Right ventricular failure has been referred to as "pulmonary blood flow inadequate to provide sufficient preload to the left ventricle." Right ventricular failure may

not be evident until after left ventricular assist pumping is initiated. The following are specific criteria indicating the potential need for a right ventricular assist device (RVAD):

1. Cardiac index less than 1.8 L/min/m² despite maximum use of conventional therapy
2. Systolic aortic blood pressure less than 90 mm Hg
3. Left atrial pressure less than 15 mm Hg despite volume loading to a right atrial pressure of 25 mm Hg
4. Hypoxia, hypercarbia, and acidosis conditions corrected

If criteria for insertion of both LVAD and RVAD are present, then use of a biventricular assist device is warranted.[39]

**VAD insertion.** In review, left ventricular failure requires a left VAD (LVAD), right ventricular failure requires a right VAD (RVAD), and biventricular failure requires use of a biventricular VAD (BiVAD).[35] In all cases, a median sternotomy is made, blood is diverted away from the natural heart, bypassing the ventricle, and returned to the patient. Actual cannula position can vary according to the surgeon's preference and the patient's condition.

Generally, with the placement of an LVAD, as seen in Fig. 12-4, blood is removed from the left atrial appendage or left atrium via a large bore, short cannula, passed through the pump, and returned via another large-bore cannula to the ascending or transverse aorta. The tip of the aortic cannula is advanced past the left subclavian artery to protect from cerebral embolization.[35] Positioning of the RVAD cannula involves removing blood from the right atrium or right atrial appendage and returning the blood into the pulmonary artery.[35] Fig. 12-5 demonstrates such a device.

In each case, the cannulae exit the skin from the sternal incision, or from separate incisions either parasternally or

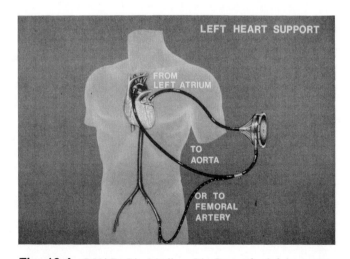

**Fig. 12-4** LVAD. Bio-Medicus Bio-Pump for left heart support. (Courtesy of Swenson/Falker Associates, Inc., Minneapolis, MN.)

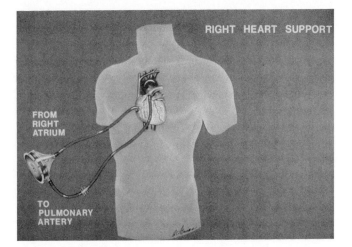

**Fig. 12-5** RVAD. Bio-Medicus Bio-Pump for right heart support.(Courtesy of Swenson/Falker Associates, Inc., Minneapolis, MN.)

infrasternally. The cannulae are then connected to the pump console via antithrombogenic tubing. In the majority of patients, the sternum is not closed and only the skin is approximated in order to avoid compression of the edematous heart and the VAD cannulae.[35] The entire surgical site is then covered with sterile towels.

**Types of ventricular assist devices.** The ventricular assist devices in current use are listed below:[6,35]

Roller
Centrifugal
Pneumatic
Electric
Hemopump
Total artificial heart

The roller, centrifugal, and pneumatic devices are more often used in the critical care setting.[56,57] The electric and hemopump are distinguished by one unique characteristic: the devices are totally implantable. The electric device rests in the upper left abdominal cavity; and the hemopump, a pencil-shaped device similar to the Archimedes' screw, resides entirely within the left ventricle.[58] The total artificial heart replaces the native heart, but only as a temporary measure until cardiac transplantation can be performed.[41]

The roller ventricular assist devices compress the blood at a manually set point and force the blood forward.[35] Roller devices typically form a portion of the cardiopulmonary bypass machines. Advantages of the roller device include simplicity of design and operation and low cost. Disadvantages are major: hemolysis of blood, need for anticoagulation therapy, poor long-term performance, and constant device supervision.[58] Potential physiologic effects seen in patients with such a device include bleeding, air emboli, and thrombus formation.

The centrifugal device uses three magnetic cones that rotate to propel the blood forward in a circular motion, thus generating centrifugal force, pressure, and flow.[59] Centrifugal devices are considered more sensitive to changes in a patient's fluid status. An increase in fluid, or preload, is reflected by an increase in the output of the device; a decrease in preload is reflected by a decrease in the output of the device. Additional advantages include simplicity of operation and low cost. Disadvantages are similar to those of the roller devices.

An important point regarding both of these ventricular assist devices is the nonpulsatile blood flow. If pulsatile blood flow is desired, an intraaortic balloon pump is inserted. Pulsatile blood flow for a patient is a major advantage from a physiologic standpoint.[35] Pulsatile blood flow provides more adequate renal perfusion, decreases systemic vascular resistance, and increases systemic circulation. In addition, pulsatile blood flow decreases blood cell trauma, reduces the need for anticoagulation therapy, lowers the incidence of thromboembolic events, and subsequently, increases the possibility of using the device for a long time.[60]

The air-driven pneumatic device provides pulsatile blood flow by puffs of air that compress a seam-free flexible sac.[39] The inflow and outflow of blood are controlled by Bjork-Shiley inlet and outlet valves. Positive pressure from the console is activated during the device's ejection phase, and negative pressure is utilized during the filling phase. On completion of the filling of the sac, a switch on the device signals the beginning of the ejection phase.[39] The device is capable of operating in three modes: (1) a fixed rate, asynchronous mode that provides a variable stroke volume during initiation and weaning of the device; (2) a synchronous mode that uses the R wave counterpulsation to synchronize the device with the heart rate to provide a variable rate of flow and stroke volume; and (3) a fill-to-empty mode that provides a variable rate of flow, but with a fixed stroke volume.[39] Disadvantages of such a device include its complexity of operation, cost of operation, and the need for FDA approval for use.[39]

### Nursing management

**Maintenance.** Optimum postoperative nursing management of a patient with a VAD involves an awareness of the patient's preoperative history, operative course, and potential complications.[35,49,61-64] After the patient is situated in the intensive care unit, a thorough nursing assessment should be performed. Nursing responsibilities include continuous patient observation, interpretation of vital signs, and determination of appropriate therapeutic interventions. Typically, one to two critical care nurses and a perfusionist assist in the care of the patient. Although the perfusionist is responsible for the operation of the device, the nurse needs to be familiar with the device and anticipate the complications that might ensue.

Care of the patient with a VAD is similar to that of

most postoperative cardiovascular surgical patients. The uniqueness of care involves managing complications. Alterations in tissue perfusion and gas exchange; the potential for bleeding, thromboembolism, infection, nutritional deficits; and ineffective patient and family coping may be encountered.

The alteration in tissue perfusion can be related to decreased myocardial contractility, dysrhythmias, acid-base imbalances, and trauma from surgery.[12,18] Goals include maintaining an adequate cardiac output as indicated by a device flow rate of 2.0 to 4.0 L/min,[54] normal vital signs, bilaterally equal pulses, and warm, pink skin. Nursing interventions to meet these goals include hemodynamic and cardiac rhythm monitoring, frequent assessment of peripheral pulses, and regulation of vasoactive medications. In the event of device console malfunction, a reserve console should be readily available.

The potential for impaired gas exchange can be related to the enforced immobilization of the patient and postoperative atelectasis.[54] Maintaining effective breathing patterns, maintaining arterial blood gases within normal limits, and preparing for eventual weaning from the ventilator are several objectives of care. Possible nursing interventions include monitoring the effects of mechanical ventilation, auscultating breath sounds frequently, performing good pulmonary toilet, utilizing the lowest percentage of oxygen to maintain adequate arterial oxygenation, and obtaining daily chest x-rays.

Bleeding can occur from the hemolysis of red blood cells, platelet destruction, or from anticoagulation therapy.[64] Anticoagulation may be recommended and is often essential to prevent the formation of thrombus in the device and circuitry. Bleeding should be prevented or controlled as evidenced by no unusual or excess bleeding from the chest tubes, nor from incisional or cannulation sites. Coagulation studies should be within normal limits. Nursing management includes monitoring the quality and quantity of all drainage; inspecting incisional and cannulation sites for abnormal bleeding, petechiae, or ecchymosis; assessing and treating coagulopathies; hemodynamic monitoring; and anticipating the need for open chest resuscitation measures. Cardiac compressions are contraindicated in any situation because this action could dislodge the cannula and lead to rapid exsanguination.[65] Therefore open chest massage is indicated in the patient who has cardiac arrest. Bleeding from accidental dislodgement of the cannula may be halted by the placement of clamps on the cannula as proximal to the patient as possible.[35]

Thrombus formation can be related to the pooling of blood in the bypassed ventricle[35] and from the device itself. Preventing the formation of thrombus is imperative, because thrombus can obstruct the inflow or outflow cannula, causing a slow or acute reduction in cardiac output.[66] Anticoagulation is accomplished by the administration of heparin or dextran once postoperative bleeding is controlled.[51]

Activated clotting times (ACTs), normally 90 to 110 seconds, are kept between 150 and 200 seconds and are monitored every hour.

Because of the multiple ports of entry and a depressed immune system, patients undergoing assist device therapy are highly susceptible to infection.[34] The goal is to avoid infection as evidenced by a normal temperature, normal white blood cell count, and no unusual or purulent drainage from any site. Interventions include monitoring and reporting temperature changes; assessing for signs and symptoms of infection; good handwashing technique; administering appropriate medications; using strict sterile techniques during procedures; placing the patient in protective isolation; providing adequate rest and nutrition to promote healing; and obtaining daily cultures of blood, wounds, and sputum.[36]

Patients requiring assist device therapy typically have nutritional deficits from a limited caloric intake and increased metabolic needs prior to device insertion.[34] Establishment of a positive nitrogen balance as evident by a stable weight and normal laboratory values is the desired goal. Beginning nasogastric tube feedings or hyperalimentation when appropriate, accurate intake and output calculations, daily weights, and the monitoring of laboratory values are important interventions to reduce the deficit.

A tremendous potential exists for ineffective coping by the patient and family because of the seriousness of the situation, knowledge deficits, poor coping abilities, or inadequate social support systems.[34,35] Goals include allowing verbalization of fears and concerns, and encouraging appropriate stress relief and grief behavior. The nurse can assist the patient and family by identifying stressors, explaining the purposes and functions of the device, encouraging questions, and providing honest answers. Additionally, encouraging the family to touch and talk to the patient and explaining the need for sedation or restraints and immobility are important components of care.

**Weaning.** Attempts to wean a patient from a VAD are typically begun after the first 24 hours of therapy.[67] A recovering ventricle should begin to show hemodynamic improvement 24 to 48 hours after the insulting event.[35] Those patients awaiting cardiac transplantation will not undergo weaning, but will continue to have evaluations of ventricular function. Evaluation of the patient's native heart may be done by portable echocardiography.

Daily assessment of the patient's response without VAD flow is done by the physician, who turns the VAD off for less than 3 minutes.[67] During the weaning process, the patient must be anticoagulated to reduce the chance of thrombus formation.[67] Generally, ACTs are kept at 200 seconds during these attempts. VAD flow rates less than 400 to 500 ml/min for prolonged periods are not recommended because of the potential for thrombus formation. During the period in which the VAD flow rate is reduced or absent, left atrial pressures are observed closely for patients with an LVAD, and right atrial pressures are monitored for patients with an RVAD.[54] A cardiac index or output may be performed at this time. If either the LAP or RAP values rise to 30 mm Hg or above, weaning is halted immediately. If, however, the patient maintains adequate LAP and RAP values, a MAP greater than 90 mm Hg, and a cardiac index greater than 2.0 L/min/m², then the VAD flow rates will be gradually reduced.[54] With the completion of VAD therapy, the device and cannulae will be removed in the operating room.

Lack of demonstrable patient contribution to total systemic blood flow after a period of 24 to 48 hours may indicate an inability of the patient to be weaned from the assist device.[68] Surviving patients usually show an average of 38% of their own ventricular function within this time period.[69] Use of a single ventricular assist device is associated with a better survival rate than use of a biventricular assist device.[57] Survival from a mechanical device is more likely if the patient underwent a primary elective cardiac procedure rather than reoperation. Age is also a factor. For patients who are 66 to 70 years of age, there is only a 12% survival rate; patients who are older than 70 years of age have only a 6% chance of survival.[44] A persistent infection also decreases survival chances.[44] Patients who were maintained on cardiopulmonary bypass for more than 7 hours before assist therapy, have persistent bleeding for more than 24 hours, and are in acute renal failure have a 100% mortality rate.[57]

## TRANSPLANTATION

Cardiac transplantation has become an acceptable therapy for patients experiencing end-stage disease refractory to medical and surgical therapy.[20,70,71] However, the inadequate supply of donors has limited the availability of this procedure, despite an increase in potential recipients. Complications of infection, rejection, and immunosuppression remain serious problems in the cardiac transplant experience.

The majority of potential recipients for cardiac transplantation have severe functional disability (New York Heart Association class IV). Dilated cardiomyopathy resulting from idiopathic, viral, or postpartum causes account for half of these disabilities. Ischemic cardiomyopathy caused by extensive arteriosclerosis accounts for the remainder.[20,70,71] Patients with this functional disability who cannot be helped with medical or surgical intervention survive only 6 to 12 months. These patients have a terminal cardiac disease with only one possible hope: cardiac transplantation.

### Recipient Selection and Evaluation

Criteria have been established to identify the patients with the best potential for physical and emotional recovery from cardiac transplantation (see the box below).[20] The selection process is lengthy and burdensome as a multitude of health care personnel carry out diagnostic procedures, examinations, and interviews (see the box on p. 440). Physiologic and psychologic support of the patient and family are crucial during this period.[72]

When the patient has been selected as a potential candidate, his name, weight, blood type, and priority classification are given to the regional organ bank and placed on the national computer (Table 12-1).[73] The patient is given a long-range beeper, if not hospitalized, for quick notification should a donor heart become available.[70] The period of waiting for a new heart has been described as the most difficult in the entire transplant experience.[71,73,74] The progression of terminal cardiac disease continues, and almost one third of patients die while waiting.[70]

The goal in working with the family and patient during this time is to provide them with factual, realistic information. Preparation will address understanding the procedure, intensive care, recovery, change in diet, exercise, and the impact of immunosuppressive therapy. The associated risks of infection and rejection need to be clearly explained.[70,72] Emotional support is vital in maintaining hope and the integrity of the family unit at this time.[73]

---

### RECIPIENT CRITERIA

**NYHA\* FUNCTIONAL CLASS IV**
**AGE <60 YEARS**

Absence of the following:

  Systemic disease/infection
  Severe pulmonary hypertension†
  Active ulcer
  Severe psychologic problems
  Compromised renal system
  Smoking

**END-STAGE IRREVERSIBLE HEART DISEASE**
**PSYCHOLOGICALLY STABLE AND COMPLIANT**

  Insulin dependent diabetes
  Recent pulmonary embolism/infarct
  Bleeding diathesis
  Cerebrovascular accident
  Compromised hepatic system
  Alcohol or drug abuse

\*NYHA, New York Heart Association.
†May result in patient referral for heart-lung transplant.

## EVALUATION PROTOCOL

Medical history
Physical examination

Laboratory tests:

| | |
|---|---|
| Fluid balance profile | Complete blood count |
| Prothrombin time | Partial prothrombin |
| Platelet count | time |
| Arterial blood gases | Liver function tests |
| Antibody screening | Blood typing |
| Human immunodeficiency | Cytomeglovirus test |
| virus | Epstein-Barr virus |
| Hepatitis B surface | Tuberculosis |
| antigen | |
| Venereal disease | |

Radiologic and nuclear scans
Pulmonary function tests
Echocardiogram
Cardiac catheterization
Psychologic consultation
Financial resources

**TABLE 12-1** Recipient status

| Status | Description |
|---|---|
| 1 | Attending school or work |
| 2 | Home bound |
| 3 | Requires nursing care at home |
| 4 | In hospital on nursing unit |
| 5 | In hospital intensive care unit (ICU) |
| 6 | In ICU on ventilator/circulatory support |
| 7 | Inactive (due to infection) |
| unos stat | Death imminent |

to augment the blood pressure. Diabetes insipidus begins when pituitary function is lost, manifesting as polyuria leading to hypovolemia. Fluid and electrolytes are given to offset the imbalances caused by this condition. Hypothermia is controlled by the use of warming lights, blankets, and warmed fluids. Endotracheal intubation and ventilation are required because of destruction of the respiratory center in the brain. Arterial blood gases and pulmonary function are closely monitored. Prophylactic antibiotics are started along with an immunosuppressive agent to prepare the heart for transplantation.[76]

Once the donor has been selected and procurement is underway, the recipient is notified and hospitalized. An initial dose of the immunosuppressive cyclosporine is given and the usual preoperative preparations are performed.[20]

## Operative Procedure

If the donor heart is to be removed and transplanted on site, two adjacent operating rooms are needed. In one, the donor heart is excised, preserving the sinoatrial node, and passed through a series of cooled saline baths. It is then transferred to the recipient's room where it is sutured in place (Fig. 12-6).[20,71]

In many instances, the donor heart must be transported to another center for transplantation. The organ is removed and placed in an iced saline solution (4° C), and topical hypothermia is provided during transport. An ischemic time for the donor heart of less than 4 hours results in satisfactory organ functioning after transplantation.[20,71]

The operative procedure is not started in the recipient until a member of the donor transplant team has directly evaluated the donor heart. Suitability of the heart is then communicated to the recipient's team, and the operation is begun. In orthotopic cardiac transplantation, the heart of the recipient is exposed via a median sternotomy. Standard cardiopulmonary bypass is initiated. The vena cavae are tied off and the aorta is clamped. The heart of the recipient is excised, leaving a right and left atrial cuff with

## Donor Selection and Procurement

Federal law now requires that all health care institutions have policies for identifying potential donors and referring them to organ procurement centers.[75,76] The individual being considered for donor selection must exhibit irreversible and total cessation of brain function. Most donors are victims of accidents resulting in neurologic damage. Donors must meet all of the following criteria:

- Less than 35 years old
- No heart disease
- No previous cardiac arrest or CPR
- No infection
- Absence of transmissible disease
- No malignancy[19,70,76]

Once the family has consented to organ donation, the cardiac status is thoroughly evaluated. A detailed history is obtained, and a physical examination is performed. The heart should be of normal size and shape by chest x-ray with normal sinus rhythm and absence of murmurs, hypertrophy, and ischemia. Cardiac catheterization may be performed to validate suspected abnormalities or coronary artery disease. If the donor heart is deemed suitable for transplantation and a recipient match is found, then plans for organ procurement can begin.[20]

Aggressive management of donors awaiting organ retrieval is essential. Most are cared for in the intensive care unit. When brain death occurs, neural control of the body is absent. Hypotension caused by loss of vasomotor tone occurs. Fluid replacement and vasoconstrictors are given

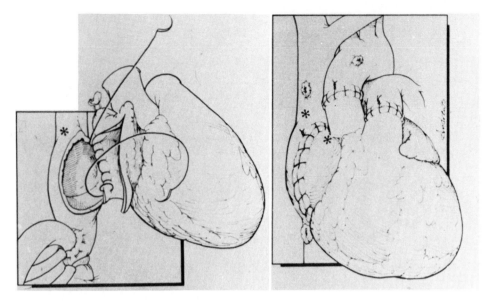

**Fig. 12-6**    Anastomosis of donor heart. (From Cooley D: Techniques in cardiac surgery, Philadelphia, 1984, WB Saunders Co.)

the sinoatrial node intact. The atrial septum, pulmonary artery, and aorta are transected distal to the semilunar valves.[20,71]

Implantation of the new heart begins with anastomosis of the left and right atria. Approximation and suturing of the aorta and pulmonary artery follows (see Fig. 12-6). At the conclusion of the grafting, it is critical to evacuate air from all the heart chambers. When the transplanted heart is warmed, it often resumes sinus rhythm. If it does not resume its pumping function, then electric defibrillation is required. Epicardial pacing wires, chest tubes, atrial/arterial lines, and venous access are placed as is usual with open-heart surgery. Isoproterenol infusion may be started to ensure an acceptable heart rate and cardiac output.[20,70,71]

## Postoperative Care

The immediate postoperative care of the transplant patient is very similar to that of any patient undergoing open-heart surgery (see the previous discussion of postoperative care in this chapter). The major exceptions are rhythm disturbances, neural control, immunosuppressive therapy, isolation, infection, and rejection.[71,76-82]

**Rhythm disturbances.** Rhythm disturbances are uncommon in the initial postoperative period if the donor heart has not been subjected to prolonged ischemia. Following transplantation, the ECG will show the appearance of activity from sinoatrial nodes of both the recipient and donor hearts. Thus there will be two P waves present in the ECG complex. The recipient's sinoatrial activity does not propagate an impulse because it is isolated from any conducting pathways. Only the sinoatrial node of the donor's heart can propagate an impulse in the donor heart. The presence of an additional P wave should be remem-

bered during rhythm interpretation to avoid misidentification of any dysrhythmia.[20,71]

**Neural control.** After cardiac transplantation, there is no longer direct neural control of the conduction system. Thus the adrenal hormones exert primary stimulation of the heart by exciting the adrenergic receptors of the donor myocardium with circulating catecholamines. Epicardial pacing wires, placed on the right atrium and ventricle, may be used to override atrial or junctional bradycardia in the early postoperative period. An isoproterenol infusion may also be used to augment the heart rate and cardiac output. It is important to remember that the denervated donor heart may be less sensitive to drugs like atropine and digoxin. Therefore all drugs given to affect cardiac performance should be carefully evaluated and adjusted to achieve the desired response.[71,80]

**Immunosuppression.** When a foreign material (antigen) gains access to the tissues of a living host, an immune response (antibody) is mounted to destroy the offending material and maintain homeostasis. This response can occur either by humoral immune mechanisms or by cell-mediated immune mechanisms. Both are derived from different types of lymphocytes.[80,82]

Lymphocytes are continually exported from the bone marrow and differentiate into T-lymphocytes and B-lymphocytes. B-lymphocytes are responsible for humoral immunity and develop into plasma cells. These cells produce and secrete antibodies. The result of the antibody-antigen reaction may be a precipitate (an agglutination that renders the cell easily phagocytosed) or a neutralization of the toxin. The humoral response produces vascular damage to the transplanted heart.[71,80,82]

Sensitized T-lymphocytes, important in cellular im-

**TABLE 12-2** Commonly used immunosuppresive drugs in cardiac transplantation

| | Azathioprine (Imuran) | Corticosteroids | Antithymocyte globulin (ATG) | Cyclosporine (Sandimmune) | Orthoclone (OKT-3) |
|---|---|---|---|---|---|
| Use in transplantation | 1962 | 1963 | 1966 | 1978 | 1985 |
| Mechanism of action | An antimetabolite that competes for and blocks specific receptors, affecting DNA and RNA synthesis and interfering with protein synthesis | Antiinflammatory properties reduce capillary permeability, vasodilatation, and edema. May also inhibit movement of T-lymphocytes from blood to graft | ATG prepared by immunizing rabbits or horses with human lymphocytes. ATG binds to T-lymphocytes and reduces their number in circulation | Acts selectively on T-lymphocytes, preventing production of effector T-cells. Does not depress bone marrow as antimetabolites. Immune activity is specific and reversible | Monoclonal antibody that blocks regeneration and functioning of $T_3$-lymphocytes. Effectively blocks both cellular and humoral immune response |
| Metabolism | Liver | Liver | — | Liver | — |
| Side effects | Bone marrow depression resulting in leukopenia, thrombocytopenia, and anemia. Recovery of bone marrow usually rapid following withdrawal or reduction of drug<br>Pancreatitis<br>Muscle-wasting in conjunction with steroids | Infection<br>Diabetes<br>GI bleeding<br>Cushingoid appearance<br>Steroid psychosis | Chills, fever<br>Hypotension<br>Anaphylaxis | Nausea, vomiting, diarrhea<br>Hepatotoxicity (elevated liver enzymes, alkaline phosphatase)<br>Nephrotoxicity (elevated BUN, creatinine clearance)<br>Hypertension | Fever, chills, nausea, vomiting, diarrhea, tremors, arthralgia, hypotension |
| Dosage | Loading: 3-5 mg/kg/day p.o.<br><br>Maintenance: Tapered to 1-2 mg/kg/day p.o. | Loading: Methylprednisone 0.5 g IV intraoperative, with 125 mg IV × 3 doses<br>Maintenance: Prednisone 100 mg p.o. every day. Taper to 0.2-0.5 mg/kg/day by 2 months | Loading: Rabbit ATG 2 mg/kg/day IM every day × 3 days, then every other day × 3 days<br>Equine ATG 10-15 mg/kg/day p.o.<br>Maintenance: Adjusted according to circulating T-cells | Loading: 14-18 mg/kg/day p.o. IV dose ⅓ of oral dose<br><br>Maintenance: 5-10 mg/kg. Adjusted to maintain therapeutic levels | 5-10 mg IV over 15 min q.d. for 10-14 days |

munity, are capable of attacking and destroying the invading antigen. Damage to the heart from this response is made evident by platelet aggregation and thrombosis.[72,80,82]

The goal of immunosuppression is to prevent graft rejection without forfeiting the host's ability to ward off infectious disease. Careful monitoring of the recipient's immune response with adjustment of pharmacologic agents to maintain therapeutic drug levels becomes a central focus in postoperative management. Table 12-2 compares the five most common drugs used today.[2,74,77-79,82]

Variations of immunosuppressive agents and protocols are currently in use. Conventional therapy includes corti-

**TABLE 12-2**  Commonly used immunosuppresive drugs in cardiac transplantation—cont'd

|  | Azathioprine (Imuran) | Corticosteroids | Antithymocyte globulin (ATG) | Cyclosporine (Sandimmune) | Orthoclone (OKT-3) |
|---|---|---|---|---|---|
| Other | Maximum tolerated level judged by absence of complications; WBC should be maintained at 500/mm$^3$ | High doses of steroids are started when rejection is diagnosed in attempt to save graft | Goal of therapy is to suppress circulating lymphocytes to less than 10% of normal (100/mm$^3$). These are assessed daily and dose adjusted. Rises above therapeutic range herald impending graft rejection. T-cells will elevate without rejection (approx. 6 wk) and this immunologic monitoring is no longer sensitive | Blood should be drawn just before drug is given to determine trough level and 2-4 hours later to determine peak levels. Levels: Blood 250-800 mg/ml. Plasma 50-300 mg/ml. Drugs that affect CYA blood levels: (1) cimetidine increases concentration; (2) phenytoin, rifampin, phenobarbital decrease concentration | Monitor T-cell marker assays, orthoclone antibody titer, endomyocardial biopsy |
| Acute rejection | Dose may be increased but in accordance with WBC, platelet count, and any clinical complications | Methylprednisone 1 g every day × 3 days | Repeat course of ATG | Dose may be increased but in accordance with serum levels and any clinical complications | As above |
| Specific nursing care | Monitoring WBC and platelets  Good oral hygiene | Anticipate multiple adverse effects of steroid therapy and plan care accordingly | Skin test prior to injection  "Z" tract technique for IM injections  Pain and inflammation from injection lessened by heat to site before and after injection, massage, exercise  Tylenol and Benedryl prior to injection to minimize anaphylactic response | Careful attention to functioning of renal and hepatic systems  Punctual lab drawing for trough and peak levels  Awareness of effects from other drugs | Pre/post medicate with steroids, acetaminophen, antihistamines  Watch for signs of volume overload or pulmonary edema. |

costeroids, azathioprine, and cyclosporine. Antithymocyte globulin and orthoclone (OKT-3) are used in rejection episodes in addition to conventional therapy.[73,77-80]

More recently orthoclone has been used postoperatively for prophylaxis of rejection as well as the drug of choice in acute rejection episodes. This drug is T-cell specific, blocking the regeneration and functioning of T$_3$-lymphocytes. Treatment is once a day and is continued for 10 to 14 days. Adverse reactions to the drug are controlled through the use of methylprednisone, acetaminophen, hydrocortisone, and diphenhydramine prior to and following administration. Cyclosporine, steroids, and azathioprine are continued during OKT-3 therapy, but their dosages may be decreased.[77,78,79]

**Isolation.** Isolation is necessary to reduce the risk of transmitting infectious organisms via personnel, equipment, and visitors while the patient is severely immunosuppressed. Following surgery, the patient is transferred to a specially equipped isolation room and remains there until endomyocardial biopsy reports and drug levels indicate an adequate immune response. At that time, isolation techniques are reduced and the patient's environment is made more natural. The type of isolation and duration of isolation vary between institutions.[20,71,80]

In preparation for the heart transplant patient, the room is vigorously cleaned with a bactericidal agent and restocked with clean supplies. Many items necessary for patient care cannot be sterilized and, therefore, should be new or made as clean as possible. All equipment must be cleansed with a bactericidal agent before being taken into the room. Traffic in the room is kept to a minimum. Everyone entering the room must undergo proper handwashing and gowning procedures.[20,71,80]

**Infection.** Infection is the leading cause of death within the first 3 months after cardiac transplantation.[80] It is also a major cause of death during the first 2 years. The majority of infections affect the pulmonary subsystem. Bacterial infections are the most common initially, and viral, fungal, and protozoan infections occur later.[71,80]

The high levels of immunosuppression given postoperatively lower the recipient's own bodily defense mechanisms.[81,82] Thus, meticulous surveillance is necessary to detect early signs and symptoms of an infectious process. Aseptic technique must be adhered to with any invasive procedure. Incisions, chest tubes, pacemaker wires, atrial lines, and intravenous lines must all be carefully monitored and cleansed. Sputum and urine cultures are obtained routinely with vigorous pulmonary care following extubation. Daily chest films and temperature ranges are monitored for signs of a beginning infectious process.[71,80]

Patients remain in protective isolation until the immunosuppression levels stabilize and signs of infection are absent.[80] The degree and duration of isolation varies between institutions and according to patient condition. Antibiotics specific to the causative organism are administered and immunosuppression is adjusted as much as possible without causing rejection. Aggressive diagnosis, intervention, and evaluation must occur to control and eradicate the infection before it becomes life-threatening.[80,81]

**Rejection.** Rejection is an expected phenomenon within the first months following cardiac transplantation.[82] It occurs when the recipient's own immune system reacts to foreign surface antigens on the donor heart. This reaction causes vascular damage, platelet aggregation, and thrombosis of the donor heart, resulting in cardiac failure and eventual cessation of function. Early diagnosis and immediate increase of immunosuppressive therapy is mandatory to reverse the rejection process.[80,82]

There are three classifications for rejection episodes. Hyperacute rejection is immediate, occurring within the first hours after transplantation. The recipient's immune system attacks the coronary arteries, resulting in ischemic organ failure. Acute rejection is observed in the first few weeks after surgery. The recipient's immune system causes necrosis with gradual donor heart destruction if not reversed with immunosuppression. Chronic rejection occurs over months and years. Atherosclerotic-like changes occur in the coronary arteries over time, resulting in diffuse disease. As a result of denervation of the donor heart, the recipient feels no chest pain. Therefore other indications must be relied on for the diagnosis of cardiac ischemia: ECG changes, hypotension, dysrhythmias, and enzyme levels.[80,82]

Clinical findings indicative of rejection include:
- Development of $S^3$ and/or $S^4$
- Weakness, fatigue, malaise
- Hypotension

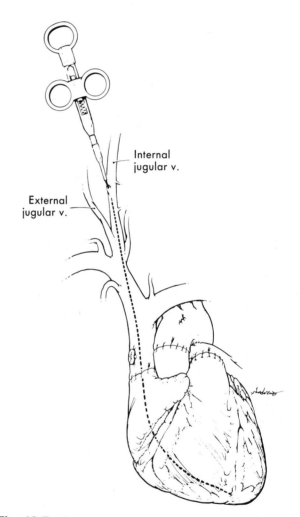

**Fig. 12-7** A myocardial biopsy obtains direct histologic confirmation of rejection. A Bioptome is passed to the apex of the right ventricle and specimens of tissue are removed. PVCs may occur as the instrument comes in contact with the endocardium. The procedure is performed with the patient under local anesthesia in the operating room or cardiac catheterization laboratory with relatively few risks. (From Cooley D: Techniques in cardiac surgery, Philadelphia, 1984, WB Saunders Co.)

Internal jugular v.

External jugular v.

- Elevated atrial pressures
- Decreased urine output
- Weight gain
- Dysrhythmias

The most reliable indicator of rejection is histologic examination of the endomyocardium via serial biopsies (Fig. 12-7). Biopsies of the right ventricle are performed via the right internal jugular vein. They are begun 5 to 7 days after transplantation, then weekly, biweekly, monthly, bimonthly, and eventually every 3 to 4 months. This schedule differs from hospital to hospital and depends on the results of the previous biopsy. Rejection is classified according to the microscopic appearance of the endomyocardial cells in the biopsy sample. Classifications are mild, moderate, or severe rejection.[20,71,80]

If rejection is moderate or severe, aggressive immunosuppressive therapy begins immediately. Initially, methylprednisone, azathioprine, and cyclosporine dosages are increased significantly. Antithymocyte globulin and/or orthoclone are considered if increasing conventional therapy is not effective. Strict protective isolation may be beneficial as the higher immunosuppressive levels pose greater risk for infection. Close monitoring is essential to adequately evaluate the effectiveness of treatment. Frequent biopsies, echocardiograms, drug level determinations, and cardiac output measurements are required to determine the course of the rejection episode. Drug dosages are adjusted carefully to potentiate the fight against rejection but prevent the potent side effects immunosuppressive drugs produce.[20,71,81] Emotional support of the patient and family are vital to achieve the hopeful outlook needed for survival of these episodes.[72,74,81]

If the acute rejection cannot be controlled medically or arteriosclerosis of chronic rejection is present, then retransplantation may be the only alternative. The patient and family need to be counseled about the benefits and risks of retransplantation. Their decision should be accepted and supported by all health personnel without judgment.[72,74]

## REFERENCES

1. American Heart Association: 1990 Heart facts, Dallas, TX, 1990, The Association.
2. Hurst JW and others: Atherosclerotic coronary heart disease: Angina pectoris, myocardial infarction, and other manifestations of myocardial ischemia. In Hurst JW and others, editors: The heart, New York, 1982, McGraw Hill Book Co.
3. Rahimtoola S and others: Ten year survival after coronary artery bypass surgery for unstable angina, N Engl J Med 308:676-681, 1983.
4. Najafi H and others: Post-myocardial ventricular aneurysm. In McCauley K and others, editors: McGoon's cardiac surgery: an interprofessional approach to patient care, Philadelphia, 1985, FA Davis Co.
5. Hurst JW and others: Atherosclerotic coronary heart disease: recognition, prognosis and treatment. In Hurst JW and others, editors: The heart, New York, 1986, McGraw Hill Book Co.
6. Grondin CM and others: Comparison of late changes in internal mammary artery and saphenous vein grafts in two consecutive series of patients 10 years after the operation, Circulation 70(suppl 1): I-208, 1984.
7. Jurado R: Preoperative evaluation and care. In Litwak R and Jurado R, editors: Care of the cardiac surgical patient, East Norwalk, CT, 1982, Appleton-Century-Crofts.
8. Franch R and others: Techniques of cardiac cath including coronary arteriography. In Hurst JW and others, editors: The heart, New York, 1986, McGraw Hill Book Co.
9. Hug CC: Anesthesia and the patient with cardiovascular disease. In Hurst JW and others, editors: The heart, New York, 1986, McGraw Hill Book Co.
10. Schoen FJ and others: Pathologic findings in postcardiotomy patients managed with a temporary left ventricular assist pump, Am J Surg 143:508, 1982.
11. McElligott MT: The person undergoing cardiac surgery. In Guzzetta CE and Dossey BM, editors: Cardiovascular nursing: bodymind tapestry, St Louis, 1984, Mosby—Year Book, Inc.
12. Guyton RA, Williams WH, and Hatcher CE: Techniques of cardiopulmonary bypass. In Hurst JW and others, editors, The heart, New York, 1986, McGraw Hill Book Co.
13. Morgan HE and Neely JR: Metabolic regulation and myocardial function. In Hurst JW and others: editors: The heart, New York, 1986, McGraw Hill Book Co.
14. Ley SJ: Fluid therapy following intracardiac operations, Crit Care Nurse 8(1):26-37, 1988.
15. Heyman, S: Effects of cardiopulmonary bypass on coagulation, Dimens Crit Care Nurs 4(2):70-80, 1985.
16. Utley JR: Pathophysiology and techniques of cardiopulmonary bypass (vol 1), Baltimore, 1982, Williams & Wilkins.
17. Lytle BW and Loop FD: Elective coronary surgery. In McCauley KM and others, editors: McGoon's cardiac surgery: an interprofessional approach to patient care, Philadelphia, 1984, FA Davis Co.
18. Weiland AP and Walker WE: Physiologic principles and clinical sequelae of cardiopulmonary bypass, Heart Lung, 15(1):34-39, 1986.
19. Browett A: Coronary artery bypass graft, Nursing (London) 3(36):26, 1989.
20. Kirklin JW and Barratt-Boyes BG: Cardiac surgery, New York, 1986, Wiley Medical Publications.
21. Jansen KJ and McFadden PM: Postoperative nursing management in patients undergoing myocardial revascularization with internal mammary artery bypass, Heart Lung 15:48, 1986.
22. Erickson RS: Mastering the ins and outs of chest drainage, Nursing 19(6):46, 1989.
23. Schultz CK and Woodall CW: Using epicardial pacing electrodes, J Cardiovasc Nurs 3(3):25, 1989.
24. Hurst JW and others: The heart, arteries and veins, New York, 1986, McGraw Hill Book Co.
25. Lazarus M, Nolasco V, and Luckette C: Cardiac arrhythmias, diagnosis and treatment, Crit Care Nurse 8:57, 1988.
26. Jaffe AS and others: Textbook of advanced cardiac life support, 1987, American Heart Association.
27. Randall EM: Recognizing cardiac tamponade, J Cardiovasc Nurs 3(3):52,1989.
28. Matthay MA and Weiner-Kronish JP: Respiratory management after cardiac surgery, Chest 95:424, 1989.
29. Schultheis AH: When and how to extubate in the recovery room, Am J Nurs 89:1040, 1989.
30. Keeler C and others: A review of infection control practices related to intravascular pressure monitoring devices (1975-1985), 16:201, 1987.
31. Shuhaiber H and others: Wound infection in cardiac surgery, J Cardiovasc Surg 28:139, 1987.
32. Norris SO: Managing postoperative mediastinitis, J Cardiovasc Surg 3(3):52, 1989.

33. Stradtman JC and Ballenger MJ: Nursing implications in sternal and mediastinal infections after open heart surgery, 16:178, 1989.
34. Brannon PHB and Towner SB: Ventricular failure: new therapy using the mechanical assist device, Crit Care Nurse 6(2):74, 1986.
35. Mulford E: Nursing perspectives for the patient receiving postoperative ventricular assistance in the critical care unit, Heart Lung 16(3)246-257, 1987.
36. Quaal SJ: Comprehensive intra-aortic balloon pumping, St Louis, 1984, Mosby–Year Book, Inc.
37. Tilkian AG and Daily EK: Intra-aortic balloon pumping, In Tilkian AG and Daily EK, editors: Cardiovascular procedures: diagnostic techniques and therapeutic procedures, 1986, St Louis, Mosby–Year Book, Inc.
38. Funk M, Gleason J, and Foell D: Lower limb ischemia related to care of the intra-aortic balloon pump, Heart Lung 18:542-552, 1989.
39. Pennock JL and others: Survival and complications following ventricular assist pumping for cardiogenic shock, Ann Surg 198(4):469-478, 1983.
40. Pennington DG: Patient selection, Ann Thorac Surg 47:77-81, 1989.
41. Pae WE and others: Long-term results of ventricular assist pumping in postcardiotomy cardiogenic shock, J Thorac Cardiovasc Surg 93:434-441, 1987.
42. Jett GK, Picone AL, and Clark RE: Circulatory support for right ventricular dysfunction, J Thorac Cardiovasc Surg 94:95-103, 1987.
43. Pae WE, Miller CA, and Pierce WS: Combined registry for the clinical use of mechanical ventricular assist pumps and the total artificial heart: third official report—1988, J Heart Transplant 8(4):277-280, 1989.
44. Schoen FJ, LaFarge CG, and Bernhard WF: Pathology and pathophysiology of temporary cardiac assist, ASAIO 8(3):174-181, 1985.
45. Zumbro GL and others: Mechanical assistance for cardiogenic shock following cardiac surgery, myocardial infarction, and cardiac transplantation, Ann Thorac Surg 44:11-13, 1987.
46. Pennock JL and others: Mechanical support of the circulation followed by cardiac transplantation, J Thorac Cardiovasc Surg 92:984-1004, 1986.
47. Hill JD: Bridging to cardiac transplantation, Ann Thorac Surg 47:167-171, 1989.
48. Olivier HF and others: The use of the biomedicus centrifugal pump in traumatic tears of the thoracic aorta, Pittsburgh, 1984, Allegheny General Hospital.
49. Ruzevich SA, Swartz MT, and Pennington DG: Nursing care of the patient with a pneumatic ventricular assist device, Heart Lung 17:399-407, 1988.
50. Pae WE Jr: Temporary ventricular support: current indications and results, Trans Am Soc Artif Intern Organs 38:4-7, 1987.
51. Park SB and others: Mechanical support of the failing heart, Ann Thorac Surg 42:627-631, 1986.
52. Pennock JL and others: Myocardial oxygen utilization during left heart bypass, Arch Surg 108:635, 1987.
53. Schaper J and others: The effects of global ischemia and reperfusion on human myocardium, quantitative evaluation by electron microscopic morphometry, Ann Thorac Surg 33:116, 1982.
54. Braunwald E and Kloner RA: The stunned myocardium: prolonged, postischemic ventricular dysfunction, Circulation 66:1145-1149, 1982.
55. Dembitsky WP and others: Temporary extracorporeal right ventricular support, J Thorac Cardiovasc Surg 91:518, 1986.
56. Pennington DG and others: Use of the Pierce-Donachy ventricular assist device in patients with cardiogenic shock after cardiac operations, Ann Thorac Surg 47:130-135, 1989.
57. Magovern GJ: Weaning and bridging, Ann Thorac Surg 47:102-107, 1989.
58. Noon GP and others: Reduction of blood trauma in roller pumps for long-term perfusion, World J Surg 9:65, 1985.
59. Magovern GJ, Park SB, and Maher TD: Use of a centrifugal pump without anticoagulants for postoperative left heart assist, World J Surg 9:25, 1985.
60. Pennington DG and others: Experience with the Pierce-Donachy ventricular assist device in postcardiotomy patients with cardiogenic shock, World J Surg 9:37-46, 1985.
61. Pierce WS: Other postoperative complications, Ann Thorac Surg 47:96-101, 1989.
62. Marchetta S and Stennis E: Ventricular assist devices, J Cardiovasc Nurs 2(2):39-55, 1988.
63. Reedy JE, Ruzevich SA, and Swartz MT: Nursing care of a patient requiring prolonged mechanical circulatory support, Prog Cardiovasc Nurs 4:1-9, 1989.
64. Copeland JG: Bleeding and anticoagulation, Ann Thorac Surg 47:88-95, 1989.
65. Gaines WE and others: The Pennsylvania State University paracorporeal ventricular assist pump: optimal methods of use, World J Surg 9:47, 1985.
66. Farrar DJ: Right heart interaction with mechanically assisted left heart, World J Surg 9:89, 1985.
67. Pennington DG and others: Seven years experience with the Pierce-Donachy ventricular assist device, J Cardiovasc Surg 96:901-911, 1988.
68. Rose DM and others: Long-term survival with partial left heart bypass following perioperative infarction and shock, J Cardiovasc Surg 83:483, 1982.
69. Litwak RS: A decade of experience with a left heart assist device in patients undergoing open intracardiac operation, World J Surg 9:18, 1985.
70. Futterman LG: Cardiac transplantation: a comprehensive nursing perspective. Part 1, Heart Lung 17:499, 1988.
71. Wallwork J: Heart and heart-lung transplantation, Philadelphia, 1989, WB Saunders Co.
72. McAleer MJ and others: Psychological aspects of heart transplantation, Heart Transplant 4:232, 1985.
73. White-Williams C: Cardiac transplantation: a post operative guide for patients, Birmingham, 1989, University of Alabama at Birmingham Publications.
74. Gunderson L: Teaching the transplant recipient, Heart Transplant 4:226, 1985.
75. Snyder LA and Peter NK: How to manage organ donation, Am Heart J 89:134, 1989.
76. Brown ME: Clinical management of organ donation, Dimens Crit Care Nurs 8:134, 1989.
77. Rogers KR, Sinott JT, and Ferguson JE: Using OKT3 to reverse allograft rejection, Heart Lung 18:490, 1989.
78. Doult LA, Nagy CS, and Collins JA: Reversing cardiac transplant rejection with orthoclone—Okt-3, Am J Nurs 89:953, 1989.
79. Ortho Multicenter Transplant Study Group: A randomized trial of OKT3 monoclonal antibody for acute rejection of cadaveric renal transplant, N Engl J Med 313:337, 1985.
80. Futterman LG: Cardiac transplantation: a comprehensive perspective. Part II, Heart Lung 17:631, 1988.
81. Laufer G: and others: Infectious complications in heart transplant recipients with combined low dose cyclosporin, azathioprine and predniscolone (triple drug) immunosuppression, Transplant Proc 21:2508, 1989.
82. Murdock DK: Rejection of the transplanted heart. Heart Lung 16:237, 1987.

# CHAPTER 13

# Cardiac Rehabilitation

Nancy Houston Miller

Technologic advances in the management of patients suffering cardiovascular diseases over the past decade have virtually revolutionized care. Innovations in both medical and surgical management, including the introduction of thrombolytic therapy and angioplasty, have been accompanied by a significant reduction in early mortality in the post–myocardial infarction population. Moreover, while there has been a burgeoning of technologic advances, the public also has become increasingly aware of the importance of a change in health behaviors or cardiovascular risk reduction.

With such changes in the early care of cardiovascular patients has come a shift and advancement in the rehabilitation of these patients. No longer are patients kept in bed and restricted from activities as they were for almost 30 years; no longer are they prevented from formally participating in moderate to high-level activity until 8 to 12 weeks postinfarction; and no longer are physicians and nurses questioning the advice they give about resumption of normal activities: all of these decisions are based on new scientific evidence of the safety of resuming such tasks early in the course of recovery for the majority of patients.

Because the goal of cardiac rehabilitation is to restore patients to their optimum physical, medical, psychologic, emotional, vocational, and economic status, it is important to review how recent changes in management and rehabilitation have affected and will continue to affect patients treated in the 1990s.

Changes in medical management have been dramatic. One such change has been the increasingly widespread application of therapies designed to restore coronary blood flow in the early hours of myocardial infarction (MI), thereby limiting the extent of infarcted myocardium. This approach has added a new dimension to coronary care, which previously was limited to therapies designed to treat the complications of an infarct rather than the underlying process. The rationale for such intervention comes from evidence that acute coronary thrombosis occurring at the site of a preexisting arteriosclerotic plaque is usually the immediate event that precipitates an MI[1] and by restoring blood flow within a critical period of time (1 to 6 hours), myocardium that would otherwise have become infarcted can now be salvaged.[2] Interventions such as thrombolytic

agents (e.g., streptokinase and tissue plasminogen activator), mechanical dilatation of an occluded or stenotic coronary vessel by percutaneous transluminal coronary angioplasty (PTCA), and acute surgical coronary artery bypass grafting (CABG) have all been used for this purpose. Thus, the end result of salvaging myocardium has had a major impact on both in-hospital survival and potential long-term survival in the months following infarction.

A second important change in management has been the recognition that clinical variables and exercise test results performed early in the course of recovery provide important prognostic information about the patient's risk of future events in the year following MI.[3] Such recognition has led to earlier interventions for high-risk patients, and recommendations for low-risk patients to resume normal activities earlier. Formerly, patients who were identified as low-risk would have been managed in an identical manner to patients identified as high-risk. The current management of these patient subsets will be discussed in the next section.

A shift in clinical management has also precipitated a shift in cardiac rehabilitation. From the 1930s until the 1960s, physicians severely restricted activities of coronary patients, especially after an MI. Patients were kept at bedrest for many days, hospitalized up to 3 to 4 weeks, and restricted from resuming normal activities often until 3 months after the event. These recommendations were based on concerns that even routine activities would cause undue stress on a damaged heart, and might precipitate further life-threatening cardiac events. Decisions were based on subjective information with little consideration given to the patient's course of recovery or to exercise testing, which was thought to be unsafe early in the postinfarction period.

In the early to middle 1970s, however, a change in management of these patients occurred as more information was acquired. Researchers began to question earlier studies, believing restrictions on activity levels were excessive and questioning the belief that all patients were at high-risk after the event. Early exercise testing provided the impetus for this change in rehabilitation management. Once it was determined to be safe in this population, early treadmill testing, performed 3 weeks after MI and then at discharge, became the standard care. Such testing provided physicians with important information about the degree of myocardial ischemia, the patient's functional capacity, and the ability of patients to resume physical activities. Likewise, hospitalization stays decreased to 7 days in many patients with uncomplicated disease, and rehabilitation programs began enrolling patients at 3 to 4 weeks after the event rather than 8 to 12 weeks. This timing facilitated the patient's return to usual activities much sooner after the cardiac event.

Although formal rehabilitation programs were developed in hospitals and community centers around the country beginning in the 1970s, it was apparent that the number of available programs was insufficient to meet the needs of the large numbers of patients with coronary heart disease. And so with the 1980s came the advent of home rehabilitation for low-risk patients. This approach continues to be tested, and methods to enhance compliance to exercise training and to modification of coronary risk factors, the cornerstone of rehabilitation efforts, continue to be explored for patients involved in home rehabilitation programs.

What does the future of cardiac rehabilitation look like in the 1990s? It is still somewhat unclear as clinical management moves ahead, but most certainly health care professionals in formal cardiac rehabilitation programs will be involved in caring for a sicker, more elderly population. And as the pendulum swings, as was the case in the 1930s through the 1960s, much is to be learned about this population's ability to exercise safely, to modify coronary risk factors, and to achieve optimum lives. In addition, critical consideration will be given to individualizing rehabilitation services to the needs of the patient. Rather than a comprehensive package of services offered to all patients, some patients will receive a very formal structured program of medically supervised training, psychologic counseling, and intensive risk factor intervention, while others will exercise on their own at home and undertake self-help methods to modify the behaviors of smoking, dietary change, weight loss, and other risk factors. Moreover, while the central focus of rehabilitation programs used to be exercise training, as younger patients experience less extensive infarctions accompanied by a shortened duration of illness and faster return to normal activities, a change in functional capacity will become less of a concern, and risk factor modification will become increasingly important. For the more elderly patient with multiple infarctions and a chronic disease state, however, medical supervision and the supportive environment of a group while undergoing exercise training may become very important.

Cardiac rehabilitation involves three basic principles. First, the patient must be evaluated early and repeatedly. Evaluation is most often provided through treadmill testing. The purposes of evaluation are to provide the basis for recommending specific activities and to identify pa-

tients in need of medication therapy or surgical treatment of complicating problems such as angina pectoris. Second, programs of exercise training must be individually prescribed to augment functional capacity. Third, intensive risk factor intervention and vocational and psychologic assessment and evaluation must be provided by members of the health care team. The remainder of this chapter will focus on the above principles.

## REHABILITATION PERIODS

It is important that the rehabilitation of patients be viewed as a continuous and logical process that begins in the hospital, most often in the coronary care unit (CCU) or intensive care unit (ICU), and extends to a lifetime program of prudent activity and risk-factor control. The efficacy of the process is compromised when such efforts are delayed weeks or months after the patient's discharge from the hospital.

For patients involved in formally structured rehabilitation programs, management is divided into four stages: (1) the in-hospital stage, which is on average 5 to 14 days for patients with an MI or undergoing coronary artery surgery; (2) the early stage after hospital discharge, generally 8 to 12 weeks; (3) the later rehabilitation stage, which is usually 4 to 6 months or longer in duration; and (4) the ongoing maintenance stage, wherein the patient seeks to continue the exercise program and a high-level of achievement in modifying risk-factors.[4] For patients who may not have access to a formally structured program it is important to consider the necessary components of rehabilitation during the in-hospital and outpatient recovery stages.

### In-hospital Rehabilitation

**Activity guidelines.** Rehabilitation begins once the patient has been stabilized and is free from life-threatening complications. For patients with uncomplicated disease, the use of the bedside commode, short walks to a private bathroom, and self-care activities such as bathing, shaving, and dressing are appropriate even in the first 24 to 48 hours. Range of motion exercises and chair-sitting counteract the deleterious effects of bedrest[5] and may forestall unwarranted fears patients have about physical activity; such fears may otherwise persist for extended periods of time after infarction. Early activity also minimizes the risk of venous thrombosis and pulmonary embolus.[6]

For most patients, gradual walking about the room and hospital corridors occurs by the third day after the event. The goal at this stage of rehabilitation is not to undertake aerobic training but to minimize physical deconditioning, prevent venous thrombosis, and enhance the overall psychologic well-being of the patient. This can best be accomplished through early ambulation.

Walking sessions within the hospital should be short (5 to 20 minutes) and of low intensity. Most often the guideline for exercise intensity is a heart rate not exceeding 20 beats/min above the resting heart rate. Multiple short walks throughout the day may be preferable to a single longer walk. Monitoring heart rate and blood pressure response to early ambulation, ECG abnormalities, and symptoms becomes important in detecting problems such as myocardial ischemia or dysrhythmias that may require immediate attention or a reduction in activity levels. Activity schedules need to be modified for those patients who experience a more complicated course involving postinfarction angina, congestive heart failure, or severe atrial or ventricular dysrhythmias. For patients who experience complications such as ventricular fibrillation or other transient dysrhythmias within the first 24 hours after MI, management is often similar to that for patients with uncomplicated disease.

In past years rehabilitation during the early stages of recovery often included carefully defined steps of gradually progressing activities. Such approaches included upper and lower body range of motion exercises, progressing to bedside dangling, chair-sitting, and eventually gradual walks of longer and longer durations occurring over several days' time. Physical therapists or nurses were responsible for employing such graduated activity guidelines. While appropriate for sicker patients, such as those with congestive heart failure, with comorbidities, and the elderly, most patients are now discharged so quickly after angioplasty, MI, and other cardiovascular events that requiring progressive steps is not feasible. The goal therefore should be to ambulate the patient as soon as possible to begin to prepare for a return to normal activities.

**Educational and psychologic needs.** Shortened hospitalizations prevent nurses, physicians, or a rehabilitation team from spending a great deal of time in providing patient education; most often this is left to the outpatient stage of recovery. Educational efforts, however, routinely begin in the hospital and should include information that is individualized and directed to patients' needs. Most often in the CCU and in the transition unit, information is provided about anatomy and physiology, procedures, and treatments. It is important to provide the following specific information before hospital discharge: (1) instructions about medications, their proper administration, and side effects; (2) activity guidelines, which provide the patient with a written prescription for exercise training; (3) recommendations for resumption of sexual activity and issues related to return to work; (4) and an introduction to coronary risk factor modification, which not only includes exercise but dietary modification and treatment of hyperlipidemia, smoking cessation, and management of hypertension, diabetes, and stress. Educational videotapes and pamphlets are often available to supplement teaching efforts. These issues will be discussed more fully in the latter part of this chapter.

Critical to the rehabilitation of the patient in any phase of recovery is the family, and especially the spouse. The spouse should be involved in all educational sessions, and attention should be paid to concerns and questions that may be quite different than those of the patient. Insufficient information about dietary management, permissible activity, and sexual activity have all been found to be sources of concern for spouses.[7] In one study spouses reported that more information at the time of hospitalization might have helped them to respond more appropriately to patients' needs.[8]

Psychologic recovery is also an important component of rehabilitation. Patients respond to a cardiac event with diverse coping mechanisms. Some patients deny the crisis event, and others exaggerate the problem, never returning to normal activities despite minimal limitations on cardiac function. For the patient suffering an MI, however, there is a normal sequence of emotional responses similar to that in Kubler-Ross's theory of grief and loss.[9] The patient may suffer anxiety, denial, depression, and anger over the event. Moreover, the spouse and family may respond with similar psychologic reactions. Such reactions should be acknowledged by rehabilitation personnel; individual interviews in the hospital with a psychologist or psychiatrist may contribute a great deal to patient management. In considering the varied responses and adaptation for patients suffering coronary heart disease, a more detailed review of psychosocial recovery is noted in Chapter 7.

**Risk stratification.** A major goal of rehabilitation in the early phase of recovery should be risk stratification. Establishing a patient's prognosis based on the results of clinical and historical information, including the physical examination and ECG findings and an exercise test performed alone or in conjunction with radionuclide scintigraphy or ventriculography, provides the basis for important management decisions. Such information is useful because the majority of second events occur early in the course of recovery, most often within 3 to 6 months.[10]

Severe left ventricular dysfunction, myocardial ischemia, and ventricular dysrhythmias are important predictors of outcome. Failure to identify these predictors may deny patients from receiving potentially life-saving therapies or may result in inappropriate decisions concerning early rehabilitation. Likewise, failure to identify low-risk patients may result in unnecessary restrictions on physical activity or delayed return to work.

DeBusk and colleagues[11] reviewed data on a cohort of patients followed for 32 months to determine medical events including death, recurrent MI, congestive heart failure, and unstable angina. Risk in the 6 months after MI was increased (8.6% versus 4.4%) for patients with history of previous MI, or angina for 2 to 3 months before the MI, and recurrent chest pain within 24 hours after admission but prior to discharge, or who had clinical characteristics that were primarily contraindications to symptom-limited treadmill testing (i.e., CHF, rest angina, severe

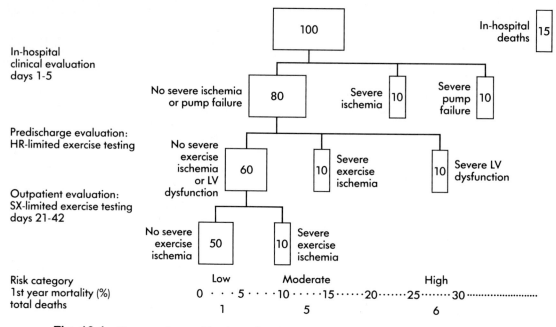

In-hospital
deaths  15

In-hospital
clinical evaluation
days 1-5

100

No severe ischemia
or pump failure  80

Severe
ischemia  10

Severe
pump
failure  10

Predischarge evaluation:
HR-limited exercise testing

No severe
exercise
ischemia
or LV
dysfunction  60

Severe
exercise
ischemia  10

Severe LV
dysfunction  10

Outpatient evaluation:
SX-limited exercise testing
days 21-42

No severe
exercise
ischemia  50

Severe
exercise
ischemia  10

| Risk category | Low | Moderate | High | |
|---|---|---|---|---|
| 1st year mortality (%) | 0 · · ·5· · · ·10· · · · ·15· · · · · ·20· · · · ·25· · · · · ·30 · · · · · · · · · · · · · · · | | | |
| total deaths | 1 | 5 | 6 | |

**Fig. 13-1**   **Prognostic stratification of patients into three risk categories (low, moderate, and high) after acute MI.** The size of each patient subset is indicated by the numbers in boxes. The stratification of patients is based on the extent of myocardial ischemia, and left ventricular (LV) dysfunction. *HR,* heart rate; *SX,* symptom. (From DeBusk R and others: N Engl J Med 314(4):162, 1986.)

cardiovascular, pulmonary, or orthopedic disease). The best treadmill test predictor was 0.2 mv or more of ST depression at a heart rate of less than 135 beats/min. Patients with such an abnormality had an event rate of 9.6% over 6 months.[11]

The ability to stratify a patient's risk allows high-risk patients with significant abnormalities to be considered for aggressive medical or surgical therapy and patients at low-risk to be cleared for early resumption of work and rehabilitation. In most reported studies at least 50% of the population is uncomplicated with an overall event rate of less than 5% in the year after MI. In this population it is doubtful that any surgical or medical intervention will improve outcome. However, 25% to 30% of all patients are high-risk patients, and those with compromised left ventricular function are most often treated medically, requiring greater attention to rehabilitation efforts. Fig. 13-1 provides an overview of the prognostic stratification of patients after acute MI.

**Treadmill test.** In stratifying risk, a treadmill exercise evaluation is performed prior to discharge or soon thereafter (1 to 2 weeks) in patients recovering from acute MI. More important than timing of the test are patient selection criteria. Clinical evidence of congestive heart failure, unstable angina, or other limiting medical conditions, such as severe obesity, peripheral vascular disease, or ECG abnormalities of atrial fibrillation or left bundle branch block, is a contraindication to testing. As noted in Fig. 13-1,

however, a large percentage of patients (80%) are eligible for exercise testing early in the course of recovery.[4] The treadmill test not only provides important prognostic information, but it also serves as a guide for decisions about resumption of physical activity, including occupational tasks, and forms the basis for an exercise prescription. Moreover, patients' confidence in their ability to perform usual activities is often reduced after an MI.[12] The treadmill test and counseling thereafter may enhance patient's perceptions of their capabilities, which in turn may affect their earlier return to normal activities.

Exercise testing elicits various ECG (ST-depression and dysrhythmias), hemodynamic (peak blood pressure and workload), and symptomatic (angina, fatigue, dyspnea) responses.[13] During the test, a 12-lead ECG should be recorded at each 2 to 3 minute stage, the blood pressure measured, and the patient's clinical status monitored. Exercise test endpoints include limiting fatigue or dyspnea; severe chest discomfort (3 on a scale of 4); a systolic fall in blood pressure of 10 mm Hg or more on a successive stage; high-grade ventricular dysrhythmias, especially 3 or more beats in a row (ventricular tachycardia); and other ECG abnormalities such as second degree or third degree heart block, atrial fibrillation, or rate-related bundle branch block. Although ischemia (ST-segment depression) has prognostic significance, it is not normally an endpoint for ending a test.

The metabolic unit (MET) is used to quantify treadmill

workloads, or an individual's physical capacity.[14] Standing quietly at rest requires 1 MET or 3.5 ml/$O_2$/kg/min. The average uncomplicated post-MI patient can complete about 7 to 8 METs of work on a symptom-limited test performed within the first 3 weeks of recovery.[15] This MET capacity is above the capacity required for almost all occupational and recreational tasks performed by patients. Thus the treadmill workload, in conjunction with other test variables, can be used to determine the safety of a return to various activities. For those patients showing prognostically significant treadmill abnormalities (i.e., low workload <5 MET, >2 mm ST-segment depression, abnormal fall in systolic blood pressure, or severe angina) further diagnostic testing and evaluation can be prescribed. For the uncomplicated patient, a recommendation for moderate exercise can be provided.

On discharge from the hospital it is recommended that patients be given explicit information about resumption of routine activities. An ideal prescription for activity includes the type, intensity, duration, and frequency of exercise, early warning signs and signals, and the components of an exercise session, all of which are discussed under the exercise training section of this chapter.

## Outpatient Recovery Period

**Early stage (up to 3 months).** The first few weeks after hospital discharge is an important time for the patient and a critical period in rehabilitation. Not only is this the period of highest mortality rates, but patients are vulnerable to anxiety over the safety of routine activities, and psychologic depression may occur in looking to the future. During this stage of recovery, rehabilitation should address the following:

1. Monitoring patient's symptoms of angina, dysrhythmias, or severe ventricular dysfunction
2. Provision for allaying psychologic fears and anxieties and fostering a positive outlook
3. Facilitating early return to work and leisure activities based on the patient's clinical status
4. Extending educational efforts with an emphasis on behavior change that was begun in the hospital

It is essential that patients have frequent contact with health care personnel, whether by telephone or face-to-face in a formal rehabilitation setting during this stage of recovery.

If cardiac rehabilitation programs exist within the hospital or community settings, patients should be enrolled in them immediately after hospital discharge. Such programs provide close medical supervision, which allows for prompt identification of complicating medical events, facilitates patients' proper interpretation of new symptoms, and provides reassurance to patients and their families. Specific attention can also be given to the spouse in this difficult time of adjustment. Although patients are given educational instructions during hospitalization, they usu-

ally do not have time or receptivity to the amount of information provided. The outpatient recovery period is a better time for learning. Therefore, adequate provision of information about cardiovascular risk reduction is critical to help patients modify their behavior during the outpatient recovery period.

In addition to providing an adequate environment for exercise training, all of the features of rehabilitation can be handled adequately when a patient has access to a formal program. If outpatient cardiac rehabilitation programs do not exist in hospitals or the community, consideration must be given to alternative methods for rehabilitation in order to address patient needs. Home rehabilitation programs using nurses and other health care personnel to manage uncomplicated patients by telephone have been shown to be effective in the outpatient recovery period.[16] The use of group educational classes, frequent contact by physician office staff, and transtelephonic ECG monitoring have also proven to be helpful when formal programs are unavailable.[17]

**Late stage (3 months and beyond).** The latter stage of the outpatient rehabilitation period is simply an extension of what was learned and undertaken on hospital discharge. Patients begin to see their limitations, if any, and a specific plan to reduce these limitations can be formulated. The specific goals continue to be enhancement of functional capacity through exercise training, identification of patients who may require intervention such as angioplasty or surgery, limitation of psychologic problems that may impede functioning, and intensive risk factor reduction to prevent future cardiac events. This process of rehabilitation continues throughout the patient's life. Although patients return to work and may achieve an optimum level of functional capacity (8 to 9 MET is often a threshold), maintenance of lifestyle changes is important, including adherence to medications, modification of diet, and continued cessation of smoking. As patients progress and learn to successfully make important lifestyle modifications, specialized assistance from the rehabilitation team may not be needed. Other patients, however, lack self-motivation and may choose to continue participation in a community program that offers a supervised maintenance program.

## EXERCISE BENEFITS AND TRAINING

Exercise training has a number of beneficial effects for the patient with coronary heart disease (CHD) who suffers an MI. Exercise aids in the management of hypertension[18] and obesity[19] and may improve glucose tolerance in patients with diabetes mellitus.[20] Moreover, exercise may improve the plasma lipid-lipoprotein profile by increasing levels of high-density lipoprotein (HDL) fraction and subfractions and reducing triglycerides.[21]

Various uncontrolled studies have reported some psychologic benefits of exercise including a reduction in anxiety and depression and improved self-esteem in patients.[22,23] However, the majority of large well-controlled studies have not shown that exercise improves psychologic status.[24]

Although there is evidence that exercise will reduce initial CHD events and mortality, whether exercise training will further reduce morbidity and mortality in patients suffering an MI is controversial.[25] Studies to date have not been large enough to test the independent effect; and because of compliance problems, the confounding effect of other CHD risk factors, and high financial costs, it is unlikely that another major research trial will ever be conducted.[26] Most of the reported randomized secondary prevention trials, however, have demonstrated a favorable trend for a lower mortality in exercising groups as compared with control groups. Therefore, in the absence of conclusive data regarding the effects of exercise training on longevity in patients after MI, the beneficial effects of an improvement in exercise capacity and the independent effects of exercise on other risk factors provide a persuasive case for exercise in cardiac rehabilitation.

## Exercise Prescription

To achieve cardiovascular conditioning, an exercise prescription should be developed considering the patient's age, past exercise history, and preferences. Exercise prescriptions are normally based on the results of the graded exercise test, taking into account the workload attained, the maximum heart rate achieved, the blood pressure response, symptoms and signs of ischemia, and dysrhythmias. The level of intensity of exercise should be low enough in the first few weeks of training to prevent undue muscle soreness or orthopedic problems.

A written exercise program should include information about the type, intensity, frequency, and duration of exercise, and indicate warning signs and symtoms of overexertion. In addition, patients should be aware of various medications that may affect their response to exercise.

Activities that promote cardiovascular conditioning involve the large dynamic muscles of the body. Such activities include brisk walking, jogging, stationary and regular cycling, swimming, stair-climbing, and selected others. These types of exercises allow the heart rate to be sustained in an appropriate intensity range to achieve cardiovascular conditioning.

**Activity intensity.** The intensity of exercise is determined by the most recent treadmill test. Although many studies in normal and coronary patients suggest that an ideal training range is an intensity sufficient to increase oxygen consumption to between 70% and 85% of maximum,[27] even patients exercising at 60% of maximum oxygen uptake ($VO_2$) will achieve conditioning benefits.[28]

One can determine the heart rate range for conditioning by adding 70% to 85% of the increment between resting heart rate and maximum heart rate to the resting heart rate.

For example, if the resting heart rate is 80 beats/min and the peak exercise heart rate is 180 beats/min, 70% of the maximum heart rate is 150 beats/min (70% of (180-80) + 80) and 85% of maximum oxygen consumption will occur at 165 beats/min (85% of (180-80) + 80). When patients count their pulse rates, they should use a 10-second interval and multiply by 6.

If patients have angina or severe ischemia (ST depression of 2 mm or greater) on an exercise test, exercise intensity should be decreased by 10 to 15 beats below the onset of angina or ischemic abnormalities.

Patients should begin an exercise program at the lower intensity threshold (i.e., 60% to 70%) for a few weeks, especially if they have not previously exercised. Signs and symptoms of overexertion should be watched for—these include excessive fatigue and shortness of breath. Any change in symptoms such as the development of angina pectoris should be reported to the physician.

Another method of monitoring the intensity of exercise is by using the Rating of Perceived Exertion Scale (Borg Scale) which corresponds to the patient's level of fatigue with increasing heart rate.[29] This 15-point scale ranging from 6 to 20 is most often used during exercise testing to measure level of comfort. Because the scale corresponds so closely to actual heart rate and is a good indicator of fatigue, it can also be used to monitor exercise training intensity provided patients are introduced appropriately to this method.

**Activity duration.** In order to achieve cardiovascular benefit, the duration of activity equates to a period of 20 to 40 minutes in which the heart rate is sustained in the target zone. Most exercise sessions begin with a warm-up period of 5 to 10 minutes during which the heart rate gradually increases, 20 to 30 minutes of a conditioning phase in the intensity threshold range, and 5 to 10 minutes of cool down when the metabolic and circulatory systems gradually return to baseline. A cool down period is essential. In formal rehabilitation programs, most occurrences of exercise-related ventricular fibrillation have developed during cool down, often in patients who were exercising beyond prescribed intensities.[30]

**Activity frequency.** Exercise must be performed on a regular basis for patients to achieve optimum cardiovascular benefit. Usually 3 to 5 days per week is optimum and may prevent risks of musculoskeletal or orthopedic injuries. If patients are exercising at a lower intensity of effort, five exercise sessions per week is preferable. Scheduling this number of exercising days also helps patients who may have problems complying with exercise sessions.

In helping the patient create an exercise prescription, appropriate consideration needs to be given to the patient's exercise preferences, goals, and personal safety. Often people begin exercise programs undertaking activities they don't necessarily enjoy and at intensities too high to permit exercise to be enjoyable. Allowing patients to become involved in planning exercise prescriptions often ensures that appropriate choices will be made, which in turn will enhance compliance and satisfaction.

## Supervised Versus Unsupervised Exercise

Unfortunately formal rehabilitation programs are available to only a small percentage of patients suffering cardiovascular disease. Most programs are located in large metropolitan areas and the majority are hospital-based. These programs provide for ongoing supervision of patients during exercise conditioning, facilitate patient education opportunities, and provide medical surveillance of patient's clinical status through contact with health care professionals.

Although the risks of exercise training in cardiovascular patients are extremely low (less than one death per 783,927 million patient man hours in a supervised setting),[31] serious problems such as ventricular fibrillation and MI do occur. In supervised programs most cardiac arrest victims are successfully resuscitated, while outside this setting such events may be uniformly lethal.

Because of a lack of availability of programs, however, or for economic and other reasons, not all patients choose to attend a formal rehabilitation program. Patients who are not in a program need to be provided with appropriate risk factor education and exercise guidelines similar to those developed for a structured formal program.

The American College of Physicians and American College of Cardiology, among others, have formulated guidelines based on research findings to indicate which patients are at particularly high risk and should require intensive surveillance in cardiac rehabilitation programs.[32,33] High-risk patients include those:

1. With left ventricular ejection fraction (LVEF) less than 30%
2. With complex dysrhythmias
3. Who demonstrate the appearance of increasing ventricular dysrhythmia with exercise
4. Whose systolic blood pressure falls 15 mm Hg or more during exercise
5. Whose graded exercise tests showed ischemia indicated by anginal pain or 2 mm or more of ST depression
6. Whose recent MI was complicated by serious ventricular dysrhythmia
7. Who are survivors of sudden cardiac death

It is estimated by these groups that approximately 25% of patients fall into this high-risk category.[34] For those patients who do not exhibit the above characteristics unsupervised activity in a home setting may be an alternative to a formal rehabilitation program. The efficacy and safety of such programs for patients suffering an uncomplicated infarction or who have undergone coronary artery surgery have been documented in the literature.[16,35] Our experience with this population of uncomplicated post-MI patients

exercising at home indicates that both functional capacity achieved at 6 months following the event and adherence are similar to that of patients enrolled in supervised cardiac rehabilitation programs.[17] The safety of home training is enhanced through patient selection, symptom-limited exercise testing prior to providing an exercise prescription, teaching patients about cautionary symptoms, and using heart rate monitors during the initial few weeks of the program to help patients learn to monitor exercise intensity. Ongoing surveillance of patients is also provided through telephone follow-up by health care professionals such as nurses. In addition, patient adherence to exercise training and other risk factors at home can be enhanced through the use of activity logs, self-monitoring charts, contracts, and self-test methods undertaken to determine improvement in exercise conditioning. Current research focuses on nurse management of multiple risk factors in patients with CHD in the year following MI. This new model of education and behavioral counseling begins in the hospital and provides for telephone follow-up and limited face-to-face counseling in the outpatient recovery stage. The behaviors of exercise, smoking cessation, and dietary and drug management of hyperlipidemia are carefully managed through home rehabilitation efforts. The success of such programs may allow a greater number of patients to receive rehabilitation services.

## MODIFICATION OF LIFESTYLE
### Managing Coronary Risk Factors

In addition to exercise, modification of coronary risk factors is an important component of rehabilitation efforts beginning during hospitalization and continuing in the outpatient stage of recovery. Many cardiac rehabilitation programs employ a multidisciplinary team in the hospital, which includes clinical nutritionists, exercise physiologists, physical and occupational therapists, and clinical psychologists in addition to physicians and nurses, to provide education about risk factor management and to carry out other rehabilitation activities. The high prevalence of coronary-prone lifestyles, of maladaptive behavioral response to environmental stresses, and acute or chronic emotional distress in coronary patients warrants the inclusion of these health professionals in the rehabilitation process on a routine basis. Other settings use only nurses and physicians to provide rehabilitation guidelines, using ancillary personnel as needed. What is critical, however, is that modification of lifestyle, which often requires changes in ingrained habits, becomes an important part of rehabilitation throughout the recovery period. Such efforts help pave the way for patients to begin to develop self-control strategies in maintaining change in behavior patterns. Management of hyperlipidemia through medications and modifications in diet, cigarette smoking, obesity, stress, and alcohol intake requires attention in secondary prevention. Modification of these lifestyle features is highlighted below.

**Diet.** A change in dietary habits may promote a reduction in serum cholesterol and triglyceride levels, blood pressure, and total body weight.[35] Moreover, those patients suffering diabetes and CHD may note an improvement in blood glucose levels.[36] Although there is no indication that a change in dietary intake of saturated fat and cholesterol has a significant impact on morbidity and mortality in those patients with established coronary heart disease, diet may significantly reduce the need for high doses of lipid-lowering and antihypertensive medications in these patients.[37]

Dietary guidelines developed by the National Cholesterol Education Program recommend that patients with cardiovascular disease and with low-density lipoprotein (LDL) cholesterol higher than 130 mg/dl begin a progressive two-stage plan to change dietary habits. The step-one diet includes a reduction in total fat to less than 30% of total daily calories, consisting of less than 10% saturated fat, less than 10% polyunsaturated fat, and remaining fat from monounsaturated fatty acids; cholesterol intake is reduced to 300 mg/day. If a step-two diet is needed, total saturated fat is further restricted to less than 7% and cholesterol to 200 mg/day. If LDL cholesterol values remain above 130 mg/dl after 6 months of dietary intervention, patients should be recommended for treatment with lipid lowering medications.[38] Dietary guidelines for the cardiovascular patient may also require sodium restriction and limiting total calorie consumption to that required to maintain ideal body weight.

Dieticians and other health care professionals can contribute to the rehabilitation of patients by analyzing dietary patterns and making specific suggestions that allow the diet to remain palatable to the individual, affordable, nutritionally adequate, and capable of achieving the desired effects. Ongoing assessment of dietary patterns at follow-up intervals may provide a means to determine if patients are able to maintain suggested dietary changes. Individual or group sessions designed to help patients with label-reading, grocery shopping, recipe modification, and cooking techniques may also support needed changes in behavior.

One dietary change important for many cardiac patients is restricting total calories to control obesity. In addition to the deleterious effects obesity has on lipoprotein levels, hypertension, and diabetes, some obese patients may experience great functional impairment and may have cardiac complications such as angina pectoris and congestive heart failure. In such cases a very low calorie diet administered under strict medical supervision may promote massive weight loss.

The National Obesity Consensus Conference considers obesity to be 20% above ideal body weight, which corresponds to a body mass index (BMI) (BMI = body weight in kg/height in meters, squared) above 26.4 for men and 25.8 for women.[39] Patients above the range should be on calorie restricted diets and provided with an appropriate exercise program for better maintenance of weight loss. A weight loss of 1 to 3 pounds per week without symptoms of ketosis can be expected for most individuals consuming 700 to 1000 calories daily.

**Serum cholesterol.** Although a change in eating habits is the first recommendation for treatment of coronary patients with elevated blood cholesterol many coronary patients will require drug therapy to achieve the recommended reduction in LDL cholesterol. Moreover, studies of patients with established coronary heart disease indicate that lowering serum cholesterol reduces the risk of subsequent coronary events, and aggressive management may actually slow the progression of coronary heart disease.[40-42] In the Coronary Drug Project, a trial of 8341 men who had suffered an MI, patients receiving nicotinic acid had a significant reduction in recurrent nonfatal MIs compared with control subjects; the reduction was still apparent 15 years after the trial.[43] Blankenhorn[42] also studied 162 men following coronary artery bypass surgery. Treatment included a diet low in fat, saturated fat, and cholesterol and a combination of colestipol and nicotinic acid or a placebo for 2 years. Atherosclerotic progression was significantly less in patients taking drugs versus placebo. Regression of the disease also occurred in 16.2% of patients treated with colestipol-niacin versus 2.4% of placebo patients (p < 0.02).[42]

The use of drugs such as the bile-acid binding resins, colestipol and cholestyramine, nicotinic acid, and gemfibrozil found to be effective in clinical trials, as well as the newer HMG CoA reductive inhibitors such as Mevinolin, may clearly affect patients' prognoses. Health care professionals, especially physicians and nurses working in rehabilitation, have an opportunity to provide education about specific medications, monitor side effects, tailor behavioral strategies to enhance compliance, and monitor ongoing problems with medications.

**Cigarette smoking.** Continued cigarette smoking is associated with recurrent fatal and nonfatal events in patients with coronary heart disease.[44,45] For example, Sparrow and associates[46] found an 18.8% mortality rate 6 years after MI in men who quit smoking compared with a 30.4% mortality in those who maintained or resumed their smoking status after infarction. Stopping smoking may reduce mortality rates by as much as 50%.[47]

In cardiac patients the rates of cessation after an event such as an MI are approximately 50% when the physician and rehabilitation team are committed to smoking cessation efforts.[48] Recidivism rates may be quite high, however, and some studies have indicated that smokers often resume their habit immediately on hospital discharge.[49]

Interventions for smoking cessation in patients with CHD have primarily consisted of physician advice; few studies have incorporated the use of behavioral modification techniques. In our recent work, however, nurses provided a relapse prevention behavioral intervention program to patients beginning in the hospital. Follow-up sessions after discharge occurred by telephone. At 1 year after MI, a biochemically confirmed cessation rate of 71% in the intervention group was found versus 45% in the usual care group, a statistically significant difference.[50]

Because smoking cessation may be the single most important lifestyle change to reduce subsequent morbidity and mortality, significant attention to smoking cessation in the hospital should be given by rehabilitation personnel. Multicomponent strategies incorporating behavioral techniques, strong physician advice, and the use of pharmacologic agents such as nicotinic gum appear to achieve the greatest long-term cessation rates.

Stress. Many patients feel that stress, often work-related, is an important factor in causing their event. While much controversy still exists over the linkage between stress, type A behavior, and CHD, with both positive and negative findings from major research studies,[51] excessive stress generally does not make people feel good. The type A behavior pattern has been the most extensively researched variable relevant to CHD. Characterized by excessive competitive drive and impatience, the component of type A that appears to be most strongly linked to CHD is hostility or anger.[52,53] It appears that other type A characteristics are of much lesser importance.

A few intervention strategies have been successful in modifying type A behavior, including hostility, in patients with CHD. Such interventions have incorporated combined exercise and cognitive behavioral programs, and stress management courses.[54,55] Further study is needed, however, to determine (1) if behavioral strategies can reduce hostility in patients with established CHD and (2) the long-term results of these interventions.

Because excessive stress and underlying hostility often make people feel uncomfortable it is important that rehabilitation personnel screen for these problems. Standard instruments such as the Cook-Medley Hostility Scale[56] or the Structured Type A Interview[54] can be employed to detect such findings. In addition, asking patients directly by interview or questionnaire to rate how stressed or angry they feel may provide insight into the need for intervention. Patients may benefit from both individual or group stress management programs, counseling with a therapist, biofeedback, and other relaxation and communication techniques.

Alcohol. Although alcohol use is not an independent risk factor for CHD it can cause major problems and lead to more difficulty with compliance to other lifestyle modifications if consumption rates are high. In patients suffering CHD, alcohol may produce atrial and ventricular dysrhythmias and impaired left ventricular functioning.[57] Alcohol in moderate doses may exert a positive effect on raising the HDL cholesterol subfraction[58]; however, heavy consumption is associated with adverse lipid and lipopro-

tein levels.[59] Moreover, heavy consumption of alcohol (more than 3 drinks per day) may increase both systolic and diastolic blood pressure.[60]

About 8% to 10% of adults consider themselves to be alcoholic, and many more may drink heavy amounts of alcohol socially. Rehabilitation personnel have the ability to adequately assess alcohol abuse by using such instruments as the CAGE questionnaire[61] or the Michigan Alcohol Screening Test (MAST).[62] Patients who receive a firm, unequivocal message about the importance of treatment and who have the support of their families are more likely to seek help. Adequate referral is appropriate to enhance both psychosocial and physical recovery.

## OTHER REHABILITATION ISSUES
### Sexual Activity

Another issue for coronary patients after an MI or coronary artery surgery is resumption of sexual activity. Although physicians, nurses, and other rehabilitation personnel view sexual activity as an important topic of discussion, the subject continues to be neglected, leaving patients with many fears and anxieties. One recent study indicates that even though patients may not be sexually active, education about this topic is of importance to them.[63]

The physiologic demands of sexual intercourse in coronary patients are relatively modest, with the average heart rate during sexual intercourse being approximately 117 beats/min.[64] If patients have undergone predischarge treadmill testing after an MI and achieved similar heart rates without significant abnormalities, they should be cleared for resumption of sexual activity at this time. If patients suffer angina pectoris, resumption may be delayed a few weeks and appropriate medications, such as long-acting nitrates, may be prescribed to be taken prior to intercourse. Prophylactic nitroglycerin may also be indicated for patients who experience angina during sexual intercourse.

In counseling, patients should be told about the physiologic effects of sexual activity on the heart, provided with specific information about timing and resumption, made aware of warning signs and symptoms that may occur during sexual activity, and appropriately referred for sexual problems, which may be long-standing. The spouse who may have many different concerns and issues should also be present for the educational session.

Sexual problems are not uncommon following an MI or coronary artery surgery. The frequency of sexual intercourse, for example, may decrease by 24% to 75% in middle-aged men following an MI.[65] The most commonly cited reasons for dysfunction are symptoms of fatigue and angina, psychologic fears that the MI has damaged the heart or fear of another MI, and medications such as beta-blocking agents and diuretics, which cause sexual impairment.[66,67] Although cardiac rehabilitation programs improve functional capacity, it is unclear whether exercise positively affects sexual functioning, interest, and desire. It is known, however, that failure to discuss this topic by health care professionals may lead to sexual dysfunction.[68]

Because patients may be reluctant to initiate discussion about this subject, it is important that rehabilitation members take an adequate sexual history, provide counseling, and refer patients to physicians, psychologists, or sexual therapists for problems such as impotence or loss of libido.

## Return to Work

Although not all patients choose to go back to work after an MI or coronary artery surgery, for many patients returning to normal activities, including work, is important. In reported studies between 49% and 93% of patients actually return to work after MI.[69,70] Factors that influence the success and timing of return to work include physical, psychosocial, demographic, and clinical characteristics.[71,72] For example, members of the older population, aged 55 to 65 years, are less likely than younger patients to return to work after MI or coronary artery surgery.[73] Patients who were unemployed in the 3 months before the event are less likely to return, which may reflect the unemployed patient's poorer health status.[74] A common misconception is that blue collar workers with coronary heart disease cannot return to work because of the physical demands of their jobs.[75] Heavy labor in this country, however, is performed by less than 20% of workers—many of whom are of younger age. Thus the percentage of people with CHD who perform heavy labor is quite small.

Rehabilitation team members can play an instrumental role in influencing the success and timing of the patient's return to work. Enhancing patients' perceptions about their health, physical capacity, and prognosis may influence their decision about returning to work. Moreover, working closely with physicians to influence their advice may be helpful.

Perceived health status in post-MI and post–coronary artery surgery patients has actually correlated with return to work independent of actual health status.[70,76] Although patients may perceive they have a poor prognosis, in reality few patients have a poor prognosis because of technologic advances over the past decade, including thrombolytic therapy. Patients who are given (1) a treadmill test early in the course of recovery to determine the prognosis, and (2) explicit advice about outcome and (3) counseling to alleviate misconceptions about occupational tasks may be significantly more likely to return to work. Rehabilitation personnel are in a unique position to provide this information as they are often involved in conducting treadmill testing and providing or reinforcing the counseling thereafter.

A physician's advice can strongly influence both the success and the timing of reemployment. In the past, the physician's perceptions about a patient's return to work were very subjective and often incorrect. In our studies, for example, physicians have overestimated the patient's likelihood of a recurrent cardiac event, including death, in the 6 months after MI. Physicians estimated the likelihood of an event to be 20%, while the actual event rate was 3.5%.[77] Patients are obviously influenced by the advice of their physicians. If the physician's views are pessimistic or if patients do not receive explicit information, they rarely resume activities quickly. Encouraging physicians to provide explicit information and to use prognostic criteria to help make decisions is important to the patient's recovery. In a recent randomized clinical trial of post-MI patients,[77] those whose physicians provided a treadmill test and explicit instructions about results, prognosis, and timing of return to work and who received reinforcement of these instructions from rehabilitation staff members actually returned to work at a median of 51 days compared with 75 days in patients receiving usual care.[77] Shortening the time of return in this case provided a substantial cost-saving to both the patient and the employer.

## SUMMARY

The goals of rehabilitation are to improve the quality of life for the patient with CHD by eliminating any physical or psychologic barriers that may impede recovery. Rehabilitation has advanced over the past 2 to 3 decades as new information has been acquired about the safety of early ambulation, exercise testing, and exercise training in this population. Modern concepts of cardiac rehabilitation now emphasize risk stratification to individualize patient management, early progressive exercise programs, and education and counseling regarding the psychologic and vocational aspects of recovery. In addition, new behavioral strategies provide support for modification of coronary risk factors in these patients. The future of rehabilitation lies in developing new methods for expansion of services to all patients; for it is only when *all* patients are provided with ways to enhance their quality of life that the goals of this field will have been met.

## REFERENCES

1. Roberts WC and Muja M: The frequency and significance of coronary arterial thrombi and other observations in fatal myocardial infarction, Am J Med 52:425, 1972.
2. Markis JE and others: Myocardial salvage after intracoronary thrombolysis with streptokinase in acute myocardial infarction, N Engl J Med 305:777, 1981.
3. DeBusk RF and others: Identification and treatment of low-risk patients after acute myocardial infarction and coronary-artery bypass graft surgery, N Engl J Med 314:161, 1986.
4. American Association of Cardiopulmonary Rehabilitation: Standards and guidelines for cardiac rehabilitation, Champaign, IL, 1990, Human Kinetics.
5. Conventino V and others: Cardiovascular responses to exercise in middle-aged men after 10 days of bed rest, Circulation 65:134, 1982.
6. Miller RR and others: Prevention of lower extremity venous thrombosis by early mobilization, Ann Intern Med 84:700, 1976.

7. Hentinen M: Need for instruction and support of wives of patients with myocardial infarction, J Adv Nurs 8:519, 1983.

8. Bramwell L: Wives' experiences in the support role after husband's first myocardial infarction, Heart Lung 15:578, 1986.

9. Kübler-Ross E: On death and dying, New York, 1969, Macmillan Publishing Co.

10. The Multicenter Post-Infarction Group: Risk stratification and survival after myocardial infarction, N Engl J Med 309:738, 1983.

11. DeBusk RF, Kraemer HC and Nash E: Stepwise-risk stratification soon after myocardial infarction, Am J Cardiol 52:1161, 1983.

12. Ewart CK and others: The effects of early post infarction exercise testing on self perception and subsequent physical activity, Am J Cardiol 51:1076, 1983.

13. DeBusk RF: Specialized testing after recent myocardial infarction, Ann Intern Med 110:470, 1989.

14. Schlant RS: Guidelines for exercise testing: a report of the American College of Cardiology/American Heart Association Subcommittee of Exercise Testing, J Am Coll Cardiol 8:725, 1986.

15. Haskell WL and DeBusk RF: Cardiovascular responses to repeated treadmill exercise testing soon after myocardial infarction, Circulation 60:1247, 1979.

16. DeBusk RF and others: Medically directed at-home rehabilitation soon after clinically uncomplicated myocardial infarction: a new model for patient care, Am J Cardiol 57:446, 1986.

17. Miller NH and others: Home versus group training for increasing functional capacity after myocardial infarction, Circulation 70:645, 1984.

18. Black HR: Nonpharmacologic therapy for hypertension, Am J Med 66:837, 1979.

19. Bjorntorp P: Exercise in the treatment of obesity, Clin Endocrinol Metab 5:431, 1976.

20. Pederson O and others: Increased insulin receptors after exercise in patients with insulin-dependent diabetes mellitus, N Engl J Med 302:886, 1980.

21. Goldberg L and others: The effects of exercise training on plasma lipids and lipoprotein levels, Med Clin North Am 69:41, 1985.

22. Dishman RK: Medical psychology in exercise and sports, Med Clin North Am 69:123, 1985.

23. Hughes JR: Psychological effects of habitual aerobic exercise: a critical review. In Forum: exercise and health, Prev Med 13:66, 1984.

24. Stern MJ and Cleary P: The National Exercise and Heart Disease Project: long-term psychological outcomes, Arch Intern Med 142:1093, 1982.

25. May GS and others: Secondary prevention after myocardial infarction: a review of long-term trials, Prog Cardiovasc Dis 24:331, 1982.

26. Oldridge NB and others: Cardiac rehabilitation after myocardial infarction, JAMA 260:945, 1988.

27. American College of Sports Medicine: Guidelines for graded exercise testing and exercise prescription, Philadelphia, 1980, Lea & Febiger.

28. Pollock ML, Foster C, and Ward A: Exercise prescription for rehabilitation of the cardiac patient, In Pollock ML and Schmidt DH, editors: Heart disease and rehabilitation, New York, 1979, John Wiley & Sons, Inc.

29. Borg G: Physical performance and perceived exertion, Lund, Sweden, Gleereys 1:63, 1962.

30. Cobb LA and others: At risk for sudden death in patients with coronary heart disease, J Am Coll Cardiol 7:215, 1986.

31. Van Camp SP and Peterson RA: Cardiovascular complications of outpatient cardiac rehabilitation programs, JAMA 256:1160, 1986.

32. American College of Physicians: Position paper on cardiac rehabilitation services, Ann Intern Med 109:671, 1988.

33. Parmley WW: President's page: American College of Cardiology position report on cardiac rehabilitation, J Am Coll Cardiol 7:451, 1986.

34. Stevens R and Hansen P: Comparison of supervised and unsupervised exercise training after coronary bypass surgery, Am J Cardiol 53:1525, 1983.

35. Conner WE and Conner SL: The dietary treatment of hypercholesterolemia. In Havel RJ, editor: The medical clinics of North America, Philadelphia, 1982, WB Saunders Co.

36. Jensen MD: The roles of diet and exercise in the management of patients with insulin dependent diabetes, Mayo Clin Proc 61:813, 1986.

37. Superko RH: The role of diet, exercise, and medication in blood lipid management of cardiac patients, Phys Sports Med 16:65, 1988.

38. National Cholesterol Education Program: Report of the National Cholesterol Education Program expert panel on detection, evaluation, and treatment of high blood cholesterol in adults, Arch Intern Med 148:38, 1988.

39. National Obesity Consensus Conference: Ann Intern Med 100:(suppl):888, 1985.

40. Castelli WP and others: Incidence of coronary heart disease and lipoprotein cholesterol levels: the Framingham study, JAMA 256:2835, 1986.

41. Brown GB and others: Niacin or lovastatin, combined with colestipol, regress coronary atherosclerosis and prevent clinical events in men with elevated apoliprotein B, Circulation 80:II-266, 1989.

42. Blankenhorn DH and others: Beneficial effects of combined colestipol-niacin therapy on coronary atherosclerosis and coronary venous bypass grafts, JAMA 257:3233, 1987.

43. Canner PL and others: Fifteen year mortality in Coronary Drug Project patients: long-term benefit with niacin, J Am Coll Cardiol 8:1245, 1986.

44. Aberg A and others: Cessation of smoking after myocardial infarction: effects on mortality after 20 years, Br Heart J 49:416, 1983.

45. Rosenberg L and others: The risk of myocardial infarction after quitting smoking in men under 55 years of age, N Engl J Med 313:1511, 1985.

46. Sparrow D, Dawber TR and Colton T: The influence of cigarette smoking on prognosis after a first myocardial infarction, J Chronic Dis 31:425, 1978.

47. Mulcahy R: Influence of cigarette smoking on morbidity and mortality after myocardial infarction, Br Heart J 49:410, 1983.

48. Schwartz JL: Review and evaluation of smoking cessation methods: the United States and Canada 1978-1985, Division of Cancer Prevention and Control, National Cancer Institute, NIH Publication No. 87-2940, 1987.

49. Baile WF and others: Rapid resumption of cigarette smoking following myocardial infarction: inverse relation to MI severity, Addict Behav 7:373, 1982.

50. Taylor CB and others: Smoking cessation after acute myocardial infarction: effects of nurse-managed intervention, Ann Intern Med 113:118, 1990.

51. Matthews KA and Haynes SG: Type A behavior pattern and coronary disease risk: update and critical evaluation, Am J Epidemiol 123:923, 1986.

52. Matthews KA and others: Competitive drive, pattern A and coronary heart disease: a further analysis of some data from the Western Collaborative Group Study, J Chronic Dis 30:489, 1977.

53. Hecker MHL and others: Coronary-prone behaviors in the Western Collaborative Group Study, Psychosom Med 2:153, 1988.

54. Friedman M and others: Alteration of type A behavior and its effects on cardiac recurrences in post myocardial infarction patients: summary results of the Recurrent Coronary Prevention Project, Am Heart J 112:653, 1986.

55. Schaeffer MA and others: Effects of occupational based behavioral counseling and exercise interventions on Type A components and cardiovascular reactivity, J Cardiopulmonary Rehab 10:371, 1988.

56. Cook WW and Medley DM: Proposed hostility and pharisaic virtue scales for the MMPI, J Appl Psychol 38:414, 1954.

57. Davidson DM: Cardiovascular effects of alcohol, West J Med 151:430, 1989.

58. Haskell WL and others: The effect of cessation and resumption of moderate alcohol intake on serum high-density-lipoprotein subfractions: a controlled study, N Engl J Med 310:805, 1984.

59. Leiber CS: To drink or not to drink? N Engl J Med 310:846, 1984.

60. Klatsky AL and others: Alcohol consumption and blood pressure: Kaiser-Permanente multiphasic health examination data, N Engl J Med 296:1194, 1977.

61. Ewing JA: Detecting alcoholism: the CAGE questionnaire, JAMA 252:1905, 1984.

62. Selzer ML: The Michigan Alcoholism Screening Test: the quest for a new diagnostic instrument, Am J Psychiatry 127:1653, 1971.

63. Baggs, JG and Karch, AM: Sexual counseling of women with coronary heart disease, Heart Lung 16:154, 1987.

64. Hellerstein HK and Friedman EH: Sexual activity and the postcoronary patient, Cardiac Rehab 3:43, 1972.

65. Mann S, Yates JE, and Raftery EB: The effects of myocardial infarction on sexual activity, J Cardiac Rehab 1:187, 1981.

66. Papadopoulos C and others: Sexual activity after coronary bypass surgery, Chest 90:681, 1986.

67. Kolman PB: Sexual dysfunction in the postmyocardial infarction patient, J Cardiac Rehab 4:334, 1984.

68. Papadopoulos C and others: Myocardial infarction and sexual activity of the female patient, Arch Int Med 143:1528, 1983.

69. Cay EL, Vetter N, and Phillip A: Return to work after a heart attack, J Psychosom Res 17:231, 1973.

70. Garrity, TF: Vocational adjustment after first myocardial infarction: comparative assessment of several variables suggested in the literature, Soc Sci Med 7:705, 1973.

71. Smith GR and O'Rourke DF: Return to work after myocardial infarction, JAMA 259:1673, 1988.

72. Nagle R, Gangola R, and Picton-Robinson, I: Factors influencing return to work after myocardial infarction, Lancet 2:454, 1971.

73. Shapiro S and others: Return to work after first myocardial infarction, Arch Environ Health 24:17, 1972.

74. Hammermeister KE and others: Effect of surgical versus medical therapy on return to work in patients with coronary artery disease, Am J Cardiol 44:105, 1979.

75. Weinblatt E and others: Return to work and work status following first myocardial infarction: Am J Public Health 2:169, 1966.

76. Gundle NJ and others: Psychosocial outcome after coronary artery surgery: a randomized clinical trial, Am J Psychiatry, 137:1591, 1980.

77. Dennis CA and others: Early return to work after uncomplicated myocardial infarction: results of a randomized trial, JAMA 260:214, 1988.

# CHAPTER 14

# Home Care of Patients with Cardiac Disease

Doris F. Glick

## PERSPECTIVES ON HOME CARE

As a consequence of recent trends in the health care system, more and more care is being provided for cardiac patients in their own homes. Patients who are treated in hospitals today tend to be more critically ill than in the past, and the severity of illness has increased among patients who are treated in their own homes. Although cardiac care is usually envisioned as technologically sophisticated, an increasing number of agencies and a diversity of providers are delivering an array of services to address the needs of patients and their families at home.

### Development of Home Care in the Health Care System

Since the beginning of recorded history, societies have recognized certain people whose designated role was to provide care for the sick at home. The earliest known visiting nurse was Phoebe, whose visits to the ill in their homes was recorded in the Bible in Paul's letters to the Romans (Romans 16:1-2). In the modern era, William Rathbone established the first visiting nurse association in Liverpool, England in 1859. Rathbone consulted his friend, Florence Nightingale, whose recommendations continue to form the conceptual basis of home health services. She recommended that care focus on the family, provision of patient teaching, and concern for environmental conditions. Nightingale believed that, in addition to the skills acquired in the hospital setting, advanced education was necessary for nurses practicing in the home setting.

In the United States, visiting nurse associations were first established in 1856 in Boston and Philadelphia. These associations formed the foundation of modern day community health nursing practice. In 1883, Lillian Wald and Mary Brewster established the Henry Street Settlement House in New York City to care for the sick poor at home.

From that time until the early 1960s, high-quality, low-cost home care services were provided by two types of agencies. Visiting nurse associations were private or voluntary nonprofit agencies that provided care for the sick at home. Public health agencies were supported by public funds and regulated through legislation at local, state and federal levels. Public health agencies focused primarily on control of communicable diseases and on health promotion and disease prevention. What home care they provided for the sick tended to focus on teaching the family or other care providers how to care for their sick member rather than on the direct provision of care. Throughout this time, home care remained a small segment of the total health care system.[1,2]

In the 1960s, the establishment of the Medicare and Medicaid systems provided some reimbursement for community health agencies to provide illness care, and the demands for home care began to increase. The most profound impact on the delivery of home care, however, occurred in the 1980s. The federal government in 1984 introduced the change from cost reimbursement to prospective payment for financing hospital services. This innovation provided significant impetus to the trend to discharge patients from hospitals much earlier in the course of their recovery.[3] Moreover, patients with many severe or acute illnesses or elective surgery were no longer admitted to a hospital. As a result, the latter part of the 1980s brought a significant increase in the severity of illness among patients being cared for at home. Frequently these patients are elderly, have multiple medical diagnoses, and require complex care. Home care services thus have become increasingly focused on illness and high technology.

Parallel to these trends, physicians have moved away from house calls. Physicians have tended to function more and more in hospital settings since the physician shortage created by World War II made home visits an inefficient means to use scarce resources. Gradually, technologic advances required medical practice to take place in hospital settings rather than in the home. Today economic incentives encourage physicians to practice in acute care institutions, and there is no formal reimbursement for physician participation in home care.[4]

Because of the changes that have occurred in health care reimbursement in recent years, and with more older and sicker patients being cared for in their own homes, there has been a notable increase in the number of home health agencies. Proprietary agencies have been established along with the nonprofit visiting nurse associations and public health departments to provide home care services. Medicare was enacted in 1966. One year later there were 1753 home health agencies certified by Medicare to provide home health services. By 1974, there were 2237 home health agencies, a 48% increase,[5] and by 1989, according to the National Association for Home Care, that number had reached 10,850.[6] This number represents a growth of 500% in 15 years.

The cost of home care accounts for an escalating proportion of the total health care budget in the United States. In 1989, expenditures of $15.9 billion for home health care accounted for 2.7% of the total health care market. According to the Health Care Financing Administration (HCFA), which oversees Medicare, expenditures for home care will continue to increase and will reach an estimated $23.2 billion by 1993. Although the annual growth in total health care expenditures is projected to be 8.5%, estimates indicate that expenditures for home care will grow at a rate of 12.1% per year.[7] Home health, thus, has become the most rapidly growing segment of the health care system.

### Scope of Home Health Services

Home care is an array of services brought to people in their own homes for the purpose of restoring health or managing illness. The focus is on family, patient teaching, home environment, multidisciplinary health care team, and return to optimum level of health. Because most patients are chronically ill and elderly, Medicare provides reimbursement to home health agencies for approximately 75% to 80% of all home care services. The remainder are reimbursed by Medicaid, private insurance companies, and in some cases, by the patients themselves. Medicare will reimburse the following services[5]:

1. Part-time or intermittent nursing care provided by or under the supervision of a registered professional nurse
2. Physical, occupational, or speech therapy
3. Medical social services under the direction of a physician
4. Part-time or intermittent services of a home health aide, as permitted by the regulations
5. Medical supplies (other than drugs and biologicals, such as serum and vaccinations) and the use of medical appliances
6. Medical services provided by an intern or resident enrolled in a teaching program in hospitals affiliated or under contract with a home health agency

### Costs and Benefits of Home Care

More comprehensive third party payment has provided impetus toward the trend to health care delivery at home. The cost of home care, even high-technology care, is usually less expensive than hospital care. According to estimates by the National Association for Home Care, the daily cost in 1987 for rather intensive treatment at home was $25 to $100 per day, versus $300 to $500 for a similar level of care in a hospital. The monthly cost for skilled

nursing care at home was $750 versus $2000 in a hospital.[7] In 1988, HCFA estimated that one third of all patients admitted to a hospital could be cared for adequately by home care.

Many people who are ill would rather be treated in their own homes. There is a trend for people to assume more responsibility for their own well-being and to be more sophisticated regarding self-care. The increasing ability of the health care system to deliver complex technical care in the home has contributed to the growing public acceptance of this mode of care. Families usually appreciate having their loved one at home with them, and patients who are cared for at home can enjoy a more normal lifestyle. They can see family and friends, sleep in their own beds, and be surrounded by things that are meaningful to them, such as pets, telephone, music, television, books, garden, and so forth. They can manage their own schedules, free from the regimented and impersonal environment of the hospital, and, perhaps most important of all, have the gratification of being in control of their own lives.[8]

Despite these benefits, home care is frequently long term and can represent a considerable emotional, social, and financial burden on the patient and family. Among people over age 65, about 30% live alone, and as many as a third of all patients receiving home health services live alone.[9] Elderly women constitute the majority of such patients.[10] Being ill at home alone can be a frightening experience for these patients who are likely to feel isolated, lonely, and worried about being able to reach help in an emergency.

Another third or more of all home health patients are cared for at home by a spouse. This caretaking spouse is likely to be elderly and female and may be feeble and in poor health. Caring for the ill spouse is an emotional and physical stressor and the patient's illness imposes stressful alterations of established roles within the marital dyad. The ability to cope varies from couple to couple and depends on the availability of family and social support systems, and on the quality of home services provided. The remainder of home health patients are cared for by other family members, such as children, siblings, parents, or significant others. One study of spouses or family who manage family members with a terminal illness found that 33% of the relatives caring for the patients were at risk of failing health status because of age or illness.[11]

Home care, thus, is frequently long term and can represent a considerable financial burden to the patient and family. While advances in medicine and refinements of high technology interventions contribute greatly to the potential for extended survival, the costs to the family of that survival may be a significant source of stress and a drain on the coping ability of the family.

### CONTINUITY OF CARE

Continuity of care is the connection and coordination of all of the health care services used by a patient. Well-planned continuity of care prevents duplication and fragmentation of services, and ensures that each patient receives the most appropriate care. It assists patients to achieve their maximum health potential with the least discomfort and stress. And, significantly, planned coordination of care reduces health care costs by assuring cost-efficient use of services.[12] Effective continuity of care requires collaboration and cooperation among all of the agencies and disciplines involved in a patient's care.

## Discharge Planning: Collaboration Among Agencies

Discharge planning facilitates the transition of patients from an acute care setting to home, by coordinating the patient's need for continuing services, equipment and supplies, family and social support, and education. It is a process that should begin at the time a patient is admitted to an acute care institution. The American Nurses' Association defines discharge planning as[13]:

. . . that part of the continuity of care process which is designed to prepare the patient or client for the next phase of care and to assist in making any necessary arrangements for that phase of care, care by family members or care by an organized health care provider.

The American Hospital Association describes discharge planning as an interdisciplinary hospital-wide process that should be provided to assist patients and their families to develop a realistic plan for posthospital care.[14] Standards have been established by the Joint Commission for Accreditation of Health Care Organizations (JCAHO) that address patients' rights to continuity of care. JCAHO site visits seek to confirm that discharge planning takes place and that its effectiveness is evaluated by the institution.[15]

Discharge planning consists of assessment of individual needs, of patient teaching, and, when ongoing care is required, assessment of the home environment, identification of a caregiver, and identification of appropriate community resources. Assessment for discharge should focus on health care needs, expected severity of illness at discharge, age, living arrangements, and anticipated need for instruction. Some patients can be identified as high-risk patients, such as those over age 65, those who live alone, those who are likely to have a decrease in their level of functioning after discharge, or those who will require complex care. When it is determined that a patient or family cannot provide the requisite self-care without assistance, referrals to home care and other appropriate community agencies should be made. Early identification of the anticipated length of stay in the hospital establishes a framework within which coordination of resources, education, and referrals must take place.[16]

The purpose of patient education is to teach self-care. Factors associated with the ability of the patient to provide adequate self-care include medical diagnosis, nursing diagnosis, functional limitations, knowledge levels and intellectual capabilities, and anxiety levels.

When a patient is not capable of self-care, a caregiver must be identified if possible. Although identification of a caregiver who is competent, able, and willing is frequently critical to the patient's well-being, locating such a person may be difficult. Caregivers may or may not be family members. Many people live alone or live with a spouse who also has health problems or functional limitations. Others may live with caregivers who work outside the home or have other responsibilities and demands on their time. Some caregivers may be poorly taught or simply unable to learn how to carry out the necessary care effectively. Although situations occur in which patients at home are neglected, improperly cared for, or even abused, in most cases caregivers in the home provide effective, dedicated, and competent care. Indeed, home caregivers are a generally unrecognized but vital link in today's health care system.

Assessment of the home environment is an important component of discharge planning. Even today, some people live without indoor plumbing and many homes have inadequate heat. The lack of a cooling system or the presence of stairs can present special problems for the cardiac patient. Factors such as space, safety, and level of repair all affect the adequacy of care at home, especially when special equipment is required.[16]

Hospital discharge planners must keep up-to-date regarding the availability of agencies that provide home health services for patients in their service area, and they should maintain close linkages with community agencies. Effective interagency collaboration helps to ease the transition from one site of care to the next for patients and their families. The discharge planners' knowledge of available community services, supplies, equipment and other resources will be crucial in determining the extent to which the patient's needs will be met after leaving the hospital.

## The Home Health Care Team: Collaboration Among Disciplines

Interdisciplinary collaboration is a necessity in the provision of home health services. No single discipline can effectively respond to all of the needs for home care, and Medicare-certified agencies are required to document interdisciplinary services. Interdisciplinary collaboration requires a comprehensive approach in which health care professionals relate effectively and cooperatively with each other. It implies effective communications, shared problem solving, and joint decision making by an integrated team.[17]

Each patient has an individualized care plan. Effective collaboration ensures that the patient's needs are met in the most appropriate manner, without overlap among disciplines. Successful interdisciplinary collaboration requires that all members of the health care team are competent practitioners in their respective disciplines. The roles and responsibilities of the disciplines involved in home health care are established by Medicare regulations, state licensing boards, and professional organizations. These disciplines and their respective responsibilities are as follows.[5]

**Physician.** Each patient who receives home health services must be under the care of a physician. Although a nurse may make an assessment visit without a physician's approval, if a plan of care is to follow, it must be certified by a physician. That is, in order for Medicare to reimburse for services, the plan of care must be certified by the physician *before* care is provided, and, if care is to continue, the plan must be recertified by the physician, in collaboration with home care professionals, at least every 60 days.

**Nurse.** The nurse receives the referral information, usually from a physician or hospital discharge planner, and makes an initial evaluation visit. At this visit the nurse interviews the patient and caregiver to determine the types and amount of services needed. Assessment includes a psychosocial and medical history, a physical examination of the patient, and an assessment of the adequacy of the environment. Medications are reviewed. The agency services are explained and the availability of insurance and/or Medicare eligibility is evaluated. Treatments may be provided if needed. Based on this initial evaluation visit, the plan of care is established.

From the first interview, the emphasis of home health nursing is on facilitating self-care. This focus is a hallmark of home nursing and represents one of the fundamental differences between home nursing and hospital nursing. Although in the hospital it is the responsibility of the nurse to provide the needed care, in the home the nurse's ultimate responsibility is to teach self-care to the patient and the family or other care provider. It is important to note that the home health nurse may be the patient's only contact with the health care system.

Subsequent nursing visits provide skilled nursing care services, teach patient care, supervise home health aides, coordinate other services, and update the plan of care as needed. The nurse serves as case manager, monitors the status of the patient, and ensures that adequate care is provided. As patient problems increase in complexity and demands for sophisticated technologic skills and services escalate, home health nurses have many demands on their attention. It is crucial that they maintain a holistic approach that includes the emotional needs and social well-being of the patient and family.

**Physical therapist.** When needed, maintenance, preventive, and restorative treatments are provided for patients in their homes by physical therapists, who have baccalaureate degrees and are licensed in the state in which they practice. Treatment may include muscle strengthening, restoration of mobility, control of spasticity, gait training, or active-passive resistive exercises. Included in the job of the physical therapist is teaching the treatment regimen to the patient and family, collaborating with other health professionals, and participating in patient care conferences.

**Occupational therapist.** Services for patients who need assistance in achieving their optimum level of functioning in activities of daily living are provided in the home by occupational therapists. These practitioners are educated at the baccalaureate level and are registered by the National Occupational Therapy Association. Occupational therapists assist patients to restore the muscle strength and mobility required for functional skills, with special focus on the upper extremities. They teach self-care activities, remove barriers, and provide adaptive equipment when needed. Like all other members of the health care team, occupational therapists are expected to collaborate with other team members and to participate in patient care conferences.

**Speech pathologist.** Patients with communication problems related to speech, language, or hearing may receive home services by a speech pathologist who holds a master's degree and is certified by the American Speech and Hearing Association. Services include evaluating speech and language abilities and teaching the patient and family how to develop optimum levels of communication. Speech pathologists may also address eating or swallowing problems.

**Social worker.** Assistance with social, emotional, and environmental factors that relate to the health and well-being of the patient and family may be provided by a social worker. In home health, the social worker usually holds a master's degree in social work. Social workers assist people to identify and use appropriate community resources. They may assist with applications for aid, be involved in crisis intervention, assist in obtaining needed equipment and supplies, or provide guidance in addressing financial problems.

**Home health aide.** Patients who need assistance with personal hygiene may receive the services of a home health aide. Supervised by the nurse, the home health aide must have experience as an aide and have special training in providing home care. Services include assistance with personal hygiene and walking, meal preparation, and light housekeeping chores. The home health aide implements the plan of care and reports to the supervising nurse.

**Homemaker.** Although similar to the home health aide, the homemaker focuses on housekeeping chores. Services include home maintenance, shopping, cooking, and companionship.

## Community Resources

In addition to the customary home health services described, most communities have some other services available to assist the ill or infirm at home. The availability of these services varies from community to community. When they do exist, the services may have long waiting lists so that they may not be able to serve all patients who could benefit.

They family caring for an ill member at home may be helped by special home care courses and materials prepared by the American Red Cross. Patient education materials that address health promotion and approaches to caring for various cardiac diagnoses are available through the American Heart Association.

Homemaker or chore services may be available through community agencies such as Senior Citizens, the Red Cross, or the Long Term Care Project. These services may also be provided by private groups or churches. Such groups may also provide transportation. Meals on Wheels is available in many communities to provide home delivered meals to the elderly or infirm. And some grocery stores and pharmacies will provide home delivery for those who need such assistance.

Medical equipment and supplies for home use are available through private vendors. Under certain conditions, Medicare will pay for some equipment used in the home. For example, for Medicare to cover the cost of a hospital bed for home use, the patient must spend at least 50% of the time in bed. Similar restrictions apply to other equipment and supplies. Many home health agencies and equipment vendors maintain a loan closet to provide supplies and equipment to patients who need but cannot afford them. Sometimes supplies are donated by private individuals or organizations.[16]

The Vial of Life Program is available in some communities: emergency information and medical history are recorded on a medical information form that is tucked into a plastic vial and stored on the right side of the top shelf of the refrigerator. A decal attached to the outside of the door of the refrigerator alerts an ambulance crew that the information is inside. Such a system is particularly useful for the elderly and for people who live alone.

Emergency electronic systems are available in many communities. An electronic device that can be activated in an emergency is either worn or placed in a strategic location in the home, such as beside the bed or in the bathroom. Activation of the system alerts an operator to call for emergency services and may also alert the patient's family or physician.[18]

In all cases, families should be instructed to post emergency numbers near their telephone. Patients should be provided with a card that describes their diagnosis and treatment, and, when relevant, the most effective means of controlling their dysrhythmias. Patients who are not homebound should be encouraged to carry this card in addition to wearing a medicalert bracelet.

A recent innovation in the provision of health services is the establishment of adult day care centers. These centers provide care for adults who are not capable of caring for themselves alone at home during the day, but who are able to leave home. This service offers respite for overburdened caretakers and those who must go to work, or to other responsibilities, during the day. Services are usually available on an hourly, daily, or weekly basis, and include nursing supervision, meals, planned activities, socialization, and assistance with bathing and other activities of daily living.

## ASSESSMENT FOR HOME CARE

Assessment for home care consists of collecting data about both the patient and the family as a basis for planning the treatment regimen to meet the patient's needs in the home setting. Included in the assessment is information about the family's ability to provide necessary care, observations about the adequacy of the home environment, and the availability of support systems and community resources.

### Family

Cardiac illness of a family member is a major life stressor for the entire family, and families vary greatly in their abilities to cope. Household routines and lifestyles are usually disrupted, and roles of the various members as they relate to each other are likely to be altered. Although it is the individual cardiac patient who initially enters the health care system, it is the family that ultimately provides the context for recovery or long-term care. The family, or lack thereof, profoundly affects the individual's response to illness and may determine whether home care is a viable option. Patients who live alone require special support and services to manage their self-care. This group is at greater risk for rehospitalization or admission to long-term care facilities than patients with caretaker families.

The concept of family is broadly defined in the health care literature. Family generally implies a social system of two or more people who coexist and who share mutual affection and mutual responsibility.[19] This definition includes traditional nuclear families, single parent families, step families, and any other couple or group who share a valued relationship characterized by commitment, mutual decision making, and shared resources. According to the U.S. Bureau of Labor statistics, the traditional family configuration of a father who is employed and a woman who stays home as wife and mother constitutes only about 13% of the households in the United States. Of the remaining households, 16% are married couples with children where both spouses work, 16% are single parent families, 23% are married couples living alone, 23% are single person households, 6% are households with extended families, and all others make up the remainder.[20]

The patient and family may not realize the full impact of the illness while the patient is in the hospital. The major adjustments must occur when the patient returns home. Frequently the patient and family must deal with issues for which they are not prepared. The degree of adjustments to the family's lifestyle will be determined by the severity of the patient's illness and the associated degree of disability, the amount of care that must be provided by others, the kind of equipment and environmental alterations that are required, and the availability and utilization of appropriate health care services. Home care frequently implies that those in the home must cope with a crisis that has no closure. The ability of family members to provide care is directly related to their levels of anxiety and their methods of coping with stress. The cultural, racial, ethnic, and religious identities of family members contribute to their health beliefs and to their style of coping with illness. The level of education affects comprehension about the disease process and determines the level at which health teaching must be provided. Families are usually able to provide effective basic health care if properly instructed by health care professionals.[21] Because families vary in their patterns of coping, assessment of the ability to cope is a first step in the provision of home care.

Several tasks have been identified that families must deal with in coping with the long-term illness of a member.[19,22] First, they must learn to manage and prevent a crisis. This is especially relevant for families of patients with cardiac disease who are at risk for life-threatening dysrhythmias or cardiac arrest. Second is the task of regimen management. The difficulty inherent in this task is contingent on the degree of modification of usual daily routine required by the patient's illness, and the extent to which this modification will have an impact on family members. The more assistance the patient requires in providing self-care, the greater the demands will be for other family members to modify their daily routines. Third is the task of symptom control. Success is contingent on the judgment of the patient and family in dealing with symptoms as they occur. Adequate teaching is necessary to allay fears and to provide information about palliative measures. The fourth task is that of dealing with temporal and role disruption. Patients suddenly spending more time at home, deprived of former activities, must find new ways to occupy their time. Moreover, the illness may bring major changes in the roles family members have in relationship to each other. Roles of economic provider, housekeeper, or decision-maker within the household may be profoundly altered by the patient's illness and may require adjustment on the part of all family members. Fifth, families must cope with the trajectory of the illness. For example, while some cardiac patients may recover, others will remain at a diminished level of health, some will slowly decline, and a few will experience sudden death. The sixth family task is to overcome social isolation. Impaired functioning, diminished energy, altered body image, and time-consuming therapeutic regimens may interfere with social relationships. In many cases, the caretaker will become isolated at home with the patient and have no respite. The final task is that of finding adequate financial resources to pay for necessary treatment, daily care, and to compensate for possible loss of income. Cardiac illness of a family member can extend over many years and may severely drain the economic resources of the family.

Home care differs from hospital care in that in the institution the roles and the realm of control of each health care provider are well defined. The hospital is their "territory" and the patient is the "guest" outsider. Health care providers control the terms and the timing of the situation. When the home is the health care setting, it is the "territory" of the household members. They are in control and have their designated roles. The home health care provider is the "guest" outsider. The patient and other members of the household control the circumstances and the timing of the care provided.

Assessment of the family should include a description of the family, including household members and members of the patient's support system who may be involved in providing care or support. Roles of each member, especially in nontraditional families, and the tasks they will assume in caring for the patient should be clarified. Family dynamics should be observed and decision makers and caretakers identified. As typical family size decreases and more women are employed outside of the home, fewer caregivers are available at home.[23] The caretaker and other family members who will be involved in the patient's day-to-day care should be assessed to determine their ability to provide the needed care.[4]

Assessment should also address environmental issues and access to care. For example, the availability of a telephone and an automobile determines the degree to which the patient and family can communicate with, and have access to, the health care system. Even today, not all households have access to these conveniences.

The ability of the family to provide care depends on their level of understanding of cardiovascular disease and of the patient's therapeutic regimen. They should understand the importance of preventing complications and know what therapeutic measures contribute to that end. They should be able to provide the patient with the necessary diet, medications, and activity and should be able to carry out necessary interventions, such as accurately monitoring pulse and blood pressure and monitoring the status of an artificial pacemaker if necessary. In some cases, it may be necessary for a caretaker to learn complex technical skills in order to manage the treatment regimen.

Household members who are willing and capable should be encouraged to learn techniques of basic cardiac life support (BCLS). Classes are frequently available through community agencies or the local affiliate of the American Heart Association or American Red Cross. Special instructions should be provided, when necessary, for resuscitating patients with a tracheostomy. The home health nurse should assess and document BCLS skills of family members and make referrals for an annual refresher course and for opportunity to practice. The client's risk for cardiac or respiratory arrest should be monitored.[24]

### Patient

Most of the need for home care results from an acute exacerbation of a chronic disease, or from a complication of a chronic disease.[25] In the majority of cases, the patient has been hospitalized prior to admission for home care. Being discharged from the hospital is an experience that is likely to be regarded with ambivalent feelings by most patients. On the one hand, patients are relieved to have survived a life-threatening cardiac crisis. On the other hand, leaving the security of the hospital may create fear and apprehension. Patients who have a major cardiac event, such as an MI, may fear a recurrence. They may wonder if recovery at home is possible, whether family members will manage to provide the necessary care, and if professional help will be available if it is needed. For many patients, the history of sudden onset of heart disease compounds these fears.

The patient's mental status, especially that of elderly patients, should be evaluated at each visit. Once survival from a cardiac event is assured, many patients become depressed. Uncertainty, worry, and a sense of loss can result in depression when the patient returns home. Symptoms may include insomnia, cognitive changes, diminished libido, restlessness, and possibly recurring thoughts of death. The problems usually diminish or disappear within 3 months as strength and feelings of well-being return.[26] In addition to psychologic disturbances, such as depression, there are many psychologic symptoms of physiologic imbalances. Side effects of medications may cause such symptoms. For example, digitalis, even at nontoxic levels, may be associated with delirium in the elderly.[27]

Assessment of the cardiac patient at home emphasizes factors that relate to controlling the disease process and modifying cardiovascular risks. The history should focus on issues most germane to management of the cardiac patient at home. The following should be addressed[28]:

1. History of symptoms, specifically:
   - Chest pain—describe onset, precipitating factors, duration, location and radiation, means of relief, and any associated symptoms
   - Weakness, faintness, headaches, dizziness
   - Cyanosis
   - Dyspnea, orthopnea
   - Palpitations
   - Edema
   - Changes in visual fields
2. History of heart disease, hypertension, or diabetes
3. Family history, especially of cardiovascular diseases and risks
4. Relationships with family and close friends, support system
5. Occupation, work environment, and relationships
6. Leisure and recreational activities
7. Exercise type and amount
8. Diet history, especially fats, salt, and total calories
9. Knowledge level about current health problems
10. Ability to carry out self-care
11. Ability to use available resources
12. Psychosocial reaction to disease status and ability to cope

Physical assessment of the cardiac patient at home should include measurement of blood pressure in both arms, sitting and standing. Readings should be taken twice, at least 10 minutes apart. Heart sounds should be evaluated for rate, rhythm, quality, and extra sounds, and radial pulse for pulse deficit. Breath sounds should be evaluated for rate, quality, and the possibility of rales. Skin color and peripheral pulses should be assessed. Abnormal signs such as peripheral edema or neck vein distention should be evaluated. Weight should be measured and, if relevant, intake and output records reviewed. The interview should evaluate for symptoms of cardiac insufficiency, such as dyspnea, orthopnea, chest pain, nausea, dizziness, decreased appetite, or excessive fatigue.[29]

Blood testing may be indicated for homebound patients for many reasons. Patients with congestive failure who are taking diuretics may have periodic electrolyte, blood urea nitrogen (BUN), and creatinine measurements. Patients on digitalis or other cardiopulmonary medications may require monitoring of serum levels. Periodic prothrombin times may be indicated for patients on anticoagulation medication.[30]

In general, all patients with cardiac disease are at risk for congestive heart failure. Homebound patients should be monitored for several cardinal signs of congestive heart failure:[31]

- Fatigue and anorexia are among the earliest signs of cardiac decompensation.
- Palpitations can be a source of great anxiety for the patient and, if dysrhythmias are frequent, can compromise cardiac output.
- Dyspnea and/or hyperpnea results from pulmonary congestion and increases the work of breathing.
- Paroxysmal nocturnal dyspnea is caused by changes in fluid dynamics and reduced cardiac output resulting from prone position. This sudden occurrence of dyspnea during sleep may be accompanied by confusion because of cerebral hypoxia. The condition may prevent the patient from getting enough rest, and it is associated with serious potential for injury, especially among the elderly.
- Orthopnea and dyspnea on exertion may occur.
- Generalized or pitting edema of the extremities occurs frequently, as does jugular venous distention and an $S_3$ heart sound.

Patients at risk for congestive failure should be advised to call their nurse or physician if (1) shoes become too tight, (2) usual tasks or activities of daily living become difficult, (3) extra sleep is needed, or (4) urination at night becomes more frequent.[31]

## THE PLAN OF CARE

The plan of care is based on the assessment data and the patient's medical and nursing diagnoses. It is a problem solving model that incorporates the patient's needs for care, the prescribed medical regimen, and the patient's and family's perceptions of the illness.

**Documentation of the treatment plan.** The home health plan of treatment must be developed and thoroughly documented to meet guidelines for Medicare reimbursement and to meet state and federal regulatory requirements for agency certification and recertification. Each patient's plan of care is developed by the nurse and must be recertified by the physician every 60 days. In addition, in order for the agency to be reimbursed for services provided, the patient must be certified to be confined to home and in need of intermittent professional skilled care.

The plan of care must include the following components[32]:

*Diagnosis*—indicates the principal medical diagnosis most closely related to the current plan of treatment. The diagnosis, expressed in the appropriate ICD-9-CM Code, may or may not relate to the most recent hospitalization of the patient, but must relate to home care services provided. In the case of multiple diagnoses, the one representing the greatest need for home care services should be used.

*Medications*—includes dose, frequency, and route for each drug. New prescriptions and changes in prescriptions must be so indicated.

*Surgical procedures*—lists those that are related to the care provided, with the date of the surgery.

*Other pertinent diagnoses*—only those that relate to the patient's plan of treatment are listed, in order of seriousness. Medicare uses these diagnoses to justify payment or denial of payment for services rendered.

*Functional limitations*—Medicare will reimburse for services only if a patient is homebound.

*Mental status*—relates to ability to function within the home.

*Nutritional requirements*—TPN may be listed here or under medications.

*Prognosis*—Medicare will continue to reimburse only if the patient's condition is improving.

*Prescriptions*—indicates the disciplines and treatments prescribed and includes the frequency of services to be provided.

Fig. 14-1 lists specific professional services, by discipline, for which Medicare will provide reimbursement. Most commercial and private health insurers have adopted Medicare guidelines as their own criteria for reimbursement decisions in home care.[33]

**Diet.** Special dietary needs of the patient at home affect the entire family. Because many of the risk factors for cardiac disease are familial, the entire family may benefit from a diet that is conducive to heart health. Family members are likely to share past dietary patterns that have put the patient at risk, and they may share unhealthy lifestyles that also include overweight, insufficient exercise, smoking behavior, and genetic predispositions. The crisis of having an ill member may motivate other members of the family to want to modify their own risk factors by changing behaviors and diet.

Decisions must be made about whether the whole family will share the patient's dietary restrictions, perhaps adding seasonings on an individual basis, or whether special food will be prepared for the cardiac patient. In general, the degree of restriction required by the patient (e.g., amount of sodium permitted) will determine the degree of impact on the rest of the household. The nurse should identify, as the target for diet teaching, the household member who does the grocery shopping, and, if different, the person who cooks the meals.

In addition to the specific dietary restrictions prescribed for an individual patient, a dietary plan for all cardiac patients should consider the following factors[29]:

- A diet that is high in fiber (such as vegetables, fruit, whole grains, and bran) will promote bowel elimination and prevent the tendency to actuate Valsalva maneuver and the discomfort of constipation. Such foods also aid in weight control, if this is a problem.
- Most cardiac patients benefit from restriction of high-sodium food in order to avoid fluid retention. Patients need to learn to avoid "hidden" salt, such as that in processed foods, pickled foods, salty snacks, and foods containing monosodium glutamate.
- Patients who are taking potassium-depleting diuretics may benefit from foods that are high in potassium, such as bananas, tomatoes, raisins and potatoes.
- Limitation of caffeine intake from coffee, tea, colas, and chocolate helps to avoid unnecessary sympathetic nervous system stimulation.
- Avoidance of cholesterol and saturated fats found in eggs, meat, cheese, and whole milk products may limit the progression of atherosclerosis. Total fat should be limited to less than 30% of total calorie intake.
- Restriction of sugar, alcohol, and total calories will aid in weight control if this is necessaary.

Patients on sodium-restricted diets may choose to use salt substitutes. Commercially available salt substitutes usually contain potassium salts. These products may safely enhance the palatability of food for most patients, and those who are taking diuretics may actually benefit from the supplemental potassium. However, patients who are already taking potassium substitutes, those on potassium-sparing diuretics, and those who may have a moderate degree of renal failure should use these products with caution. In these circumstances, serum potassium levels might be monitored, or nonpotassium salt substitutes used instead.[30]

Patients are much more likely to comply with long-term dietary restrictions if prior eating preferences and cultural and religious aspects of diet are incorporated into the diet plan. Modifications of familiar foods will be much more palatable to most people than a diet based on new and different foods. In addition the family's economic constraints and the availability of foods must be considered in the diet plan. It is futile to recommend fresh fruits or

**TREATMENT CODES FOR PROFESSIONAL SERVICES REQUIRED**

### Skilled Nursing

| | | | | |
|---|---|---|---|---|
| A 1 | Skilled Observation (Inc. V.S., Response to Med., etc.) | | A15 | Teach Ostomy or Ileo conduit care |
| | | | A16 | Teach Nasogastric Feeding |
| A 2 | Foley Insertion | | A17 | Reinsertion Nasogastric Feeding Tube |
| A 3 | Bladder Instillation | | A18 | Teach Gastrostomy Feeding |
| A 4 | Open Wound Care/Dressing | | A19 | Teach Parenteral Nutrition |
| A 5 | Decubitus Care - Stage 3,4,5 | | A20 | Teach Care of Trach |
| A 6 | Venipuncture | | A21 | Adm. Care of Trach |
| A 7 | Restorative Nursing | | A22 | Teach Inhalation Rx |
| A 8 | Post Cataract Care | | A23 | Teaching Care of Any Indwelling Catheter |
| A 9 | Bowel/Bladder Training | | A24 | Teach Adm. of Injection |
| A10 | Chest Physio (Inc. Postural drainage) | | A25 | Teach Diabetic Care |
| | | | A26 | Disimpaction/F.U. Enema |
| A11 | Adm. of Vitamin B/12 | | A27 | Other (Spec. under Orders) |
| A12 | Adm. Insulin | | A28 | Wound Care/Dressing - Closed Incision/Suture Line |
| A13 | Adm. Other IM/Subq. | | A29 | Decubitus Care - Stage 1, 2 |
| A14 | Adm. IV's/Clysis | | | |

### Physical Therapy

| | | | | |
|---|---|---|---|---|
| B 1 | Evaluation | | B 7 | Ultra Sound |
| B 2 | Therapeutic Exercise | | B 8 | Electro Therapy |
| B 3 | Transfer Training | | B 9 | Prosthetic Training |
| B 4 | Home Program | | B10-B14 | Reserved |
| B 5 | Gait Training | | B15 | Other (Specify under Orders) |
| B 6 | Chest Physiotherapy | | | |

### Speech Therapy

| | | | | |
|---|---|---|---|---|
| C 1 | Evaluation | | C 6 | Aural rehabilitation |
| C 2 | Voice Disorders Treatments | | C 7 | Reserved |
| C 3 | Speech Articulation Disorders Treatments | | C 8 | Nonoral Communication |
| C 4 | Dysphagia Treatments | | C 9 | Other (Specify under Orders) |
| C 5 | Language Disorders Treatments | | | |

### Occupational Therapy

| | |
|---|---|
| D 1 | Evaluation |
| D 2 | Independent Living/Daily Living Skills (ADL Training) |
| D 3 | Muscle Re-education |
| D 4 | Reserved |
| D 5 | Perceptual Motor Training |
| D 6 | Fine Motor Coordination |
| D 7 | Neuro-development Treatment |
| D 8 | Sensory Treatment |
| D 9 | Orthotics/Splinting |
| D10 | Adaptive Equipment (fabrication and training) |
| D11 | Other (Specify under Orders) |

### Medical Social Services

| | |
|---|---|
| E 1 | Assessment of Social and Emotional Factors |
| E 2 | Counseling for Long Range Planning and Decision Making |
| E 3 | Community Resources Planning |
| E 4 | Short Term Therapy |
| E 5 | Reserved |
| E 6 | Other (Specify under Orders) |

### Home Health Aids

| | | | | |
|---|---|---|---|---|
| F 1 | Tub/Shower Bath | | F 8 | Assist with Ambulation |
| F 2 | Partial/Complete Bed Bath | | F 9 | Reserved |
| F 3 | Reserved | | F10 | Exercises |
| F 4 | Personal Care | | F11 | Prepare Meal |
| F 5 | Reserved | | F12 | Grocery Shop |
| F 6 | Catheter Care | | F13 | Wash Clothes |
| F 7 | Reserved | | F14 | Housekeeping |
| | | | F15 | Other (Spec. under Orders) |

(From HCFA Medicare Home Health Agency Manual, Transmittal No. 203)

**Fig. 14-1**  Treatment codes for professional services required. (From HCFA Medicare Home Health Agency Manual, Transmittal No. 203.)

seafood, for example, if they are either unaffordable or unavailable.

## Medications

Patients with cardiac problems frequently must comply with complex regimens for medication administration at home. The extent and accuracy of compliance is related to several factors in the home situation. Noncompliance may occur because the patient or caregiver does not understand how or when the drugs are to be taken. They may not understand why the drugs are important. They may not be able to remember to take them or they may be confused. Patients may resist taking a medication because they are experiencing side effects that they find difficult to discuss with their physician or nurse (such as decreased libido associated with antihypertensives). Some patients may be noncompliant because they cannot manage the cost of the drugs, and some patients, especially the elderly, may have difficulty opening the containers.

The home medication regimen begins with a nursing evaluation of the potential of the patient or caregiver to administer the necessary medications. Special consideration should be given to cognitive ability, motivation, dexterity, financial resources, and ability to obtain refills. The patient should be evaluated for the effects of the medications, possible side effects, and potential for misuse of over-the-counter drugs. Patients taking antihypertensives, for example, should be warned against using over-the-counter antihistamines without first consulting their physician.

Teaching addresses individual needs. The nurse should emphasize the importance of taking the prescribed drugs and should instruct the patient about the correct dose, route, and time. The patient should be taught the action of the drug and the possible side effects. Audiovisual aids are helpful and most patients benefit from written materials aimed at the individual's level of understanding.

Patients who must take frequent doses of medications usually benefit from dispenser boxes that can be labeled and prefilled on a weekly basis. These can be purchased at a pharmacy or may be made from egg cartons that are cut and pasted to accommodate the dosage schedule required (e.g., tid, qid). Others may prefer a calendar or tally sheet that can be checked off. Such assistance is frequently appreciated even by fully cognizant patients or caretakers who must deal with a repetitious daily routine and many other demands on their attention.[29]

Patients who are taking digitalis should be taught to monitor their own pulse and to identify changes in rate or rhythm. They should be advised to withhold the digitalis and notify the physician if the rate drops below 60 or if a regular pulse becomes irregular or an irregular pulse changes. Patients should be aware of the signs and symptoms of digitalis toxicity: anorexia, nausea, vomiting, diarrhea, or visual changes. It should be noted that patients taking diuretics are at increased risk of digitalis toxicity because of potassium depletion.

Some patients who have been hospitalized with a cardiovascular diagnosis are discharged on anticoagulant therapy. Home care includes assessing for signs of overdose such as severe bruising, bleeding gums, nosebleeds, blood in the urine, tarry stools, headaches, or visual or motor changes, and patients on this therapy should be taught these warning signs. Patients should be advised to use electric razors rather than sharp blades, to use soft toothbrushes, and to avoid cuts or trauma. Aspirin should not be used by these patients.[34]

## Pain Management

Pain experienced by the cardiac patient at home is likely to be either the pain of angina related to myocardial ischemia or the postoperative pain of a sternal incision. In some instances, it may be necessary to differentiate between these two sources of pain. Patients often describe the pain of angina as aching, squeezing, burning, tightness, or choking. It frequently radiates to the shoulder, arm, neck, or jaw. Ischemic pain may be accompanied by nausea, epigastric burning, diaphoresis, fatigue, anxiety, or palpitations. Incisional pain, on the other hand, is likely to occur only with deep breaths or movement. A history that describes the pain, its usual patterns, precipitating factors, and methods of relief may be useful to the nurse in evaluating the type of pain and planning the appropriate intervention.

The pain of angina is relieved by measures that enhance myocardial oxygenation, either by improving delivery of oxygen to the myocardium or by decreasing its demand for oxygen. This can be accomplished by having the patient rest in a head-up position, either sitting or in a semi-Fowler's position. Lying prone increases venous return and consequently myocardial wall tension and consumption of oxygen. If rest alone does not relieve the pain, sublingual nitroglycerin may be administered at 5-minute intervals up to three times. Nitroglycerin causes vasodilatation, which decreases venous return and subsequent coronary workload and increases myocardial oxygen supply as a result of dilatation of the coronary vessels. The patient should be advised that if three doses of nitroglycerine do not relieve the pain, the physician or an ambulance should be contacted immediately. Patients should be warned that nitroglycerine may cause headaches, and they should be cautioned to remain seated when taking nitroglycerine in order to avoid syncope and falls. This is especially critical for patients who live alone and those with osteoporosis.

The patient, or the caretaker, should understand that nitroglycerine has a short shelf life and needs to be replaced about every 3 months. It should be kept in a dark bottle and refrigerated to prevent rapid deterioration. The patient may carry a few days supply, and household members should know where the tablets are stored.

Other coronary vasodilators may be prescribed for some patients. For example, long-acting nitrates in the form of patches or slow-release capsules may be used to promote more consistent coronary artery vasodilatation. The patient should know how to use these properly. A beta adrenergic blocker such as propranolol, which decreases myocardial oxygen consumption, may be prescribed to decrease the frequency of anginal attacks.[34]

Prevention of angina pain, especially that of stable angina, may be possible if precipitating factors can be identified. The possible influence of diet (especially caffeine), smoking, emotional stress, exercise, temperature changes, blood pressure levels, and diabetic control should be evaluated. Interventions may then be devised that assist the patient either to avoid the precipitating factor or to learn to handle the situation more effectively. These may entail lifestyle changes that may or may not be acceptable to the patient and appropriate to the situation. Measures that may be helpful include increasing aerobic capacity by regular moderate exercise, learning to better cope with stress, stopping cigarette smoking, eating smaller meals more frequently, weight reduction, avoiding temperature extremes, and learning to pace daily activities.

When pain is caused by incisional discomfort resulting from cardiac surgery, the patient may exhibit rapid, shallow respirations, which attempt to ease the discomfort. Ineffective breathing patterns may result. These patients should have analgesics prescribed to be used if necessary to prevent severe discomfort. The analgesics may be taken ahead of time to better enable the patient to do deep breathing exercises. This is a problem of limited duration that will be resolved when the chest heals.[35]

## Activity and Rest

Patients must be homebound in order for home care to be reimbursed by third party payers; therefore, by definition, they are likely to have limited activity tolerance. Prior hospitalization and immobility from prolonged bedrest may result in decreased physical work capacity, evidenced by hyperventilation and decreased cardiac reserve. Other possible effects of immobility are diminished vasomotor reflex, increased potential for thromboembolism, nitrogen and protein loss, and loss of skeletal muscle mass. The activity level of a homebound cardiac patient may be further curtailed by signs and symptoms of overexertion, such as shortness of breath or chest pain, by anxiety and misunderstanding, or by another complicating diagnosis such as diabetes, arthritis, or chronic pulmonary disease.

In general, a patient should be encouraged to exercise to the extent tolerated. Physical activity assists in overcoming the deconditioning effects of immobility, increases aerobic capacity, contributes to the relief of anxiety and depression, and helps to improve self-esteem and body image.[35]

Initial assessment of activity tolerance focuses on ability to perform normal activities of daily living without distress. Other activities such as climbing stairs or performing light household chores contribute to the patient's daily well-being. Blood pressure and pulse may be monitored before and after exercise to determine tolerance levels. Decrease of blood pressure by more than 20 mm Hg, increase of pulse by more than 20% of the resting rate or a rate above 120, or the development of chest pain are indications that the activity level should be decreased.

In general, activity levels should be increased gradually, according to the individual's diagnosis and potential for cardiac rehabilitation. If the patient is not participating in a cardiac rehabilitation program, the plan of treatment should include specific guidelines for home care in regard to heart rate limits, specific activities, and precautions.

Activities should be planned to allow for periods of rest and relaxation between activities. For the more severely ill and debilitated patients, this schedule may necessitate pacing activities of daily living. Patients should know how to assess their own level of fatigue. Isotonic exercises such as lifting, and activities that involve holding the arms over the head for a long while, such as curling one's own hair, should be avoided. Quiet, leisure activities such as watching TV, listening to music, working at a computer, or reading should be encouraged. As tolerance for activity increases, walking gradually increasing distances may be advisable. Patients should be cautioned to avoid extremes of temperatures, such as walking outside in very hot or cold weather.[29,35]

## Sexual Activity

Patients with cardiac disease, both men and women, are prone to sexual dysfunction. Problems such as decreased libido, impotence, or orgasmic dysfunction may be caused by medications, organic problems, anxiety, depression, or poor self-esteem. For patients who have had a cardiac crisis, such as an MI or bypass surgery, these sexual problems may be exacerbated by the lack of knowledge and by the reluctance of health care professionals to deal with this issue.

Cardiac patients may have a variety of fears: death during sexual intercourse, inadequate sexual performance, another infarction caused by sexual activity, and diminished sexual ability caused by illness and aging. They may fear that medical advice will prohibit sexual activity. These fears may become heightened when information about sexuality is omitted from extensive patient teaching protocols. Yet few patients are sufficiently comfortable to approach the physician or nurse with these concerns.

Some drugs frequently prescribed for cardiac patients have side effects that affect sexual functioning. The likelihood of problems varies among individuals, contingent on such factors as dosage of the drug, possible interactions with other drugs or foods, the weight of the patient, rates of absorption and excretion, and compliance with the medication regimen. The most common drugs causing sexual problems are the antihypertensives. The thiazide diuretics, spironolactone, methyldopa, guanethidine, and furosemide have been associated with impotence, diminished libido, impaired arousal, and retarded ejaculation.[35] While most of the available information on sexual side effects of drugs comes from studies of men, similar problems have been reported in women.

Previous sexual patterns should be taken into consideration when advising cardiac patients about return to sexual activity. This advising requires an ongoing professional relationship with the patient, good rapport and trust, and a nonjudgmental attitude. It should be noted that, although sexual response may become slower with advancing age, there is no physiologic reason for sexual activity to cease because of age.

Sexual partners are likely to have many of the same fears as the cardiac patient, and they may try to avoid sexual activities in order to protect the patient. It may be helpful, therefore, to include the patient's partner when providing information about return to sexual functioning.

Marital coitus is physiologically equivalent to activities such as a brisk walk or climbing a flight of stairs. It has been equated to 5 METs of work on an exercise stress test. Advice to patients should be based on consultation with the physician. Generally, patients who can sustain a heart rate of 110 to 120 with no shortness of breath or anginal pain may resume sexual activity. These patients are most likely to be those who have experienced an MI or cardiac surgery and whose recovery is not complicated by cardiac failure or dysrhythmias.

Patients should be advised to resume sexual activity gradually, and only after activities such as walking moderate distances or climbing stairs can be done comfortably. Sexual activity causes the least amount of stress when it occurs in familiar surroundings with the usual partner. Gradual foreplay helps the heart prepare for coitus. The patient should assume comfortable positions during sexual activity, avoiding positions that cause isometric muscle contractions. Activity should be slowed or stopped if chest pain or shortness of breath occurs. Sexual activity should be avoided soon after eating because food intake diverts blood flow to the gastrointestinal organs. Likewise, alcohol, which decreases cardiac output, should be avoided. The cardiac patient and sexual partner should be encouraged to communicate their feelings about sex openly and frankly with each other. Such candid sharing helps to avoid misunderstandings and false impressions that frequently occur under these circumstances.[35]

### Psychosocial Considerations

Some families have a tendency to overprotect their ill member. Although all family members are prone to this behavior, it is frequently seen in wives of cardiac patients. These families become overindulgent in providing care, make decisions without involving the patient, and become overly cautious in their efforts to limit the patient's behavior. Acting out fear and anxiety, such families become overbearing and are a hinderance to the patient's sense of self-control. Some patients may rebel against this treat-

ment, behave recklessly, and take unnecessary chances in order to regain a sense of control over their lives. Others may become more dependent than their condition warrants and succumb to a sense of hopelessness.

Loss of personal control and a sense of powerlessness results from the disabling effects of both the aging process and chronic illness. The perception of control over one's life is critical to self-management of a chronic illness. Control enhances the ability to recover from illness, or to maintain well-being and prevent deterioration. Control is the belief that individuals can influence the events in their lives and can manipulate some parts of their environments.

Perceived control may enhance the patient's ability to cope with illness and its possible complications. Families should be helped to understand that the patient's sense of control may be augmented by planning his or her own daily activities, rather than having others plan the day. Daily scheduling, however, may have to revolve around the treatment regimen and can become problematic when the patient depends on a caretaker to perform these activities.[36]

Knowledge and understanding contribute to a sense of control. Patient teaching that provides information about the illness and its symptoms and management can modify the sense of loss of control that is associated with anxiety about the unknown. Likewise, the provision of anticipatory guidance can help the patient and caretaker prepare for unfamiliar trajectories.

Patients should always be included in decisions that relate to their care. Caretakers should be assisted to understand that the patient's ability to cope is directly related to participation in decisions and the resulting sense of control over daily life.

## HOME CARE FOR CARDIAC PATIENTS WITH SPECIAL NEEDS

In no other area are the changes in health care more obvious than in the complexity and sophistication of medical technology that has been introduced into the home health arena. Recent advances in cardiac treatment have placed special demands on the home health team for expertise to manage complex and technical interventions in the home and to educate patients and caregivers to handle complicated therapeutic regimens.

### Holter Monitor

A Holter monitor may be worn for 12 to 24 hours to record an ambulatory ECG while the patient engages in normal daily activities. Such recording is helpful in detecting and documenting intermittent dysrhythmias or those that occur only during certain daily activities.

The home health provider should explain to the patient and family the reasons for the procedure, answer questions, and help to reduce anxiety about the equipment. The patient, or if necessary the caregiver, should keep a log of all activities and events that occur while the monitor is in place, and any symptoms or sensations that may arise. The patient should be encouraged to carry on with normal daily activities, except for showering. The recorder should be protected from water and should not be dropped. Any electrodes that come loose should be reapplied and taped in place. It is important to confirm that the patient understands where to go to have the monitor removed at the designated time.[24]

## Pacemaker

A permanent artificial pacemaker may be inserted for patients who have a permanent dysfunction of the cardiac conduction system that cannot be controlled by drugs. Such complex heart block may be secondary to MI, surgery, or trauma. Patients with rhythm disturbances such as severe bradycardia, sick sinus syndromes, or Stokes-Adams attacks may also be candidates for pacemaker insertion in order to maintain normal rate and adequate cardiac output.

Pacemaker insertion is a surgical procedure that takes place in the hospital. Although teaching begins at that time, anxiety, problems in communication, or hearing deficits may limit patient understanding about pacemaker function and care. Teaching is thus a major priority for home care after pacemaker insertion. Teaching begins with assessment of patient and family levels of anxiety and understanding.

The patient will probably return home from the hospital without a dressing on the suture line. The area should be checked by the home health nurse for redness, drainage, or pain, any of which would indicate an infection of the incision or the subcutaneous pocket. The patient should be assessed for presence of prepacemaker symptoms such as chest pain, dyspnea, dizziness, or edematous ankles.

The patient should be on bedrest for 48 to 72 hours following pacemaker insertion to avoid electrode dislodgment. After that time, newly formed tissue will secure the electrode to the endocardium. Incision discomfort, if present, will be mild and acetaminophen is likely to provide sufficient relief.

Vigorous motion, especially of the arms, should be avoided for 6 weeks to prevent displacement of the electrode. After 6 weeks all normal activity, including sexual activity, may be resumed. The patient may swim and engage in sports, but activities such as contact sports that could cause chest trauma should be avoided.

The patient and the caretaker must know how to take a resting pulse, for 1 full minute each day and to record it. Ideally this measurement should be done with the patient seated on the side of the bed before rising each morning. The patient and caretaker should know the normal rate of the pacemaker and understand that heart rate may exceed that rate, but any heart rate below that rate may indicate a failing generator and should be reported. A physician may request that a magnet be placed over the generator while the heart rate is counted. The magnet puts the pacemaker in a fixed-rate mode so that the heart rate indicates the pacemaker function. A slight decrease of the rate is likely. This technique carries a slight risk of triggering ventricular dysrhythmias and should never be done by the patient alone.

Patients who live long distances from their physician or clinic, or those who have difficulty traveling, may have their pacemakers checked via telephone. For this to be accomplished, the patient must be provided with a special telephone transmitter. The transmitter has wrist electrodes that convert heart impulses to electronic signals that can be transmitted via the telephone. The call comes from the pacemaker clinic to the patient at a prearranged time, and the patient puts on the wrist electrodes and turns on the transmitter; a record of the patient's ECG can be printed out at the clinic. Many clinics have 24-hour service available so that patients can call at any time if they have problems or are concerned about the status of their pacemaker functioning.

A fixed-rate pacemaker may be checked by placing a transistor radio tuned to 55 or 550 AM directly over the generator. A magnet will be needed for placement over the generator of a demand pacemaker. Clicks will be heard from the radio that correspond to the pacemaker rate. If the pacemaker leads are intact, a pulse should be felt with each click. A click without a corresponding pulse may indicate a problem with the leads. Conversely, a pulse without a click indicates that the heart is beating without pacemaker stimulation.

Patients with permanent pacemakers should be taught to avoid exposure to electromagnetic fields that could interfere with pacemaker function. For example, malfunctioning engines, power tools and equipment, dental equipment, and inadequately shielded microwave ovens can affect pacemaker function. Some radio frequencies, especially 3.5 MHz and 28.5 MHz used by ham or citizen band radio operators, can cause problems. Generally, well-maintained household appliances are safe. Work and specialized settings should be evaluated on an individualized basis, because the degree of risk varies with the type of signal generated by the electric device and the type of artificial pacemaker used. Patients should know that if a device causes symptoms, such as fainting or dizziness, they should immediately move away from the source. They should also understand that electronic metal detectors, such as those used in airports and libraries, will be triggered by a pacemaker, but pacemaker function will not be affected.[24]

## Supplemental Oxygen

Patients with chronic hypoxemia may require administration of oxygen at home. Typically these patients suffer from inadequate cardiac output and/or chronic obstructive pulmonary disease. Many home health patients suffer from a combination of cardiac and respiratory problems. Oxygen is available for home use in cylinders, oxygen concentrators, or liquid oxygen systems. Home oxygen use requires a physician's prescription.

Oxygen cylinders are the most common mode for home oxygen use. These stationary tanks weigh about 150 pounds and are 5 feet high. A gauge indicates the amount of oxygen remaining in the tank. Such a cylinder, used at a flow rate of 2 L/min, will last about 50 hours.

Oxygen concentrators, available in floor or tabletop models, concentrate oxygen that is removed from the room air. This is the most expensive mode of delivery unless the patient requires large amounts of oxygen. Rental and use of this system equals the cost of about 8 to 10 cylinders per month. If an oxygen concentrator is used, an oxygen cylinder should be kept at hand in case of a power failure.

Patients who are mobile may be provided with a liquid oxygen system. Large stationary units weighing about 70 pounds store oxygen under pressure as a liquid. Smaller portable canisters can be refilled from these home units. The portable unit lasts up to 16 hours and may be carried with the patient away from home.

Most commonly oxygen is administered via nasal cannula, rather than a mask, because it does not have to be removed for the patient to eat or drink. Generally hypoxemia caused by cardiac insufficiency is relieved by oxygen at 1 to 2 L/min by nasal cannula. A cannula delivers oxygen at a concentration of approximately 24% to 44%. A humidifier should always be attached to the tank to moisturize the dry oxygen gas.

Assessment of the patient requiring home oxygen should include cardiovascular and respiratory history, with attention to smoking and environmental irritants. Blood gases should be evaluated before oxygen therapy is begun. Periodic assessment by the home health nurse should include respiratory status and periodic monitoring of arterial blood gases. Assessment should include signs of dyspnea, tachycardia, and indications of hypoxia such as dizziness, restlessness, or confusion. The nasal mucosa should be checked for irritation from the nasal prongs. Signs of oxygen toxicity may be similar to those of hypoxia. It is important that the family and the patient understand that the oxygen should be used as directed, and that an increased amount may be harmful.

Safety teaching must be a high priority for home care when oxygen is in use. The oxygen should be stored and used at least 10 feet away from open flames, such as gas stoves, heaters, or wood burners. No one should smoke within 10 feet of the equipment. Any electric equipment that is used near the oxygen system should be grounded with a 3-pronged plug. Electric appliances such as razors and hair dryers should not be used near the oxygen. Wool blankets and clothing or night clothes made of nylon should not be used, to avoid sparks from static electricity. Aerosols should not be used in the area.

Home care for a patient using oxygen is likely to require some financial counseling for the patient and family. It must be determined if, and how much of, the cost of the oxygen and equipment will be paid by a third party payer such as Medicare. The cost of the different types of equipment should be compared, and the options of renting or purchasing the equipment should be considered. In addition, the home must have adequate storage space. Oxygen cylinders require storage away from heat, sunlight, and flammable materials. Liquid oxygen should be stored in a well-ventilated area because small amounts are likely to escape.

Family members must be taught how to use and maintain the equipment and how to safely store the oxygen. They must know when to reorder oxygen cylinders.[24]

## DYING AT HOME

In recent years there has been a trend toward allowing the elderly and hopelessly ill to die at home. This trend parallels other changes that have occurred in the health care system. Hospitals today have become oriented toward more intensive care of the critically ill and, for many patients, this high-technology environment is no longer warranted. For many chronically ill or dying patients, palliative care is the best that can be offered. These patients need comfort, communication, and competent caregivers. Often this kind of care can best be provided at home where the patient can experience a comfortable life for as long as possible. When death is inevitable, it can occur in familiar surroundings with the support of family and friends.[4]

The trend has occurred in the context of major changes in the way health care is funded. Dying at home, especially when the illness is long term, is a more economically feasible alternative than hospitalization. The hospice movement has provided momentum to this trend, and Medicare now provides benefits for hospice care. The hospice movement in the United States is grounded on the work of Dame Cicely Saunders, the English nurse and physician who, in 1968, founded St. Christopher's Hospice in London. Hospice is a concept that aims to provide palliative, symptomatic care rather than aggressive treatment. The goal is to relieve pain and keep the patient comfortable and conscious. Care might be provided in the patient's home or in a hospice setting; in either case, the atmosphere is relaxed and homelike.[37] Care is provided by a team of professionals and volunteers who address the needs of the patient and family for physical caring and emotional, spiritual, social, and financial assistance.

Because of the manner in which hospice care is funded, the majority of patients who participate in the program are cancer patients. In order to be eligible for reimbursement for hospice care, the patient must have a prognosis of death within less than 6 months. While such a prognosis is possible for many cancer patients, the course of cardiac disease is usually less predictable. Thus, although more people die of cardiac disease than any other cause, death is more likely to be sudden and unplanned, and few cardiac patients participate in a hospice program.

The unexpectedness of cardiac death frequently places a family in a sudden crisis for which they are not prepared. The family facing the potential or actual loss of a member will experience the grief process before they can reach a renewed equilibrium. Grief is intense emotional suffering that a person feels as a result of being deprived of something that is valued. This may be the loss of a significant person, a valued object, or a part of oneself, or it may be a developmental loss. Engle described three stages of grief and mourning that a family is likely to experience: (1) shock and disbelief, (2) awareness of the loss, and (3) restitution.[38]

Initially when a loss occurs, especially if it is unanticipated, family members are likely to be stunned and disorganized. Emotions may be paralyzed and people may feel out of contact with reality as they go about making necessary arrangements. Soon the loss will become real and each person in his own way will feel anguish, pain, anger, and denial. People may feel varying degrees of helplessness and hopelessness. If family members blame themselves for the death of a loved one they may feel guilty; others may direct anger at health care providers for not saving the patient. Finally, restitution begins, and families begin to accept the reality of their loss and learn new ways of coping. Ultimately family equilibrium is restored as other family members take over the roles formerly belonging to the deceased member.

When life-threatening situations provide time, family members may prepare for the loss of a member. Facing potential of loss, people experience anticipatory grief. In this circumstance, the loss may be rehearsed, in fantasy, many times. This process may sometimes help people to deal with the real loss when it actually occurs.[20]

Patients who realize they are approaching their own death also experience the grief process. Kubler-Ross identified five stages of grief likely to be experienced by a patient: (1) denial and isolation, (2) anger, (3) bargaining, (4) depression, and (5) acceptance.[39]

When death seems inevitable, it may be appropriate to provide anticipatory guidance for the patient and family. In addition, the caretaker should be given emergency phone numbers and instructions for handling an emergency. The home care team should be aware of local regulations regarding the handling of a home death. This information can be obtained from the local police department or from the medical examiner's office.

If death occurs during a home visit, rescue procedures should be initiated according to policy. The physician should be notified. The health care providers should stay with the family until the body has been removed, providing support, offering assistance in contacting the funeral director, and assisting and supporting the family while the body is removed.[40]

The family's religious orientation should be accepted and supported. Some religions require ritual acts associated with the death process. These rituals include special rites or anointing of the sick, or they may require special washing and handling of the body after death. These requirements should be known and the wishes of the family respected.

## RESEARCH NEEDS

Home care presents researchers with many challenges. Home health research generally aims to find improved ways to assure cost-effective delivery of high-quality health care. Research needs fall into three areas: quality of care, financing, and technology.

As more agencies are established to meet needs for illness care at home, more and more elderly people will depend on this mode of health care delivery. It is estimated that 4 million Americans, most of whom are elderly, require assistance in performing activities of daily living.[41] At the same time, there is much emphasis on the use of complex technology in home settings. As this trend evolves, quality assurance systems are needed to promote the delivery of safe, high-quality care for all patients. Such systems must focus on the delivery of safe, competent and sophisticated care for the acutely ill, as well as on the delivery of appropriate and compassionate care for the chronically ill and aged.

Studies are needed to establish the most effective treatment protocols for home care of patients with specific cardiac diagnoses. Norms are needed as a basis for decision making for elderly patients with advanced disease who need supportive care and for those who can be rehabilitated. Likewise, for younger patients, criteria are needed regarding the most appropriate type and amount of home care to maximize potential for long-range positive outcomes. Studies are needed that examine ways to enhance potential for self-care. Examination of patterns of referral can contribute to better determination of the most effective site of care at various levels of severity of illness.

As discussed earlier, the financing of care is a critical issue in the health care system. Regulations governing reimbursement are restrictive and they limit the type and amount of care that people receive. The government is faced with the quandary of how to reconcile budget constraints, lower taxes, and decreased government spending with public demands for health care and increasing health care costs.[4] The health care system is faced with the challenge of finding ways to provide the best quality care for the least cost. Some of these issues present ethical questions that cannot be directly answered by research. For example, what portion of the burden of the cost of care should fall on the consumer and what portion should be borne by government? On the other hand, research must provide information that forms the context in which these decisions are made. Studies are needed to find the most cost-effective means of providing care for patients with common diagnoses. The outcomes of care and long-range consequences must be evaluated. For example, at what point in the course of an illness can patients be discharged from a service without increasing their risk of relapse and readmission? What are the most effective referral patterns? Finally, studies are needed to determine the most effective models for interagency and interdisciplinary cooperation to ensure continuity of services without duplication.

As technologic advances enhance the in-hospital management of serious illnesses, adaption of these technologies for home use must be sought through research. Sophisticated technology used in the home must be cost-effective and must be designed simply enough to be managed by families and nonprofessional caretakers. Studies are needed that address how to efficiently provide equipment for home use and how to effectively train home care users. Special attention should be given to providing safe, compassionate, and humane care in the home while maintaining cost-effective services and appropriate utilization of technologic advances.

## REFERENCES

1. Keating SB and Kelman GB: Home health care nursing: concepts and practice, Philadelphia, 1988, JB Lippincott Co.
2. Lancaster J: History of community health and community health nursing. In Stanhope M and Lancaster J, editors: Community health nursing: process and practice for promoting health, St Louis, 1988, Mosby–Year Book, Inc.
3. Report to Congress: Impact of the medicare hospital prospective payment system, Washington DC, 1986 Annual Report, Health Care Financing Administration.
4. Haddad AM: High tech home care: a practical guide, Rockville, MD, 1987, Aspen Publication.
5. Garvey E and Logue JH: The community health nurse in home health and hospice care. In Stanhope M and Lancaster J, editors: Community health nursing: process and practice for promoting health, St Louis, 1988, Mosby–Year Book, Inc.
6. Home health care: profile, Am Nurse 22(2):24, 1990.
7. Selby TL: Home health care finds new ways of caring: skilled RNs meet patient needs as agencies flourish, Am Nurse 22(2):1, 1990.
8. Malloy C: Overview of acute care nursing in the home. In Malloy C and Hartshorn J, editors: Acute care nursing in the home: a holistic approach, Philadelphia, 1989, JB Lippincott Co.
9. Cafferata GL: Marital status, living arrangements, and the use of health services by elderly persons, J Gerontol 42(6):613, 1987.
10. Glick DF: An analysis of the relationship between utilization of home health services and nursing diagnosis as a measure of patient health problems, unpublished doctoral dissertation, University Park, 1987, Pennsylvania State University.
11. Wilkes E: Dying now, Lancet, 1(8383):950-952, 1984.
12. Steffl BM and Eide I: Discharge planning handbook, 1981, Charles B Slack, Inc.
13. Continuity of care and discharge planning program, New York, 1975, American Nurses Association.
14. Guidelines: discharge planning, Chicago, 1984, American Hospital Association.
15. The joint commission 1990: accreditation manual for hospitals, Chicago, 1989, Joint Commission on Accreditation of Healthcare Organizations.
16. Smith CD: Discharge planning. In Malloy C and Hartshorn J, editors: Acute care nursing in the home: a holistic approach, Philadelphia, 1989, JB Lippincott Co.
17. Mariano C: The case for interdisciplinary collaboration, Nurs Outlook 37(6):285-288, 1989.
18. Harris MD: Home care. In Caliandro G and Judkins BL, editors: Primary nursing practice, Glenview, IL, 1988, Scott, Foresman & Co.
19. Hanson SMH: Family nursing and chronic illness. In Wright LM and Leahey M, editors: Families and chronic illness, Springhouse, PA, 1987, Springhouse Corp.
20. Bozett FW: Family nursing and life threatening illness. In Leahey M and Wright LM, editors: Families and life-threatening illness, Springhouse, PA, 1987, Springhouse Corp.
21. Orem DE: Nursing concepts of practice, New York, 1980, McGraw-Hill Book Co.
22. Stauss AL and Glasser BG: Chronic illness and quality of life, St Louis, 1975, Mosby–Year Book, Inc.
23. Seigel H: Nurses improve hospital efficiency through risk assessment model at admission, Nurs Manage 19(10):38-46, 1988.
24. Walsh J, Persons CB, and Wieck L: Manual of home health care nursing, Philadelphia, 1987, JB Lippincott Co.
25. Folden SL: Caring for older homebound adults: a chronic illness perspective, J Home Health Care Pract 2(1):57-62, 1989.
26. Friedman JA: Home health care, New York, 1986, WW Norton & Co, Inc.
27. Goldberg PB and Roberts J: Rational drug regimens for the elderly patient, Med Clin North Am 67(2):323, 1983.
28. Caliandro G: Adults with coronary artery disease. In Caliandro G and Judkins BL, editors: Primary nursing practice, Glenview, IL, 1988, Scott Foresman & Co.
29. Rovinski CA and Zastocki DK: Home care: a technical manual for the professional nurse, Philadelphia, 1989, WB Saunders Co.
30. Babitz LE and Kahn ML: Cardiac disease. In Bernstein LH, Grieco AJ, Dete MK, editors: Primary care in the home, Philadelphia, 1987, JB Lippincott Co.
31. McGurn W: People with cardiac problems: nursing concepts, Philadelphia, 1981, JB Lippincott Co.
32. Marrelli TM: Handbook of home health standards and documentation guidelines for reimbursement, St Louis, 1988, Mosby–Year Book, Inc.
33. HCFA Medicare home health agency manual, transmittal No 203, Washington, DC, 1987, Health Care Financing Administration.
34. Gaul AL: Cardiovascular disease. In Hogstel MD, editor: Home nursing care for the elderly, Bowie, MD, 1985, Brady Communications Co.
35. Pratt N: Alterations in circulation. In Malloy C and Hartshorn J, editors: Acute care nursing in the home: a holistic approach, Philadelphia, 1989, JB Lippincott Co.
36. Miller JF and Oertel CB: Powerlessness in the elderly: preventing hopelessness. In Miller JF, editor: Coping with chronic illness: overcoming powerlessness, Philadelphia, 1983, FA Davis Co.
37. Miller MC: Spirituality, beliefs, values and practices. In Malloy C and Hartshorn J, editors: Acute care nursing in the home: a holistic approach, Philadelphia, 1989, JB Lippincott Co.
38. Engle GL: Psychological development in health and disease, Philadelphia, 1962, WB Saunders Co.
39. Kubler-Ross E: On death and dying, New York, 1969, Macmillan Publishing Co.
40. Stewart R: Manual of community and home health nursing, Boston, 1987, Little, Brown & Co.
41. NCHSR home health research, National center for health services research program note, Sept 1989.

# Index

Page numbers in italics indicate illustrations; t indicates tables.

# Fast and Effective. From Mosby–Year Book.

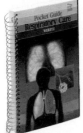

**NEW!**
**POCKET GUIDE TO RESPIRATORY CARE**
Pamela Becker Weilitz, RN, MSN
1991 (0-8016-0189-4)

This portable spiral-bound reference provides essential clinical information on care of the patient with respiratory alterations in acute, extended care, and home-care settings. Content includes assessment, laboratory data and diagnostic procedures, significant findings, and nursing implications.
* Provides important information about frequently used respiratory therapy equipment and mechanical ventilators, to enable nurses to check functioning and troubleshoot problems.
* Includes separate chapters on pulmonary rehabilitation and home health care, plus illustrated exercises to assist in educating the patient.

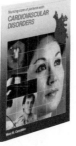

**CARDIOVASCULAR DISORDERS**
Mary M. Canobbio, RN, MN
1990 (0-8016-1405-8)
*Clinical Nursing Series, Volume 1*

Comprehensive and beautifully illustrated in full color, this new title presents state-of-the-art information on all aspects of care for patients with cardiovascular disorders.
* Illustrations commissioned specifically for this title clarify cardiac structure, function, and related pathology. The illustrations also serve as effective patient teaching tools.
* Numerous patient teaching guides are written for the patient and are designed to be easily reproduced.

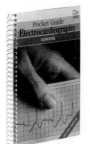

**POCKET GUIDE TO ELECTROCARDIOGRAPHY**
**2nd Edition**
Mary Boudreau Conover, RN, BS
1990 (0-8016-6247-8)

The second edition of this unique pocket guide presents complete electrocardiographic information in a concise, easy-to-use format.
* The nursing-oriented organization for each arrhythmia chapter includes a brief overview of anatomy and physiology, ECG characteristics, pathophysiology, nursing implications, variations and differential diagnosis, and treatment.
* Each chapter is preceded by an illustration of the heart, with arrhythmia sites highlighted in a second color.

*To order ask your bookstore manager or call toll-free 800-426-4545.*
*We look forward to hearing from you soon.*

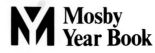

NMA045